Therapeutic roles of selective COX-2 inhibitors

Therapeutic roles of selective COX-2 inhibitors

Edited by

JOHN R VANE and REGINA M BOTTING

The William Harvey Research Institute, St Bartholomew's & The Royal London School of Medicine & Dentistry, London, United Kingdom

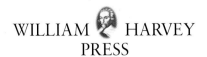
WILLIAM HARVEY PRESS

Distributors

Gazelle Book Services Limited, Falcon House, Queen Square, Lancaster LA1 1RN.

A catalogue record for this book is available from the British Library.

ISBN 0 9534039 1 2

Published in the United Kingdom by William Harvey Press, St Bartholomew's and the Royal London School of Medicine and Dentistry, Charterhouse Square, London EC1M 6BQ, UK.

Designed and Typeset by Cambridge Photosetting Services, Cambridge.

Printed and bound in Great Britain by Burlington Press, Foxton, Cambridge.

Contents list

List of contributors

Victoria Allport and Phillip Bennett
Institute of Reproductive and Development Biology, Imperial College
School of Medicine, Hammersmith Hospital, Du Cane Road,
London W12, UK

Leslie R Ballou, Clark M Blatteis and Rajendra Ragow
Department of Medicine & Biochemistry, University of Tennessee,
VA Med Ctr (151), 1030 Jefferson Ave, Memphis TN 38104, USA

Alan Bennett
Academic Department of Surgery, The Rayne Institute, Guy's, King's and
St Thomas' School of Medicine, King's College, London, SE5 9NU, UK

Leslie J Crofford
Division of Rheumatology, The University of Michigan Medical Center,
1150 W Medical Center Drive, Ann Arbor, MI 48109-0680, USA

Frank Degner, Stephan Lanes, Joanne van Ryn and Ralf Sigmund
Boehringer Ingelheim GmbH, CD Therapeutic Area 1, Binger Strasse 173,
Ingelheim am Rhein D 55216, Germany

Raymond N DuBois
Department of Medicine, Vanderbilt University Medical Center,
GI: MCN C-2104, 1161 21st Ave South, Nashville,
TN 37232-2279, USA

Garret A FitzGerald and Carlo Patrono
Department of Pharmacology, University of Pennsylvania,
153 Johnson Pavilion, 3620 Hamilton Walk, Philadelphia,
PA 19104-6084, USA

Luis Alberto García Rodríguez and Sonia Hernández-Diaz
CEIFE, C/Almirante 28 2°, Madrid 28004, Spain

Raymond C Harris
Division of Nephrology, Vanderbilt University Medical Center,
S-3223 Medical Center North, Nashville, TN 37232-2372, USA

Chris J Hawkey
Division of Gastroenterology, The University of Nottingham,
University Hospital Queen's Medical Centre, Nottingham NG7 2UH, UK

PC Isakson, RG Kurumbail, J Gierse, K Seibert and TJ Maziasz
Pharmacia Corporation, Mail Zone BB2B, 700 Chesterfield Parkway
North, St Louis, MO 63198, USA

Richard A Jones
Shire Pharmaceuticals Ltd, East Anton, Andover,
Hampshire SP10 5RG, UK

Zunaid Karim and Paul Emery
Rheumatology & Rehabilitation Research Unit, University of Leeds School
of Medicine, 36 Clarendon Road, Leeds LS2 9NZ, UK

JB Lefkowith, KM Verburg and GS Geis
Pharmacia Corporation, 4901 Searle-Parkway, Skokie, IL 60077, USA

Jane A Mitchell and Salome J Stanford
Unit of Critical Care Medicine, Royal Brompton Hospital,
Sydney Street, London SW3 6NP, UK

**Briggs Morrison, Thomas J Simon, Lisa DeTora
and Rhoda Sperling**
Merck Research Laboratories, 126 E Lincoln Ave, RY32-629,
PO Box 2000, Rahway, NJ 07065-7345, USA

Michel Pairet
Boehringer Ingelheim GmbH, Department of Pulmonary Research,
Binger Strasse 173, Ingelheim am Rhein D 55216, Germany

Guilio Maria Pasinetti
Department of Psychiatry, Neuroinflammation Research Center,
Mount Sinai Medical School, One Gustave L Levy Place,
New York, NY 10029-6574, USA

Carol C Pilbeam and Yosuke Okada
Department of Medicine, University of Connecticut Healthcare,
Farmington, CT 06030, USA

Petpiboon Prasit, Denis Riendeau and Chi Chung Chan
Merck Frosst Centre for Therapeutic Research, PO Box 1005,
Pointe-Claire, Dorval, Quebec H9R 4P8, Canada

Ari Ristimäki, Kirsi Narko, Outi Nieminen and Kirsi Saukkonen
Department Obstetrics & Gynaecology, Helsinki University Central
Hospital, Haartmaninkatu 2, Helsinki 00029, Finland

Daniel L Simmons and Joel E Wilson
Department of Chemistry & Biochemistry, Brigham Young University,
C100 Benson Science Building, PO Box 25700, Provo,
UT 84602-5700, USA

John R Vane and Regina M Botting
The William Harvey Research Institute, St Bartholomew's & the Royal
London School of Medicine & Dentistry, Charterhouse Square,
London EC1M 6BQ, UK

Timothy D Warner
Department of Cardiovascular & Inflammation Research, The William
Harvey Research Institute, St Bartholomew's & the Royal London School
of Medicine & Dentistry, Charterhouse Square, London EC1M 6BQ, UK

Brendan JR Whittle
The William Harvey Research Institute, St Bartholomew's & the Royal
London School of Medicine & Dentistry, Charterhouse Square,
London EC1M 6BQ, UK

Derek Willoughby, Toby Lawrence and Paul Colville-Nash
Department of Experimental Pathology, William Harvey Research Institute,
St Bartholomew's & the Royal London School of Medicine & Dentistry,
Charterhouse Square, London EC1M 6BQ, UK

Tony L Yaksh and Camilla Svensson
Department of Anesthesiology 0818, University of California, San Diego,
9500 Gilman Dr, La Jolla, CA 92093, USA

Acknowledgements

Grateful thanks are extended to Jenny Maclagan and Sandra Hewerdine for their co-ordination of the production of this volume, to the Copy Editor, Bob Carling, to the Picture Editor, Sheila Betts and to the Proof Reader, Annmarie Hedges.

Preface

Throughout history, man has sought herbal remedies and some have stood the test of time to become useful medicines. Plants containing salicylate such as myrtle, spiroea and willow are outstanding for their extensive use, in many different cultures worldwide, first documented more than 4000 years ago.

Salicylate was synthesised in 1859 and the acetyl derivative, aspirin was patented in 1897. The use of aspirin as an antipyretic, analgesic and anti-inflammatory drug burgeoned throughout the world. Today it is estimated that 45,000 tons of aspirin are consumed each year, an amount which would be far greater but for the development of many congeners, collectively termed non-steroid anti-inflammatory drugs (NSAIDs). These all shared the common therapeutic actions of aspirin but also its toxic actions, particularly gastric erosion.

The long sought biochemical mechanism through which NSAIDs exert both their therapeutic and toxic effects was established in 1971, when Vane showed that all NSAIDs suppressed the synthesis of prostaglandins by inhibition of the cyclooxygenase enzyme which converts arachidonic acid into the unstable hydroperoxide, prostaglandin G_2, the precursor of the physiologically and pathologically important prostanoids.

The common mechanism for both the therapeutic and toxic actions of NSAIDs suggested that the toxicity of these drugs would never be divorced from efficacy. However, the discovery of a cyclooxygenase induced during inflammation and encoded by a gene different from that of the constitutive enzyme (COX-1) raised the possibility that selective inhibition of the induced enzyme (COX-2) might result in therapeutic benefit without the previously inevitable gastrotoxicity.

Measurement of the relative inhibitory action of existing NSAIDs against the two COX enzymes indicated that those with high activity on the induced enzyme compared with the constitutive COX-1, were less toxic than those that inhibited both enzymes. Proof of concept was achieved when, following description of the crystal structures of the two enzyme isoforms, novel compounds were synthesised tailored to penetrate the active site of COX-2 with minimal action on COX-1. In clinical trials with thousands of patients, they were equally efficacious to established NSAIDs but with significantly less gastrotoxicity.

This development of selective COX-2 inhibitors is a milestone in the treatment of rheumatoid disease, reducing pain and swelling without the frequently life-threatening gastrointestinal perforations, ulcers and bleeds. But the focus of research on COX-2 selective inhibitors is now far wider than rheumatology.

COX-2 enzyme is present in numerous malignant tumours (but not in adjacent normal tissue) and trials are underway to evaluate the possible beneficial effects of COX-2 selective inhibitors in colon cancer. Furthermore, a possible involvement with Alzheimer's dementia has emerged since experimental studies with mice, genetically prone to overexpress neuronal COX-2 have shown increased intensity of ß-amyloid protein in the brain, and preliminary clinical studies suggest that NSAIDs slow the progression of early dementia in Alzheimer's patients. Such results have stimulated the initiation of formal clinical trials with NSAIDs in patients with questionable to mild dementia.

The continued research on the actions and mode of action of salicylate and other NSAIDs has clearly resulted in improvement in therapy, yet we are possibly just at the threshold of understanding the pathophysiological significance of cyclooxygenase enzymes and of the clinical applications of selective inhibitors. This volume, with contributions from established leaders in the diverse aspects of the field, provides background information for clinicians and interested scientists. In addition, it may provide a stimulus for specialists in dissociated fields to extend further knowledge of the importance of prostanoids, and the enzymes associated with their synthesis, in health and disease.

John R Vane & Regina M Botting

Abbreviations

AA	arachidonic acid, eicosatetraenoic acid
Aβ	β-amyloid
ACE	angiotensin converting enzyme
AD	Alzheimer's disease
AMPA	2-amino-3,3-hydroxy-5-methyl-isoxasol-4-yl propionic acid
AP-1	activator protein-1
APC	adenomatous polyposis coli gene
APP	amyloid precursor protein
AS	ankylosing spondylitis
AT_{1a} and AT_{1b}	angiotensin type 1a and 1b
AVP	arginine vasopressin
b.i.d.	twice a day
BMD	bone mineral density
bp	base pairs
BSA	bovine serum albumin
BV	blood vessels
cAMP	cyclic adenosine monophosphate
CAPK	ceramide-activated protein kinase
CDK	cyclin-dependent kinase
CHO	Chinese hamster ovary cells
CI	confidence interval
CLASS	celecoxib long-term arthritis safety study
CNS	central nervous system
COX	cyclooxygenase enzyme
CRE	cyclic adenosine monophosphate response element
Cx	connexin
DP	prostaglandin D_2 receptor
DRG	dorsal root ganglion
DSS	dextran sodium sulphate
EAA	excitatory amino acid
ECM	extracellular matrix
EGF	epidermal growth factor
EMSA	electrophoretic mobility shift assays

EP	prostaglandin E_2 receptor
FAP	familial adenomatous polyposis
FGF-2	fibroblast growth factor
FP	prostaglandin F_2 receptor
FSH	follicle stimulating hormone
5-FU	5-fluorouracil

G_i and G_s	inhibitory and stimulatory G proteins
GFR	glomerular filtration rate
GI	gastrointestinal
GM-CSF	granulocyte–macrophage-colony stimulating factor
GR	glucocorticoid receptor
GSH	glutathione
GSK	glycogen synthase kinase-3

HCG	human chorionic gonadotrophin
12-HETE	12-hydroxyeicosatetraenoic acid
HGF	hepatocyte growth factor
HHT	hydroxyheptadecatrienoic acid
hmWBA	human modified whole-blood assay
HO-1	haem oxygenase-1
H-PGDS	haematopoietic-prostaglandin D synthase
HSF-1	heat shock factor 1
HSP	heat shock protein
HUVEC	human umbilical vein endothelial cells
hWBA	human whole-blood assay

IC_{50}	concentration that reduces effect by 50%
ICAM-1	adhesion molecule
ID_{50}	dose that reduces effect by 50%
IκB	inhibitor kappa B protein
IL	interleukin (e.g. IL-6, IL-1, IL-10)
IFN	interferon (e.g. IFN-γ)
IP	prostaglandin I_2 receptor
i.p.	intraperitoneal
i.t.	intrathecal
i.v.	intravenous

JG	juxtaglomerular
JGA	juxtaglomerular apparatus
JUNK	c-Jun kinase

KSR	kinase suppressor of *Ras*

LCA	leukocyte common antigen
LTB_4	leukotriene B_4
LDL	low-density lipoprotein
L-NAME	L-Nitro arginine methyl ester
LOX	lipoxygenase
L-PGDS	lipocalin-prostaglandin D synthase
LPS	lipopolysaccharide
LUC	luciferase
M-CSF	macrophage-colony stimulating factor
2-MAC	2-macroglobulin
MAPK	mitogen activated protein kinases
MDA	malondialdehyde
MI	myocardial infarction
Min	multiple intestinal neoplasia gene
MN	mononuclear cells
6-MNA	6-methoxy 2-naphthylacetic acid
MR	mineralocorticoid receptor
MS	multiple sclerosis
NF-κB	nuclear factor-kappa B
NK1	neurokinin 1
NMDA	N-methyl-D-aspartate
NOS-1 and NOS-2	nitric oxide synthase 1 and 2
iNOS	inducible nitric oxide synthase
eNOS	endothelial nitric oxide synthase
nNOS	neuronal nitric oxide synthase
NSAIDs	non-steroid (or non-steroidal) anti-inflammatory drugs
NTX	N-telopeptide cross-link excretion
OA	osteoarthritis
ODN	oligodeoxynucleotides
o.d.	once-daily dosing
OVLT	organum vasculosum lamina terminalis (of hypothalamus)
PAF	platelet activating factor
PCR	polymerase chain reaction
PD	potential difference
PDGF	platelet-derived growth factor
PG	prostaglandin (e.g. PGD_2, PGE_1, PGE_2, $PGF_{2\alpha}$, PGG_2, PGH_2)
PGDH	prostaglandin dehydrogenase

PGHS	prostaglandin H_2 synthase, prostaglandin endoperoxide synthase
PGI_2	prostacyclin
$cPLA_2$, $sPLA_2$	cytosolic and secretory phospholipases
PMA	phorbol myristate acetate
PMN	polymorphonuclear leukocytes
p.o.	by mouth (*per os*)
PPAR	peroxisome proliferator-activated receptor
p.p.m.	parts per million
PTH	parathyroid hormone
PUB, PUBs	upper GI perforations, ulcers and bleeds
q.i.d.	four times a day
RA	rheumatoid arthritis
RT-PCR	reverse transcriptase-polymerase chain reaction
SAPK	stress-activated protein kinase
SAR	structure activity relationship
SEM	standard error of the mean
SLE	systemic lupus erythematosus
SP	substance P
SR-A	class A scavenger receptor
SSRE	shear stress response element
STAT	signal transducer of activated T cells
t.i.d.	three times a day
TG	tubuloglomerular
TGF-1	transforming growth factor-1
TNF	tumour necrosis factor
TNFR	tumour necrosis factor receptor
TP	thromboxane A_2 receptor
TRANCE	tumour necrosis factor-related activation induced cytokine
TXA_2 and TXB_2	thromboxane A_2 and B_2
TXAS	thromboxane A_2 synthase
UGI	upper gastrointestinal
UV	ultraviolet
VEGF	vascular endothelial growth factor
VIGOR	'Vioxx' gastrointestinal outcomes research

1 | Formation and actions of prostaglandins and inhibition of their synthesis

John R.Vane and Regina M. Botting

William Harvey Research Institute, Charterhouse Square, London EC1M 6BQ

Seventy years ago two American gynaecologists, Kurzrok and Lieb[1], showed that isolated strips of human uterus relax or contract when exposed to human semen, thus heralding the discovery of a most versatile group of local hormones. Some years later, Goldblatt[2] in England and von Euler[3] in Sweden reported that seminal fluid contained activity that contracted uterine smooth muscle and also caused a fall in blood pressure. Von Euler identified the active principle as a lipid-soluble acid, which he named 'prostaglandin' (PG) because he thought it originated from the prostate gland[4]. Technical advances allowed in the 1960s the characterization of the PGs as a family of lipid compounds with a unique structure. PGE_1 and $PGF_{1\alpha}$ were isolated in crystalline form[5] and proved to be 20-carbon unsaturated carboxylic acids with a cyclopentane ring[6]. In 1964 Bergström and co-workers[7] synthesized PGE_2 using arachidonic acid and an enzyme preparation from ram seminal vesicles, thus demonstrating these organs as the true source of PGs in the semen.

PGs and related compounds are some of the most prevalent of autacoids and have been detected in every tissue and body fluid except in red blood cells. As local hormones, they produce in minute concentrations an incredibly broad spectrum of effects that modulate almost every biological function. They derive mostly from the 20-carbon fatty acid, arachidonic acid ($C20:4\omega6$) and almost 100 different derivatives have been identified to date, including lipoxins[8] and isoprostanes[9].

The PGs are pivotal to inflammatory responses, as evidenced by the anti-inflammatory effects of drugs that interfere with their synthesis such as the steroid and non-steroid anti-inflammatory drugs (NSAIDs). The discovery 10 years ago of a second cyclooxygenase (COX-2), inducible by cytokines,

1

has led to an important clarification of our understanding of the roles of PGs as mediators of inflammation. In general, inflammation induces COX-2, which makes PGs locally, whereas COX-1 is a housekeeping enzyme responsible for modulating physiological events. The fact that COX-2 is an enzyme induced over a few hours means that tissue and fluid levels of COX and of PGs may have to be re-evaluated, for many of the studies were made before COX-2 and all its ramifications were discovered.

STRUCTURE OF PROSTAGLANDINS

The eicosanoids derive from 20-carbon essential fatty acids: eicosatrienoic, eicosatetraenoic (arachidonic or AA) and eicosapentaenoic (EPA) acids. The PGs derived from them differ by the substituents on the cyclopentane ring and the subscripts indicate the number of double bonds in the side chain. PGs of the 3 series, for example PGI_3, derive from EPA and are more abundant in fish and marine animals. EPA is an important constituent of fish oils and the different pharmacological properties of the derived eicosanoids, as compared with prostacyclin (PGI_2) and thromboxane (TXA_2) from arachidonic acid, are the basis of its promotion as a health food.

 Arachidonic acid has four double bonds and leads to the important physiologically active PGs such as PGD_2, PGE_2, $PGF_{2\alpha}$, PGI_2 and TXA_2 (Figure 1). Eicosatrienoic acid contains three double bonds, but there is little evidence that the derived PGs, such as PGE_1, or PGI_1 play a role in humans, although PGE_1 has been found in human semen.

SYNTHESIS OF PROSTAGLANDINS

Prostaglandins are formed from arachidonic acid by way of unstable endoperoxide intermediates by a dimeric enzyme with two active sites in the same enzyme protein, prostaglandin endoperoxide synthase (PGHS) or cyclooxygenase (COX). The COX and peroxidase activities together catalyse the insertion of oxygen and rearrangement of the carbon skeleton of the substrate, arachidonic acid, to form the endoperoxides PGG_2 and then PGH_2 (Figure 1)[10]. PGH_2 acts as a substrate for different synthases to form the more stable primary PGs (see below).

TWO CYCLOOXYGENASE ENZYMES

Over the years, there were various suggestions that there was a second COX enzyme. As early as 1972, Smith and Lands[11], and Flower and Vane[12], speculated on the existence of isoenzymes. In 1980, Whittle et al.[13] discussed the selectivity of enzymes in different tissues to explain the lack of toxicity of salicylate on the stomach. Lin et al.[14] reported maximal increases in the levels

Figure 1 The arachidonic acid cascade.

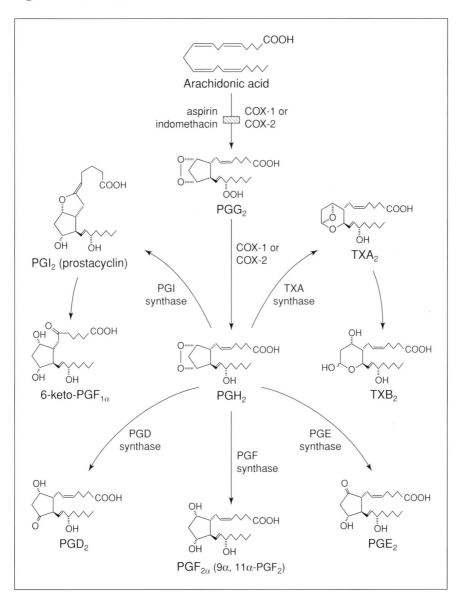

of PGE$_2$ synthesis and of COX mRNA, but no increase in COX protein, in NIH-3T3 cells 3 h after stimulation with recombinant platelet-derived growth factor (rPDGF). They speculated that rPDGF was inducing the expression of a second COX originating from a separate gene.

As often happens before a new discovery is properly defined, many pharmacologists and biochemists reported an inducible COX without knowing that they were working with a different enzyme. Needleman and his colleagues[15] demonstrated COX induction in a perfused rabbit kidney in which ureteric obstruction 72 h before removal had set up an inflammatory reaction. There was a progressive increase in the release of PGE_2 in response to a fixed dose of bradykinin, which could be prevented by treatment with the protein synthesis inhibitors actinomycin D or cycloheximide. Aspirin inhibited PG release in the initial stages of the kidney perfusion process, but was less effective as the perfusion continued. The authors concluded that the progressive increase in PG release depended on *de novo* synthesis of cyclooxygenase enzyme in the ureter-obstructed kidney[15].

Treatment of human umbilical vein endothelial cells (HUVEC) in culture with interleukin-1 (IL-1), tumour necrosis factor (TNF) [16] or phorbol ester for 24 h induced an increase of PGI_2 synthesis[17] and expression of COX mRNA[18] as well as COX protein[19]. Prostacyclin levels reached a maximum 12 h after exposure to TNF[16] or phorbol ester[18], and 24 h after stimulation with IL-1[19]. The stimulation of eicosanoid biosynthesis was abolished by cycloheximide or actinomycin D, whereas the induction of COX mRNA by IL-1α was potentiated with cycloheximide, which is characteristic of the regulation of transcription for immediate-early genes[20]. Interestingly, increased COX enzyme levels leading to increased PG synthesis were also reported in murine smooth muscle and osteoblastic cells treated with epidermal growth factor (EGF) [21,22], in 3T3 cells treated with PDGF[23], in human amnion cells treated with EGF[24], and in human dermal fibroblasts stimulated with IL-1[25]. The induction of COX synthesis by IL-1 in human dermal fibroblasts was reported to be a transcriptional as well as a post-transcriptional event[26]. In rat vascular smooth muscle cells, COX mRNA levels were enhanced by EGF and transforming growth factor (TGF)-β, but suppressed completely by dexamethasone.

In 1989, Rosen et al.[27] were studying the regulation of COX in cultures of epithelial cells from trachea and found an increase in activity of COX during prolonged cell culture. The increase in activity was not associated with an increase in 70 kDa COX protein nor by increased mRNA of 2.8 kb. They did find a second mRNA of 4.0 kb and suggested that their evidence was consistent with the 4.0 kb mRNA being derived from a distinct COX-related gene that encoded for a protein with COX activity.

Needleman and his group[28-30] continued their earlier work and reported that bacterial lipopolysaccharide (LPS) increased the synthesis of PGs in human monocytes *in vitro* and in mouse peritoneal macrophages *in vivo*. This increase, but not the basal level of enzyme, was inhibited by dexamethasone and associated with *de novo* synthesis of new COX protein. This reinforced the concept of 'multiple COX pools – constitutive and stimulated – possibly under different regulatory controls'[31].

THE DISCOVERY OF CYCLOOXYGENASE-2

The breakthrough discovery of a different COX came from molecular biologists outside the field of PGs. Simmons and his colleagues[32,33] were studying early response genes and discovered an inducible second form of COX in chicken embryo cells. It was encoded by a 4.1 kb mRNA similar in size to that reported by Rosen et al.[27]. They cloned the gene, deduced the protein structure and found it homologous to COX, but to no other known protein. Independently, Herschmann and his colleagues[34] found a similar gene in the mouse, as later did Simmons et al.[35], O'Banion et al.[36] and Sirois and Richards[37]. Thus, there are two distinct enzymes, COX-1 and COX-2. Both enzymes have a molecular weight of 70–71 kDa and the amino acid sequence of the inducible COX-2 shows a 60% homology with the sequence of the constitutive enzyme COX-1. The mRNA for inducible COX-2 approximates 4.5 kb and that of the constitutive COX-1, 2.8 kb. The inhibition by glucocorticoids of the expression of COX-2 is an additional aspect of the anti-inflammatory actions of the corticosteroids, which are also mediated by the release of lipocortin[38]. The levels of COX-2, normally very low in cells, are tightly controlled by a number of factors including cytokines, intracellular messengers and by the availability of substrate.

The overall field is still in a rapid phase of development, but some generalizations can be made. The constitutive isoform, COX-1 is ubiquitous and has clear physiological functions. Its activation leads, for instance, to the production of PGI_2 which, when released by the vessel wall (but see later), is vasodilator and anti-thrombogenic[39] and is cytoprotective when released by the gastric mucosa[40]. The second isoform, COX-2, is inducible in a number of cells by proinflammatory stimuli[41]. Since COX-2 is induced by inflammatory stimuli and by cytokines in migratory and other cells it was attractive to suggest, as Vane and others did in 1993[42,43], that the anti-inflammatory actions of NSAIDs are due to the inhibition of COX-2, whereas the unwanted side effects, such as irritation of the stomach mucosa and toxic effects on the kidney, are due to inhibition of the constitutive enzyme COX-1. This very important hypothesis[44] is now well supported, not only by a wealth of data on COX-2 inhibitors in animal tests, but also by the better tolerability in humans of selective COX-2 inhibitors (see below).

Whereas the side effects on the stomach are clearly connected to inhibition of COX-1, those on the kidney are more complex. We now know that the macula densa and the thick ascending loop of Henle (TALH) contain small amounts of constitutive COX-2 and that its products probably regulate the renin–angiotensin system (see R.Harris, Chapter 9). The side effects of NSAIDs in causing fluid and sodium retention are probably due to inhibition of COX-2 in the kidney, whereas the effects on glomerular filtration rate (GFR) are due to inhibition of COX-1[45]. Apart from its role in inflammation, induced COX-2 also has physiological functions, such as in ovulation and childbirth[46,47].

RELEASE OF PROSTAGLANDINS

Because PGs are not stored, concentrations found in tissues or exudates represent new synthesis and release. Release by chemicals, such as bradykinin, is immediate and transient (through COX-1), whereas release by a trauma, such as inflammation, is slow and long-lasting (through COX-2). The arachidonic acid substrate is liberated from membrane phospholipids by activation or induction of phospholipase A_2.

The measurement of PG concentrations in tissues is complicated by the fact that any chemical or physical disturbance of cells 'turns on' PG production[48] so that, for instance, in homogenized tissues, PG concentrations represent the capacity of the tissue to generate PGs rather than the tissue content. Recognition of this fact led to the development of a standard 'vortex' mixing to measure the capacity of tissues to generate PGs[49].

PROSTAGLANDIN SYNTHASES

Although the existence of PGHS or COX has been recognized since the 1960s, the synthase enzymes that convert the endoperoxide products of COX into the primary prostaglandins, PGE_2, PGD_2, $PGF_{2\alpha}$, PGI_2 and TX have been characterized relatively recently.

PGE synthase

An inducible PGE synthase[50] was recently identified. This is a 15–16 kDa glutathione-dependent, membrane-associated protein that is upregulated by IL-1β and downregulated by phenobarbitone. The 2 kb mRNA is strongly expressed in the cancer cell lines A549 and HeLa and in human placenta, prostate gland, testis, breast and bladder. Several other tissues, including small intestine and colon, express PGE synthase mRNA, but less strongly. The PGE synthase gene spans 14.8 kb and is localized to the same chromosome as the genes for PGD synthase and COX-1. PGE synthase and COX-2 are likely to be co-induced by cytokines such as IL-1β, so that PGE_2 biosynthesis may depend on the activity of both of these enzymes[51-53].

However, two separate glutathione-dependent PGE synthases with different tissue and subcellular distributions have been reported. A cytosolic PGE synthase, found mainly in brain, may predominantly convert PGH_2 derived from COX-1 into PGE_2, whereas a microsomal PGE synthase induced during the inflammatory response may be functionally linked with COX-2 in preference to COX-1[54].

PGF synthase

A 36.8 kDa cytosolic enzyme was isolated from bovine and human lungs and from bovine liver, which catalyses not only the reduction of PGH_2 to $PGF_{2\alpha}$, but also reduces PGD_2 to $9\alpha,11\beta$-PGF_2 (refs 55,56). In the liver, this enzyme also oxidizes various substrates, such as endogenous steroid compounds and $9\alpha,11\beta$-PGF_2, although in the lungs it functions primarily as a PGF synthase.

PGD_2 released by mast cells may exacerbate bronchoconstriction in allergic asthma[57] (see later), so the PGF synthase expressed in lung lymphocytes may influence the pathogenesis of allergic lung diseases[56] by modulating the metabolism of PGD_2.

PGD synthases

In the early 1960s large amounts of a protein named β-trace were found that appeared to be specific to the human cerebrospinal fluid (CSF)[58,59]. Thirty years later[60] β-trace was found to be identical in structure to lipocalin-PGD synthase (L-PGDS), one of the two enzymes synthesizing PGD_2 from PGH_2. The lipocalins are members of a superfamily of lipophilic ligand-carrier proteins binding, among others, retinoids or thyroid hormones[61,62]. L-PGDS is localized mainly in the leptomeninges, choroid plexus and oligodendrocytes of the central nervous system (CNS) and circulates in the CSF, as β-trace, through the ventricular system and extracellular spaces of the brain[63]. The PGD_2 produced by this enzyme in the adult brain is thought to act as a neurohormone to induce sleep[64] or hyperalgesia[65]. However, in immature rat brain or chick spinal cord, immunoreactivity for L-PGDS is also detected in developing neurons where PGD_2 may function as a neurotransmitter[66]. In addition to its role in the brain and spinal cord, L-PGDS is also distributed in auditory and ocular tissues, in male genital organs and in the cardiovascular system, where production of anti-aggregatory PGD_2 may protect against formation of atherosclerotic plaques[67].

The other enzyme synthesizing PGD_2, haematopoietic-PGD synthase (H-PGDS) has the same molecular weight of 26 kDa as L-PGDS, but it is biochemically and immunologically different[68]. H-PGDS is an isoenzyme of glutathione (GSH) S-transferase and requires GSH for the reaction with PGH_2 (ref. 69). Rat H-PGDS is most strongly expressed in the spleen and moderately so in oviduct, thymus, bone marrow and ileum[70], while the human enzyme is expressed strongly in placenta, less so in lung and weakly in brain. The induction of H-PGDS may be involved in mast cell maturation[71] and also in megakaryocytic differentiation[72].

Thromboxane synthase

Investigation of TXA_2 synthase (TXAS) came soon after the discovery of TXA_2 itself in 1975[73], for it was hoped that inhibition of this enzyme would lead to the development of effective anti-platelet drugs. TXAS was initially purified from human platelets[74]. It is a 58.8 kDa, membrane-bound protein attached to the endoplasmic reticulum[75], consisting of 533 amino acids and converts PGH_2 to TXA_2, which degrades chemically within 30 s to TXB_2, the stable hydrolysis product[75,76]. The size of the TXAS mRNA from human platelets is approximately 2.2 kb. TXAS activity is also found in many other tissues such as lung, kidney and spleen, as well as in macrophages and fibroblasts. 50–70% of the total products of the conversion of PGH_2 to TXA_2 consist of malondialdehyde (MDA) and hydroxyheptadecatrienoic acid (HHT) in a 1:1:1 ratio with TXA_2 (measured as its metabolite, TXB_2), although possible functions for these other products are unknown.

TXAS contains one haem group in each molecule and its primary structure, determined from the nucleotide sequence of its cDNA, shows a 34–36% similarity to the amino acid sequences of cytochrome P450 (CYP450) enzymes. However, TXAS has no monooxygenase activity. Nucleotide sequencing[77] demonstrated that the human gene encoding TXAS spans over 75 kb, and studies of tissue distribution found high concentrations of the 2.2 kb mRNA in platelets, peripheral blood leukocytes, spleen, lung and liver, with smaller amounts in kidney, placenta and thymus. The TXAS gene contains potential binding sites for several transcription factors, including a cAMP response element that may regulate its expression; however, studies of the enzyme have been hampered until recently by the low yields of recombinant protein obtained in expression systems[78]. Interestingly, dexamethasone, which suppresses the expression of COX-2, increased TXAS enzyme protein levels, whereas treatment with phorbol ester induced TXAS mRNA in cultured HE cells[79]. After platelets, blood monocytes have the highest content of TXAS[80] while no enzyme was found in human neutrophils (see below).

Prostacyclin synthase

In 1976, Vane and his colleagues discovered that blood vessels made a previously unknown prostanoid that they called PGX[39] and later renamed PGI_2 (ref. 81). This is a bicyclic eicosanoid with a short chemical half-life of approximately 3 min at physiological pH, which degrades to the inactive substance 6-keto-$PGF_{1\alpha}$. Production of PGI_2 by cultured cells from vessel walls shows that endothelial cells are the most active producers of PGI_2 (ref. 82).

Salmon and Flower[83] developed the assay for PGI_2 synthase (PGIS). Subsequently, the enzyme was purified from bovine aorta by DeWitt and Smith[84] and, like TXAS, found to be a haemoprotein with optical and electron paramagnetic resonance spectra characteristic of the P450 monooxygenases[85]. PGIS is predominantly expressed in vascular endothelial and smooth muscle cells[86]. Cloning and sequence analysis of the cDNA from aortic endothelial cells[87] established that the amino acid sequence of PGIS was about 32% homologous with the sequences of the P450 enzymes, but shared only 16%

common identity with the structure of TXAS[88]. This membrane-bound enzyme is made up of 500 amino acids and has a molecular weight of about 57 kDa. The mRNA for bovine PGIS[87] is 2.7 kb in size, whereas human aortic endothelial cells contain a major mRNA of 6 kb and minor mRNAs of 3.2, 2.5 and 1.7 kb[89]. PGIS mRNA is expressed in many human tissues particularly in ovary, heart, skeletal muscle, lung and prostate gland. In the rat, PGIS mRNA is most strongly expressed in smooth muscle cells of the arteries, bronchi and uterus but also detected in other cell types such as fibroblasts in heart myocardium, lung parenchyma cells and kidney inner medulla tubular and interstitial cells[90].

The gene encoding human PGIS is about 60 kb long[91] and contains a responsive site for shear stress and a site for nuclear factor-κB (NF-κB), which can be activated by TNF-α[92]. In bovine endothelial cells, TNF-α stimulates the generation of PGI_2 (ref. 93) and increases levels of PGIS mRNA and enzyme protein 4–12 h after the start of treatment[87,94]. Shear loading applied to HUVECs in culture increased production of 6-keto-$PGF_{1\alpha}$, the stable metabolite of PGI_2, as well as doubling the expression of the mRNAs for PGIS and COX-2 after 6 h of treatment. No increase in phospholipase A_2 (PLA_2) mRNA was observed, but COX-1 mRNA increased 1.4-fold after 1 h application of shear stress and then remained constant for 12 h[95].

PROSTAGLANDIN RECEPTORS

The nomenclature for prostaglandin receptors includes the letter 'P' for 'prostaglandin' with a prefix of 'E', 'I', 'F', 'D' or 'T' to signify prostaglandin E, I, F, D or thromboxane.

Receptors for prostaglandin E_2 (EP)

So far, four EP receptors have been identified. EP_1 is present in smooth muscle cells and mediates contraction of some smooth muscle (including gastrointestinal smooth muscle).

EP_2 is found in smooth muscle and other cells. It mediates relaxation of smooth muscle and is coupled to a G_s protein to stimulate adenylate cyclase, thereby raising intracellular cAMP levels. EP_2 is important for *in vivo* fertilization, as $EP_2^{-/-}$ mice ovulated normally but the ova failed to become fertilized[96]. EP_2 also mediates arterial dilation and salt-sensitive hypertension. An infusion of PGE_2, which is normally hypotensive, raised blood pressure in $EP_2^{-/-}$ mice and $EP_2^{-/-}$ mice fed a high salt diet became hypertensive while there was no change in systolic blood pressure of control animals[97].

EP_3 is widely distributed and mediates contraction of smooth muscle (including vascular smooth muscle), platelet shape change, inhibition of stomach acid secretion, inhibition of autonomic transmitter release and inhibition of fat cell lipolysis. PGE_2 also mediates fever generation through the EP_3 receptor since deletion of the EP_3 gene in mutant mice abolishes the febrile response to PGE_2 as well as to LPS and IL-1[98].

EP_4 is important for the closure of the ductus arteriosus in neonate mice. Most $EP_4^{-/-}$ neonates die within 72 h after birth and histological examination of these animals showed that the ductus arteriosus remained open. Thus, normal function of the EP_4 receptor is required to mediate neonatal adaptation of the cardiovascular system[99,100].

The differences between these four EP receptors should provide the medicinal chemist with opportunities for design of receptor antagonists that can distinguish between separate activities of PGE_2.

Receptor for prostaglandin I₂ (IP)

IP is found on platelets and it is involved in inflammatory responses. It stimulates adenylate cyclase through a G_s protein and its activation results in elevation of intracellular cAMP levels. This is also the mechanism for the relaxant action of prostacyclin on vascular smooth muscle[101,102]. Mutant mice with a deleted gene for expression of the IP receptor suffer from an increased susceptibility to thrombosis and reduced responses to inflammation and pain[103].

Receptor for thromboxane A₂ (TP)

TP mediates contraction of all vascular and airway smooth muscle by TXA_2. Stimulation of the TP receptor on platelets leads to their aggregation and deletion of the TP gene greatly prolongs bleeding time in mice[104]. TP receptors are coupled through regulatory G proteins to increased intracellular phosphoinositol hydrolysis. Antagonists for the TP receptor on platelets are of interest to inhibit platelet aggregation and prevent further thrombosis after myocardial infarction.

Receptor for prostaglandin F₂α (FP)

Prostaglandin $F_{2\alpha}$ is involved in reproductive processes such as ovulation, luteolysis and parturition. In most species, except primates and humans, FP stimulation in ovarian luteal cells by $PGF_{2\alpha}$ initiates parturition by abolishing release of progesterone. Homozygous FP-deficient mice became pregnant but failed to go into labour. Thus, mice lacking the FP gene are unable to give birth[105]. In humans, the induction of COX-2 in the amniotic membranes and uterine wall at parturition leads to the production of $PGF_{2\alpha}$ and PGE_2 that contract the smooth muscle to expel the uterine contents (see P. Bennett, Chapter 11).

Receptor for prostaglandin D₂ (DP)

DP receptors are present in the brain, as well as in some vascular smooth muscle and in blood platelets. They are coupled to adenylate cyclase through a G_s protein and stimulation results in formation of cAMP. Deletion of the

DP gene prevents inflammatory cell migration into the site of allergen challenge in sensitized mice, suggesting that PGD_2 released from lung mast cells may have a pathological role in allergic asthma[106].

PHYSIOLOGICAL AND PATHOLOGICAL FUNCTIONS OF PROSTAGLANDINS

Inflammation

Prostaglandin E_2 is found in synovial fluid of arthritic joints of patients at a concentration of approximately 20 ng ml^{-1} (ref. 107). It is the major PG involved in inflammation and pain since antibodies to PGE_2 inhibit pain and inflammation (Figure 2) in the rat model of carrageenan-induced paw oedema[108,109]. Carrageenan-induced hyperalgesia in the rat paw was also reversed by administration of SC58635, a selective COX-2 inhibitor, demonstrating PGE_2 synthesis by the COX-2 enzyme in this animal model[110]. Both PGE_2 and PGI_2 have been detected in inflammatory lesions. There may well be species differences, for inflammation is suppressed in mice in which the receptor for PGI_2 has been deleted[103]. It is likely, therefore, that both PGE_2 and PGI_2 contribute to the development of inflammatory erythema and pain[111].

Pain

Prostaglandin E_2 is hyperalgesic, so that it does not cause pain when applied to an unprotected blister base on a human forearm, but potentiates pain induced by bradykinin or histamine[112]. Ferreira concluded that the pain-producing action of inflammatory mediators such as bradykinin or histamine was potentiated when PGs sensitized chemical receptors on primary afferent nerve terminals. PGI_2 rather than PGE_2 may be involved in short-lasting hyperalgesia because it was more potent than PGE_2 in producing hyperalgesia in both the rat and dog models[113]. PGI_2 is mainly responsible for the stretching response to an intraperitoneal (i.p.) injection of zymosan in mice[114] and IP receptor-deficient mice showed greatly reduced nociceptive responses to i.p. administration of dilute acetic acid[103]. The stretching response to acetic acid is mediated mainly by COX-1 since it is abolished in COX-1$^{-/-}$ mice[115]. Thus, both PGE_2 and PGI_2 can sensitize nociceptors on sensory nerve terminals to painful stimulation.

Fever

Fever is caused by release of PGE_2 by inflammatory mediators in blood vessels of the hypothalamus[116]. LPS from infecting organisms stimulates formation of the cytokine IL-1, which in turn stimulates the synthesis of PGE_2 close to the organum vasculosum lamina terminalis (OVLT) region of the hypothalamus. The EP$_3$ receptor mediates the pyretic action of PGE_2

Figure 2 Anti-inflammatory (a) and analgesic (b) activity of monoclonal anti-PGE$_2$ antibody (2B5). Rats were treated with either 2B5 (▲) or MOPC21 protein (control for 2B5) (■) 18 h before or indomethacin (●) or vehicle (○) 1 h before injection of 1% carrageenan in saline into the hind paw. 2B5 and indomethacin reduced carrageenan-induced paw oedema and hyperalgesia. (Modified from ref. 109 with permission.)

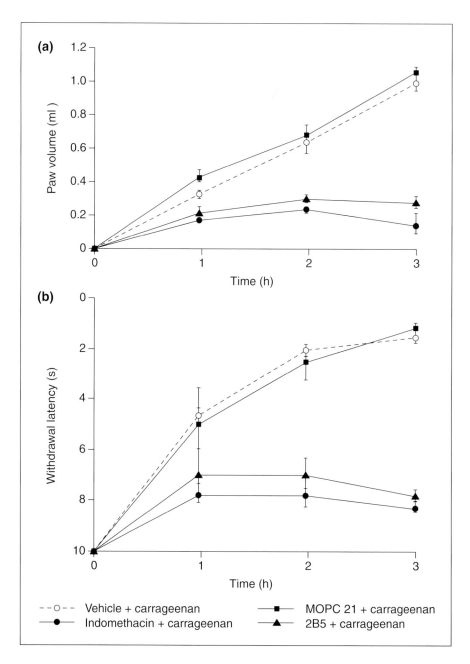

since mutant mice lacking this receptor do not develop fever with PGE_2, IL-1 or LPS[98] (see above). Pyretic PGE_2 is produced by COX-2 because selective COX-2 inhibitors abolish fever in several species, including humans[117,118].

Li et al.[117] tested the effects of LPS in producing a fever in knockout mice. Wild-type, and COX-1[+/-] and COX-1[-/-] mice all responded to LPS within 1 h with a 1°C rise in core temperature – the fever gradually abated over the next 4 h. By contrast, COX-2[+/-] and COX-2[-/-] mice displayed no temperature rise after LPS. Thus, COX-2 is necessary for the fever produced by LPS. A corollary of this finding is that there is unlikely to be a COX-3 through which paracetamol brings down a fever. Recently, Oates et al.[119] showed that in HUVECs in culture, paracetamol inhibits COX-2 with an IC_{50} of 66 μM, well within the therapeutic range in humans. Furthermore, the selective COX-2 inhibitor rofecoxib is a potent antipyretic agent in man[120].

In the immune system

Mouse macrophages stimulated with inflammatory mediators to induce COX-2 release PGE_2 and PGI_2, whereas stimulated human monocytes and macrophages secrete large amounts of TXA_2 together with PGE_2 (refs 121,122). Neutrophils make moderate amounts of PGE_2, while mast cells produce PGD_2 almost exclusively[123]. No known prostanoids are made by lymphocytes, although both COX-1 and COX-2 have been detected in these cells[124]. Release of PGE_2 by macrophages may act as a negative feedback control mechanism, reducing further activation and producing inhibition of immune function.

PGE_2 also inhibits interleukin-2 (IL-2) and interferon-γ (IFN-γ) production from T lymphocytes[125] as well as IL-1 and TNF-α release from macrophages[126-128]. However, immature cells of the immune system are stimulated by PGE_2. For example, PGE_2 induces immature thymocytes and B lymphocytes to differentiate and acquire the functional characteristics of mature cells[129].

It has been suggested that PGE_2 produced by tumour cells accounts for the depression of the immune system associated with cancer. Large amounts of PGs are produced by tumour cells[130], which induce a generalized state of immunodeficiency[131]. This immunosuppression was prevented in tumour-bearing mice with inhibitors of PG synthesis such as indomethacin[132]. Treatment of rheumatoid arthritis with aspirin-like drugs leads to inhibition of PG formation and thus to removal of the immunosuppressant effect of these eicosanoids. Another consequence of removing the suppression of immune processes by PGs may be the enhancement of cartilage breakdown seen with NSAIDs *in vitro* and *in vivo*[133,134].

Cyclopentenone PGs such as 15-deoxy-PGJ_2, may exert anti-inflammatory activity by inhibiting inhibitor kappa B (IκB) kinase and promoting the resolution of chronic inflammation[135,136].

In the gastrointestinal tract

PG synthesis can be demonstrated in every part of the gastrointestinal (GI) tract. In rat tissues, using vortex generation, the rank order of PGI_2 synthesis as determined by bioassay techniques was greatest in gastric muscle and forestomach, followed by gastric mucosa, colon, rectum, ileum, caecum, duodenum, jejunum and oesophagus[137]. A striking demonstration of the 'cytoprotective' action of prostanoids was the finding that gastric damage induced by topical application of strong acids, hypertonic solutions or ethanol in rats, could be reduced by coadministration of various PGs[138-140].

The cytoprotective action is complex and depends on a combination of several mechanisms:

1. Both PGE_2 (acting on the EP_3 receptor) and PGI_2 (acting on the IP receptor) reduce secretion of gastric acid, even histamine-stimulated acid secretion, by the parietal cells of the stomach. This action is species-dependent since PGI_2 is more active than PGE_2 in anaesthetized rat, conscious dog and in the monkey, while PGE_2 is a more potent inhibitor of acid secretion in the stomach of the anaesthetized dog[139,141-145].
2. Intravenous infusions of PGE_2 or PGI_2 exerted a direct vasodilator action on the gastric mucosa[142]. Increases in gastric mucosal blood flow could be beneficial in maintaining the functional integrity of the gastric tissue[144].
3. Intragastric administration of PGE_2 to humans stimulates the release of viscous mucus[146] that could play a defensive role against mucosal injury[147]. PGE_2 is synthesized by epithelial and smooth muscle cells in the stomach. Other than providing a physical barrier, mucus may act to create an unstirred layer of secreted bicarbonate[148] and hence help to neutralize hydrogen ions diffusing back from the lumen into the mucosa. PGE_2 stimulates bicarbonate secretion via the EP_3 receptor, so that application of acid induces more severe damage to the stomach mucosa in $EP_3^{-/-}$ than in wild-type mice[149].

In the cardiovascular system

PGE_2 potently relaxes vascular smooth muscle accounting for the characteristic vasodilation (EP_2 receptor) leading to the erythema seen in acute inflammation[150]. The effect of vasodilatation is to increase blood flow through inflamed tissues that augments the extravasation of fluid, thus facilitating oedema formation[151].

Pulsatile pressure releases PGI_2 from isolated arteries[152], which is likely to be an important release mechanism for PGI_2 *in vivo*. The shear stress induced by laminar, but not by turbulent flow upregulates COX-2 in endothelial cells[153] and very likely PGIS as well[95] (see above). Recent work in humans with selective COX-2 inhibitors shows that most of the PGI_2 made by endothelial cells derives from induced COX-2[45,154]. To measure PGI_2

production in the whole body, the metabolite 2,3-dinor-6-keto-$PGF_{1\alpha}$ in the urine was estimated[155].

PGI_2 potently inhibits aggregation of blood platelets (IP receptors), an effect mediated by stimulation of platelet adenylate cyclase, which results in accumulation of cAMP[156]. PGI_2 induces vasodilation by relaxing the smooth muscle of the blood vessel walls[101]. A deficiency in PGI_2 formation in blood vessel walls occurs in atherosclerosis and diabetes, whereas its overproduction is associated with endotoxic shock[157]. Thus, adequate PGI_2 production may be important in preventing the development of thrombosis and atherosclerosis. In a model of thrombosis in which vascular endothelial cells were damaged, IP$^{-/-}$ mice showed a greater tendency for thrombus formation than normal controls[102,158].

Blood platelets contain only COX-1, which converts arachidonic acid to the potent pro-aggregatory and vasoconstrictor eicosanoid TXA_2 the major COX product formed by platelets. TXA_2 has a half-life at body pH and temperature of 30 s, breaking down to the inactive TXB_2 (ref. 159). It was proposed in 1976 that PGI_2 and TXA_2 represent the opposite poles of a homeostatic mechanism for regulation of haemostasis *in vivo*[160]. TP$^{-/-}$ mice have greatly prolonged bleeding times demonstrating the importance of TXA_2 in haemostasis[103].

In the kidney

The cortex of normal kidneys produces mainly PGE_2 and PGI_2 with very small amounts of TXA_2 (ref. 161). The renal medulla produces mostly PGE_2 for which it has a synthetic capacity approximately $20\times$ that of the cortex[162]. PG levels in the urine are generally regarded as reflecting production of PGs by the kidneys[163]. PGE_2 and PGI_2 are vasodilators in the kidney and intrarenal infusions increase renal blood flow. PGs are also natriuretic, inhibiting tubular sodium reabsorption and, in the TALH, they reduce chloride transport. Glomerular epithelial and mesangial cells have the synthetic capacity to form both PGI_2 and PGE_2. These prostanoids are therefore uniquely situated to influence renal blood flow, GFR and the release of renin. Both PGI_2 and PGE_2 synthesized in the renal cortex are important stimulators of renin release[164]. PGI_2 formed by COX-2 in mesangial cells may directly stimulate renin secretion since upregulation of COX-2 has been observed in the macula densa following salt deprivation[165].

Different nephron segments synthesize a distinctive spectrum of arachidonic acid metabolites that behave as either modulators or mediators of the actions of hormones on tubular function[166,167]. Studies on rabbit medullary cells in the mTALH revealed that the principal pathway of arachidonic acid metabolism in this segment of the nephron is via CYP450 and not COX-1[168]. Thus, the major CYP450-derived arachidonic acid products synthesized by the rabbit mTALH are 19- and 20-hydroxyeicosatetraenoates (HETEs) and

20-COOH HETE, a metabolite of 20-HETE[167]. However, some COX-2 protein is also expressed constitutively in unstimulated mTALH cells and COX-2 expression increases after treatment with TNF or phorbol myristate acetate (PMA)[169]. In addition, the products of CYP450 interact with TNF formed by mTALH cells and with angiotensin II to regulate ion transport in cells of the mTALH[170].

Maintenance of kidney function both in animal models of disease states and in patients with congestive heart failure, liver cirrhosis or renal insufficiency, is dependent on vasodilator PGs. These patients are, therefore, at risk of renal ischaemia when PG synthesis is reduced by NSAIDs. Synthesis of PGE_2 is mainly by COX-1, although as mentioned above, there are discrete cells in the macula densa that contain constitutive COX-2[165,171]. PGI_2, made by constitutive COX-2 may drive the renin–angiotensin system[171]. Schneider and Stahl[172] have reviewed this rapidly evolving field.

Fitzgerald's group[45] compared the renal effects of the non-selective COX inhibitor indomethacin with those of the selective COX-2 inhibitor rofecoxib and with placebo in healthy older adults over 2 weeks of treatment. Both active regimes were associated with a transient but significant decline in urinary sodium excretion during the first 72 h. The GFR was decreased by indomethacin but not changed significantly by rofecoxib. Thus, acute sodium retention by NSAIDs in healthy adults is mediated by inhibition of COX-2, whereas depression of GFR is due to inhibition of COX-1.

The urinary excretion of the PGI_2 metabolite, 2,3-dinor-6-keto-$PGF_{1\alpha}$ was decreased by both rofecoxib and indomethacin, but not by placebo[45]. The implication of this is that the endothelial cell uses COX-2 to make prostacyclin – this enzyme is possibly induced by the shear stress in the arterial wall, rather than being present constitutively.

In the lungs

PGs have potent actions on bronchiolar tone and on the diameter of the pulmonary blood vessels. The airways of most species, including humans, contract to $PGF_{2\alpha}$, TXA_2 and PGD_2, whereas PGE_2 and PGI_2 are weak bronchodilators. PGD_2 and $PGF_{2\alpha}$ potently constrict the airways in asthmatic patients and potentiate the constrictor responses to other spasmogens[173,174]. The concentrations of PGD_2 and $PGF_{2\alpha}$ in bronchoalveolar lavage fluid of asthmatic subjects were tenfold higher than in control non-asthmatic and atopic individuals[175]. Excretion of the stable metabolite of TXA_2 increases after allergen challenge[176]. Thus, raised levels of bronchoconstrictor PGs in the lungs may contribute to allergic bronchospasm during asthmatic attacks. Pulmonary blood vessels are constricted by $PGF_{2\alpha}$ and TXA_2, but in some species they dilate to PGE_2. PGI_2 is a potent vasodilator of the pulmonary circulation in humans and other species.

Blood levels of PGI_2 increase 15- to 20-fold in anaesthetized patients with artificial ventilation. This endothelium-derived PGI_2 is well placed to function as a local vasodilator and to prevent the formation of microthrombi[177]. PGI_2 may be important in regulating pulmonary vascular tone during chronic hypoxia. Overexpression of PGIS in lung epithelium of transgenic mice prevented development of pulmonary hypertension after exposure to hypobaric hypoxia[178], while lungs of patients with severe pulmonary hypertension expressed lower levels of PGIS than those of control subjects[179].

Mediators of inflammation such as bradykinin, histamine and 5-hydroxytryptamine release PGs from lung tissue. Histamine releases $PGF_{2\alpha}$ from human lung fragments by stimulating H_1 receptors. Lungs of asthmatics produce more histamine than normal lungs, which correlates with the greater number of mast cells found in asthmatic lungs[180]. Proinflammatory cytokines such as IL-1β and TNF-α are present in the inflamed airways of asthmatic patients[181] and induce COX-2 expression in lung epithelial cells, airway smooth muscle, pulmonary endothelial cells and alveolar macrophages[182]. In the carrageenan-induced pleurisy model of inflammation, levels of COX-2 in the cell pellets of pleural exudate increased maximally 2 h after the injection of carrageenan[183]. This was accounted for by induction of COX-2 in 100% of mast cells, in 65% of resident mononuclear leukocytes and in 8% of extravasated neutrophils present in the exudate[184].

Inflammatory stimuli cause differential release of PGs from various regions of the lungs. Human cultured pulmonary epithelial cells stimulated with LPS, IL-1β, TNF-α or a mixture of cytokines synthesize mainly PGE_2 together with smaller amounts of $PGF_{2\alpha}$, PGI_2 and TXA_2. This PG production can be suppressed by dexamethasone[185]. Thus, PGE_2 is the main product of COX-2 induced in lung epithelial cells[186,187] and *in vitro* studies in animals suggest that epithelial PGE_2 may protect against bronchoconstriction induced by bradykinin, tachykinins and endothelin[188-192]. Endogenous PGE_2 may therefore be bronchoprotective in asthma and may act as an endogenous anti-inflammatory factor[193]. Aspirin-induced asthma may be triggered by increased release of leukotrienes from inflammatory cells caused by removal of the inhibitory influence of PGE_2, a major product of COX-2 in airways[194-196].

The true role of PGs in asthma is unclear. The non-selective NSAIDs have very little effect on airway function in most patients with asthma except to make the disease worse in aspirin sensitive asthmatics. Perhaps the actions of the bronchoconstrictor PGs are counterbalanced by the protective dilator action of PGE_2. It remains to be seen whether selective COX-2 inhibitors will be beneficial in allergic asthma. However, mast cells, by producing PGD_2 in response to an allergic challenge[197] may have a pathological role in allergic asthma. Disruption of the gene encoding the DP receptor in ovalbumin-sensitized mice[106], prevented the infiltration of cytokine-responsive cells into the lungs. This suggests that PGD_2 released from mast cells stimulates production of cytokines and chemokines by an action on DP receptors, which leads to recruitment of inflammatory cells into the lungs.

Because it was found in non-inflamed rat lungs, a physiological role has been proposed for lung constitutive COX-2[198]. COX-2 is present in vascular smooth muscle cells of normal rat lungs as well as in lung macrophages and mast cells. Arachidonic acid perfused through isolated rat lungs forms TXA_2 and causes vasoconstriction that is blocked dose-dependently with selective COX-2 inhibitors, suggesting a physiological role for COX-2 in the regulation of pulmonary blood flow[198].

In reproduction

Human seminal fluid contains high concentrations of several PGs, including PGE_2, PGE_1, PGE_3 and $PGF_{2\alpha}$ (ref. 199), perhaps to relax corporeal smooth muscle. These PGs may also facilitate conception by stimulating contractions of the cervix, fallopian tubes and uterus. PGE_1 given by injection into the corpus cavernosum has been used as a treatment for impotence.

$EP_2^{-/-}$ female mice give birth to unusually small litters because of problems with ovulation and fertilization[200], emphasizing the importance of PGE_2 in reproductive processes. PGE_2 is involved in ripening of the cervix prior to labour and can itself induce labour at any stage of pregnancy. It is made, together with $PGF_{2\alpha}$, by both COX-1 and COX-2 in the pregnant uterus, fetal membranes and umbilical cord. COX-2 mRNA in the amnion and placenta increases considerably immediately before and after the start of labour[201]. In rodents, $PGF_{2\alpha}$ activity, made by the induction of COX-2, is required for commencement of parturition, because mutant mice lacking the gene for the FP receptor are unable to give birth (see above). The action of $PGF_{2\alpha}$ on the FP receptor of the corpus luteum induces luteolysis, which terminates progesterone production and hence triggers parturition since, in the absence of progesterone, the uterus becomes more sensitive to oxytocin[105]. Analogues of $PGF_{2\alpha}$ are, in fact, used to synchronize oestrus and to produce luteolysis in farm animals.

In the brain

COX-1 is found in neurons throughout the brain but it is most abundant in the forebrain[202,203] where PGs may be involved in complex integrative functions, such as control of the autonomic nervous system and in sensory processing. COX-2 mRNA is induced in brain tissue and in cultured glial cells by pyrogenic substances such as LPS, IL-1 or TNF[116,204,205]. However, low levels of COX-2 protein and COX-2 mRNA have been detected in neurons of the forebrain without previous stimulation by proinflammatory stimuli[202,203,206]. These 'basal' levels of COX-2 are particularly high in neonates and are probably induced by nervous activity. Intense nerve stimulation, leading to seizures, induces COX-2 mRNA in discrete neurons of the hippocampus[207], whereas acute stress raises levels in the cerebral cortex[202]. COX-2 mRNA is also constitutively expressed in the spinal cord of normal rats and may be involved with processing of nociceptive stimuli[208]. Endogenous, fever-producing PGE_2 is thought to originate from COX-2 induced by LPS or IL-1 in endothelial cells lining the blood vessels of the hypothalamus[204].

Thus, PGE_2 is synthesized in the human brain, as well as PGD_2, which has a rather limited distribution. Large amounts of PGD_2 are found in the brains of mammals[209,210] and in mast cells but practically nowhere else. In addition to PGD_2, PGD synthase and 15-hydroxy-PGD_2 dehydrogenase, which metabolizes PGD_2, have been identified in mammalian brains[211,212]. In young rodents, PGD synthase is localized in neurons, whereas in adult animals it is mainly restricted to oligodendrocytes[213]. The reason for this selective distribution and the significance of PGD_2 in the brain is unknown.

PGD_2 and PGE_2 have opposing actions in sleep and temperature regulation. Microinjections of PGD_2 into the preoptic area of the rat brain induce normal sleep[214], whereas PGE_2 infused into the region of the posterior hypothalamus causes wakefulness[215]. Similarly, administration of PGD_2 lowers body temperature[216], and PGE_2 has a pyretic action[217]. It is interesting that patients with systemic mastocytosis fall deeply asleep after periods of production of large amounts of PGD_2 by their mast cells[218].

DRUGS THAT INHIBIT COX-1 AND COX-2

The activities of the NSAIDs are through inhibition of COX. When COX-2 was discovered, a search for selective COX-2 inhibitors was instigated, so as to avoid the gastric side effects of the older NSAIDs, which are due to concomitant inhibition of COX-1.

Structural basis for COX-2 selectivity

The inducible enzyme, COX-2 is very similar in structure and catalytic activity to the constitutive COX-1. The three dimensional structures of both enzymes consist of three independent folding units: an epidermal growth factor-like domain; a membrane-binding section; and an enzymic domain[219-221] (Figure 3a). However, the residues that form the substrate binding channel, the catalytic sites and the residues immediately adjacent are all identical except for two small variations. The primary sequence difference in the active site itself is the valine (V) 523 side chain in COX-2, which is smaller by a single methyl group than the isoleucine side chain that it replaces in COX-1. This opens up access to a side pocket off the main substrate channel in COX-2 allowing the enzyme inhibitor to react with arginine (R) 513, which replaces histidine in COX-1[222] (Figure 3b). Support for this suggestion can be deduced from the results obtained with the recently described mutant of COX-1 with

Figure 3 (a) X-ray crystal structure of human COX-2 with a COX-2-selective inhibitor in the active site. (b) X-ray crystal structure of the active site of human COX-2 showing the orientation of a COX-2-selective inhibitor.

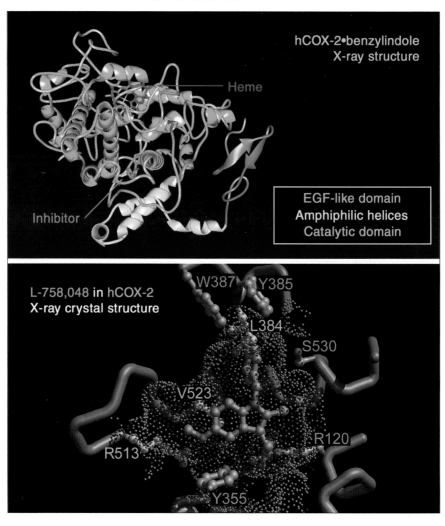

isoleucine 523 substitution for valine and histidine 513 substitution for arginine, which exhibited increased binding of selective COX-2 inhibitors and decreased binding of COX-1 inhibitors, as predicted. Surprisingly, unlike native COX-2, this mutant did not show increased 15-HETE production after acetylation with aspirin[223]. Another sequence difference is situated outside but close to the active site and can indirectly influence its conformation. The large residue, phenylalanine 503, in COX-1 is replaced by the smaller leucine in COX-2. This allows leucine (L) 384 which borders the active site to re-orientate its methyl side chain out of the active site and thus leave more space available for a larger inhibitor molecule in COX-2 than in COX-1 (Figure 3b). This change does not produce a mutant with increased selectivity for COX-2 inhibitors, but it may explain the COX-2 selective inhibitory action of large molecules such as meloxicam or etodolac.

In spite of the differences between the two isoenzymes, the extensive overall structural and biochemical similarity between COX-1 and COX-2 must be reiterated. Both use the same endogenous substrate, arachidonic acid, and form the same products by the same catalytic mechanism. X-ray crystallography on arachidonic acid complexed to an ovine COX-1 shows that arachidonic acid is bound in an extended L-conformation in the active site with the carboxylate group interacting with Arg 120. Substitution of Arg 120 with glutamine causes a 1000-fold increase in the K_m, which emphasizes the importance of the ionic bond between arachidonic acid and Arg 120 as a major contributor to high affinity binding. The 13proS hydrogen becomes aligned with tyrosine (Y) 385 leaving ample space for the first O_2 insertion to C-11 and facilitating bridging of the incipient 11-hydroperoxyl radical to C-9 to form the endoperoxide. However, the ω end of arachidonic acid must then undergo a subsequent conformational rearrangement so C-12 can react with C-8 to form the cyclopentane ring[224] (Figure 4).

The design of selective COX-2 inhibitors

Two brilliant scientists led the field, racing with their teams to design selective COX-2 inhibitors. Tony Ford-Hutchinson, then at Merck Frosst in Canada, and Phil Needleman, then Research Director at Monsanto Searle (now Pharmacia), committed substantial resources to the projects. The results were the marketing within 10 years of rofecoxib (Vioxx®) by Merck and of celecoxib (Celebrex®) by Searle. Meanwhile, it turned out that some NSAIDs already on the market were selective COX-2 inhibitors, including etodolac, nimesulide and meloxicam.

All these drugs have less adverse effects on the GI tract than the standard comparators such as diclofenac and piroxicam, but the best studied in extensive clinical trials are meloxicam[225-228], celecoxib[229] and rofecoxib[230,231] (see F. Degner et al., J. B. Lefkowith et al. and B. Morrison et al., Chapters 23, 21 and 25). Rofecoxib and celecoxib are effective analgesics in man for moderate to severe pain following tooth extraction[232-233].

The Celecoxib Long-term Arthritis Safety Study (CLASS)[229] was a double-blind, randomized controlled trial in 8059 patients with osteoarthritis (OA) or rheumatoid arthritis (RA), comparing celecoxib with ibuprofen or diclofenac. The use of anti-thrombotic doses of aspirin was allowed. The incidence rates of ulcer complications and symptomatic ulcers for celecoxib versus NSAIDs were 2.08% versus 3.54% ($P = 0.02$). No difference was noted in the number of cardiovascular events, including myocardial infarction,

Figure 4 Mechanistic sequence for converting arachidonic acid (AA) to PGG$_2$. Abstraction of the 13-pro$S$ hydrogen by the tyrosyl radical leads to the migration of the radical to C-11 on AA. Attack of molecular oxygen, coming from the base of the COX channel, occurs on the side antrafacial to hydrogen abstraction. As the 11R-peroxyl radical swings over C-8 for an R-side attack on C-9 to form the endoperoxide bridge, C-12 is brought closer to C-8 via rotation about the C-10/C-11 bond allowing the formation of the cyclopentane ring. The movement of C-12 also positions C-15 optimally for addition of a second molecule of oxygen, formation of PGG$_2$, and the migration of the radical back to Tyr[385]. Y = Tyr = tyrosine. (Reproduced from ref. 224 with permission.)

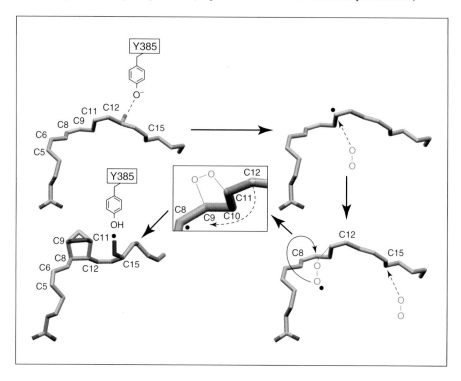

between the two groups. In the subgroup of patients taking aspirin as well as celecoxib, the incidence of severe adverse events was no better than in the comparator group (4.7% versus 6.0%; $P = 0.49$).

The 'Vioxx' Gastrointestinal Outcomes Research (VIGOR)[230], comparing rofecoxib with naproxen in patients with RA, reported fewer serious GI symptoms with rofecoxib (2.1% with rofecoxib versus 4.5% with naproxen), but a higher incidence of heart attacks (0.4% with rofecoxib versus 0.1% with naproxen). As patients taking aspirin were excluded from the VIGOR study, this result may reflect the ability of naproxen to inhibit platelet aggregation.

Interestingly, thrombosis of the feet and lungs was reported in four patients with connective tissue disorders after treatment with celecoxib. Reduced synthesis of PGI_2 by endothelial COX-2 may have precipitated this condition in subjects already suffering from circulatory diseases. At therapeutic doses neither celecoxib nor rofecoxib inhibit TXA_2 synthesis by COX-1 in platelets, thus preserving intact aggregatory mechanisms unopposed by the anti-aggregatory action of PGI_2[234]. Post-marketing surveillance will show the frequency with which thrombosis is associated with administration of selective COX-2 inhibitors such as celecoxib or rofecoxib.

Early selective cyclooxygenase-2 inhibitors

Meloxicam, nimesulide and etodolac were identified in the 1980s as potent anti-inflammatory drugs with low ulcerogenic activity in the rat stomach. In some instances this was also shown to parallel low activity against PG synthesis in the rat stomach. After the characterization of the COX-2 gene, these three drugs were each found selectively to inhibit COX-2 rather than COX-1 (see Table 1).

Meloxicam, which has selectivity towards COX-2 of about five in the human whole-blood assay (hWBA), is marketed around the world for use in RA and OA. In double-blind trials[225-228] in many thousands of patients with OA, meloxicam in doses of 7.5 mg or 15 mg o.d. compared in efficacy with standard NSAIDs such as naproxen 750–1000 mg, piroxicam 20 mg or diclofenac 100 mg. Both doses of meloxicam produced significantly fewer

Table 1 The COX-2/COX-1 ratios for some NSAIDs and selective COX-2 inhibitors in whole-blood assays in different laboratories. The data from Warner et al.[248] is for the modified whole-blood assay (a) and for the usual whole-blood assay (b).

Drug	Warner et al.[248] (a)	Warner et al.[248] (b)	Patrignani et al.[247]	Brideau et al.[286]	Pairet et al.[245]	Glaser[236]
Ketoprofen	5.1	61	1.7	5.4		
Flurbiprofen	10.0	73	1.0	14.6		
Indomethacin	10.0	80	0.53	2.88	0.82	5.7
Piroxicam	0.1	3.3	0.32	11.8	1.1	
Naproxen	3.8	3.0	1.67	9.5		13.1
Ibuprofen	2.6	0.9	2.0	6.3		
6-MNA*	2.6	>5	0.67			
Diclofenac	0.3	0.5		0.36	0.39	1.5
Etodolac	0.1	0.2				0.09
Nimesulide	0.038	0.19	0.006			
Meloxicam	0.04	0.37	0.009		0.08	
Celecoxib	0.3	0.7			0.029	
NS-398	0.0061	0.051	0.006	0.09		0.00003
SC-58125		<0.01	0.007	<0.033	0.027	<0.001
L-745,337	<0.01	<0.01	0.007	<0.3		
Rofecoxib	0.0049	0.013				

*6-methoxy 2-naphthylacetic acid

GI adverse effects than the standard NSAIDs ($P < 0.05$). Discontinuation of treatment due to GI side effects was also significantly less frequent with meloxicam. Perforations, ulcerations and bleeding (PUBs) occurred in fewer meloxicam-treated patients than in patients treated with piroxicam, diclofenac or naproxen. Moreover, the frequency of adverse events with meloxicam was significantly less ($P < 0.05$) when compared with piroxicam and naproxen. These large-scale clinical trials with a selective COX-2 inhibitor add weight to the concept that the sparing of COX-1 inhibition reduces gastric damage. These clinical results have been reinforced by a meta-analysis based on the published literature, showing for meloxicam a 50% reduction in the incidence of PUBs compared with standard NSAIDs[228]. Meloxicam is well tolerated by NSAID-sensitive individuals whose adverse reactions are manifested by urticaria or angioedema[235]. Whether it precipitates asthma in aspirin sensitive-asthmatics remains to be determined.

Etodolac is marketed in Europe and North America for the treatment of OA and RA. It has about fivefold selectivity for COX-2 in human whole blood[236]. In healthy human volunteers, etodolac twice daily did not suppress gastric mucosal PG production and caused less gastric damage than naproxen[237]. Patients with OA or RA obtained relief from symptoms with etodolac equal to other commonly used NSAIDs, but with a lower incidence of serious GI toxicity[238].

Nimesulide is currently sold in Europe and South America for the relief of pain associated with inflammatory conditions. It is a selective inhibitor of COX-2 with about fivefold greater potency against this enzyme than against COX-1 in the hWBA (Table 1). In limited clinical trials for its use in acute and chronic inflammation in patients it was more effective than placebo or had comparable anti-inflammatory activity to established NSAIDs[239]. Interestingly, nimesulide was shown to be safe for use in aspirin-sensitive asthmatics. Several recent studies in NSAID-intolerant asthmatic patients demonstrated that therapeutic doses of nimesulide did not induce asthmatic attacks, while high doses (400 mg) only precipitated mild attacks in 10% of patients[240]. Perhaps aspirin-induced asthma is associated with COX-1 inhibition? Interestingly, COX-2 is the constitutive and dominant form of the enzyme in human cultured lung epithelial cells[241]. A recent epidemiological study[242] identified 1505 patients with upper GI tract bleeding. It showed nimesulide to have a similar relative risk to that of naproxen (4.4 times control) and more than diclofenac (2.7 times control). Clearly, other factors are also involved, such as frequency of dosage, etc. As with other NSAIDs, nimesulide is used in different dosages and when these are separated, the higher doses give a much higher relative risk. Other actions of nimesulide, demonstrated *in vitro*, such as inhibition of neutrophil function[243] and quenching of free radicals[244], may contribute to its anti-inflammatory effect.

ASSAYING ASPIRIN-LIKE DRUGS ON THE TWO ENZYMES

In vitro assays

Mitchell et al.[42] were the first to measure the relative effects of NSAIDs on both COX-1 and COX-2. They showed a wide variation of activity on COX-1, which paralleled the extent of side effects on the stomach. Recently, several methods have been published to determine the difference in activities of NSAIDs on COX-1 and COX-2. These range from isolated enzymes (now usually recombinant human enzymes) through whole-cell preparations *in vitro* to the hWBA (see ref. 245 for discussion of relative merits and T. Warner et al., Chapter 4). The isolated enzyme assays give the highest ratios for COX-2:COX-1. For instance, meloxicam has a ratio of 100 (ref. 246), whereas celecoxib and rofecoxib have ratios of more than 1000 in favour of COX-2. However, such assays do not take into account the avid, but variable, binding of most of these drugs to plasma protein and other aspects of the kinetics of drug–enzyme interaction and of drug distribution.

Human whole-blood assays

It is now generally accepted that the hWBA *in vitro*, first described by Patrono and colleagues[247] best reflects *in vivo* activity in man. The activity of compounds on COX-1 is measured in the platelets of the blood sample and that on COX-2 in white cells induced over 24 h to express COX-2 by LPS or a cytokine. An improvement by Warner et al.[248] reduces the time to measure COX-2 effects down to 1.5 h (see Table 1).

The advantages of these methods are that they use human cells that, importantly, are in a physiological environment (plasma), which automatically takes any protein binding of the test drug into account. What is more, the assays give reproducible results between various laboratories. For significant differences between drugs, changes in ratio of an order of magnitude are needed. Interestingly, the ratios change substantially in this assay. In our hands[248], for example, meloxicam has a ratio in favour of COX-2 of about five, celecoxib is hardly different at ten, whereas rofecoxib has a ratio of > 60 (see Table 1).

Ex vivo assays

The same whole-blood assays can be used to measure the effects of NSAIDs *ex vivo*. Giuliano et al. gave volunteers etodolac, meloxicam, nimesulide, nabumetone or naproxen for 4 days[249]. They measured the effects of these drugs on COX-1 and COX-2 in the modified whole-blood assay[248]. Meloxicam and nimesulide were clearly COX-2 selective, with a smaller selectivity for etodolac and nabumetone. Naproxen was not COX-2 selective but was strongly selective for COX-1.

Clinical trials (*in vivo* studies)

For the recent clinical trials on celecoxib, meloxicam and rofecoxib, traditional NSAIDs were chosen as comparators. These included diclofenac, piroxicam, naproxen and ibuprofen. These three selective COX-2 inhibitors are as potent as standard NSAIDs in reducing inflammation in RA and OA, but each of the clinical trials using meloxicam[225-228], celecoxib[229] or rofecoxib[230,231] have demonstrated unequivocally that they incur fewer serious gastric side effects. This is the ultimate aim of using selective COX-2 inhibitors – not to increase their potency but to increase their safety.

Correlation between selectivity in whole-blood assays and clinical results

The purpose of making tests outside the body is to try to predict the effects of a drug on COX-1 and COX-2 in patients. Most NSAIDs are used at concentrations that give an 80% or more inhibition of COX-2 and this is the explanation of their therapeutic effects. Measurement of the inhibition of COX-1 in platelets in the whole-blood assay is an attempt to predict whether the drug will adversely affect the stomach through inhibition of gastric COX-1.

In the platelet there is an overproduction of TXA_2, so that to achieve a functional effect (inhibition of platelet aggregation), COX-1 has to be inhibited by more than 90%. Thus, the levels of inhibition of thromboxane formation by COX-1 in platelets found with selective COX-2 inhibitors (sometimes up to 50–60%) have no effect on function, i.e. aggregation.

We do not know how much inhibition of COX-1 in the stomach is needed to cause functional effects (mucosal damage), but it is reasonable to assume that, like many other biological systems (including platelets), there will also be a 'safety margin' or overproduction by COX-1 of PGE_2 or PGI_2 for protection of the stomach mucosa. Thus, chronic inhibition of this COX-1 by say, up to 60%, may not lead to mucosal damage.

The clinical trial results with celecoxib, meloxicam and rofecoxib all show a substantial reduction of serious adverse events over the comparator NSAIDs. These clinical results reinforce the concept that selective COX-2 inhibitors are safer drugs, in that they spare COX-1. However, there appears to be no measurable difference in the degree of reduction of adverse events, even though the three drugs display different degrees of inhibition of COX-1 in platelets in the whole-blood assay.

From these results, it can be concluded that differences in the small effects of these three drugs on COX-1 in platelets in the hWBA do not predict differences in adverse events on the stomach. Rather, the conclusion can be drawn that COX-1 in the stomach overproduces the protective PGs and small differences in inhibition of COX-1 by the selective COX-2 inhibitors will not reflect differences between the drugs in causing adverse effects in the patient. This is in contrast to the non-selective COX inhibitors such as indomethacin and naproxen, where inhibition of COX-1 at therapeutic doses is sufficient to cause a major inhibition of platelet function and an increase in GI adverse events is evident.

GENE DELETION STUDIES

Cyclooxygenase-1-deficient mice

It was hoped that the relative roles of COX-1 and COX-2 would be clarified by breeding mutant mice lacking the genes to produce mRNA and protein for these enzymes. However, these studies have yielded some unexpected results.

As expected, mice with a non-functional COX-1 gene had blood platelets that did not aggregate to arachidonic acid. Moreover, fetuses born to homozygous COX-1 null animals did not survive, probably because their ductus arteriosus remained patent after birth. But most surprising was the finding that animals without the COX-1 gene did not spontaneously develop stomach ulcers[250]. This has been explained by an adaptation process whereby increased production of nitric oxide or calcitonin gene related peptide have taken over the cytoprotective role of the absent PGs.

Both COX-1 and COX-2 may be required for GI mucosal defence. COX-1$^{-/-}$ or COX-2$^{-/-}$ mice were more susceptible to colonic injury with dextran sodium sulphate (DSS) than wild-type mice but the administration of a selective COX-2 inhibitor exacerbated the mucosal injury with DSS in COX-1$^{-/-}$ mice[251]. Similarly, neither the selective COX-1 inhibitor SC-560 nor the selective COX-2 inhibitor celecoxib administered to rats produced gastric damage, even though SC-560 reduced both gastric PGE$_2$ synthesis and gastric blood flow. However, the combination of SC-560 with celecoxib resulted in gastric erosions in all rats. Celecoxib, but not SC-560, increased leukocyte adherence to the vascular endothelium of the GI microcirculation. Thus, inhibition of the activity of both COX-1 and COX-2 may be necessary to cause gastric damage[252]. This work is awaiting confirmation.

Cyclooxygenase-2-deficient mice

Deletion of the COX-2 gene resulted in female mice which were infertile because they did not ovulate[47]. Thus, COX-2 appears to be essential for ovulation in mice. However, ovulation was restored in these animals[253] by treatment with PGE$_2$ or IL-1β, demonstrating the role of PGE$_2$ in ovulation. In addition, the young male and female animals showed arrested development of the kidneys[46,254]. Rodent kidneys develop fully only after birth, and COX-2 appears to be important in this process. Failure to develop mature kidneys shortened the life span of the COX-2-gene null mice to approximately 8 weeks. This retardation of renal cortical development could be mimicked in mice and rats by chronic administration of a selective COX-2 inhibitor during pregnancy until weaning[255]. However, this developmental defect may have been overcome by cross-breeding the original COX-2$^{-/-}$, C57BL/6 mice with a DBA/1 strain[114]. The animals of this mixed strain live a full life span and their kidneys appear to develop normally (L. Ballou, personal communication).

Unexpectedly, inflammation in the COX-2 gene-deleted mice was not affected. However, only an acute inflammatory response was measured that almost certainly involved COX-1 rather than COX-2[250].

A study which demonstrated the involvement of COX-2 in colon cancer yielded some interesting results. Mice with a mutation of the adenomatous polyposis coli (*APC*) gene develop large numbers of intestinal polyps and represent a model of human familial adenomatous polyposis (FAP). Some of the polyps in FAP patients and in the mouse model develop into malignant tumours. Deletion of the COX-2 gene or administration of a selective COX-2 inhibitor in animals already lacking an *APC* gene, reduced the number of polyps by 90%[256]. Thus, selective COX-2 inhibitors may be a valuable treatment for tumours expressing COX-2.

NOMENCLATURE

Merck and Searle refer to their new COX-2 inhibitors as 'specific', arguing that at therapeutic doses, there is only inhibition of COX-2 and not of COX-1. Pharmacologists use the word 'specific' far more rigorously, and 'selective' is a more appropriate description.

Similarly, some scientists and clinicians refer to celecoxib and rofecoxib as the 'coxibs' rather than referring to them as 'NSAIDs'. This is also incorrect, since 'coxibs' is a WHO definition (like oxicams) which says nothing about their pharmacology or selectivity towards COX-2.

Of course, there is nothing new about COX-2 inhibitors, for we have been using them for many years. All of the NSAIDs are COX-2 inhibitors – that is how they work in inflammation. What is new is that now we have drugs that do not concomitantly inhibit COX-1, so they have less GI toxicity. Perhaps a more accurate and descriptive term would be 'COX-1 sparing drugs'[257].

FUTURE THERAPEUTIC USES FOR SELECTIVE COX-2 INHIBITORS

Premature labour

PGs, in particular PGF$_{2\alpha}$, induce uterine contractions during labour. NSAIDs such as indomethacin will delay premature labour by inhibiting the production of PGs, but will at the same time cause early closure of the ductus arteriosus and reduce urine production by the fetal kidneys[258]. The delay in the birth process is probably due to inhibition of COX-2 since mRNA for COX-2 increases substantially in the amnion and placenta immediately before and

after the start of labour[201], whereas the side effects on the fetus are due to inhibition of COX-1. One cause of preterm labour could be an intrauterine infection resulting in release of endogenous factors that increase PG production
by upregulating COX-2[259]. Nimesulide reduces PG synthesis in isolated fetal
membranes and has been used successfully for a prolonged period to delay
premature labour without manifesting the side effects of indomethacin on the
fetus[258].

Colon cancer

Epidemiological studies, beginning with the early study of Kune et al. in
1988[260], have established a strong link between ingestion of aspirin and a
reduced risk of developing colon cancer[261,262]. Sulindac also caused reduction
of PG synthesis and regression of adenomatous polyps in 11 out of 15 patients
with FAP, a condition in which many colorectal polyps develop spontaneously
with eventual progression to tumours[263]. Treatment with combined therapy
of a non-selective COX inhibitor and an inhibitor of EGF receptor kinase may
have advantages over monotherapy with either drug alone. *Min* mice, which
normally develop multiple intestinal polyps, were almost completely protected
from adenoma formation by treatment with both sulindac and EKB-569, an
EGF receptor kinase inhibitor[264].

That COX activity is involved in the process leading to colon cancer is
supported by the demonstration that COX-2 but not COX-1 is highly
expressed in human and animal colon cancer cells as well as in human
colorectal adenocarcinomas[265,266]. The number of years that patients survived
after a diagnosis of colon cancer was related to tumour size and the extent of
COX-2 expression in the tumour cells. Staining for COX-2 was more extensive in the larger tumours found in more advanced stages of the disease[267].
Further support for the close connection between COX-2 and colon cancer
has come from studies in the mutant *APC* mouse, which is a model of FAP
in humans. The spontaneous development of intestinal polyposis in these mice
was strongly reduced either by deletion of the COX-2 gene or by treatment
with a highly selective COX-2 inhibitor[256,268,269]. Nimesulide also reduced the
number and size of intestinal polyps in *Min* mice[270]. Furthermore, the development of azoxymethane-induced colon tumours over a year was inhibited in
celecoxib-fed rats[271]. A clinical trial of celecoxib in patients with FAP has
shown a 30% reduction in polyps[272] and this indication for the drug has been
allowed by the Food and Drug Administration, USA.

Azoxymethane-induced colon carcinogenesis appears to be mediated by
PGE_2 acting on EP_1 receptors, since the number of azoxymethane-induced
aberrant crypt foci (ACF) in the colon of $EP_1^{-/-}$ mice decreased by 40% compared with that for wild-type mice. ONO-8711, a selective EP_1 antagonist
also reduced, by 30%, the number of ACF that developed in azoxymethane-
treated wild-type mice[273].

The antineoplastic action of COX-2 inhibitors may involve additional inhibition of host-derived COX-2. Tumours implanted in COX-2$^{-/-}$ mice developed more slowly and were less vascular than tumours grown in COX-1$^{-/-}$ or wild-type mice. Stromal supporting cells of these tumours produced less angiogenic factors, such as vascular endothelial growth factor, leading to reduced vascularization of the neoplasms[274].

There is much speculation about the mechanism of the antineoplastic effects of COX-2 inhibitors. It has been proposed that they cause apoptosis of tumour cells[275] perhaps by raising their intracellular level of unesterified arachidonic acid[276]. Addition of exogenous arachidonic acid increased apoptosis in colon cancer and other cell lines, while overexpression of COX-2 blocked apoptosis, the reduction of cell death being inversely correlated with the level of COX-2 in the cell[276]. COX-2 may modulate cellular processes through production of PGI_2 and activation of peroxisome proliferator-activated receptor δ (PPARδ). However, it is not clear if PPARδ play a causal or protective role in the development of colorectal cancer. When this is known, modulators of this pathway may have therapeutic potential in humans[277].

However, recent findings suggest that the antineoplastic action of NSAIDs may not be dependent on inhibition of COX-2 or COX-1, since NSAIDs cause apoptosis of fibroblasts deficient in both enzymes[278]. Resolution of this mechanism will be a key issue for the successful use of selective COX-2 inhibitors in colon and other cancers. γ-Tocopherol is a potent inhibitor of COX-2 in some human cells. Perhaps this relatively non-toxic agent will demonstrate anti-inflammatory and anti-cancer activity and prevent these diseases at physiological concentrations[279].

Alzheimer's disease

The connection between COX and Alzheimer's disease (AD) has been based mostly on epidemiology because of the lack of a relevant animal model of the disease. A number of studies have shown a significantly reduced odds ratio for AD in those taking NSAIDs as anti-inflammatory therapy[280-282]. The Baltimore Longitudinal Study of Aging[283], with 1686 participants, showed that the risk of developing AD is reduced among users of NSAIDs, especially those who have taken the medications for 2 years or more. No decreased risk was evident with paracetamol (acetaminophen) or aspirin use. However, aspirin was probably taken in a dose too low to have an anti-inflammatory effect. The protective effect of NSAIDs is consistent with evidence of inflammatory activity in the pathophysiology of AD. There is a strong interest in COX-2 in AD, and increased expression of COX-2 has been shown in the frontal cortex of brains from Alzheimer's patients[284].

In a recent study, prolonged treatment with ibuprofen reduced the number of amyloid plaques laid down in the brains of amyloid protein precursor transgenic mice. The mechanism of this inhibition appeared to be a reduction in the brain content of the soluble Aβ peptide that aggregates to form amyloid plaques[285].

CONCLUSIONS

Selective inhibitors of COX-2 clearly provide important advances in the therapy of inflammation. Conventional NSAIDs are associated with GI side effects, which include ulceration of the stomach, sometimes with subsequent perforation and deaths estimated at several thousand a year in the USA alone. Selective COX-2 inhibitors have substantially reduced side effects on the stomach. Already, the published extensive clinical results with meloxicam, rofecoxib and celecoxib show this improved safety and tolerability, with a reduction in serious adverse events of about 50% when compared with conventional NSAIDs.

In addition to their beneficial actions in inflammatory diseases, these drugs may be useful in the future for the prevention of colon cancer, Alzheimer's disease or premature labour.

Finally, the suppression of PGI_2 release from endothelial cells by 'specific' COX-2 inhibitors[45,153] suggests the possibility of interference with the cardiovascular system. However, COX-2 inhibitors have been in use for many years since this is how the NSAIDs produce their therapeutic effects. Thus, the 'selective COX-2' inhibitors will do nothing different to PGI_2 production than a conventional NSAID, although the PGI_2–TX balance may be changed because of their lack of effect on platelet COX-1.

New side effects of the selective COX-2 inhibitors, if any, may arise from the fact that they cross the blood–brain barrier far more easily than do the conventional carboxy acid NSAIDs.

REFERENCES

1. Kurzrok R, Lieb CC. Biochemical studies of human semen. II. Action of semen on the human uterus. *Proc Soc Exp Biol Med.* 1930;28:268–72.
2. Goldblatt MW. Properties of human seminal plasma. *J Physiol (Lond).* 1935;84:208–18.
3. von Euler US. Zur Kenntnis der pharmakologischen Wirkung von nativsekreten und extracten männlicher accessorischer Geschlechtsdrüsen. *Arch Exp Path Pharmak.* 1934;175:78–84.
4. von Euler US. On specific vasodilating and plain muscle stimulating substances from accessory genital glands in man and certain animals (prostaglandin and vesiglandin). *J Physiol.* 1936;88:213–34.
5. Bergström S, Ryhage R, Samuelsson B, Sjövall J. The structure of prostaglandin E, F_1 and F_2. *Acta Chem Scand.* 1962;16:501–2.
6. Bergström S, Ryhage R, Samuelsson B, Sjövall J. Prostaglandins and related factors, 15. The structures of E_1, $F_{1\alpha}$, and $F_{1\beta}$. *J Biol Chem.* 1963;238;3555–64.

7. Bergström S, Danielsson H, Samuelsson B. The enzymatic formation of prostaglandin E$_2$ from arachidonic acid. Prostaglandins and related factors 32. *Biochim Biophys Acta.* 1964;90:207–10.

8. Serhan CN. Lipoxins and aspirin-triggered 15-epi-lipoxins. In: Gallin JI, Snyderman R, editors. *Inflammation: Basic Principles and Clinical Correlates.* Philadelphia: Lippincott Williams & Wilkins; 1999:373–85.

9. Pratico D, Barry OP, Lawson JA, Adiyaman M, Hwang S-W, Khanapure SP et al. IPF$_{2\alpha}$-1: an index of lipid peroxidation in humans. *Proc Natl Acad Sci USA.* 1998;95:3449–54.

10. Smith WL, Marnett LJ, DeWitt DL. Prostaglandin and thromboxane biosynthesis. *Pharmac Ther.* 1991;49:153–79.

11. Smith WL, Lands WEM. Oxygenation of polyunsaturated fatty acids during prostaglandin biosynthesis by sheep vesicular gland. *Biochemistry.* 1972;11:3276–85.

12. Flower RJ, Vane JR. Inhibition of prostaglandin synthetase in brain explains the antipyretic activity of paracetamol (4-acetamidophenol). *Nature.* 1972;240:410–1.

13. Whittle BJR, Higgs GA, Eakins KE, Moncada S, Vane JR. Selective inhibition of prostaglandin production in inflammatory exudates and gastric mucosa. *Nature.* 1980;284:271–3.

14. Lin AH, Bienkowski MJ, Gorman RR. Regulation of prostaglandin H synthase mRNA levels and prostaglandin biosynthesis by platelet-derived growth factor. *J Biol Chem.* 1989;164:17379–83.

15. Morrison AR, Moritz H, Needleman P. Mechanism of enhanced renal biosynthesis in ureter obstruction. Role of *de novo* protein synthesis. *J Biol Chem.* 1978;253:8210–2.

16. Kawakami M, Ishibashi S, Ogawa H, Murase T, Takaku F, Shibata S. Cachectin/TNF as well as interleukin-1 induces prostacylin synthesis in cultured vascular endothelial cells. *Biochem Biophys Res Commun.* 1986;141:482–7.

17. Rossi V, Breviario F, Ghezzi P, Dejana E, Mantovani A. Prostacyclin synthesis induced in vascular cells by interleukin-1. *Science.* 1985;229:174–6.

18. Wu KK, Hatzakis H, Lo SS, Seong DC, Sanduja SK. Stimulation of *de novo* synthesis of prostaglandin G/H synthase in human endothelial cells by phorbol ester. *J Biol Chem.* 1988;263:19043–7.

19. Maier JAM, Hla T, Maciag T. Cyclooxygenase is an immediate-early gene induced by interleukin-1 in human endothelial cells. *J Biol Chem.* 1990;265:10805–8.

20. Shaw G, Kamen R. A conserved AU sequence from the 3(untranslated region of GM-CSF mRNA mediates selective degradation. *Cell.* 1986;46:659–67.

21. Bailey JM, Muza B, Hla T, Salata K. Restoration of prostacyclin synthase in vascular smooth muscle cells after aspirin treatment: regulation by epidermal growth factor. *J Lipid Res.* 1985;26:54–61.

22. Yokota K, Kusaka M, Ohshima T, Yamamoto S, Kurihara N, Yoshino T et al. Stimulation of prostaglandin E$_2$ synthesis in cloned osteoblastic cells of mouse (MC3T3-E1) by epidermal growth factor. *J Biol Chem.* 1986;261:15410–5.

23. Habenicht AJR, Goerig M, Grulich J, Rothe D, Gronwald R, Loth U et al. Human platelet-derived growth factor stimulates prostaglandin synthesis by activation and by rapid *de novo* synthesis of cyclooxygenase. *J Clin Invest.* 1985;75:1381–7.

24. Casey ML, Korte K, MacDonald PC. Epidermal growth factor stimulation of prostaglandin PGE$_2$ biosynthesis in amnion cells. *J Biol Chem.* 1988;263:7846–54.

25. Raz A, Wyche A, Siegel N, Needleman P. Regulation of fibroblast cyclooxygenase synthesis by interleukin-1. *J Biol Chem.* 1988;263:3022–8.

26. Raz A, Wyche A, Needleman P. Temporal and pharmacological division of fibroblast cyclooxygenase expression into transcriptional and translational phases. *Proc Natl Acad Sci USA.* 1989;86:1657–61.

27. Rosen GD, Birkenmeier TM, Raz A, Holtzman MJ. Identification of a cyclooxygenase-related gene and its potential role in prostaglandin formation. *Biochem Biophys Res Commun.* 1989;164:1358–65.

28. Honda A, Raz A, Needleman P. Induction of cyclo-oxygenase synthesis in human promyelocytic leukemia (HL-60) cells during monocytic or granulocytic differentiation. *Biochem J.* 1990;272:259–62.

29. Fu J-Y, Masferrer JL, Seibert K, Raz A, Needleman P. The induction and suppression of prostaglandin H_2 synthase (cyclooxygenase) in human monocytes. *J Biol Chem.* 1990;265:16737–40.

30. Masferrer JL, Zweifel BS, Seibert K, Needleman P. Selective regulation of cellular cyclooxygenase by dexamethasone and endotoxin in mice. *J Clin Invest.* 1990;86:1375–9.

31. Seibert K, Masferrer JL, Jiyi F, Honda A, Raz A, Needleman P. The biochemical and pharmacological manipulation of cellular cyclooxygenase (COX) activity. *Adv Prostaglandin Thromboxane Leukotriene Res.* 1990;21:45–51.

32. Simmons DL, Levy DB, Yannoni Y, Erikson RL. Identification of a phorbol ester-repressible *v-src*-inducible gene. *Proc Natl Acad Sci USA.* 1989;86:1178–82.

33. Xie W, Chipman JG, Robertson DL, Erikson RL, Simmons DL. Expression of a mitogen-responsive gene encoding prostaglandin synthase is regulated by mRNA splicing. *Proc Natl Acad Sci USA.* 1991;88:2692–6.

34. Kujubu DA, Fletcher BS, Varnum BC, Lim RW, Herschman HR. TIS10, a phorbol ester tumor promoter-inducible mRNA from Swiss 3T3 cells, encodes a novel prostaglandin synthase/cyclooxygenase homologue. *J Biol Chem.* 1991;266:12866–72.

35. Simmons DL, Xie W, Chipman J, Evett G. Multiple cyclooxygenases: cloning of a mitogen-inducible form. In: Bailey M, editor. *Prostaglandins, Leukotrienes, Lipoxins and PAF.* London: Plenum Press; 1991:67–68.

36. O'Banion MK, Sadowski HB, Winn V, Young DA. A serum- and glucocorticoid-regulated 4-kilobase mRNA encodes a cyclooxygenase-related protein. *J Biol Chem.* 1991;266:23261–7.

37. Sirois J, Richards JS. Purification and characterisation of a novel, distinct isoform of prostaglandin endoperoxide synthase induced by human chorionic gonadotropin in granulosa cells of rat preovulatory follicles. *J Biol Chem.* 1992;267:6382–8.

38. Flower RJ, Rothwell NJ. Lipocortin-1: cellular mechanisms and clinical relevance. *Trends Pharmacol Sci.* 1994;15:71–6.

39. Moncada S, Gryglewski R, Bunting S, Vane JR. An enzyme isolated from arteries transforms prostaglandin endoperoxides to an unstable substance that inhibits platelet aggregation. *Nature.* 1976;263:663–5.

40. Whittle BJR, Boughton-Smith NK, Moncada S, Vane JR. Actions of prostacyclin (PGI_2) and its product 6-oxo-$PGF_{1\alpha}$ on the rat gastric mucosa *in vivo* and *in vitro*. *Prostaglandins.* 1978;15:955–68.

41. Xie W, Robertson DL, Simmons DL. Mitogen-inducible prostaglandin G/H synthase: a new target for nonsteroidal antiinflammatory drugs. *Drug Dev Res.* 1992;25:249–65.

42. Mitchell JA, Akarasereenont P, Thiemermann C, Flower RJ, Vane JR. Selectivity of nonsteroidal anti-inflammatory drugs as inhibitors of constitutive and inducible cyclooxygenase. *Proc Natl Acad Sci USA.* 1993:90;11693–7.

43. Meade EA, Smith WL, DeWitt DL. Differential inhibition of prostaglandin endoperoxide synthase (cyclooxygenase) isozymes by aspirin and other non-steroidal anti-inflammatory drugs. *J Biol Chem*. 1993;268:6610–4.
44. Vane JR. Towards a better aspirin. *Nature*. 1994;367:215–6.
45. Catella-Lawson F, McAdam B, Morrison BW, Kapoor S, Kujubu D, Antes L et al. Effects of specific inhibition of cyclooxygenase-2 on sodium balance, hemodynamics, and vasoactive eicosanoids. *J Pharmacol Exp Ther*. 1999;289:735–41.
46. Dinchuk JE, Car BD, Focht RJ, Johnston JJ, Jaffee BD, Covington MB et al. Renal abnormalities and an altered inflammatory response in mice lacking cyclooxygenase II. *Nature*. 1995;378;406–9.
47. Lim H, Paria BC, Das SK, Dinchuk JE, Langenbach R, Trzaskos JM et al. Multiple female reproductive failures in cyclooxygenase 2-deficient mice. *Cell*. 1997;91:197–208.
48. Piper PJ, Vane JR. The release of prostaglandins from lung and other tissues. *Ann NY Acad Sci USA*. 1971;180:353–85.
49. Boughton-Smith NK, Whittle BJR. Stimulation and inhibition of prostacyclin formation in the gastric mucosa and ileum in vitro by anti-inflammatory agents. *Br J Pharmacol*. 1983;78:173–80.
50. Jakobsson P-J, Thorén S, Morgenstern R, Samuelsson B. Identification of human prostaglandin E synthase: a microsomal, glutathione-dependent, inducible enzyme, constituting a potential novel drug target. *Proc Natl Acad Sci USA*. 1999;96:7220–5.
51. Naraba H, Murakami M, Matsumoto H, Shimbara S, Ueno A, Kudo I et al. Segregated coupling of phospholipases A_2, cyclooxygenases, and terminal prostanoid synthases in different phases of prostanoid biosynthesis in rat peritoneal macrophages. *J Immunol*. 1998;160:2974–82.
52. Matsumoto H, Naraba H, Murakami M, Kudo I, Yamaki K, Ueno A et al. Concordant induction of prostaglandin E_2 synthase with cyclooxygenase-2 leads to preferred production of prostaglandin E_2 over thromboxane and prostaglandin D_2 in lipopolysaccharide-stimulated rat peritoneal macrophages. *Biochem Biophys Res Commun*. 1997;230:110–4.
53. Brock T, McNish R, Peters-Golden M. Arachidonic acid is preferentially metabolised by cyclooxygenase-2 to prostacyclin and prostaglandin E_2. *J Biol Chem*. 1999;274:11660–6.
54. Kudo I, Tanioka T, Nakatani Y, Semmyo N, Naraba H, Ueno A et al. Identification of two distinct PGE_2 synthases that display different functional coupling with two cyclooxygenases. Abstracts of 11th International Conference on Advances in Prostaglandin and Leukotriene Research, Florence, Italy, June 4–8, 2000, p23.
55. Kuchinke W, Barski O, Watanabe K, Hayaishi O. A lung type prostaglandin F synthase is expressed in bovine liver: cDNA sequence and expression in *E. coli*. *Biochem Biophys Res Commun*. 1992;183:1238–46.
56. Suzuki-Yamamoto T, Nishizawa M, Fukui M, Okuda-Ashitaka E, Nakajima T, Ito S et al. cDNA cloning, expression and characterization of human prostaglandin F synthase. *FEBS Lett*. 1999;462:335–40.
57. Lewis RA, Soter NA, Diamond PT, Austen KF, Oates JA, Roberts II LJ. Prostaglandin D_2 generation after activation of rat and human mast cells with anti-IgE. *J Immunol*. 1982;129:1627–31.
58. Clausen J. Proteins in normal cerebrospinal fluid not found in serum. *Proc Soc Exp Biol Med*. 1961;107:170–2.

59. Hochwald GM, Thorbecke GJ. Use of an antiserum against cerebrospinal fluid in demonstration of trace proteins in biological fluids. *Proc Soc Exp Biol Med.* 1962;109:91–5.

60. Hoffmann A, Conradt HS, Gross G, Nimtz M, Lottspeich F, Wurster U. Purification and chemical characterisation of β-trace protein from human cerebrospinal fluid: its identification as prostaglandin D synthase. *J Neurochem.* 1993;61:451–6.

61. Nagata A, Suzuki Y, Igarashi M, Eguchi N, Toh H, Urade Y et al. Human brain prostaglandin D synthase has been evolutionarily differentiated from lipophilic-ligand carrier proteins. *Proc Natl Acad Sci USA.* 1991;88:4020–4.

62. Beuckmann CT, Aoyagi M, Okazaki I, Hiroike T, Toh H, Hayaishi O et al. Binding of biliverdin, bilirubin and thyroid hormones to lipocalin-type prostaglandin D synthase. *Biochemistry.* 1999;38:8006–13.

63. Urade Y, Kitahama K, Ohishi H, Kaneko T, Mizuno N, Hayaishi O. Dominant expression of mRNA for prostaglandin D synthase in leptomeninges, choroid plexus and oligodendrocytes of the adult rat brain. *Proc Natl Acad Sci USA.* 1993;90:9070–4.

64. Urade Y, Hayaishi O. Prostaglandin D$_2$ and sleep regulation. *Biochim Biophys Acta.* 1999;1436:606–15.

65. Eguchi N, Minami T, Shirafuji N, Kanaoka Y, Tanaka T, Nagata A et al. Lack of tactile pain (allodynia) in lipocalin-type prostaglandin D synthase-deficient mice. *Proc Natl Acad Sci USA.* 1999;96:726–30.

66. Urade Y, Fujimoto N, Kaneko T, Konishi A, Mizuno N, Hayaishi O. Postnatal changes in the localisation of prostaglandin D synthetase from neurons to oligodendrocytes in the rat brain. *J Biol Chem.* 1987;262:15132–6.

67. Urade Y, Hayaishi O. Prostaglandin D synthase: structure and function. *Vitam Horm.* 2000;58:89–120.

68. Urade Y, Fujimoto N, Ujihara M, Hayaishi O. Biochemical and immunological characterisation of rat spleen prostaglandin D synthetase. *J Biol Chem.* 1987;262:3820–5.

69. Thomson AM, Meyer DJ, Hayes JD. Sequence, catalytic properties and expression of chicken glutathione-dependent prostaglandin D$_2$ synthase, a novel class Sigma glutathione S-transferase. *Biochem J.* 1998;333:317–25.

70. Ujihara M, Urade Y, Eguchi N, Hayashi H, Ikai K, Hayaishi O. Prostaglandin D$_2$ formation and characterization of its synthetases in various tissues of adult rats. *Arch Biochem Biophys.* 1988;260:521–31.

71. Murakami M, Matsumoto R, Urade Y, Austen KF, Arm JP. cKit ligand mediates increased expression of cytosolic phospholipase A$_2$, prostaglandin endoperoxide synthase-1, and hematopoietic prostaglandin D$_2$ synthase and increased IgE-dependent prostaglandin D$_2$ generation in immature mouse mast cells. *J Biol Chem.* 1995;270:3239–46.

72. Mahmud I, Ueda N, Yamaguchi H, Yamashita R, Yamamoto S, Kanaoka Y et al. Prostaglandin D synthase in human megakaryoblastic cells. *J Biol Chem.* 1997;272:28263–6.

73. Hamberg M, Svensson J, Samuelsson B. Thromboxanes: a new group of biologically active compounds derived from prostaglandin endoperoxides. *Proc Natl Acad Sci USA.* 1975;72:2994–8.

74. Haurand M, Ullrich V. Isolation and characterization of thromboxane synthase from human platelets as a P-450 enzyme. *J Biol Chem.* 1985;260:15059–67.

75. Nüsing R, Schneider-Voss S, Ullrich V. Immunoaffinity purification of human thromboxane synthase. *Arch Biochem Biophys*. 1990;280:325–30.

76. Yokoyama C, Miyata A, Ihara H, Ullrich V, Tanabe T. Molecular cloning of human platelet thromboxane A synthase. *Biochem Biophys Res Commun*. 1991;178:1479–84.

77. Miyata A, Yokoyama C, Ihara H, Bandoh S, Takeda O, Takahashi E et al. Characterization of the human gene (*TBXAS1*) encoding thromboxane synthase. *Eur J Biochem*. 1994;224:273–9.

78. Hsu P-Y, Tsai A-L, Kulmacz RJ, Wang L-H. Expression, purification and spectroscopic characterization of human thromboxane synthase. *J Biol Chem*. 1999;274:762–9.

79. Nanayama T, Hara S, Inoue H, Yokoyama C, Tanabe T. Regulation of two isozymes of prostaglandin endoperoxide synthase and thromboxane synthase in human monoblastoid cell line U937. *Prostaglandins*. 1995;49:371–82.

80. Nüsing R, Ullrich V. Immunoquantitation of thromboxane synthase in human tissues. *Eicosanoids*. 1990;3:175–80.

81. Johnson RA, Morton DR, Kinner JH. The chemical structure of prostaglandin X (prostacyclin). *Prostaglandins*. 1976;12:915–28.

82. Weksler BB, Marcus AJ, Jaffe EA. Synthesis of prostaglandin I_2 (prostacyclin) by cultured human and bovine endothelial cells. *Proc Natl Acad Sci USA*. 1977;74:3922–6.

83. Salmon JA, Flower RJ. Preparation and assay of prostacyclin synthase. *Meth Enzym*. 1982;86:91–9.

84. DeWitt DL, Smith WL. Purification of PGI_2 synthase by immunoaffinity chromatography: evidence that the enzyme is a hemoprotein. *J Biol Chem*. 1983;258:3285–93.

85. Ullrich V, Graf H. Prostacyclin and thromboxane synthase as P450 enzymes. *Trends Pharmacol Sci*. 1984;5:352–5.

86. Smith WL, DeWitt DL, Allen ML. Bimodal distribution of the prostaglandin I_2 synthase antigen in smooth muscle cells. *J Biol Chem*. 1983;258:5922–6.

87. Hara S, Miyata A, Yokoyama C, Inoue H, Brugger R, Lottspeich F et al. Isolation and molecular cloning of prostacyclin synthase from bovine endothelial cells. *J Biol Chem*. 1994;269:19897–903.

88. Tanabe T, Ullrich V. Prostacyclin and thromboxane synthases. *J Lipid Mediators Cell Signalling*. 1995;12:243–55.

89. Miyata A, Hara S, Yokoyama C, Inoue H, Ullrich V, Tanabe T. Molecular cloning of human prostacyclin synthase. *Biochem Biophys Res Commun*. 1994;200:1728–34.

90. Tone Y, Inoue H, Hara S, Yokoyama C, Hatae T, Oida H et al. The regional distribution and cellular localization of mRNA encoding rat prostacyclin synthase. *Eur J Cell Biol*. 1997;72:268–77.

91. Wang L-H, Chen L. Organization of the gene encoding human prostacyclin synthase. *Biochem Biophys Res Commun*. 1996;226:631–7.

92. Donald R, Ballard DW, Hawiger J. Proteolytic processing of NF-kappa B/I kappa B in human monocytes. ATP-dependent induction by pro-inflammatory mediators. *J Biol Chem*. 1995;270:9–12.

93. Murakami M, Kudo I, Inoue K. Molecular nature of phospholipase A_2 involved in prostacyclin I_2 synthesis in human umbilical vein endothelial cells. Possible participation of cytosolic and extracellular type II phospholipase A_2. *J Biol Chem*. 1993;258:839–44.

94. Siegle I, Nüsing R, Brugger R, Sprenger R, Zecher R, Ullrich V. Characterization

of monoclonal antibodies generated against bovine and porcine prostacyclin synthase and quantitation of bovine prostacyclin synthase. *FEBS Lett.* 1994;347:221–5.

95. Okahara K, Sun B, Kambayashi J. Upregulation of prostacyclin synthesis-related gene expression by shear stress in vascular endothelial cells. *Arterioscler Thromb Vasc Biol.* 1998;18:1922–6.

96. Tilley SL, Audoly LP, Hicks EH, Kim HS, Flannery PJ, Coffman TM et al. Reproductive failure and reduced blood pressure in mice lacking the EP_2 prostaglandin E_2 receptor. *J Clin Invest.* 1999;103:1539–45.

97. Kennedy CRJ, Zhang Y, Brandon S, Guan Y, Coffee K, Funk CD et al. Salt-sensitive hypertension and reduced fertility in mice lacking the prostaglandin EP_2 receptor. *Nature Med.* 1999;5:217–20.

98. Ushikubi F, Segi E, Sugimoto Y, Murata T, Matsuoka T, Kobayashi T et al. Impaired febrile response in mice lacking the prostaglandin E receptor subtype EP_3. *Nature.* 1998;395:281–4.

99. Nguyen M, Camenisch T, Snouwaert JN, Hicks E, Coffman TM, Anderson PA et al. The prostaglandin receptor EP_4 triggers remodelling of the cardiovascular system at birth. *Nature.* 1997;390:78–81.

100. Segi E, Sugimoto Y, Yamasaki A, Aze Y, Oida H, Nishimura T et al. Patent ductus arteriosus and neonatal death in prostaglandin receptor EP_4-deficient mice. *Biochem Biophys Res Commun.* 1998;246:7–12.

101. Oliva D, Nicosia S. PGI_2 receptors and molecular mechanisms in platelets and vasculature: state of the art. *Pharmacol Res Commun.* 1987;19:735–65.

102. Namba T, Oida H, Sugimoto Y, Kakizuka A, Negishi M, Ichikawa A et al. cDNA cloning of a mouse prostacyclin receptor: multiple signaling pathways and expression in thymic medulla. *J Biol Chem.* 1994;269:9986–92.

103. Murata T, Ushikubi F, Matsuoka T, Hirata M, Yamazaki A, Sugimoto Y et al. Altered pain perception and inflammatory response in mice lacking prostacyclin receptor. *Nature.* 1997;388:678–82.

104. Thomas DW, Mannon RB, Mannon PJ, Latour A, Oliver JA, Hoffman M et al. Coagulation defects and altered hemodynamic responses in mice lacking receptors for thromboxane A_2. *J Clin Invest.* 1998;102:1994–2001.

105. Sugimoto Y, Yamasaki A, Segi E, Tsuboi K, Aze Y, Nishimura T et al. Failure of parturition in mice lacking the prostaglandin F receptor. *Science.* 1997;277:681–3.

106. Matsuoka T, Hirata M, Tanaka H, Takahashi Y, Murata T, Kabashima K et al. Prostaglandin D_2 as a mediator of allergic asthma. *Science.* 2000;287:2013–7.

107. Higgs GA, Vane JR, Hart FD, Wojtulewski JA. Effects of anti-inflammatory drugs on prostaglandins in rheumatoid arthritis. In: Robinson HJ, Vane JR, editors. *Prostaglandin Synthetase Inhibitors.* New York: Raven Press; 1974:165–73.

108. Mnich SJ, Veenhuizen AW, Monahan JB, Sheehan KC, Lynch KR, Isakson PC et al. Characterization of a monoclonal antibody that neutralizes the activity of prostaglandin E_2. *J Immunol.* 1995;155:4437–44.

109. Portanova JP, Zhang Y, Anderson GD, Hauser SD, Masferrer JL, Seibert K et al. Selective neutralization of prostaglandin E_2 blocks inflammation, hyperalgesia and interleukin 6 production *in vivo. J Exp Med.* 1996;184:883–91.

110. Zhang Y, Shaffer A, Portanova J, Seibert K, Isakson PC. Inhibition of cyclo-oxygenase-2 rapidly reverses inflammatory hyperalgesia and prostaglandin E_2 production. *J Pharmacol Exp Ther.* 1997;283:1069–75.

111. Higgs EA, Moncada S, Vane JR. Inflammatory effects of prostacyclin (PGI_2) and 6-oxo-$PGF_{1\alpha}$ in the rat paw. *Prostaglandins.* 1978;16:153–62.

112. Ferreira SH. Prostaglandins, aspirin-like drugs and analgesia. *Nature.* 1972;240:200–3.

113. Ferreira SH, Nakamura M, Abreu Castro MS. The hyperalgesic effects of prostacyclin and PGE$_2$. *Prostaglandins.* 1978;16:31–7.

114. Doherty NS, Beaver TH, Chan KY, Coutant JE, Westrich GL. The role of prostaglandins in the nociceptive response induced by intraperitoneal injection of zymosan in mice. *Br J Pharmacol.* 1987;91:39–47.

115. Ballou LR, Botting RM, Goorha S, Zhang J, Vane JR. Nociception in cyclooxygenase isozyme-deficient mice. *Proc Natl Acad Sci USA.* 2000;97:10272–6.

116. Cao C, Matsumura K, Yamagata K, Watanabe Y. Cyclooxygenase-2 is induced in brain blood vessels during fever evoked by peripheral or central administration of tumor necrosis factor. *Mol Brain Res.* 1998;56:45–56.

117. Li S, Wang Y, Matsumura K, Ballou LR, Moreham SG, Blatteis CM. The febrile response to lipopolysaccharide is blocked in cyclooxygenase-2$^{-/-}$ mice. *Brain Res.* 1999;825:86–94.

118. Schwartz J, Mukhopadhyay S, McBride K, Jones T, Adcock S, Sharp P et al. Antipyretic activity of a selective cyclooxygenase (COX-2) inhibitor, MK-0966. *Clin Pharmacol Ther.* 1998;63:167.

119. Oates JA, Marnett LJ, Boutaud O. The antipyretic action of acetaminophen: inhibition of the cyclooxygenase activity of endothelial cells treated with IL-1. Abstracts of 11th International Conference on Advances in Prostaglandin and Leukotriene Research, Florence, Italy, June 4–8, 2000; p37.

120. Schwartz JI, Chan C-C, Mukhopadhyay S, McBride KJ, Jones TM, Adcock S et al. Cyclooxygenase-2 inhibition by rofecoxib reverses naturally occurring fever in humans. *Clin Pharmacol Ther.* 1999;65:653–60.

121. Tripp CS, Leahy KM, Needleman P. Thromboxane synthase is preferentially conserved in activated mouse peritoneal macrophages. *J Clin Invest.* 1985;76:898–901.

122. Fels OAS, Pawlowski NA, Abraham EL, Cohn ZA. Compartmentalized regulation of macrophage arachidonic acid metabolism. *J Exp Med.* 1986;163:752–7.

123. Stenson WF, Parker CW. Metabolites of arachidonic acid. *Clin Rev Allergy.* 1983;1:369–84.

124. Pablos JL, Santiago B, Carreira PE, Galindo M, Gomez-Reino JJ. Cyclooxygenase-1 and -2 are expressed by human T cells. *Clin Exp Immunol.* 1999;115:86–90.

125. Betz M, Fox BS. Prostaglandin E$_2$ inhibits the production of Th1 lymphokines but not Th2 lymphokines. *J Immunol.* 1991;146;108–13.

126. Kunkel SL, Chensue SW, Phan SH. Prostaglandins as endogenous mediators of interleukin 1 production. *J Immunol.* 1986;136:186–92.

127. Kunkel SL, Wiggins RC, Chensue SW, Larrick J. Regulation of macrophage tumour necrosis factor production by prostaglandin E$_2$. *Biochem Biophys Res Commun.* 1986;137:404–10.

128. Kunkel SL, Spengler M, May MA, Spengler R, Larrick J, Remick D. Prostaglandin E$_2$ regulates macrophage-derived tumor necrosis factor gene expression. *J Biol Chem.* 1988;263:5380–4.

129. Parker CW. Leukotrienes and prostaglandins in the immune system. *Adv Prostaglandin Thromboxane Leukotriene Res.* 1986;16:113–34.

130. Bennett A, Del Tacca M, Stamford IF, Zebro T. Prostaglandins from tumors of human large bowel. *Br J Cancer.* 1977;35:881–4.

131. Plescia OJ, Smith A, Grinwich K. Subversion of the immune system by tumor cells and the role of prostaglandins. *Proc Natl Acad Sci USA.* 1975;72:1848–52.

132. Pollard M, Luckert PH. Treatment of chemically induced intestinal cancers with indomethacin. *Proc Soc Exp Biol Med.* 1981;167:161–4.

133. Desa FM, Chander CL, Moore AR, Howat DW, Corry DG, Willoughby DA. The effect of indomethacin on cartilage breakdown. *Agents Actions.* 1989;27:485–7.

134. Pettipher ER, Henderson B, Edwards JCW, Higgs GA. Indomethacin enhances proteoglycan loss from articular cartilage in antigen-induced arthritis. *Br J Pharmacol.* 1988;94:341P.

135. Rossi A, Kapahi P, Natoll G, Takahashi T, Chen YI, Karin M et al. Anti-inflammatory cyclopentenone prostaglandins are direct inhibitors of IκB kinase. *Nature.* 2000;403:103–8.

136. Straus DS, Pascual G, Li M, Welch JS, Ricote M, Hsiang C-H et al. 15-Deoxy-$\Delta^{12,14}$-prostaglandin J$_2$ inhibits multiple steps in the NF-κB signaling pathway. *Proc Natl Acad Sci USA.* 2000;97:4844–9.

137. Whittle BJR, Salmon JA. In: Turnberg LA, editor. *Intestinal Secretion.* Welwyn Garden City: Smith Kline and French Publications; 1983:69–73.

138. Robert A, Nezamis JE, Phillips JP. Inhibition of gastric acid secretion by prostaglandins. *Am J Dig Dis.* 1967;12:1073–6.

139. Robert A, Nezamis JE, Lancaster C, Hanchar AJ. Cytoprotection by prostaglandins in rats – prevention of gastric necrosis produced by alcohol, HCl, NaOH, hypertonic NaCl and thermal injury. *Gastroenterology.* 1979;77:433–43.

140. Miller TA. Protective effects of prostaglandins against gastric mucosal damage: current knowledge and proposed mechanisms. *Am J Physiol.* 1983;245:G601–23.

141. Robert A. In: Glass GJ, editor. *Progress in Gastroenterology*, Vol III. New York: Grune and Stratton, 1977:777–801.

142. Konturek SJ, Robert A, Hancher AJ, Nezamis JE. Comparison of prostacyclin and prostaglandin E$_2$ on gastric acid secretion, gastrin release and mucosal blood flow in dogs. *Dig Dis Sci.* 1980;25:673–9.

143. Gerkens JF, Gerber JC, Shand DG, Branch RA. Effect of PGI$_2$, PGE$_2$ and 6-keto-PGF$_{1\alpha}$ on canine gastric blood flow and acid secretion. *Prostaglandins.* 1978;16:815–23.

144. Whittle BJR, Boughton-Smith NK, Moncada S, Vane JR. Actions of prostacyclin (PGI$_2$) and its product 6-oxo-PGF$_{1\alpha}$ on the rat gastric mucosa *in vivo* and *in vitro*. *Prostaglandins.* 1978;15:955–68.

145. Shea-Donohue T, Nompleggi D, Myers L, Dubois A. A comparison of effects of prostacyclin and the 15(S),15-methyl analogs of PGE$_2$ and PGF$_{2\alpha}$ on gastric parietal and non-parietal secretion. *Dig Dis Sci.* 1982;27:17–22.

146. Johansson C, Kollberg B. Stimulation by intragastrically administered E$_2$ prostaglandins of human gastric mucus output. *Eur J Pharmacol.* 1979;9:229–32.

147. Allen A, Garner A. Mucus and bicarbonate secretion in the stomach and their possible role in mucosal protection. *Gut.* 1980;21:249–62.

148. Bahari HMM, Ross IN, Turnberg LA. Demonstration of a pH gradient across the mucus layer on the surface of human gastric mucosa *in vitro*. *Gut.* 1982;23:513–6.

149. Takeuchi K, Ukawa H, Kato S, Furukawa O, Araki H, Sugimoto Y et al. Impaired duodenal bicarbonate secretion and mucosal integrity in mice lacking prostaglandin E-receptor subtype EP$_3$. *Gastroenterology.* 1999;117:1128–35.

150. Solomon LM, Juhlin L, Kirchenbaum ME. Prostaglandins on cutaneous vasculature. *J Invest Dermatol.* 1968;51:280–2.

151. Williams TJ, Peck MJ. Role of prostaglandin-mediated vasodilatation in inflammation. *Nature.* 1977;270:530–2.

152. Quadt JFA, Voss R, Ten-Hoor F. Prostacyclin production of the isolated pulsatingly perfused rat aorta. *J Pharmacol Methods*. 1982;7:263–70.

153. Topper JN, Cai J, Falb D, Gimbrone Jr MA. Identification of vasular endothelial genes differentially responsive to fluid mechanical stimuli: cyclooxygenase-2, manganese superoxide dismutase, and endothelial cell nitric oxide synthase are selectively up-regulated by steady laminar shear stress. *Proc Natl Acad Sci USA*. 1996;93:10417–22.

154. McAdam BF, Catella-Lawson F, Mardini IA, Kapoor S, Lawson JA, FitzGerald GA. Systemic biosynthesis of prostacyclin by cyclooxygenase (COX)-2: The human pharmacology of a selective inhibitor of COX-2. *Proc Natl Acad Sci USA*. 1999;96:272–7.

155. Fitzgerald DJ, Catella F, FitzGerald GA. Platelet activation in unstable coronary disease. *N Engl J Med*. 1986;315:983–9.

156. Tateson JE, Moncada S, Vane JR. Effects of prostacyclin (PGX) on cyclic AMP concentrations in human platelets. *Prostaglandins*. 1977;13:389–97.

157. Nawroth PP, Stern DM, Kaplan KL, Nossel HL. Prostacyclin production by perturbed bovine aortic endothelial cells in culture. *Blood*. 1984;64:801–6.

158. Ushikubi F, Sugimoto Y, Ichikawa A, Narumiya S. Roles of prostanoids revealed from studies using mice lacking specific prostanoid receptors. *Jpn J Pharmacol*. 2000;83:279–85.

159. Needleman P, Moncada S, Bunting S, Vane JR, Hamberg M, Sammuelsson B. Identification of an enzyme in platelet microsomes which generates thromboxane A_2 from prostaglandin endoperoxides. *Nature*. 1976;261:558–60.

160. Moncada S, Needleman P, Bunting S, Vane JR. Prostaglandin endoperoxide and thromboxane generating systems and their selective inhibition. *Prostaglandins*. 1976;12:323–9.

161. Farman N, Pradelles P, Bonvalet JP. PGE_2, $PGF_{2\alpha}$, 6-keto-$PGF_{1\alpha}$, and TXB_2 synthesis along the rabbit nephron. *Am J Physiol*. 1987;252:F53–9.

162. Zusman RM, Keiser HR. Prostaglandin biosynthesis by rabbit renomedullary interstitial cells in tissue culture. Stimulation by angiotensin II, bradykinin and arginine vasopressin. *J Clin Invest*. 1977;60:215–23.

163. Patrono C, Dunn MJ. The clinical significance of inhibition of renal prostaglandin synthesis. *Kidney Int*. 1987;32:1–12.

164. Osborn JL, Kopp UC, Thames MD, DiBona GF. Interactions among renal nerves, prostaglandins and renal arterial pressure in the regulation of renin release. *Am J Physiol*. 1984;247:F706–13.

165. Harris RC, McKanna JA, Akai Y, Jacobson HR, Dubois RN, Breyer MD. Cyclooxygenase-2 is associated with the macula densa of rat kidney and increases with salt restriction. *J Clin Invest*. 1994;94:2504–10.

166. Carroll MA, Sala A, Dunn CE, McGiff JC, Murphy RC. Structural identification of cytochrome P450-dependent arachidonate metabolites formed by rabbit medullary thick ascending limb cells. *J Biol Chem*. 1991;266:12306–12.

167. Omata K, Ibraham NG, Schwartzman ML. Renal cytochrome P-450-arachidonic acid metabolism: localization and hormonal regulation in SHR. *Am J Physiol*. 1992;262:F591–9.

168. Schwartzman M, Ferreri NR, Carroll MA, Songu-Mize E, McGiff JC. Renal cytochrome P450-related arachidonate metabolite inhibits $(Na^+–K^+)$ATPase. *Nature*. 1985;314:620–2.

169. Ferreri NR, An SJ, McGiff JC. Cyclooxygenase-2 expression and function in the medullary thick ascending limb. *Am J Physiol*. 1999;277:F360–8.

170. Ferreri NR, McGiff JC, Vio CP. Cyclooxygenase is expressed functionally in the renal thick ascending limb via angiotensin II stimulation of tumour necrosis factor-α. In: Vane JR, Botting R, editors. *Clinical Significance and Potential of Selective COX-2 Inhibitors*. London: William Harvey Press; 1998:109–19.

171. Harris RC. The macula densa: recent developments. *J Hypertension.* 1996;14:815–22.

172. Schneider A, Stahl RAK. Cyclooxygenase-2 (COX-2) and the kidney: current status and potential perspectives. *Nephrol Dial Transplant* 1998;13:10–12.

173. Hardy CC, Robinson C, Tattersfield AE, Holgate ST. The bronchoconstrictor effect of inhaled prostaglandin D_2 in normal and asthmatic men. *N Engl J Med.* 1984;311:210–3.

174. Fuller RW, Dixon CMS, Dollery CT, Barnes PJ. Prostaglandin D_2 potentiates airway responses to histamine and methacholine. *Am Rev Respir Dis.* 1986;133:252–4.

175. Liu MC, Bleecker ER, Lichtenstein LM, Kagey Sobotka A, Niv Y, McLemore TL et al. Evidence for elevated levels of histamine, prostaglandin D_2 and other bronchoconstricting prostaglandins in the airways of subjects with mild asthma. *Am Rev Respir Dis.* 1990;142:126–32.

176. Sladek K, Dworski R, FitzGerald GA, Buitkus KL, Block FJ, Marney Jr SR et al. Allergen-stimulated release of thromboxane A_2 and leukotriene E_4 in humans. Effect of indomethacin. *Am Rev Respir Dis.* 1990;141:1441–5.

177. Bakhle YS, Ferreira SH. Lung metabolism of eicosanoids. In: Fishman A, Fisher AB, editors. *Handbook of Physiology*. Bethesda, MD: American Physiological Society; 1985:365–86.

178. Geraci MW, Gao B, Shepherd DC, Moore MD, Westcott JY, Fagan KA et al. Pulmonary prostacyclin synthase overexpression in transgenic mice protects against development of hypoxic pulmonary hypertension. *J Clin Invest.* 1999;103:1509–15.

179. Tuder RM, Cool CD, Geraci MW, Wang J, Abman SH, Wright L et al. Prostacyclin synthase expression is decreased in lungs from patients with severe pulmonary hypertension. *Am J Respir Crit Care Med.* 1999;159:1925–32.

180. Holgate ST. The pathophysiology of bronchial asthma and targets for its drug treatment. *Agents Actions.* 1986;18:281–7.

181. Barnes PJ. Cytokines as mediators of chronic asthma. *Am J Respir Crit Care Med.* 1994;150:S42–9.

182. Mitchell JA, Larkin S, Williams TJ. Cyclooxygenase-2: regulation and relevance in inflammation. *Biochem Pharmacol.* 1995;50:1535–42.

183. Tomlinson A, Appleton I, Moore AR, Gilroy DW, Willis D, Mitchell JA et al. Cyclooxygenase and nitric oxide synthase isoforms in rat carrageenin-induced pleurisy. *Br J Pharmacol.* 1994;113:693–4.

184. Hatanaka K, Harada Y, Kawamura M, Ogino M, Saito M, Katori M. Cell types expressing COX-2 in rat carrageenin-induced pleurisy. *Jpn J Pharmacol.* 1996;71(Suppl I):304P.

185. Mitchell JA, Belvisi MG, Akarasereenont P, Robbins RA, Kwon O-J, Croxtall J et al. Induction of cyclo-oxygenase-2 by cytokines in human pulmonary epithelial cells: regulation by dexamethasone. *Br J Pharmacol.* 1994;113:1008–14.

186. Newton R, Kuitert LME, Bergmann M, Adcock IM, Barnes PJ. Evidence for the involvement of NFκB in the transcriptional control of cyclooxygenase-2 gene expression by interleukin-1β. *Biochem Biophys Res Commun.* 1997;237:28–32.

187. Springall DR, Meng Q-H, Redington AE, Howarth PH, Polak JM. Inflammatory genes in asthmatic airway epithelium: suppression by corticosteroids. *Eur Respir J.* 1995;8(Suppl 19):44S.

188. Frossard N, Stretton CD, Barnes PJ. Modulation of bradykinin responses in airway smooth muscle by epithelial enzymes. *Agents Actions*. 1990;31:204–9.

189. Frossard N, Rhoden KJ, Barnes PJ. Influence of epithelium on guinea pig airway responses to tachykinins: role of endopeptidase and cyclooxygenase. *J Pharmacol Exp Ther*. 1989;248:292–8.

190. Devillier P, Acker M, Advenier C, Regoli D, Frossard N. Respiratory epithelium releases relaxant prostaglandin E_2 through activation of substance P (NK_1) receptors. *Am Rev Respir Dis*. 1991;139:A351.

191. Battistini B, Filep J, Sirois P. Potent thromboxane-mediated in vitro bronchoconstrictor effect of endothelin in guinea pig. *Eur J Pharmacol*. 1990;178:141–2.

192. Goldie RG, Fernandes LB, Farmer SG, Hay DWP. Airway epithelium-derived inhibitory factor. *Trends Pharmacol Sci*. 1990;11:67–70.

193. Pavord ID, Tattersfield AE. Bronchoprotective role for endogenous prostaglandin E_2. *Lancet*. 1995;344:436–8.

194. Szczeklik A. Aspirin-induced asthma as a viral disease. *Clin Allergy*. 1988;18:15–20.

195. Szczeklik A. Prostaglandin E and aspirin-induced asthma. *Lancet*. 1995;345:1056.

196. Kuitert LM, Newton R, Barnes NC, Adcock IM, Barnes PJ. Eicosanoid mediator expression in mononuclear and polymorphonuclear cells in normal subjects and patients with atopic asthma and cystic fibrosis. *Thorax*. 1996;51:1223–8.

197. Lewis RA, Austen KF. Mediation of local homeostasis and inflammation by leukotrienes and other mast cell-dependent compounds. *Nature*. 1981;293:103–8.

198. Ermert L, Ermert M, Althoff A, Merkle M, Grimminger F, Seeger W. Vasoregulatory prostanoid generation proceeds via cyclooxygenase-2 in non-inflamed rat lungs. *J Pharmacol Exp Ther*. 1998;286:1309–14.

199. Samuelsson B. Isolation and identification of prostaglandins from human seminal plasma. 18. Prostaglandins and related factors. *J Biol Chem*. 1963;238:3229–34.

200. Hizaki H, Segi E, Sugimoto Y, Hirose M, Saji T, Ushikubi F et al. Abortive expansion of the cumulus and impaired fertility in mice lacking the prostaglandin E receptor subtype EP_2. *Proc Natl Acad Sci USA*. 1999;96:10501–6.

201. Gibb W, Sun M. Localization of prostaglandin H synthase type 2 protein and mRNA in term human fetal membranes and decidua. *J Endocrinol*. 1996;150:497–503.

202. Yamagata K, Andreasson KI, Kaufman EW, Barnes CA, Worley PF. Expression of a mitogen-inducible cyclooxygenase in brain neurons; regulation by synaptic activity and glucocorticoids. *Neuron*. 1993;11:371–86.

203. Breder CD, Dewitt D, Kraig RP. Characterization of inducible cyclooxygenase in rat brain. *J Comp Neurol*. 1995;355:296–315.

204. Cao C, Matsumura K, Yamagata K, Watanabe Y. Endothelial cells of the brain vasculature express cyclooxygenase-2 mRNA in response to systemic interleukin-1β: a possible site of prostaglandin synthesis responsible for fever. *Brain Res*. 1996;733:263–72.

205. Breder CD, Saper CB. Expression of inducible cyclooxygenase mRNA in the mouse brain after systemic administration of bacterial lipopolysaccharide. *Brain Res*. 1996;713:64–9.

206. Cao C, Matsumura K, Yamagata K, Watanabe Y. Induction by lipopolysaccharide of cyclooxygenase-2 mRNA in rat brain; its possible role in the febrile response. *Brain Res*. 1995;697:187–96.

207. Marcheselli VL, Bazan NG. Sustained induction of prostaglandin endoperoxide synthase-2 by seizures in hippocampus. *J Biol Chem*. 1996;271:24794–9.

208. Beiche F, Scheuerer S, Brune K, Geisslinger G, Goppelt-Struebe M. Up-regulation of cyclooxygenase-2 mRNA in the rat spinal cord following peripheral inflammation. *FEBS Lett.* 1996;390:165–9.

209. Ogorochi T, Narumiya S, Mizuno N, Yamashita K, Miyazaki H, Hayaishi O. Regional distribution of prostaglandins D_2, E_2 and $F_{2\alpha}$ and related enzymes in post-mortem human brain. *J Neurochem.* 1984;43:71–92.

210. Narumiya S, Ogorochi T, Nakao K, Hayaishi O. Prostaglandin D_2 in rat brain, spinal cord and pituitary: basal level and regional distribution. *Life Sci.* 1982;31:2093–103.

211. Watanabe K, Shimizu T, Iguchi S, Wakatsuka H, Hayashi M, Hayaishi O. An NADP-linked prostaglandin D dehydrogenase in swine brain. *J Biol Chem.* 1980;225:1779–82.

212. Tokumoto H, Watanabe K, Fukushima D, Shimizu T, Hayaishi O. An NADP-linked 15-hydroxyprostaglandin dehydrogenase specific for prostaglandin D_2 from swine brain. *J Biol Chem.* 1982;257:13576–80.

213. Urade Y, Fujimoto N, Kaneko T, Konisho A, Mizuno N, Hayaishi O. Postnatal changes in the localisation of prostaglandin D synthetase from neurons to oligodendrocytes in the rat brain. *J Biol Chem.* 1987;262:15132–6.

214. Ueno R, Ishikawa Y, Nakayama T, Hayaishi O. Prostaglandin D_2 induces sleep when microinjected into the preoptic area of conscious rats. *Biochem Biophys Res Commun.* 1982;109:576–82.

215. Hayaishi O. Molecular mechanisms of sleep-wake regulation: roles of prostaglandins D_2 and E_2. *FASEB J.* 1991;5:2575–81.

216. Ueno R, Narumiya S, Ogorochi T, Nakayama T, Ishikawa Y, Hayaishi O. Role of prostaglandin D_2 in the hyperthermia of rats caused by bacterial lipopolysaccharide. *Proc Natl Acad Sci USA.* 1982;79:6093–7.

217. Milton AS, Wendlandt S. Effects on body temperature of prostaglandins of the A, E and F series on injection into the third ventricle of unanaesthetised cats and rabbits. *J Physiol (Lond).* 1971;218:325–6.

218. Roberts JL II, Sweetman BJ, Lewis RA, Austen KF, Oates JA. Increased production of prostaglandin D_2 in patients with systemic mastocytosis. *N Engl J Med.* 1981;303:1400.

219. Luong C, Miller A, Barnett J, Chow J, Ramesha C, Browner MF. Flexibility of the NSAID binding site in the structure of human cyclooxygenase-2. *Nature Struct Biol.* 1996;3:927–33.

220. Kurumbail RG, Stevens AM, Gierse JK, McDonald JJ, Stegeman RA, Pak JY et al. Structural basis for selective inhibition of cyclooxygenase-2 by anti-inflammatory agents. *Nature.* 1996;384:644–8.

221. Picot D, Loll PJ, Garavito RM. The X-ray crystal structure of the membrane protein prostaglandin H_2 synthase-1. *Nature.* 1994;367:243–9.

222. Wong E, Bayly C, Waterman HL, Riendeau D, Mancini JA. Conversion of prostaglandin G/H synthase-1 into an enzyme sensitive to PGHS-2-selective inhibitors by a double His[513] to Arg and Ile[523] to Val mutation. *J Biol Chem.* 1997;272:9280–6.

223. Mancini JA, O'Neill GP, Bayly C, Vickers PJ. Mutation of serine 516 in human prostaglandin G/H synthase-2 to methionine or aspirin acetylation of this residue stimulates 15-R-HETE synthesis. *FEBS Lett.* 1994;342:33–7.

224. Malkowski MG, Ginell SL, Smith WL, Garavito RM. The productive conformation of arachidonic acid bound to prostaglandin synthase. *Science.* 2000;289:1933–7.

225. Hawkey C, Kahan A, Steinbrück K, Alegre C, Baumelou E, Bégaud B et al. Gastrointestinal tolerability of meloxicam compared to diclofenac in osteoarthritis patients. *Br J Rheumatol*. 1998;37:937–45.

226. Dequeker J, Hawkey C, Kahan A, Steinbrück K, Alegre C, Baumelou E et al. Improvement in gastrointestinal tolerability of the selective cyclooxygenase (COX)-2 inhibitor, meloxicam, compared with piroxicam: results of the safety and efficacy large-scale evaluation of COX-inhibiting therapies (SELECT) trial in osteoarthritis. *Br J Rheumatol*. 1998;37:946–51.

227. Distel M, Meuller C, Bluhmki E, Fries J. Safety of meloxicam: a global analysis of clinical trials. *Br J Rheumatol*. 1996;35:68–77.

228. Schoenfeld P. Gastrointestinal safety profile of meloxicam: a meta-analysis and systematic review of randomized controlled trials. Proceedings of a Symposium 'Rationalizing Cyclooxygenase Inhibition for Optimization of Efficacy and Safety Profiles'. *Am J Med*. 1999;107(Suppl 6A):48S–54S.

229. Silverstein FE, Faich G, Goldstein JL, Simon LS, Pincus T, Whelton A et al. Gastrointestinal toxicity with celecoxib vs nonsteroidal anti-inflammatory drugs for osteoarthritis and rheumatoid arthritis: the CLASS study: a randomised controlled trial. Celecoxib Long-term Arthritis Safety Study. *J Am Med Assoc*. 2000;284:1247–55.

230. Bombardier C, Laine L, Reicin A, Shapiro D, Burgos-Vargas R, Davis B et al. Comparison of upper gastrointestinal toxicity of rofecoxib and naproxen in patients with rheumatoid arthritis. *N Engl J Med*. 2000;343:1520–8.

231. Langman MJ, Jensen DM, Watson DJ, Harper SE, Zhao PL, Quan H et al. Adverse upper gastrointestinal effects of rofecoxib compared with NSAIDs. *J Am Med Assoc*. 1999;282:1929–33.

232. Hubbard RC, Mehlisch DR, Jasper DR, Nugent MJ, Yu S, Isakson PC. SC-58635, a highly selective inhibitor of COX-2, is an effective analgesic in an acute post-surgical pain model. *J Invest Med*. 1996;44:293A.

233. Ehrich EW, Dallob A, De Lepleire I, Van Hecken A, Riendeau D, Yuan W et al. Characterization of rofecoxib as a cyclooxygenase-2 isoform inhibitor and demonstration of analgesia in the dental pain model. *Clin Pharmacol Ther*. 1999;65:336–47.

234. Crofford LJ, Oates JC, McCune WJ, Gupta S, Kaplan MJ, Catella-Lawson F et al. Thrombosis in patients with connective tissue diseases treated with specific cyclooxygenase 2 inhibitors. A report of four cases. *Arthritis Rheum*. 2000;43:1891–6.

235. Quarantino D, Romano A, Di Fonso M, Papa G, Perrone MR, D'Ambrosio FP et al. Tolerability of meloxicam in patients with histories of adverse reactions to nonsteroidal anti-inflammatory drugs. *Ann Allergy Asthma Immunol*. 2000;84:613–7.

236. Glaser KB. Cyclooxygenase selectivity and NSAIDs: cyclooxygenase-2 selectivity of etodolac (Lodine). *Inflammopharmacology*. 1995;3:335–45.

237. Laine L, Sloane R, Ferretti M, Cominelli F. A randomised double-blind comparison of placebo, etodolac and naproxen on gastrointestinal injury and prostaglandin production. *Gastrointest Endosc*. 1995;42:428–33.

238. Cummings DM, Amadio Jr P. A review of selected newer nonsteroidal anti-inflammatory drugs. *Am Fam Physician*. 1994;49:1197–202.

239. Lücker PW, Pawlowski C, Friederich I, Faiella F, Magni E. Double-blind, randomized, multi-centre clinical study evaluating the efficacy and tolerability of

nimesulide in comparison with etodolac in patients suffering from osteoarthritis of the knee. *Eur J Rheumatol Inflamm.* 1994;14:29–38.

240. Senna GE, Passalacqua G, Andri G, Dama AR, Albano M, Fregonese L et al. Nimesulide in the treatment of patients intolerant of aspirin and other NSAIDs. *Drug Safety.* 1996;14:94–103.

241. Asano K, Lilly, CM, Drazen JM. Prostaglandin G/H synthase-2 is the constitutive and dominant isoform in cultured human lung epithelial cells. *Am J Physiol.* 1996;271:126–31.

242. Garcia Rodriguez LA, Cattaruzzi C, Troncom MG, Agostinis L. Risk of hospitalization for upper gastrointestinal tract bleeding associated with ketorolac, other nonsteroidal anti-inflammatory drugs, calcium antagonists, and other antihypertensive drugs. *Arch Intern Med.* 1998;158:33–9.

243. Capecchi PL, Ceccatelli L, Beermann U, Lahgi Psini F, Di Perri T. Inhibition of neutrophil function in vitro by nimesulide. Preliminary evidence of an adenosine-mediated mechanism. *Arzneimittel-Forsch.* 1993;43:992–6.

244. Maffei Facino R, Carini M, Aldini G, Saibene L, Morelli R. Differential inhibition of superoxide, hydroxyl and peroxyl radicals by nimesulide and its main metabolite 4-hydroxynimesulide. *Arzneimittel-Forsch.* 1995;45:1102–9.

245. Pairet M, van Ryn J, Mauz A, Schierok H, Diederen W, Turck D et al. Differential inhibition of COX-1 and COX-2 by NSAIDs: a summary of results obtained using various test systems. In: Vane J, Botting J, editors. *Selective COX-2 Inhibitors. Pharmacology, Clinical Effects and Therapeutic Potential.* Lancaster: Kluwer Academic Publishers/London: William Harvey Press; 1998;27–46.

246. Churchill L, Graham A, Shih C-K, Pauletti D, Farina PR, Grob PM. Selective inhibition of human cyclooxygenase-2 by meloxicam. *Inflammopharmacology.* 1996;4;125–35.

247. Patrignani P, Panara MR, Greco A, Fusco O, Natoli C, Iacobelli S et al. Biochemical and pharmacological characterization of the cyclooxygenase activity of human blood prostaglandin endoperoxide synthases. *J Pharmacol Exp Ther.* 1994;271:1705–10.

248. Warner TD, Giuliano F, Vojnovic I, Bukasa A, Mitchell JA Vane JR. Nonsteroid drug selectivities for cyclo-oxygenase-1 rather than cyclo-oxygenase-2 are associated with human gastrointestinal toxicity: a full in vitro analysis. *Proc Natl Acad Sci USA.* 1999;96:7563–8.

249. Guiliano F, Vojnovic I, De Nucci G, Warner TD. Cyclooxygenase selectivity of non-steroidal anti-inflammatory drugs (NSAIDs) in humans: *ex vivo* evaluation. *Br J Pharmacol.* 2000;129 (Suppl):99P.

250. Langenbach R, Morham SG, Tiano HF, Loftin CD, Ghanayem BI, Chulada PC et al. Prostaglandin synthase 1 gene disruption in mice reduces arachidonic acid-induced inflammation and indomethacin-induced gastric ulceration. *Cell.* 1995;83:483–92.

251. Morteau O, Morham SG, Sellon R, Dieleman LA, Langenbach R, Smithies O et al. Impaired mucosal defense to acute colonic injury in mice lacking cyclooxygenase-1 or cyclooxygenase-2. *J Clin Invest.* 2000;105:469–78.

252. Wallace JL, McKnight W, Reuter BK, Vergnolle N. NSAID-induced gastric damage in rats: requirements for inhibition of both cyclooxygenase 1 and 2. *Gastroenterology.* 2000;119:706–14.

253. Davis BJ, Lennard DE, Lee CA, Tiano HF, Morham SG, Wetsel WC et al. Anovulation in cyclooxygense-2-deficient mice is restored by prostaglandin E_2 and interleukin-1β. *Endocrinology.* 1999;140:2685–95.

254. Morham SG, Langenbach R, Loftin CD, Tiano HF, Vouloumanos N et al. Prostaglandin synthase 2 gene disruption causes severe renal pathology in the mouse. *Cell.* 1995;83:473–82.

255. Kömhoff M, Wang J-L, Cheng H-F, Langenbach R, McKanna JA, Harris RC et al. Cyclooxygenase-2-selective inhibitors impair glomerulogenesis and renal cortical development. *Kidney Int.* 2000;57:414–22.

256. Oshima M, Dinchuck JE, Kargman SL, Oshima H, Hancock B, Kwong E et al. Suppression of intestinal polyposis in $Apc^{\Delta716}$ knockout mice by inhibition of cyclooxygenase 2 (COX-2). *Cell.* 1996;87:803–9.

257. Vane JR, Warner TD. Nomenclature for COX-2 inhibitors. *Lancet.* 2000;356:1373–4.

258. Sawdy R, Slater D, Fisk N, Edmonds DK, Bennett P. Use of a cyclo-oxygenase type-2 selective non-steroidal anti-inflammatory agent to prevent preterm delivery. *Lancet.* 1997;350:265–6.

259. Spaziani EP, Lantz ME, Benoit RR, O'Brien WF. The induction of cyclooxy-genase-2 (COX-2) in intact human amnion tissue by interleukin-4. *Prostaglandins.* 1996;51:215–23.

260. Kune GA, Kune SA, Watson LF. Colorectal cancer risk, chronic illnesses, operations and medications: case control results from the Melbourne Colorectal Cancer Study. *Cancer Res.* 1988;48:4399–404.

261. Thun MJ, Manboodiri MM, Heath CWJ. Aspirin use and reduced risk of fatal colon cancer. *N Engl J Med.* 1991;325:1593–6.

262. Luk GD. Prevention of gastrointestinal cancer – the potential role of NSAIDs in colorectal cancer. *Schweiz Med Wochenschr.* 1996 126:801–12.

263. Matsuhashi N, Nakajima A, Fukushima Y, Yazaki Y, Oka T. Effects of sulindac on sporadic colorectal adenomatous polyps. *Gut.* 1997;40:344–9.

264. Torrance CJ, Jackson PE, Montgomery E, Kinzler KW, Vogelstein B, Wissner A et al. Combinatorial chemoprevention of intestinal neoplasia. *Nature Med.* 2000;6:1024–8.

265. Kutchera W, Jones DA, Matsunami N, Groden J, McIntyre TM, Zimmerman GA et al. Prostaglandin H synthase 2 is expressed abnormally in human colon cancer: evidence for a transcriptional effect. *Proc Natl Acad Sci USA.* 1996;93:4816–20.

266. Gustafson-Svärd C, Lilja I, Hallböök O, Sjödahl R. Cyclooxygenase-1 and cyclooxygenase-2 gene expression in human colorectal adenocarcinomas and in azoxymethane induced colonic tumours in rats. *Gut.* 1996;38:79–84.

267. Sheehan KM, Sheahan K, O'Donoghue DP, MacSweeney F, Conroy RM, Fitzgerald DJ et al. The relationship between cyclooxygenase-2 expression and colorectal cancer. *J Am Med Assoc.* 1999;282:1254–7.

268. Eberhart CE, Coffey RJ, Radhika A, Giardiello FM, Ferrenbach S, DuBois RN. Up-regulation of cyclooxygenase 2 gene expression in human colorectal adenomas and adenocarcinomas. *Gastroenterology.* 1994;104:1183–8.

269. Sheng H, Shao J, Kirkland SC, Isakson P, Coffey RJ, Morrow J et al. Inhibition of human colon cancer cell growth by selective inhibition of cyclooxygenase-2. *J Clin Invest.* 1997;99:2254–9.

270. Nakatsugi S, Fukutake M, Takahashi M, Fukuda K, Isoi T, Taniguchi Y et al. Suppression of intestinal polyp development by nimesulide, a selective cyclooxy-genase-2 inhibitor, in *Min* mice. *Jpn J Cancer Res.* 1997;88:1117–20.

271. Kawamori T, Rao CV, Seibert K, Reddy BS. Chemopreventive activity of cele-coxib, a specific cyclooxygenase-2 inhibitor, against colon carcinogenesis. *Cancer Res.* 1998;58:409–12.

272. Steinbach G, Lynch PM, Phillips RK, Wallace MH, Hawk E, Gordon GB et al. The effect of celecoxib, a cyclooxygenase-2 inhibitor, in familial adenomatous polyposis. *N Engl J Med.* 2000;342:1946–52.

273. Watanabe K, Kawamori T, Nakatsugi S, Ohta T, Ohuchida S, Yamamoto H et al. Role of the prostaglandin E receptor subtype EP$_1$ in colon carcinogenesis. *Cancer Res.* 1999;5093–6.

274. Williams CS, Tsujii M, Reese J, Dey SK, DuBois RN. Host cyclooxygenase-2 modulates carcinoma growth. *J Clin Invest.* 2000;105:1589–94.

275. Simmons DL, Botting RM, Robertson PM, Madsen ML, Vane JR. Induction of an acetaminophen-sensitive cyclooxygenase with reduced sensitivity to nonsteroid anti-inflammatory drugs. *Proc Natl Acad Sci USA.* 1999;96:3275–80.

276. Cao Y, Pearman AT, Zimmerman GA, McIntyre TM, Prescott SM. Intracellular unesterified arachidonic acid signals apoptosis. *Proc Natl Acad Sci USA.* 2000;97:11280–5.

277. Gupta RA, Tan J, Krause WF, Geraci MW, Willson TM, Dey SK et al. Prostacyclin-mediated activation of peroxisome proliferator-activated receptor δ in colorectal cancer. *Proc Natl Acad Sci USA.* 2000;97:13275–80.

278. Zhang X, Morham SG, Langenbach R, Young DA. Malignant transformation and antineoplastic actions of nonsteroidal anti-inflammatory drugs (NSAIDs) on cyclooxygenase-null embryo fibroblasts. *J Exp Med.* 1999;190:451–9.

279. Jiang Q, Elson-Schwab I, Courtemanche C, Ames BN. γ-Tocopherol and its major metabolite, in contrast to α-tocopherol, inhibit cyclooxygenase activity in macrophages and epithelial cells. *Proc Natl Acad Sci USA.* 2000, 97:11494–9.

280. McGeer PL, McGeer EG. The inflammatory response system of brain: implications for therapy of Alzheimer and other neurodegenerative diseases. *Brain Res Rev.* 1995;21:195–218.

281. Cochran FR, Vitek MP. Neuroinflammatory mechanisms in Alzheimer's disease: new opportunities for drug discovery. *Expert Opin Invest Drugs.* 1996;5:449–55.

282. Breitner JCS. The role of anti-inflammatory drugs in the prevention and treatment of Alzheimer's disease. *Annu Rev Med.* 1996;47:401–11.

283. Stewart WF, Kawas C, Corrada M, Metter EJ. Risk of Alzheimer's disease and duration of NSAID use. *Neurology.* 1997;48:626–32.

284. Pasinetti GM, Aisen PS. Cyclooxygenase-2 expression is increased in frontal cortex of Alzheimer's disease brain. *Neuroscience.* 1998;87:319–24.

285. Lim GP, Yang F, Chu T, Chen P, Beech W, Teter B et al. Ibuprofen suppresses plaque pathology and inflammation in a mouse model for Alzheimer's disease. *J Neurosci.* 2000;20:5709–14.

286. Brideau C, Kargman S, Liu S, Dallob AL, Ehrich EW, Rodger IW et al. A human whole blood assay for clinical evaluation of biochemical efficacy of cyclooxygenase inhibitors. *Inflamm Res.* 1996;45:68–74.

2 | Cyclooxygenase-2 specific inhibitors: structural and functional aspects of isozyme inhibition

P. C. Isakson,[1] R. G. Kurumbail,[2] J. Gierse,[2]
K. Seibert[2] and T. J. Maziasz[1]

*[1]Pharmacia Corporation, 4901 Searle Parkway, Skokie,
IL 60077, USA, and [2]Pharmacia Corporation, Mail Zone BB2B,
700 Chesterfield Parkway North, St Louis, MO 63198, USA.*

CONSTITUTIVE AND INDUCED CYCLOOXYGENASE ACTIVITY

Cyclooxygenase (COX), also referred to as prostaglandin H_2 synthase (PGHS), was first characterized in the 1970s, and a second inducible isoform of COX was identified in the early 1990s[1-3]. The distribution of COX-1 and COX-2 under basal conditions has been well characterized by numerous tissue localization studies. Northern blotting, immunohistochemical localization and *in situ* hybridization analyses in rodents have revealed that, under basal conditions, the COX-1 isoform can be found in nearly all tissues, including the gastrointestinal (GI) tract, platelets and endothelial cells, and in the renal medullary collecting ducts and interstitium[4]. COX-2 has been detected under basal conditions only in the brain, kidney, and in small quantities in the lung, liver and stomach[5].

Given the broad distribution of the COX-1 isoform under basal conditions, it can be assumed that COX-1 plays a significant role in maintaining a variety of homeostatic functions. COX activity, via the synthesis of prostaglandins (PG) and thromboxane (TX), has been implicated in the mediation of platelet function and blood clotting, the regulation of blood flow through the kidneys, maintenance of the gastric mucosa, bone metabolism, nerve growth and development, wound healing, ovulation and initiation of labour, and immune responses[6]. While it is clear that COX-1 is the predominant isoform in platelets and GI mucosa, the role of each isoform in other processes such as bone metabolism and central nervous system (CNS) function is less clear and the subject of much current research. COX-2 is the product of an immediate-early gene (IEG) that is highly restricted under basal conditions and rapidly induced during inflammatory processes[4]. Early studies on enzyme inhibition indicated that the non-steroid anti-inflammatory drugs (NSAIDs, or aspirin-like drugs) inhibited both COX isoforms[7]. The strong association of COX-2 with inflammation and COX-1 with physiological processes led to the hypothesis that specific inhibition of COX-2 would provide the thera-peutic benefits of NSAIDs in inflammation and pain without mechanism-based side effects on the GI tract, platelets and kidney. This led to the search for specific inhibitors of COX-2 using a rational, molecularly targeted approach. The first such agent to test this hypothesis and to be approved for use was celecoxib, followed shortly by rofecoxib. In this chapter we will review structural and kinetic features of specific COX-2 inhibition and some of the properties of celecoxib.

STRUCTURAL HOMOLOGY OF THE TWO CYCLOOXYGENASE ENZYMES

The COX-1 and COX-2 isoforms are structurally similar, comprising two distinct functional (peroxidase and cyclooxygenase) active sites[8]. Both have a molecular weight of 71 kDa and are composed of approximately 600 amino acids[9]. There is a 63% sequence homology[10] and a 77% similarity[11] between the amino acids of the two isoforms.

X-ray crystallography data have demonstrated that the overall topology of the enzymes is not affected by the minor variations in the amino acid residues observed between the two isoforms[12] and that the structures of both murine and human COX-2 can be superimposed on COX-1[12-14]. The tertiary struc-tures of both isoforms comprise three distinct folding units: an N-terminal epidermal growth factor (EGF) domain, a membrane-binding motif, and the C-terminal catalytic domain containing the cyclooxygenase and peroxidase active sites[12,14]. The cyclooxygenase active site is located at the end of a long, narrow hydrophobic channel[15].

STRUCTURAL BASIS FOR SELECTIVITY OF COX-2 INHIBITORS

Despite the high degree of structural homology between COX-1 and COX-2, there are important differences with regard to substrate and inhibitor selec-tivity. These functional differences appear to be the result of relatively minor structural variations.

One notable difference between the two isoforms is the substitution of valine for isoleucine at residue 523, which lines the cyclooxygenase channel in COX-2. Valine is smaller than isoleucine, allowing the COX-2 specific inhibitors access to a side pocket that is located off the main substrate channel[10] (Figure 1). Access to this side pocket is restricted by the presence of the larger isoleucine moiety found in the COX-1 isoform. Site-directed mutagenesis studies support the role of the 523 substitution in COX-2 specific inhibition. When valine is mutated to isoleucine at the 523 position on the COX-2 isoform, COX-2 specific inhibitors are less able to bind and inhibit prostaglandin H$_2$ (PGH$_2$) formation[10,11].

It has also been suggested that the valine substitution at position 434 may play a role in COX-2 specific inhibition by increasing access to the side pocket[12]. Another difference between the isoforms is the presence of a 17 amino acid sequence at the N-terminus of the COX-1 isoform. This sequence is absent in COX-2. Similarly, an 18 amino acid sequence is found at the C-terminus of the COX-2 isoform that is not present in COX-1. The significance of these changes is unknown. Also, it should be noted that the C-terminal sequence observed in the COX-2 isoform does not change the last four amino acid residues present in both isoforms[16]. This homologous, four amino acid sequence regulates the signal for attachment to the endoplasmic reticulum[16,17].

Figure 1 Structural basis for selectivity between COX-1 and COX-2 isoforms. Reproduced with permission from ref. 33.

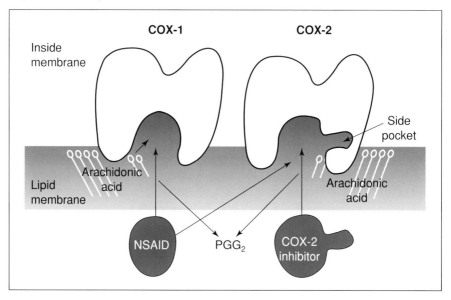

STRUCTURAL ASPECT OF THE INHIBITORY ACTION OF CELECOXIB ON COX-2

Celecoxib is a 1,5-diaryl pyrazole-based compound (Figure 2), which exhibits marked selectivity for COX-2 in human recombinant-enzyme assays. Structure activity studies of the 1,5-diaryl pyrazole series of COX-2 specific inhibitors have demonstrated the importance of the *p*-sulphamoylphenyl group in COX-2 inhibition and *in vivo* efficacy. Similarly, the trifluoromethyl or difluoromethyl groups at the 3-position of the pyrazole provided optimal potency and selectivity, as did substituents on the phenyl moiety at the 5-position of the pyrazole ring[18].

The binding of SC-558, a celecoxib prototype, to the COX-2 isoform has been investigated using X-ray crystallography. Like celecoxib, SC-558 is a 1,5-diaryl pyrazole-based compound comprising a central pyrazole ring and sulphonamide group attached to one of the aryl rings[12]. However, the bromide moiety in SC-558 has been substituted for a methyl group in celecoxib[18]. The phenylsulphonamide moiety appears to be the primary determinant for COX-2 selectivity in the diaryl heterocyclic class of inhibitors.

The phenylsulphonamide moiety binds in a pocket within the channel that leads from the membrane to the cyclooxygenase active site (Figure 3). As described above, this pocket is more accessible in COX-2 than in COX-1, as a result of the 523 substitution. In COX-2, the smaller valine side chain, together with the conformational changes at Tyr 355, provides access to the hydrophobic section of the pocket. Kurumbail et al.[12] also suggest that the 434 substitution facilitates access to this pocket. At position 434, the side chain of the hydrophobic residue rests against Phe 518, forming a molecular gate that spans the pocket. This gate is closed in COX-1 as a result of the larger side chain on isoleucine. However, the smaller valine side chain in COX-2 provides enough room for the gate to open, and thus allows the sulphonamide group to enter the pocket. A third substitution may also

Figure 2 Chemical structure of celecoxib.

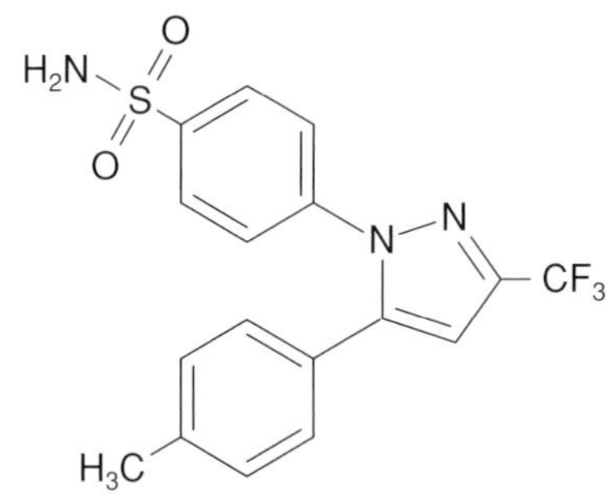

Figure 3 COX-2 active site with celecoxib prototype. Derived from data in ref. 12.

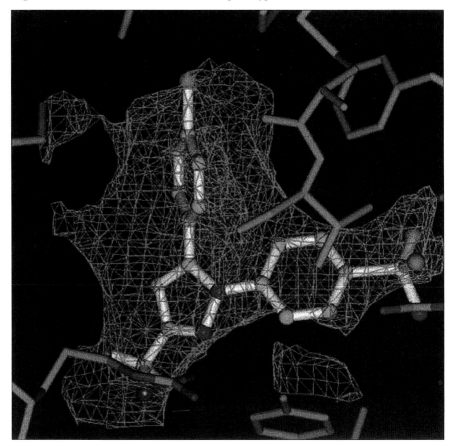

contribute to the COX-2 specificity. At position 513, arginine in COX-2 is substituted for histidine in COX-1, and superposition of the two isoforms predicts that the imidazole ring of histidine would not extend enough to bind with the sulphonamide group[12]. It appears that one of the consequences of these amino acid differences in the side pocket of COX-1 and COX-2 is to create an optimal environment in COX-2 for forming hydrogen bonding interactions with a sulphonamide or methylsulphone containing compound.

KINETIC BASIS FOR SELECTIVE INHIBITION OF COX-2

The inhibition kinetics of celecoxib has been characterized using the oxygen uptake, peroxidase, and prostaglandin E_2 (PGE_2) ELISA assays[19]. Similar IC_{50} values were obtained for COX-1, using the three assays; however, IC_{50}

values determined for COX-2 varied considerably depending on the assay and were comparable with the concentration of enzyme present in each assay. This finding suggests that celecoxib is acting as an active-site titrant with high affinity for COX-2. Celecoxib demonstrated 155–3200-fold selectivity for COX-2 over COX-1, depending on the assay.

In the absence of preincubation, celecoxib displayed initial, competitive inhibition with COX-2 ($K_I = 11$–15 μM). Subsequently, celecoxib exhibited slow, time-dependent kinetics resulting in potent inhibition ($K_{inact} = 0.03$–0.5 s^{-1})[19]. These time-dependent kinetics have been attributed to the molecular complexity associated with the binding of the inhibitor to the pocket[12]. The K_I values obtained in this study suggest that celecoxib exhibits stronger binding during the time-dependent phase than in the initial, competitive phase. In contrast, celecoxib has a different mechanism of action with respect to COX-1, displaying simple, competitive inhibition. This may be due to its inability to access the restricted pocket in this isoform or to weaker overall interactions between the enzyme and the inhibitor[12,19]. This hypothesis is supported by studies using the V523I mutant of COX-2, which is competitively inhibited by the diaryl heterocyclic compounds[12].

ANALYSIS OF CYCLOOXYGENASE SPECIFICITY

The degree to which a pharmacological agent inhibits either COX-1 or COX-2 is frequently represented in terms of its IC$_{50}$ (i.e. the concentration necessary to inhibit 50% of COX activity *in vitro*). Selectivity for COX-2 refers to the separation of concentration–response curves for COX-1 and COX-2 inhibition *in vitro*. For COX-2 selective agents the curve representing COX-1 inhibition is right-shifted to higher doses in relation to the curve for COX-2 inhibition. The differential inhibition of both COX isoforms is often reported as the ratio of IC$_{50}$s for COX-1 and COX-2. However, as discussed below, there is little scientific validity in calculating ratios of IC$_{50}$ values.

The relevance of *in vitro* assays for evaluating inhibition of COX isozymes is limited by a lack of consensus as to the most appropriate (i.e. predictive) set of assay conditions. There are currently four known mechanisms of inhibition of COX isozymes[19]. With certain mechanisms, the results of *in vitro* enzyme assays are inherently dependent on variables such as enzyme and substrate concentration, presence or absence of membranes, and time and order of addition of substrate and inhibitor[20]. The variability of *in vitro* assays is demonstrated by the remarkably divergent values for COX-1/COX-2 inhibition ratios reported in the literature for 6-methoxy 2-naphthylacetic acid (6-MNA), the active metabolite of nabumetone (Table 1). These 'selectivity' ratios vary by up to two orders of magnitude, even in studies using the same source of enzymes.

In the case of celecoxib, ratios of 150 to over 3000 have been obtained with

Table 1 Selectivity ratios reported with active metabolite of nabumetone

Drug	Ratio of $IC_{50}s$ COX-1/COX-2	In vitro assay system	Reference
6-MNA	7	mouse enzymes	21
6-MNA	1.5	human enzymes	22
6-MNA	0.7	human enzymes	23
6-MNA	0.08	human enzymes*	–

*K. M. Verburg, T. J. Maziasz, E. Weiner et al., unpublished data.

varying assays in the same laboratory[19]. It is evident from these data that *in vitro* assays can support widely varying conclusions on the COX-selectivity of a given drug. Thus, while a high degree of selectivity *in vitro* is an important preliminary criterion, it is only one aspect of the data needed to establish a compound as a selective COX-2 inhibitor.

There has also been considerable debate concerning the validity of IC_{50} ratios for characterizing COX-2 selectivity. Difficulties with this manipulation of *in vitro* data arise from the complex mechanisms by which non-selective or selective COX-2 inhibitors inhibit COX-1 and COX-2[19]. Most conventional NSAIDs, including diclofenac and indomethacin, inhibit both isozymes in a time-dependent, pseudo-irreversible fashion first described by Rome and Lands[24]. Although a competitive (i.e. rapidly reversible, low affinity, high micromolar) inhibition is present, the potency of these drugs as inhibitors increases due to a time-dependent transition to high-affinity (low nanomolar) inhibition. Selectivity for COX-2 is achieved by agents that retain both the competitive and the high-affinity, time-dependent binding to COX-2, but only the low-affinity, competitive binding to COX-1[25,26]. Thus, it is evident that lowering substrate concentration will favour the competitive kinetic component over the time dependent component, resulting in lower apparent selectivity for COX-2 than is seen with higher substrate concentrations[27]. Whether these low substrate concentrations reflect what occurs in relevant cells *in vivo* is highly speculative. Conventional NSAIDs, in contrast, inhibit both COX isozymes by the same mechanism, resulting in non-selective, or concomitant, inhibition of COX-1 and COX-2 at any level of drug. The differences in mechanisms of isozyme inhibition and the lack of common kinetic constants lead to concentration–response curves that vary in shape, making comparison of *in vitro* potencies unreliable[19]. Thus, comparison of $IC_{50}s$ does not necessarily provide meaningful information regarding the COX-2 selectivity of an agent.

LIMITATIONS OF CYCLOOXYGENASE ASSAYS

A commonly used method for assessing COX activity introduced by Patrono and colleagues is the human whole-blood assay (hWBA)[28], wherein whole blood is collected from individuals treated with a COX inhibitor or control. COX-1 activity is assessed by allowing the blood to clot, which rapidly releases large quantities of TXA_2 generated via platelet COX-1. COX-2 activity is assessed by adding bacterial endotoxin to heparinized blood, then measuring PGE_2 formation produced by activated monocytes. The assay can be modified when testing compounds in vitro[27]. The major advantage of this assay is that drugs are evaluated in relevant cell populations, platelets and monocytes. However, it has limitations that should be acknowledged. First, it is not a direct measure of COX-2 activity, since the enzyme must first be induced in monocytes by lipopolysaccharide, a process that takes several hours. Second, the fundamental conditions for assessing COX-1 and COX-2 activity differ markedly in terms of time (seconds versus hours) and, potentially, the substrate concentration at the site. Finally, as already discussed, there are limitations in comparing enzyme IC_{50} values that reflect distinct kinetic mechanisms.

In vitro studies have been useful for providing insight into enzymatic mechanisms and the basis for the clinical toxicity of conventional NSAIDs. However, any in vitro assessment of activity is in essence a surrogate marker for a clinical effect and, as such, is only useful in so far as the assessment accurately predicts a clinical response in humans. Our preference has been to assess COX inhibitory activity using an in vitro system where assay conditions for COX-1 and COX-2 are identical, which has allowed the rigorous kinetic analyses described above[19]. However, with the inherent limitations of in vitro assay systems, greater reliance must be placed on in vivo assays and ultimately clinical data to assess fully the pharmacological activity of COX specific inhibitors.

Measurement of PG concentrations in whole animals can be used as physiological surrogates (i.e. biomarkers) for the activity of COX-1 or COX-2 in vivo; moreover, inhibition of both isozymes can be assessed in the same animal[29]. Examples of results obtained with this assay are shown in Figure 4. Celecoxib was found to be a potent inhibitor of COX-2 (half-maximal inhibitory dose, ID_{50}, of 0.2 mg kg^{-1}); in contrast, it is a poor inhibitor of PG production from COX-1, even at doses as high as 200 mg kg^{-1} (P. C. Isakson, unpublished observation).

While this approach provides less biased assessment of COX inhibition than in vitro assays, it is still not correct to measure selectivity by comparing ratios of ED_{50} values. This is because comparison of potencies of different agents using dose–response curves requires that the slopes of the individual curves be parallel[30]. As can be seen in Figure 4, the shapes of dose–response curves obtained with various drugs often do not meet this requirement, much in the same manner encountered with in vitro enzyme assays. Thus, quantitative comparisons of COX-2 selectivity for drugs with different mechanisms based on ED_{50} values are also questionable.

Figure 4 Assessment of inhibition COX-1 and COX-2 *in vivo* using prostaglandins (K. M. Verburg, T. J. Maziasz, E. Weiner, et al., unpublished data).

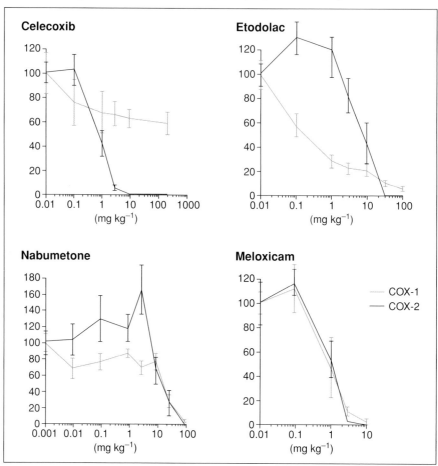

DEFINITION OF A COX-2 SPECIFIC INHIBITOR

In light of the high degree of variability and questionable validity of the *in vitro* assay systems discussed above, *in vivo* data also need to be considered when evaluating COX-2 specificity. The demonstration of decreased GI toxicity and anti-platelet effects in patients at maximally effective doses is necessary definitively to characterize an agent as COX-2 specific.

PRECLINICAL CELECOXIB DATA

It is now evident from a number of studies that COX-2 specific inhibitors have efficacy in traditional animal models of inflammation and arthritis equivalent to non-specific COX inhibitors, the NSAIDs (Table 2). For example, celecoxib achieved effects similar to that of indomethacin and naproxen in rodent models of inflammation and/or pain[18]. However, unlike conventional NSAIDs, celecoxib exhibited neither acute GI toxicity in rats at doses up to 200 mg kg^{-1} nor chronic GI toxicity at doses up to 600 mg kg^{-1} over ten days[17]. The conventional NSAIDs displayed severe toxicity at these doses.

In the adjuvant-induced arthritis model of chronic inflammation, celecoxib administered twice daily for ten days reduced oedema associated with foot-pad injection of *Mycobacterium butyricum*[18]. Celecoxib resulted in an 80–85% decrease in paw swelling, suggesting that the induction of COX-2 is largely responsible for the inflammatory response observed in this model of rheumatoid arthritis[31].

Prophylactic administration of celecoxib reduced paw volume and withdrawal latency to thermal stimuli in the carrageenan-induced acute inflammation and pain model[18,32]. SC-560, a potent and selective inhibitor of COX-1, had no effect on the onset of either hyperalgesia or oedema, suggesting that the inflammatory response observed in this model is associated with the COX-2 isoform[32]. Oral celecoxib (30 mg kg^{-1}), but not SC-560, also resulted in a reduction of PGE$_2$ in cerebrospinal fluid to baseline levels[32].

CONCLUSIONS

The development of celecoxib was the result of a rational approach to new drug discovery, i.e. specifically targeting a molecular entity thought to be

Table 2 *In vivo* effects of celecoxib and comparator NSAIDs

Model	Parameter	ED_{50} (mg kg^{-1} orally)			
		Celecoxib	Indomethacin	Naproxen	Piroxicam
Adjuvant-induced arthritis	Inflammation (chronic)	0.37	0.11	0.94	0.15
Carrageenan-induced paw oedema	Inflammation (acute)	7.1	1.15	1.6	2.4
Carrageenan-induced hyperalgesia	Analgesia	34.5	4.1	66% (at 10 mg kg^{-1})	52% (at 10 mg kg^{-1})
Acute gastric toxicity[a]	Gastric damage[b]	No effect[c]	7	255	2.9

[a]ED_{50} defined as the dose at which 50% of the animals showed no gastric damage
[b]Microscopic assessment
[c]At single doses up to 200 mg kg^{-1}
ED_{50} = dose producing 50% inhibition
(Reproduced from ref. 18.)

important in disease, in this case the enzyme COX-2, by medicinal chemistry approaches, then rigorously evaluating the hypothesis in animal models and finally in humans. The latter is detailed in a subsequent chapter (J. B. Lefkowith et al., Chapter 21).

REFERENCES

1. Xie W, Chipman JG, Robertson DL, Erikson RL, Simmons DL. Expression of a mitogen-responsive gene encoding prostaglandin synthase is regulated by mRNA splicing. *Proc Natl Acad Sci USA.* 1991;88:2692–6.
2. Kujubu DA, Fletcher BS, Varnum BC, Lim RW, Herschman HR. TIS10, a phorbol ester tumor promoter-inducible mRNA from Swiss 3T3 cells, encodes a novel prostaglandin synthase/cyclooxygenase homologue. *J Biol Chem.* 1991;266:12866–72.
3. O'Banion MK, Sadowski HB, Winn V, Young DA. A serum- and glucocorticoid-regulated 4-kilobase mRNA encodes a cyclooxygenase-related protein. *J Biol Chem.* 1991;266:23261–7.
4. Crofford L. COX-1 and COX-2 tissue expression: implications and predictions. *J Rheumatol.* 1997;(Suppl 49)24:15–9.
5. Lipsky PE. Role of cyclooxygenase-1 and -2 in health and disease. *Am J Orthop.* 1999;28(Suppl 3):8–12.
6. DuBois R, Abramson S, Crofford C, Gupta R, Simon, L, Van de Putte L et al. Cyclooxygenase in biology and disease. *FASEB J.* 1998;12:1063–73.
7. Mitchell JA, Akarasereenont P, Thiemermann C, Flower RJ, Vane JR. Selectivity of nonsteroidal antiinflammatory drugs as inhibitors of constitutive and inducible cyclooxygenases. *Proc Natl Acad Sci USA.* 1994;90:11693–7.
8. Hawkey CJ. COX-2 inhibitors. *Lancet.* 1999;353:307–14.
9. Smith WL, Garavito RM, DeWitt DL. Prostaglandin endoperoxide H synthases (cyclooxygenases)-1 and -2. *J Biol Chem.* 1996;271:33157–60.
10. Vane JR, Bakhle YS, Botting RM. Cyclooxygenases 1 and 2. *Annu Rev Pharmacol Toxicol.* 1998;38:97–120.
11. Gierse JK, McDonald JJ, Hauser SD, Rangwala SH, Koboldt CM, Seibert K. A single amino acid difference between cyclooxygenase-1 (COX-1) and -2 (COX-2) reverses the selectivity of COX-2 specific inhibitors. *J Biol Chem.* 1996;271:15810–4.
12. Kurumbail RG, Stevens AM, Gierse JK, McDonald JJ, Stegeman RA, Pak JY et al. Structural basis for selective inhibition of cyclooxygenase-2 by anti-inflammatory agents. *Nature.* 1996;384:644–8.
13. Luong C, Miller A, Barnett J, Chow J, Ramesha C, Browner MF et al. Flexibility of the NSAID binding site in the structure of human cyclooxygenase-2. *Nature Struct Biol.* 1996;3:927–33.
14. Picot D, Loll PJ, Garavito M. The X-ray crystal structure of the membrane protein prostaglandin H_2 synthase. *Nature.* 1994;367:243–49.
15. Garavito RM. The three-dimensional structure of cyclooxygenases. In: Vane J, Botting J, Botting R, editors. *Improved Non-steroid Anti-inflammatory Drugs: COX-2 Enzyme Inhibitors.* Dordrecht: Kluwer Academic Publishers; 1996: 29–43.
16. Ren Y, Loose-Mitchell, DS, Kulmacz RJ. Prostaglandin H synthase-1: evaluation of C-terminus function. *Arch Biochem Biophys.* 1995;316:751–7.

17. Ren Y, Walker C, Loose-Mitchell DS, Deng J, Ruan K-H, Kulmacz RJ. Topology of prostaglandin H synthase-1 in the endoplasmic reticulum membrane. *Arch Biochem Biophys*. 1995;301:205–14.

18. Penning TD, Talley JJ, Bertenshaw SR, Carter JS, Collins PW, Doater S et al. Synthesis and biological evaluation of the 1,5 diarylpyrazole class of cyclooxygenase-2 inhibitors: identification of 4-[5-(4-methylphenyl)-3-(trifluoromethyl)-1H-pyrazol-1-yl] benzenesulfonamide (SC-58635, celecoxib). *J Med Chem*. 1997;40:1347–65.

19. Gierse JK, Koboldt CM, Walker MK, Seibert K, Isakson PC. Kinetic basis for selective inhibition of cyclooxygenases. *Biochem J*. 1999;339:607–14.

20. Frölich JC. A classification of NSAIDs according to the relative inhibition of cyclooxygenase isoenzymes. *Trends Pharmacol Sci*. 1997;18:30–4.

21. Meade EA, Smith WL, DeWitt DL. Differential inhibition of prostaglandin endoperoxide synthase cyclooxygenase isozymes by aspirin and other non-steroidal anti-inflammatory drugs. *J Biol Chem*. 1993;268:6610–4.

22. Laneuville O, Breuer DK, Dewitt DL, Hla T, Funk CD, Smith WL. Differential inhibition of human prostaglandin endoperoxide H synthases-1 and -2 by non-steroidal anti-inflammatory drugs. *J Pharmacol Exp Ther*. 1994;271:927–34.

23. Battistini B, Botting R, Bakhle YS. COX-1 and COX-2: Toward the development of more selective NSAIDs. *Drug News and Perspectives*. 1994;7:501–12.

24. Rome LH, Lands WEM. Structural requirements for time-dependent inhibition of prostaglandin biosynthesis by anti-inflammatory drugs. *Proc Natl Acad Sci USA*. 1975;72:4863–5.

25. Copeland RA, Williams JM, Giannaras J, Nurnberg S, Covington J, Pinto D et al. Mechanism of selective inhibition of the inducible isoform of prostaglandin G/H synthase. *Proc Natl Acad Sci USA*. 1994;91:11202–6.

26. Gierse JK, Hauser SD, Creely DP, Koboldt C, Rangwala SH, Isakson PC et al. Expression and selective inhibition of the constitutive and inducible forms of human cyclooxygenase. *Biochem J*. 1995;305:479–84.

27. Warner T, Giuliano F, Vojnovic I, Bukasa A, Mitchell J, Vane J. Nonsteroid drug selectivities for cyclo-oxygenase-1 rather than cyclo-oxygenase-2 are associated with human gastrointestinal toxicity: a full *in vitro* analysis. *Proc Natl Acad Sci USA*. 1999;96:7563–8.

28. Patrignani P, Panara MR, Greco A, Fusco O, Natoli C, Iacobelli S et al. Biochemical and pharmacological characterization of the cyclooxygenase activity of human blood prostaglandin endoperoxide synthases. *J Pharmacol Exp Ther*. 1994;271:1705–12.

29. Masferrer J, Zweifel B, Manning PT, Hauser SD, Leahy KM, Smith WG et al. Selective inhibition of inducible cyclooxygenase 2 *in vivo* is anti-inflammatory and non-ulcerogenic. *Proc Natl Acad Sci USA*. 1994;91:3228–32.

30. Tallarida RJ, Jacob LS. Construction of dose-response curves: statistical considerations. In: Tallarida RJ, editor. *The Dose–Response Relation in Pharmacology*. New York: Springer-Verlag; 1979:85–110.

31. Tindall E. Celecoxib for the treatment of pain and inflammation: the preclinical and clinical results. *J Am Osteopath Assoc*. 1999;99(Suppl):S13–7.

32. Smith CJ, Zhang Y, Koboldt CM, Muhammad J, Zweifel BS, Shaffer A et al. Pharmacological analysis of cyclooxygenase-1 in inflammation. *Proc Natl Acad Sci USA*. 1998;95:13313–8.

33. Adelizzi RA. COX-1 and COX-2 in health and disease. *J Am Osteopath Assoc*. 1999;99(Suppl):S7–12.

3 | Discovery of Vioxx® (rofecoxib)

PETPIBOON PRASIT, DENIS RIENDEAU AND
CHI C. CHAN
*Merck Frosst Centre for Therapeutic Research, PO Box 1005,
Pointe Claire-Dorval, Quebec H9R 4P8, Canada.*

By 1992, the excitement generated by the discovery of the inducible form of cyclooxygenase, COX-2, reached its peak. In January of that year, the Keystone Winter Prostaglandin Conference devoted an entire session to the topic. Galbraith et al. from Dupont described an experimental agent DuP 697 (1; Figure 1) as a compound with potent anti-inflammatory activity but with a superior gastrointestinal (GI) profile in animal models as compared with standard non-steroid anti-inflammatory drugs (NSAIDs)[1]. They postulated that this agent could be working through the selective inhibition of COX-2 that had been described by earlier speakers in the session, including Herschman and Simmons. In particular, they described the ability of DuP 697 to inhibit the synthesis of prostaglandins (PGs) in lipopolysaccharide (LPS)-induced human monocytes and interleukin (IL)-1-induced human fibroblasts and its lack of potency against human platelet-derived thromboxane[2]. In July 1992, at the Prostaglandins and Related Compounds Conference in Montreal, Canada, Futaki et al. from Taisho described a structurally distinct compound, NS-398, and its *in vivo* and *ex vivo* activity profiles[3,4]. In the *in vivo* assays, such as rat paw oedema, NS-398 was equipotent to the dual COX inhibitor indomethacin. However, NS-398 was less potent than indomethacin in its ability to inhibit the synthesis of PGs *ex vivo* from rat tissues such as stomach mucosa and kidney. These properties, though not proven, pointed to the fact that its potential mechanism of action was through the selective inhibition of COX-2.

From the drug development point of view, since these agents demonstrated anti-inflammatory activity with GI sparing profiles, it became critical to confirm that compounds such as DuP 697 or NS-398 preferentially inhibit COX-2 over COX-1 and this would therefore confirm the COX-2 hypothesis.

Figure 1 Structures of prototype COX-2 inhibitors.

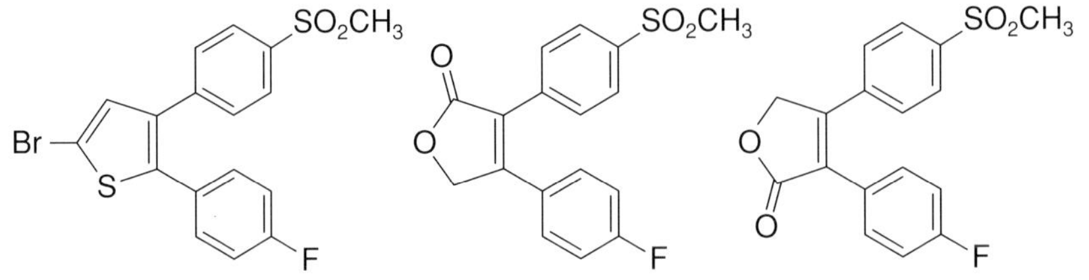

The corollary is that the therapeutic properties of NSAIDs are due to the inhibition of the inducible enzyme (COX-2) and the toxicity of NSAIDs is due to the inhibition of the constitutive enzyme (COX-1). Therefore selective COX-2 inhibitors should be anti-inflammatory, analgesic and antipyretic, with an improved GI safety profile.

IDENTIFICATION OF LEAD COX-2 INHIBITORS

At Merck Frosst, the process of cloning the human cDNA of COX-2 began in mid-June 1992. Fortuitously, the U937 and osteosarcoma cell lines were rapidly identified as cell lines that selectively express the COX-1 and COX-2 enzymes respectively. These two cell lines allowed us to evaluate the relative selectivity of various agents without having to express the enzymes themselves. Subsequently, the Merck Frosst group cloned and purified human COX-2 from a recombinant baculovirus system[5]. A number of standard NSAIDs and NS-398 were evaluated. As expected, most of the NSAIDs on the market were found to be non-selective. In contrast, NS-398 was found to be very selective. Under the assay conditions, NS-398 had an IC_{50} of 10 nM for the production of PGE_2 in the COX-2-expressing osteosarcoma cells and only 10% inhibition at 10 μM in the COX-1-expressing U937 cells. These data prompted us to examine other compounds that were claimed in the literature to be GI-sparing such as nimesulide[6], flosulide[7], DuP 697[1], FK 3311[8], T-614[9] and a number of others. Interestingly, nimesulide was sold in some European and South American countries as an anti-inflammatory agent at the time. Except for DuP 697, the other compounds mentioned above can be classified as being structurally similar. They are sulphanilides with an acidic hydrogen that can be converted into sodium salts, which, in general, makes this class of compounds intrinsically more bioavailable. DuP 697, on the other hand, is a rigid, lipophilic molecule containing a methylsulphonyl group. All the above-mentioned compounds, except FK 3311 which was inactive, exhibited varying degrees of COX-2 inhibition selectivity.

The following sections of this review deal with various *in vitro* and *in vivo* assays that were used throughout the development programme. Suffice it to say that these assays were set up and tuned on an ongoing basis as the programme progressed. The structure activity relationship (SAR) studies that led to the identification of rofecoxib will follow and the last section will summarize the preclinical profile of rofecoxib.

IN VITRO ASSAYS: ENZYME AND CELL-BASED ASSAYS

A large variety of *in vitro* systems using cell lines, tissue extracts and recombinant enzymes have been described for the evaluation of the selectivity of inhibition of COX-2 over COX-1. It is now apparent that the selectivity of inhibition observed for COX-2 (typically expressed as the ratio of IC_{50} values for the inhibition of COX-2 and COX-1) varies depending on the type of assay and conditions used for the measurement of COX activity. Nevertheless, the different *in vitro* assays have been extremely useful in the identification of lead inhibitors with selectivity for COX-2 and in eliminating COX-2 inactive compounds, as well as guiding the medicinal chemistry effort.

As mentioned previously, an initial objective in our COX-2 programme was rapidly to identify sources of COX-2 and COX-1 activity and to develop assays for each of the isoforms. Osteosarcoma cells and undifferentiated U937 cells provided cell line models for the expression of COX-2 and COX-1, respectively[10]. These cells had been used extensively in our leukotriene biosynthesis inhibitor and phospholipase A_2 (PLA_2) inhibitor programmes and prior experiments had revealed several differences between these cells, including the ability of osteosarcoma cells to produce large amounts of PGE_2 when grown to confluence. Reverse transcriptase polymerase chain reaction (RT-PCR) and immunoblot analyses confirmed the inducibility of COX-2 in osteosarcoma cells and demonstrated the selective expression of COX-1 by U937 cells. The production of PGE_2 by osteosarcoma cells and U937 cells following arachidonic acid stimulation provided initial assays for the evaluation of the selectivity of COX-2 inhibition against COX-1.

In order to evaluate the inhibitory effects of the compounds against COX-1 from human tissue, kidney microsomes were used. Although the kidney expresses both COX isoforms, COX-1 is the predominant form and the production of PGE_2 by human kidney microsomes was found to be useful as a screening assay for human COX-1. This assay can also be performed with rat and dog kidney preparations, the two species used for safety studies.

The osteosarcoma cells provided a source of RNA for the cloning of the COX-2 cDNA and overexpression of the enzyme in mammalian[11] and insect cells[12,13] in order to develop additional assays and to supply sufficient amounts of the enzymes for purification and characterization. Stably transfected Chinese hamster ovary (CHO) cells overexpressing human COX-2 and COX-1 provided new whole-cell assays for the evaluation of inhibitor potency and selectivity[14]. This assay offers the advantage of permitting the comparison of the effects of inhibitors against COX-1 and COX-2 in the same cell vector and also of reducing the variability associated with the inducibility of COX-2 in osteosarcoma cells.

In order to develop a method that would allow the rank ordering of potency of very weak inhibitors of COX-1, a specially sensitive assay was set up with U937 microsomes using the lowest practically usable arachidonic acid concentration (0.1 μM) that would give stimulation of PGE_2 production[15]. In this situation, the inhibitors show a higher inhibitory potency than in platelet and other assays due to the competition with subsaturating substrate concentrations. This may be of relevance *in vivo* where, in certain tissues, there may be limited amounts of arachidonic acid.

Enzyme inhibition studies

Studies with purified recombinant COX-1 and COX-2 revealed significant differences between the mechanism of inhibition of the two enzymes. The prototypes NS-398 and DuP 697 were found to be time-dependent and slowly reversible inhibitors of COX-2 and rapidly reversible competitive inhibitors of COX-1[16,17]. In addition, both the intact inhibitor and the active enzyme can be recovered from the inhibited enzyme, indicating that the mechanism of inhibition does not involve any irreversible covalent inactivation[18]. In agreement with the competitive nature of the COX-1 inhibition, the inhibitory effects on purified human COX-1 vary with the arachidonic acid concentration and can be detected with the highly selective inhibitors only at low concentrations of the arachidonic substrate.

Whole-blood assay

As already discussed, the observed selectivity of inhibition of COX-2 versus COX-1 can vary according to assay conditions such as differences in pre-incubation times or substrate concentrations. Thus, it was of importance to identify assays that would more accurately reflect the *in vivo* situation than those with purified enzymes or cell lines. Whole-blood assays present the advantage of measuring COX activities with locally derived substrate and in the presence of plasma proteins which can affect the concentration of free drug, which, in turn, will affect the apparent potency[19,20]. For COX-1, the release of platelet thromboxane B_2 (TXB_2) following clotting of the blood is used as a measure of activity. For COX-2, the blood is incubated with bacterial LPS to induce COX-2 protein synthesis and the increase in PGE_2 production following LPS-challenge corresponds to COX-2 activity. In whole blood, the potency of inhibition of COX-2 and the selectivity for COX-2 are often reduced as compared with other *in vitro* assays. Thus, whole-blood assays represent more stringent tests to assess the selectivity of COX-2 inhibition. NS-398 and DuP 697 show ten- and 20-fold selectivity for COX-2, respectively, in these assays and are more selective than traditional NSAIDs (see Table 1). The *in vitro* whole blood data can be directly compared with *ex vivo* assays performed with whole blood from volunteers who have received different doses of COX-2 inhibitors. In clinical trials, the inhibition of LPS-stimulated PGE_2 production was found to correlate with the plasma concentration of the COX-2 inhibitors.

ANTI-INFLAMMATORY, ANALGESIC AND ANTI-PYRETIC EFFECTS

Many of the commonly used *in vivo* models of inflammation, pain and pyresis were already in place at Merck at the initiation of the COX-2 inhibitor programme. These preclinical models, such as the carrageenan-induced rat paw oedema assay, carrageenan-induced rat hyperalgesia assay and adjuvant-induced arthritis in rats, are models used to evaluate the effectiveness of currently used NSAIDs. Thus, these are appropriate models to test the efficacy of COX-2 inhibitors since the COX-2 hypothesis proposes that COX-2 inhibitors would have the same therapeutic effects as conventional NSAIDs. In general the efficacy of NSAIDs in these rodent models are in line with their clinical doses[21,22]. An additional non-human primate model of pyresis[23] was set up to test the efficacy of COX-2 inhibitors to complement the rodent models.

Table 1 Inhibition of COX-1 and COX-2 in whole-blood assays (IC_{50}, μM)

	COX-1	COX-2	Ratio COX-1:COX-2
Ketoprofen	0.02	1.1	0.02
Piroxicam	0.76	9.0	0.1
Sulindac sulphide	1.0	10	0.1
Naproxen	7.8	74	0.1
6-MNA	29	154	0.2
Ibuprofen	4.8	24	0.2
Indomethacin	0.2	0.5	0.4
Ketolorac	0.36	0.86	0.4
Meloxicam	1.4	0.7	2
Diclofenac	0.1	0.05	2
Mefenamic acid	4.6	2.2	2
Etodolac	9.0	3.7	2
Nimesulide	4.1	0.6	7
NS-398	4.8	0.5	10
DuP 697	1.2	0.06	20
Flosulide	32	0.8	40

GASTROINTESTINAL EFFECTS

Traditionally, the GI side effects of NSAIDs are examined in short-term studies by scoring the GI tract for the presence of drug-induced bleeds, erosions, lesions and ulcers in postmortem animals. This is a very sensitive and practical method to detect GI side effects of NSAIDs, due to their prominent effect on the GI tract. However, in the development of COX-2 inhibitors, this method proved to be less useful because COX-2 inhibitors in general do not cause detectable bleeds or ulcers in animals, even at high multiples of their efficacious doses. Scoring the stomach using the traditional method will only give a cut-off level, as reported for the COX-2 inhibitor L-745,337[24]. It does not give a quantitative end-point to differentiate whether one COX-2 inhibitor is better than another. Furthermore, this method is not suitable for use in larger animals such as non-human primates, where it cannot be conducted on a routine basis. Therefore, there is a need to establish a more sensitive and measurable end-point to assess the GI effects of COX-2 inhibitors in animals, particularly in non-human primates, without sacrificing the animals at the end of the studies.

The faecal ^{51}chromium (^{51}Cr) excretion assay was adopted for the study of the ulcerogenic potential of COX-2 inhibitors. This technique is quantitative, sensitive and detects the integrity of the entire GI tract. It is also used in clinical trials with conventional NSAIDs[25,26] and, in fact, with a COX-2 inhibitor[27]. In this assay, ^{51}Cr-labelled red blood cells were injected intravenously into animals and the amount recovered in the faeces after a 24–48 h collection period was used as an index for GI permeability. An adaptation of this technique, which is even more sensitive, was later used where ^{51}Cr–EDTA complex was given orally and the amount of urinary ^{51}Cr–EDTA was used as an index. In the pathogenesis of GI lesions, a breakdown in GI integrity, manifested as an increase in GI permeability, often precedes the formation of lesions. Thus, it would be appropriate to measure the effects of COX-2 inhibitors on GI permeability to compare the ulcerogenic potential of COX-2 inhibitors. As discussed below, inhibitors with an array of selectivity ratio on COX-2/COX-1 showed differential activities in the ^{51}Cr-faecal excretion assay.

Standard NSAIDs, including some of the more selective ones such as etodolac, meloxicam, diclofenac (as judged by the whole cell or whole-blood assays), showed a marked increase in the GI permeability in this assay[28]. In particular, under chronic conditions, diclofenac, for example, produced a marked increase in the ^{51}Cr leakage at doses not much higher than its therapeutic dose. In a comparative study conducted in-house, NS-398, DuP 697 and indomethacin (as a positive control) were given to rats at 30 mg kg^{-1}, 30 mg kg^{-1} and 10 mg kg^{-1}, respectively, either in a single dose or, in the case of NS-398, chronically for 5 days. Upon scoring the gastric tissues for ulcers, as expected it was found that indomethacin was ulcerogenic. NS-398 or DuP 697, on the other hand, did not cause detectable gastric ulcers, which is consistent with their reduced COX-1 inhibitory activity. Subsequent studies using the ^{51}Cr-faecal excretion assay have confirmed the larger margin of GI safety observed with NS-398 and DuP 697. However, at higher doses there appeared to be a slight loss of the GI integrity as judged by leakage of the ^{51}Cr, suggesting that there was an opportunity for improvement.

The results were consistent with the fact that the reduced GI toxicity correlated with the reduced COX-1 inhibition. The critical question became how much selectivity is required in the next generation of anti-inflammatory drugs to make it a significant clinical advance. Some of the very interesting and provoking questions that never arose in the NSAID area can now be asked of this 'new mechanism' since the GI toxicity is potentially no longer a dose limiting factor with specific COX-2 inhibitors. This raises questions such as what would be the effect of a prolonged 'around the clock' inhibition of COX-2, which was not previously possible. Will COX-2 inhibitors be as effective clinically as non-selective COX-1/COX-2 inhibitors? In other words, is there any component of pain, inflammation and fever associated with COX-1? The upside is that since these agents are potentially safer, they may be used to treat, or even used prophylactically, for the prevention of diseases in which COX-2 has been shown to be upregulated, for example, colon cancer and Alzheimer's disease. The obvious downside would be that these inhibitors would lack the cardioprotective effect provided by concomitant COX-1 inhibition afforded by the dual inhibitors, for which aspirin is an excellent example.

CHEMISTRY

A number of strategies were pursued in the search for the safe and effective clinical candidate. Both classes of compounds, NS-398 and DuP 697, were used as starting points of optimization. With the aid of molecular modelling, structural biology and X-ray crystallography, attempts were made at trying to remove COX-1 inhibitory activity from dual inhibitors such as indomethacin, flurbiprofen and diclofenac. However, it is beyond the scope of this article to describe all the avenues that were pursued. This article will focus exclusively on the discovery of Vioxx® (rofecoxib, MK-0966).

Apparently, the development program of DuP 697 (1; Figure 1) at Dupont did not progress beyond the clinic because there was a long lasting metabolite, X-6882, in which the bromine atom of DuP 697 is replaced by a thiomethyl-sulphonyl moiety. The SAR of this molecule was extensively studied and can be summarized as follows[29,30].

The methylsulphonyl group is extremely important for both COX-2 potency and selectivity. The only other functionality that confers such properties on this class of molecule is the sulphonamide SO_2NH_2. However, there are pros and cons with using either the sulphone or the sulphonamide as the head group. Sulphonamides are more potent at inhibiting COX-1 than the corresponding sulphones, thus making the sulphonamides, in general, less selective. In addition, some sulphonamides are associated with sulphonamide allergy which will require such labelling. The advantage of the sulphonamides, however, is that they tend to be more bioavailable than the corresponding sulphones. In addition, it is possible to make prodrugs of sulphonamides such as acylsulphonamides, where sodium salts can be made and can potentially be administered as an i.v. solution that has an added advantage in certain clinical settings. In any event, the sulphone/sulphonamide moiety has to be at the *para* position of the phenyl ring. The *ortho* and *meta* isomers are inactive. Replacing the phenyl ring with other aromatic heterocycles, both five and six-membered as well as having additional substituents on the phenyl ring were briefly explored but yielded inferior compounds.

The central thiophene ring can be replaced by a wide variety of cyclic groups that do not have to be aromatic. It appeared that the role of the thiophene ring here is simply to act as a template to anchor the two phenyl rings in a rigid conformation. The essential characteristic of the ring is that the atoms of the cycle bearing the phenyl rings have to be sp^2 in character. The ring size can be six, five, four and even simply a double bond. Thus cyclobutanones[31], cyclopentenes[32], cyclopentanones[33], furanones[34] and pyridines[35], for example, fit the description and as such can act as templates for this class of inhibitors. Ring sizes larger than six members have not been explored. However, fused ring systems such as benzofuran, benzothiophene, indene and others[36] have been reported.

Presumably the lower phenyl group fits into a lipophilic pocket of the active site. This is probably the most promiscuous site on the molecule. Although this site can accommodate wide-ranging substituents, some tuning of selectivity is also possible here. For instance, a substitution at the *para* position of the phenyl ring, even with a small group such as a fluorine atom, usually gave an enhancement of the COX-1 inhibitory potency. In contrast, a similar substitution of the fluorine atom at the *meta* position of the phenyl ring reduces the potency against COX-1 . Neither of these changes affects the COX-2 inhibitory activity greatly and thus, in general, compounds with a *meta* substitution in the lower phenyl ring are more selective than the corresponding *para* substituted ones.

With respect to DuP 697, it was found that the bromine atom was not essential for the inhibition of COX-2. In fact, the corresponding desbromo compound was more selective than DuP 697 itself, albeit less potent on the COX-2 enzyme. The trend observed is that smaller substituents at this position tend to give lower COX-1 inhibitory activity and therefore higher selectivity for COX-2. The final point about this series of compounds, particularly the thiophenes, is that they suffered from poor bioavailability.

In fact DuP 697 appeared to be the most bioavailable compound of the series.

With all this SAR information in hand, we made a conscious decision to work on those compounds with methylsulphonylphenyl as the head group instead of the more bioavailable sulphonamide series. This decision, as stated earlier, was primarily based on the superior selectivity profile of the methyl-sulphonylphenyl class as well as the potential allergy labelling issue associated with sulphonamides. The major issue for this series was, therefore, how to improve the oral bioavailability. Attempts to replace the thiophene template by a number of heterocycles, such as various thiophene isomers, oxazoles, indoles, thiazoles, etc., although resulting in potent and selective COX-2 inhibitors, did not provide a significant increase in oral absorption in most cases. It occurred to us that since the thiophene core can potentially be replaced by a number of heterocycles, aromatic or otherwise, could it also be replaced by a five-membered lactone, a butenolide, moiety? If it could, then potentially the lactone ring can be opened up to provide the hydroxyacid pro-drug that may then be administered as a sodium salt. Following this rationale, the two possible lactones (2 and 3; Figure 1) were prepared. Only the lactone (3; Figure 1) was found to be active and selective for COX-2 (Table 2). Attempts to open the lactone moiety with aqueous base resulted in the destruction of the molecule, presumably through base-catalysed self-conden-sation. Fortuitously, however, the neutral lactone was found to be quite bioavailable. Given to rats at 20 mg kg^{-1}, it gave a C_{max} as high as 39 μM, which was unprecedented for the methylsulphonylphenyl class of compounds up to this point. With this level of absorption, it was not unexpected that the compound exhibited significant anti-inflammatory and anti-pyretic activities. In the rat paw oedema model, this prototype lactone has an ED$_{50}$ of 2.0 mg kg^{-1} (5% Tween 80 as vehicle) and an ED$_{50}$ of 1.3 mg kg^{-1} in the rat pyresis model, which compares favourably with indomethacin.

Although 3 in Figure 1 is a relatively selective and orally active COX-2 inhibitor, it was felt desirable to enhance its COX-2 selectivity further. As with other COX-2 inhibitors of the tricyclic class, a substituent at the 4-position on the lower phenyl ring increases COX-1 activity and thus is detrimental to the selectivity. For example, 3 (X = 4-fluorine, entry a, Table 3) is more potent in the COX-1 assay than entry b (X = H). This is generally true for other *para*

Table 2 Cyclooxygenase inhibitory activities of lactone 3 and indomethacin (IC$_{50}$, μM)

	COX-2 Whole blood	COX-1 Whole blood	Ratio	COX-2 Whole cell	COX-1 Whole cell	Ratio
Indomethacin	0.5	0.2	0.4	0.03	0.02	0.7
Lactone 3	0.6	10	17	0.01	4.7	470

Table 3 *In vitro* data of representative cyclooxygenase-2 inhibitors (IC_{50}, μM)

	Human whole blood COX-2	Human whole blood COX-1	Whole cells (CHO) COX-2	Whole cells (CHO) COX-1
a	0.6	10	0.01	4.7
b	0.5	19	0.02	> 15
c	1.8	86	0.02	> 50
d	0.9	13	0.03	> 50
e	> 33	nd	> 5.0	nd
f	0.8	5.8	nd	nd
Indomethacin	0.4	0.2	0.03	0.02

substituents such as halogens, methyl, methoxy and others. It is worth noting that these changes do not greatly affect their potencies against COX-2. Moreover, by moving these substituents from the 4- to the 3-position (entry c) or by adding substituents at both the 3- and 4-positions (entry d), the COX-1 inhibitory activity is reduced, again without dramatically affecting the inhibitory activity against COX-2. This trend is consistent with the fact that the COX-1 active site is sterically more demanding than that of COX-2[37], making it more sensitive to changes to the substitution pattern. Sulphonamido derivatives were also briefly investigated but, as expected (entry f), the compounds in this series were deemed to have unacceptable levels of COX-1 inhibitory activity. A number of sulphonamido compounds indeed caused significant increase in the ^{51}Cr-faecal excretion assay for GI integrity. Some heterocycles can be used to replace the lower phenyl ring of the lactone (entry e) but in general, these compounds, particularly the unsubstituted ones, demonstrate a decrease in COX-2 inhibitory potency.

VIOXX® (rofecoxib)

Of the large number of compounds prepared and examined, the compound with the best overall profile proved to be entry b (now designated as rofecoxib, MK-0966 or Vioxx®). A summary of the effect of rofecoxib in a large number of different *in vitro* assays is presented in Table 4.

Table 4 Potency of rofecoxib in *in vitro* assays (IC$_{50}$)

Assays	Rofecoxib	Indomethacin
PGE$_2$ production by osteosarcoma cells(COX-2)	26 ± 10 nM (n = 5)	21 ± 6 nM (n = 7)
PGE$_2$ production by U937 cells (COX-1)	> 50 μM (n = 4)	7 ± 1 nM (n = 5)
PGE$_2$ production by CHO [COX-2] cells	18 ± 7 nM (n = 6)	27 ± 6 nM (n = 12)
PGE$_2$ production by CHO [COX-1] cells	> 15 μM (n = 3)	18 ± 2 μM (n = 9)
PGE$_2$ production by LPS-induced human mononuclear cells (COX-2)	45 ± 7 nM (n = 11)	57 ± 14 nM (n = 18)
PGE$_2$ production by LPS-induced rat mononuclear cells (COX-2)	41 ± 10 nM (n = 10)	
PGE$_2$ production by human kidney microsomes	14 μM (n = 4)	0.1-0.4 μM (n = 8)
PGE$_2$ production by rat kidney microsomes	> 30 μM (n = 3)	0.3 ± 0.1 μM (n = 3)
PGE$_2$ production by dog kidney microsomes	> 30 μM (n = 2)	~0.3 μM (n = 2)
PGE$_2$ production by U937 microsomes (low substrate)	2.0 ± 0.5 μM (n = 7)	19.8 ± 0.2 nM (n = 23)
Purified human COX-2	0.34 ± 0.07 μM (n = 2)	0.6 ± 0.1 μM (n = 16)
Purified human COX-1 (low substrate)	26.3 ± 6.4 μM (n = 11)	n.d.
Coagulation-induced TXB$_2$ production in human whole blood (COX-1)	18.8 ± 0.9 μM (n = 211)	0.19 ± 0.02 μM (n = 36)
LPS-induced PGE$_2$ production in human whole blood (COX-2)	0.53 ± 0.02 μM (n = 614)	0.44 ± 0.07 μM (n = 34)

Rofecoxib's *in vivo* activities in animal models in comparison with indomethacin are summarized in Table 5. It is essentially equipotent to indomethacin in most models of pain and inflammation. However, it is significantly less ulcerogenic (see below). A comparison of the *in vitro* potency, in the whole-blood assays performed under the same conditions, of rofecoxib and other COX-2 inhibitors that have progressed beyond the preclinical stage are summarized in Table 6. Rofecoxib exhibited superior COX-2 selectivity as compared with celecoxib[38] and JTE-522[39]. The superior selectivity of rofecoxib over celecoxib in the whole-blood assay has been confirmed independently by others[40]. The latter two compounds, celecoxib and JTE-522, possess a sulphonamido as opposed to the methylsulphonyl moiety that is

Table 5 Comparison of rofecoxib and indomethacin in various *in vivo* assays (ED50, mg kg⁻¹)

	Rofecoxib	*Indomethacin*
Rat paw oedema	1.5	2.0
Rat pyresis	0.2	1.1
Rat paw hyperalgesia	1.0	1.5
Adjuvant arthritis	0.7 (b.i.d.)	0.2

Table 6 Comparison of rofecoxib and other inhibitors in human whole-blood assays (IC$_{50}$, μM)

	Rofecoxib	*Celecoxib*	*JTE-522*	*Meloxicam*	*Diclofenac*
COX-2	0.53	0.87	42% @ 33 μM	0.70	0.05
COX-1	19	6.7	46% @ 100 μM	1.4	0.1
Ratio	36	7.6		2	2

found in rofecoxib. The reason behind the choice of the sulphonamide is presumably to circumvent the oral absorption issue faced by the methylsulphone series, which was solved, in our case, by the selection of the furanone as the template.

Meloxicam and diclofenac are also included in Table 6 as examples of the more selective standard NSAIDs as measured by whole-blood assay. However, both meloxicam and diclofenac inhibit COX-1 at therapeutic doses. On the other hand, it has been shown in humans that the oral administration of 1 g of rofecoxib, approximately 20–80 times the recommended therapeutic doses, did not affect the thromboxane production *ex vivo* in the COX-1 human whole-blood assay[20].

The reduced incidence of the GI effects of rofecoxib, consistent with its reduced COX-1 inhibitory activity, was demonstrated in a number of ways. Using a highly stringent model of GI integrity, i.e. the use of ^{51}Cr-labelled red blood cells to probe the intestinal permeability, rofecoxib did not show any ^{51}Cr leakage at a daily oral dose of 200 mg kg⁻¹ (100 mg kg⁻¹ b.i.d.), for 5 days in either rats or squirrel monkeys. In contrast, a single dose of a non-selective inhibitor such as diclofenac or indomethacin at 10 mg kg⁻¹ caused a significant increase in ^{51}Cr excretion. In a pilot safety study, oral dosing of rofecoxib to rats at 300 mg kg⁻¹ for 14 days did not produce GI lesions, whereas a single dose of indomethacin at 3 mg kg⁻¹ produced clearly visible gastric lesions. The superior GI profile of rofecoxib, in contrast to conventional NSAIDs, has also been confirmed in clinical trials using ^{51}Cr as a marker for GI integrity[27], or using upper GI tract endoscopic findings (perforation, ulcers and bleeds) as an endpoint[41,42].

Given that the ED_{50} of rofecoxib is approximately 1 mg kg^{-1} in a number of animal models, this translates into an unprecedented therapeutic index of > 300. Moreover, the compound exhibits excellent pharmacokinetics and dose proportionality in a number of species, including rats, dogs, mice and squirrel monkeys.

CONCLUSIONS

In summary, a potent, selective and orally active COX-2 inhibitor, rofecoxib, has been discovered. It possesses an *in vivo* therapeutic window of > 300-fold in animal models which is consistent with the *in vitro* data. It also demonstrates that the selective inhibition of COX-2, and not both isoforms, is sufficient for the reduction of pain, inflammation and fever in animal models and humans. It is currently the most selective COX-2 inhibitor on the market. The improved gastric safety profile of rofecoxib over standard NSAIDs should allow for long-term prophylactic use in otherwise healthy individuals with a known genetic susceptibility to certain chronic diseases such as Alzheimer's disease and colon cancer. The compound was proposed as a development candidate in December 1993, approximately 15 months after the programme started. It was first introduced into humans in November 1994 and was approved by the USA's Food and Drug Administration and launched in the USA in May 1999 for the treatment of acute pain in addition to osteoarthritic pain. It is now widely available in many European countries, Canada and Australia.

ACKNOWLEDGEMENTS

We would to thank all the people involved in the COX-2 program throughout Merck, a lot of whom are mentioned in the references.

Address all correspondence to: Petpiboon Prasit, Merck Frosst Centre for Therapeutic Research, PO Box 1005, Pointe Claire-Dorval, Quebec H9R 4P8, Canada.

REFERENCES

1. Galbraith R. DuP 697 as an agent which may be a selective cyclooxygenase inhibitor. *Winter Prostaglandin Conference*, Keystone, CO, USA, January 1992; Abs.
2. Gans K, Galbraith R, Roman R, Haber S, Kerr J, Schmidt W et al. Anti-inflammatory and safety profile of DuP 697, a novel orally effective prostaglandin synthesis inhibitor. *J Pharmacol Exp Ther.* 1990;254;180–7.
3. Futaki N, Hamasaka Y, Takahashi S, Arai I, Higuchi S, Otomo S. Pharmacological studies of NS-398; a newly synthesized NSAID with selective inhibition of prostaglandin synthesis in inflamed tissue, *The 8th International Conference on Prostaglandins and Related Compounds*, July 1992; Abs 389.

4. Futaki N, Yoshikawa K, Hamasaka Y, Arai I, Higuchi S, Iizuka H et al. NS-398, A novel NSAID with potent analgesic and antipyretic effects which cause minimal stomach lesions. *Gen Pharmacol.* 1993;24:105–10.

5. Cromlish WA, Payette P, Culp SA, Ouellet M, Percival MD, Kennedy BP. High level expression of active human cyclooxygenase-2 in insect cells. *Arch Biochem Biophys.* 1994;314:193–9.

6. Weissenbach R. Clinical trial with Nimesulide, a new non-steroid anti-inflammatory agent, in rheumatic pathology. *J Int Med Res.* 1981;9:349–52.

7. Weisenberg-Boettcher I, Schweizer A, Green JR, Seltenmeyer Y, Muler K. The pharmacological profile of CGP28238, a highly potent anti-inflammatory compound. *Agents Actions.* 1989;26:240–2.

8. Nakamura K, Tsuji K, Konishi N, Matsuo M. Studies on antiinflammatory agents. III. Synthesis and pharmacological properties of metabolites of 4′-acetyl-2′-(2,4-difluorophenoxy) methanesulfonanilide (FK3311). *Chem Pharm Bull.* 1993;41:2050–2.

9. Tanaka K, Shimotori T, Makino S, Aikawa Y, Inaba T, Yoshida C et al. Pharmacological studies of the new antiinflammatory agent 3-formylamino-7-methylsulfonylamino-6-phenoxy-4H-1-benzopyran-4-one. First communication: antiinflammatory, analgesic and other related properties. *Arzneimittel-Forschung.* 1992;42:935–44.

10. Wong E, DeLuca C, Boily C, Charleson S, Cromlish W, Denis D et al. Characterization of autocrine inducible prostaglandin H synthase-2 (PGHS-2) in human osteosarcoma cells. *Inflamm Res.* 1997;46:51–59.

11. O'Neill GP, Mancini JA, Kargman S, Yergey J, Kwan MY, Falgueyret JP et al. Overexpression of human prostaglandin G/H synthase-1 and -2 by recombinant vaccinia virus: inhibition by nonsteroidal anti-inflammatory drugs and biosynthesis of 15-hydroxy eicosatetraenoic acid. *Mol Pharmacol.* 1994;45:245–54.

12. Percival MD, Ouellet M, Vincent CJ, Yergey JA, Kennedy BP, O'Neill GP. Purification and characterization of recombinant human cyclooxygenase-2. *Arch Biochem Biophys.* 1994;315:111–8.

13. Cromlish WA, Kennedy BP. Selective inhibition of cyclooxygenase-1 and -2 using intact insect cell assays. *Biochem Pharmacol.* 1996;52:1777–85.

14. Kargman S, Wong E, Greig GM, Falgueyret JP, Cromlish W, Ethier D et al. Mechanism of selective inhibition of human prostaglandin G/H synthase-1 and -2 in intact cells. *Biochem Pharmacol.* 1996;52:1113–25.

15. Riendeau D, Charleson S, Cromlish W, Mancini JA, Wong E, Guay J. Comparison of the cyclooxygenase-1 inhibitory properties of nonsteroidal anti-inflammatory drugs (NSAIDs) and selective COX-2 inhibitors, using sensitive microsomal and platelet assays. *Can J Physiol Pharmacol.* 1997;75:1088–95.

16. Copeland RA, Williams JM, Giannaras J, Nurnberg S, Covington M, Pinto D et al. Mechanism of selective inhibition of the inducible isoform of prostaglandin G/H synthase. *Proc Natl Acad Sci USA* 1994;91:11202–6.

17. Ouellet M, Percival MD. Effect of inhibitor time-dependency on selectivity towards cyclooxygenase isoforms. *Biochem J.* 1995;306:247–51.

18. Chan CC, Boyce S, Brideau C, Charleson S, Cromlish W, Ethier D et al. Rofecoxib [Vioxx, MK-0966; 4-(4′-methylsulfonylphenyl)-3-phenyl-2-(5H)-furanone]: a potent and orally active cyclooxygenase-2 inhibitor. Pharmacological and biochemical profiles. *J Pharmacol Exp Ther.* 1999;290:551–60.

19. Brideau C, Kargman S, Liu S, Dallob AL, Ehrich EW, Rodger IW et al. A human

whole blood assay for clinical evaluation of biochemical efficacy of cyclooxygenase inhibitors. *Inflamm Res.* 1996;45:68–74.

20. Ehrich EW, Dallob A, De Lepeleire I, Van Hecken A, Riendeau D, Yuan W et al. Characterization of rofecoxib as a cyclooxygenase-2 isoform inhibitor and demonstration of analgesia in the dental pain model. *Clin Pharmacol Ther.* 1999;65:336–47.

21. Otterness IG, Bliven ML. Laboratory models for testing NSAIDs. In: Lombardino JG, editor. *NSAIDs.* New York: John Wiley; 1985;111–252.

22. Mukherjee A, Hale VG, Borga O, Stein R. Predictability of the clinical potency of NSAIDs from the preclinical pharmacodynamics in rats. *Inflamm Res.* 1996;45:531–40.

23. Chan CC, Panneton M, Taylor AM, Therien M, Rodger IW. A selective inhibitor of cyclooxygenase-2 reverses endotoxin-induced pyretic responses in non-human primates. *Eur J Pharmacol.* 1997;327:221–5.

24. Chan CC, Boyce S, Brideau C, Ford-Hutchinson AW, Gordon R, Guay D et al. Pharmacology of a selective cyclooxygenase-2 inhibitor, L-745,337: a novel non-steroidal anti-inflammatory agent with an ulcerogenic sparing effect in rat and non-human primate stomach. *J Pharmacol Exp Ther.* 1995;274:1531–7.

25. Leese P. Comparison of the effects of etodolac SR and naproxen on gastro-intestinal blood loss. *Curr Med Res Opin.* 1992;13:13–20.

26. Warrington SJ, Debbas NM, Farthing M, Horton M, Johnston A, Thillainayagam A et al. Lornoxicam, indomethacin and placebo: comparison of effects on faecal blood loss and upper gastrointestinal endoscopic appearances in healthy men. *Postgrad Med J.* 1990;66:622–6.

27. Sigthorsson G, Crane R, Simon T, Hoover M, Quan H, Bolognese J et al. COX-2 inhibition with rofecoxib does not increase intestinal permeability in healthy subjects. A double-blind, crossover study comparing rofecoxib with placebo and indomethacin. *Gut* 2001; in press.

28. Riendeau D, Percival MD, Boyce S, Brideau C, Charleson S, Cromlish W et al. Biochemical and pharmacological profile of a tetrasubstituted furanone as a highly selective COX-2 inhibitor. *Br J Pharmacol.* 1997;121:105–17.

29. Leblanc Y, Gauthier JY, Ethier D, Guay J, Mancini J, Riendeau D et al. Synthesis and biological evaluation of COX-2 and COX-1 inhibitors. *Bioorg Med Chem Letts.* 1995;5:2123–8.

30. Gauthier JY, Leblanc Y, Black WC, Chan CC, Cromlish W, Gordon R et al. Synthesis and biological evaluation of 2,3-diarylthiophenes as selective COX-2 inhibitors. Part II: replacing the heterocycle *Bioorg Med Chem Letts.* 1996;6:87–92.

31. Friesen RW, Dube D, Fortin R, Frenettte R, Prescott S, Cromlish W et al. Novel 1,2-diarylcyclobutenes: selective and orally active COX-2 inhibitors. *Bioorg Med Chem Letts* 1996;6:2677–82.

32. Reitz DB, Huang HC, Li JJ, Garland DJ, Manning RE, Anderson GD et al. Selective cyclooxygenase inhibitors:novel 4-spiro 1,2-diarylcyclopentenes are potent and orally active COX-2 inhibitors *Bioorg Med Chem Letts* 1995;5:867–72.

33. Black C, Brideau C, Chan C.C, Charleson S, Chauret N, Claveau D et al. 2,3-Diarylcyclopentenones as orally active, highly selective COX-2 Inhibitors *J Med Chem.* 1998;42:1274–81.

34. Prasit P, Wang Z, Brideau C, Chan CC, Charleson S, Cromlish W et al. The discovery of rofecoxib [MK 966, Vioxx, 4-(4′-methylsulfonylphenyl)-3-phenyl-2(5H)-furanone], an orally active cyclooxygenase-2-inhibitor. *Bioorg Med Chem Letts.* 1999;9:1773–8.

35. Friesen RW, Brideau C, Chan CC, Charleson S, Deschenes D, Dube D et al. 2-Pyridinyl-3-(4-methylsulfonyl) phenyl-pyridines: selective and orally active cyclooxygenase-2 inhibitors. *Bioorg Med Chem Letts.* 1998;8:2777–82.
36. Prasit P, Riendeau D. Selective cyclooxygenase-2 inhibitors. *Ann Rep Med Chem.* 1997;32:211–20.
37. Wong E, Bayly C, Waterman HL, Riendeau D, Mancini JA. Conversion of prostaglandin G/H synthase-1 into an enzyme sensitive to PGHS-2-selective inhibitors by a double His513–Arg and Ile523–Val mutation. *J Biol Chem.* 1997;272:9280–6.
38. Penning TD, Talley JJ, Bertenshaw, SR, Carter, JS, Collins PW, Docter S et al. Synthesis and biological evaluation of the 1,5-diarylpyrazole class of cyclooxygenase-2 inhibitors: identification of 4-[5-(4-methylphenyl)-3-(trifluoromethyl)-1H-pyrazol-1-yl] benzenesulfonamide (SC-58635, celecoxib). *J Med Chem.* 1997;40:1347–65.
39. Masaki M, Matsushita M, Wakitani K. Inhibitory effects of JTE-522, a novel prostaglandin H synthase-2 inhibitor, on adjuvant-induced arthritis bone changes in rats. *Inflamm Res.* 1998;4:187–92.
40. Warner TD, Giuliano F, Vojnovic I, Bukasa A, Mitchell JA, Vane JR. Nonsteroid drug selectivities for cyclo-oxygenase-1 rather than cyclo-oxygenase-2 are associated with human gastrointestinal toxicity: a full in vitro analysis. *Proc Natl Acad Sci USA.* 1999;96:7563–8.
41. Laine L, Harper S, Simon T, Bath R, Johanson J, Schwartz H et al. A randomized trial comparing the effect of rofecoxib, a cyclooxygenase 2-specific inhibitor, with that of ibuprofen on the gastroduodenal mucosa of patients with osteoarthritis. Rofecoxib Osteoarthritis Endoscopy Study Group. *Gastroenterology.* 1999;117:776–83.
42. Langman MJ, Jensen DM, Watson DJ, Harper SE, Zhao PL, Quan H et al. Adverse upper gastrointestinal effects of rofecoxib compared with NSAIDs. *J Am Med Assoc.* 1999;282:1929–33.

4 | Test systems for inhibitors of cyclooxygenase-1 and cyclooxygenase-2

TIMOTHY D. WARNER,[1] MICHEL PAIRET[2] AND JOANNE VAN RYN[2]

[1]*Department of Cardiac, Vascular and Inflammation Research, The William Harvey Research Institute, St Bartholomew's and the Royal London School of Medicine and Dentistry, Charterhouse Square, London EC1M 6BQ, UK and* [2]*Department of Respiratory Research, Boehringer Ingelheim Research and Development, Birkendorfer Strasse 65, 88397 Biberach a/d Riss, Germany.*

Since the early 1970s it has been established that the non-steroid anti-inflammatory drugs (NSAIDs) owe their therapeutic and side effects to inhibition of cyclooxygenase (COX). Indeed, up until the early 1990s it was believed that both therapeutic and side effects were explained by inhibition of a single COX enzyme – inhibition of COX at inflammatory sites explaining the therapeutic actions of NSAIDs and inhibition of COX in platelets, the kidney and the gastrointestinal (GI) tract explaining the side effects[1-3]. With the discovery of two isoforms of COX, COX-1 being the so-called 'house-keeping' or constitutive isoenzyme found under physiological conditions in most tissues, and COX-2[4,5] being the inducible isoform found particularly during inflammatory processes, this old hypothesis has been refined[1-3]. It is now widely believed that inhibition of COX-1 accounts for the side effects, whilst inhibition of COX-2 accounts for the therapeutic benefits of NSAIDs[1-3,6].

The discovery of two COX isoforms was a major stimulant to research efforts – clearly, selective inhibitors of COX-2 had the potential to retain the anti-inflammatory effects of the NSAIDs while having much reduced side effects. To aid in the development of such compounds, numerous *in vitro* assays have been developed to allow comparisons to be made of the relative activities of NSAIDs as inhibitors of COX-1 and COX-2[7]. Researchers have often taken the direct approach of using these assays to construct inhibitor curves for test compounds against the activities of COX-1 or COX-2 within their experimental systems. These inhibitor curves have then been used to calculate IC_{50} values (the concentration of drug required to inhibit the production of prostanoids by 50%) for both COX-1 and COX-2. From these IC_{50} values IC_{50} ratios are derived, i.e. the ratio between the concentration of drug required to inhibit COX-1 and that required to inhibit COX-2 – it is the IC_{50} ratio that has been widely used as a descriptor of the COX-2 selectivity of a drug. Generally IC_{50} ratios are used in such a way that low numbers are associated with selectivity towards COX-2 and high numbers with selectivity towards COX-1. However, as discussed below, we must go beyond this simple approach if we are to make intelligent use of data generated by these *in vitro* assays.

This review will consider the strengths and weaknesses of the various assays and, drawing upon experience from clinical use, assess the predictive values of *in vitro* tests.

IN VITRO ASSAYS

Many *in vitro* assay systems have been developed to investigate the COX-2 selectivity of NSAIDs. These have been reviewed in detail elsewhere[7] but in broad terms these test systems can be classified into three groups: assays using animal enzymes, cells, or cell lines, which were the first to be developed[6,8–12]; assays using human recombinant enzymes, cell lines, or blood cells (mainly platelets and monocytes), which are the current standards[12–28]; and newly developed models using those human cells that are targets for the anti-inflammatory and adverse effects of NSAIDs[29–34]. These targets include human gastric mucosa cells, chondrocytes and synoviocytes.

Apart from variations in the sources of the COX enzymes there are wide variations in the experimental conditions in these various assays. For example, arachidonic acid can come from both endogenous (often in cell-based assays) and exogenous sources (in isolated enzyme or broken-cell assays). It is important to remember that the potencies of some NSAIDs, particularly those that act as competitive substrate inhibitors[35], are influenced by the supply of arachidonic acid. Also, expression systems and cell transfection targets vary considerably, including even non-mammalian cells such as those from insects. Other experimenters have used cells that express the COX enzymes constitutively, following stable transfection with the recombinant enzymes, to avoid the problems associated with variability in the types and concentrations of inducing agents used. As well as substrate, the time of incubation of the test drug with the COX enzyme systems can have a strong influence on the apparent potencies of drugs. In particular, a number of NSAIDs and newer COX-2 selective agents inhibit COX-2 in a time-dependent manner[35,36].

Another important factor is the protein concentration present in the medium. This is a critical issue for NSAIDs, which bind avidly to plasma proteins such that within the circulation, for instance, the level of free drug is usually only a few per cent of the total concentration in the blood.

The advantages and drawbacks of each individual test system have been analysed elsewhere[7] and will not be discussed in detail in this review. However, from what is now known, it is clear: that an ideal assay should use native human enzymes that are present in whole cells; that the cells used should be target cells for the anti-inflammatory and adverse effects of NSAIDs; that COX-2 should be induced, thereby simulating an inflammatory process, rather than being constitutively expressed; that prostaglandin (PG) synthesis should be measured from arachidonic acid released from endogenous stores rather than from exogenously added arachidonic acid; and that the protein concentration in the medium should also closely mimic plasma protein concentration. The above relates, of course, to assays in which we are attempting to predict the clinical effects of novel NSAIDs. However, clearly, if one wishes to investigate, for instance, interactions between NSAIDs and the active site of COX then isolated enzyme studies would be of much more use.

EXPLOITING DATA FROM *IN VITRO* ASSAYS

The IC_{50} values of COX-1 and COX-2 inhibition obtained in *in vitro* assays are often used to calculate selectivity ratios. Unfortunately, it has often been difficult to relate data derived by different assays. Even on the simplest level, comparisons of data from different assays have shown wide variations in inhibitor ratios, even for individual compounds. The reasons for these variations have been discussed in detail elsewhere[7] but, as outlined above, include wide variations in protein concentrations in assay media, variations in incubation times and variations in substrate supply. Indeed, even variations in species have been reported to be associated with marked differences in the potencies of compounds in *in vitro* assays[37]. Secondly, calculating selectivity ratios by dividing the IC_{50} value for COX-2 by the IC_{50} value for COX-1 (the lower the ratio, the greater the COX-2 selectivity; the higher the ratio, the greater the COX-1 selectivity) is a very simplistic approach. It relies upon concentration curves being parallel, and takes little account of the plasma concentrations of drugs achieved following therapeutic dosing. Furthermore, if two drugs have similar selectivity ratios but very different slopes to their inhibitor curves the conclusions we can draw must be very different. In simple terms, steep curves allow a better dissociation between COX-1 and COX-2 inhibition than flat curves[7]. So, even though COX-2 selectivity can be expressed by selectivity ratios derived from *in vitro* assays we must be very cautious before extrapolating to clinical conditions.

HUMAN WHOLE-BLOOD ASSAY

For many of the reasons discussed above, the human whole-blood assay (hWBA) appears to offer many advantages over other *in vitro* tests. In this assay, COX-1 activity is assessed by the release of prostanoids from platelets following stimulation of human whole-blood clotting, while COX-2 activity is assessed by the release of prostanoids from white blood cells (principally monocytes) over about 18 h following incubation of the whole blood with bacterial lipopolysaccharide (Figure 1). The hWBA has many advantages: intact human cells are used, which are target cells for the anti-inflammatory effects (monocytes) and side effects (platelets) of NSAIDs; plasma proteins are present; the whole blood used for both assays is taken from the same volunteer (or patient) at the same time, allowing a direct comparison of the results from each assay; the assay can be performed using blood from volunteers (or patients) who have been treated previously with NSAIDs (*ex vivo* assay).

The main drawback of the hWBA is that since COX-2 has to be induced, different incubation times are used for COX-1 and COX-2. In addition, cell types other than platelets and monocytes, such as gastric mucosal cells and synoviocytes, would of course be more representative of target cells for the therapeutic or adverse effects of NSAIDs. Despite these reservations, results obtained by different laboratories using the hWBA have demonstrated similar rank orders for COX-2 selectivity[7]. Standard NSAIDs range from being

Figure 1 Confocal microscopy showing expression of COX-2 (green coloration) in human white blood cells induced by incubation with bacterial lipopolysaccharide (LPS) (10 µg ml^{-1}) for 18 h.

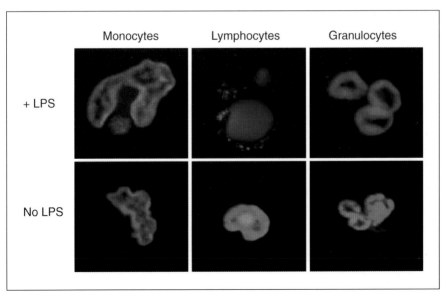

COX-1-selective to being approximately equally effective on both isoenzymes with diclofenac having the most favourable profile. Compounds such as etodolac, nimesulide, and meloxicam followed by celecoxib, flosulide, DuP 697, NS-398, rofecoxib, L-745,337, SC-58125 and DFP show increasing selectivity for COX-2. Unfortunately, the hWBA does not work so well for highly COX-2 selective compounds, such as DFP – taking into account the level of plasma binding of the drugs there is often insufficient free drug to permit any inhibition of COX-1 to be detected. For the further characterization of such compounds, assays of COX-1 activity in the presence of very low levels of arachidonic acid substrate have been developed[38,39]. Clearly, although these assays are useful in producing numbers relating to COX-1 inhibition, the hWBA may still better reflect the fact that these compounds are almost without effect on COX-1 in normal physiological systems.

A further development of the hWBA has been to mix A549 human cells, already induced to express COX-2, with aliquots of human whole blood (human modified whole-blood assay, hmWBA)[28]. In this way the COX-1 and COX-2 assays can be conducted over identical time courses (Figure 2). As for the standard hWBA, the hmWBA has been used to generate ratios for the COX-1/COX-2 selectivities of a wide range of NSAIDs and newer COX-2 selective agents. As discussed above, the comparison of the activities of NSAIDs at the IC_{50} level is not easily justified. NSAIDs are used therapeutically at doses that produce more than a 50% reduction in prostanoid formation. Indeed, a survey of the literature[28] established that for diclofenac[40], etodolac[41], indomethacin[42,43], fenoprofen[42], flurbiprofen[44], ketoprofen[42], ketorolac[43,45], meclofenamate[42], meloxicam[46], naproxen[47], nimesulide[48],

Figure 2 Schematic diagram of the human modified whole-blood assay (hmWBA) relying upon COX-1 contained within the platelets and COX-2 contained within A549 cells preinduced by incubation with interleukin-1β for 24 h.

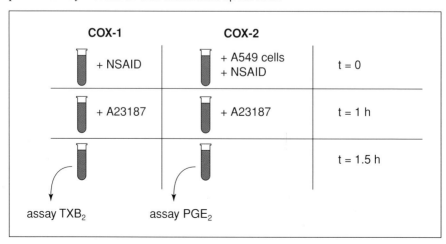

piroxicam[49], sulindac[50] and tolmetin[42] the steady-state plasma concentrations of these drugs, as well as the peak concentrations of aspirin[42], would produce $89 \pm 2\%$ inhibition of COX-2 (n = 15). Comparison of the potencies of the NSAIDs against COX-1 and COX-2 at the IC_{80} value, therefore, appears more appropriate. Further comparisons of the relative activities of all these NSAIDs as inhibitors of human COX-1 versus COX-2 to their likelihood of inducing GI toxicity[51,52] supports the idea that it is inhibition of COX-1 rather than inhibition of COX-2 that underlies the gastrotoxic effects of the NSAIDs (Figure 3)[2]. A further analysis of the data generated by the hmWBA shows an interesting comparison (Figure 4). This displays the extent of COX-1 inhibition produced by individual NSAIDs at concentrations that cause 80% inhibition of COX-2. This analysis essentially provides the answer to the important question: *if an NSAID is used at levels sufficient to inhibit COX-2 by 80%, i.e. to produce some therapeutic effect, by how much will COX-1 be inhibited?* As can be seen, the classical NSAIDs produce inhibitions of around 80% or more. This implies that even for a drug such as diclofenac, which is more than fourfold selective for COX-2 in terms of IC_{80} values, therapeutically relevant selectivity will be very difficult to achieve, i.e. the concentration of

Figure 3 Relationship for NSAIDs between relative activities against COX-1 versus COX-2 (IC_{80} ratios[28]) and risk of producing gastrointestinal toxicity[52].

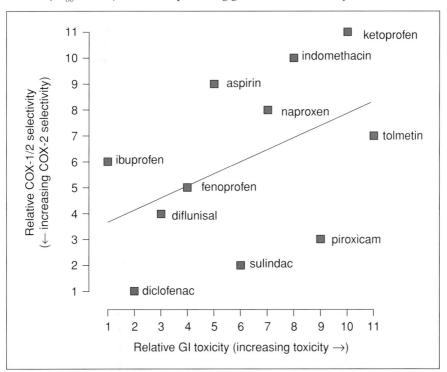

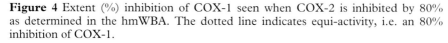

Figure 4 Extent (%) inhibition of COX-1 seen when COX-2 is inhibited by 80% as determined in the hmWBA. The dotted line indicates equi-activity, i.e. an 80% inhibition of COX-1.

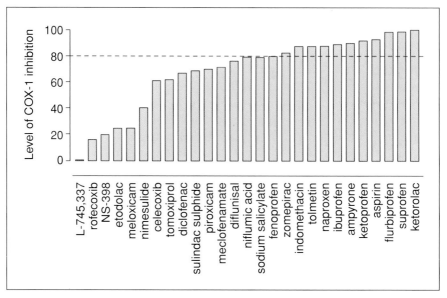

diclofenac necessary to produce 80% inhibition of COX-2 will produce almost 70% inhibition of COX-1. To extend this line of reasoning it is also clear that when relative selectivities differ by only slight amounts, other variables, such as ingested dose and plasma half-life, will have a particular influence on NSAID toxicity. This may well be especially true for piroxicam, which in the hmWBA was not found to be notably COX-1-selective despite its well-established GI toxicity. Piroxicam, however, has a much longer elimination half-life (30 – 70 h)[49] than other NSAIDs and plasma half-life has been previously correlated with GI toxicity[53].

OTHER ASSAYS

Alternative and newer *in vitro* assays are always being developed. On the face of it, test systems that appear the most interesting are those using human cells such as gastric mucosa cells, chondrocytes or synoviocytes that are target cells for the anti-inflammatory or adverse effects of NSAIDs. These generate similar data to those seen with human recombinant enzymes and the hWBA[30–32,34,54] and it can be shown that the data from such assays correlate with the idea that increased COX-2 selectivity is associated with reduced GI toxicity[33], although these assays still have the problem that they do not mimic well the drug binding to proteins seen *in vivo*. One must therefore be careful when trying to draw conclusions about the effects on tissue PG formation by comparing potencies against tissue and whole-blood prostanoid formation[55]. Potentially in the future, as we gain more understanding of the processes underlying the interactions between inhibitors and the COX enzymes, molecular modelling may be used to bypass some of the routine work of *in vitro* selectivity assays[36].

IN VIVO RELEVANCE OF *IN VITRO* RESULTS

Clearly the purpose of *in vitro* tests is to predict the usefulness of NSAIDs *in vivo*. In particular, following the idea that inhibition of COX-2 explains efficacy and inhibition of COX-1 explains side effects, will a drug be efficacious without causing side effects? Unfortunately, however, the effective concentrations found in many *in vitro* assays can often not be compared with therapeutic concentrations since drug binding to proteins cannot be accurately taken into account. So for most assays one cannot go beyond selectivity ratios. The exception is clearly the human whole-blood assay, since the presence of plasma allows a better representation of *in vivo* interactions. From these assays we can map blood therapeutic concentrations derived by pharmacokinetic studies (assuming drug concentrations in red cells are negligible and the haematocrit is 45%) and compare them with the concentrations of drug required to inhibit COX-1 and COX-2 in *in vitro* assays. Such composite figures have been derived from the hmWBA, examples being those for diclofenac (Figure 5), meloxicam (Figure 6) and rofecoxib (Figure 7). These models are interesting because, as mentioned above, they show that the blood concentrations of drug following therapeutic dosing fit the idea that approximately 80% inhibition of COX-2 is associated with efficacy. Thus, the three drugs shown (diclofenac, meloxicam and rofecoxib) are established to be efficacious at standard doses and are demonstrated here to produce similar inhibition of COX-2. However the level of COX-1 inhibition varies greatly (from approximately 70% to approximately 10%). Once again, this supports the idea that it is inhibition of COX-2 that underlies the efficacious actions of COX inhibitors. Clearly, if inhibition of COX-1 was required for drugs to be efficacious, diclofenac would be considerably more efficacious than either meloxicam or rofecoxib. These simulations also underline the fact that administration of compounds with lower relative selectivities for COX-2, such as etodolac, nimesulide and meloxicam at high doses (i.e. supratherapeutic), will result in moderate increases in COX-2 inhibition but notably larger increases in COX-1 inhibition.

It should be stressed that a drawback of such simulations is that drug concentrations in the joints are not taken into account. Even though one can produce models to compare simulated COX-1 inhibition in blood with simulated COX-2 inhibition in synovial fluid[56] these will never replace, nor be as good as, experimental data obtained in human pharmacological

Figure 5 Inhibition by diclofenac of COX-1 (●) and COX-2 (○) determined in hmWBA[28]. Greyed bar indicates concentrations achieved *in vivo* following ingestion of therapeutic doses.

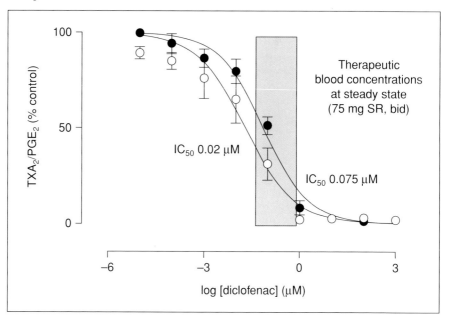

Figure 6 Inhibition by meloxicam of COX-1 (●) and COX-2 (○) determined in hmWBA[28]. Greyed bar indicates concentrations achieved *in vivo* following ingestion of therapeutic doses.

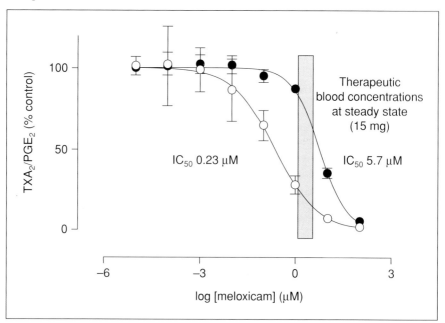

Figure 7 Inhibition by rofecoxib of COX-1 (●) and COX-2 (○) determined in hmWBA[28]. Greyed bar indicates concentrations achieved *in vivo* following ingestion of therapeutic doses.

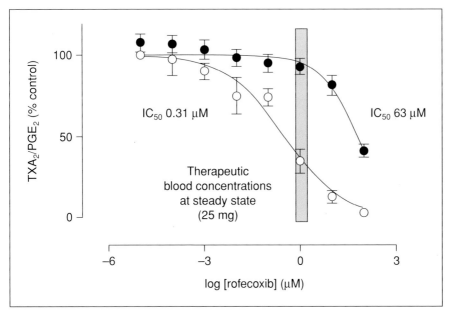

HUMAN PHARMACOLOGY STUDIES

studies, which investigate the differential inhibition of prostanoid synthesis in target tissues.

The most relevant markers of COX-1 and COX-2 activity *in vivo* would be PGE_2 or PGI_2 production by the gastric mucosa, and PGE_2 production by sites of inflammation, most notably the inflamed synovium. Indeed, similar models have been developed for use in experimental animals. However, for practical reasons, such studies are more difficult to perform in humans, since target tissues are not easily obtained. Furthermore, PG production can be stimulated when tissues are harvested. Despite these reservations there are a number of studies that appear promising[57–61]. Generally the differential inhibition of COX-1 and COX-2 by NSAIDs is studied in humans by *in vivo* pharmacological studies. The effects of repeated administration of anti-inflammatory doses on COX-2 activity measured in a whole-blood assay *ex vivo*, or on markers of COX-1 activity such as platelet aggregation, plasma thromboxane B_2 (TXB_2) concentrations or urinary excretion of PGE_2, are usually investigated. Of these, serum TXB_2 appears to be the most sensitive measure of COX-1 inhibition by a drug because platelet aggregation does not appear affected until plasma TXB_2 is reduced by more than 95%[62]. Studies performed with several non-selective 'standard' NSAIDs showed a close relationship between plasma drug concentrations and inhibition of serum TXB_2[63-67] (most likely to be COX-1 inhibition) and inhibition of synovial PGE_2 (most likely to be COX-2 inhibition)[57,61]. Similar results have been found with studies looking at COX-2 selective inhibitors. For example, using an *ex vivo* whole-blood assay, nimesulide, in a dose of 100 mg twice daily, exhibited either a 50% inhibition[24] or no inhibition[68] of platelet TXB_2 synthesis. Such a wide discrepancy may be explained by the steep plasma concentration curves and relatively high peak plasma levels of the compound, i.e. concentrations that inhibit COX-1 to a significant extent may be temporarily reached at peak levels but not at other times. Indeed, 200 mg of nimesulide b.i.d. has been found to reduce urinary excretion of PGE_2 markedly, suggesting that, at this dose, the COX-1 sparing effect had vanished[69]. Single oral dosing with 100 mg nimesulide resulted in 50% and 90% inhibitions of COX-1 and COX-2, as assessed *ex vivo* up to 6 h[70]. Even at 24 h COX-2 activity was still inhibited by 49% although COX-1 was un- affected. Interestingly, these results show that despite nimesulide having in the same studies a 20-fold selectivity *in vitro*, therapeutic plasma levels of nimesulide following oral dosing are still sufficient to produce detectable inhibition of COX-1. Indeed, this idea is supported by the analysis shown in Figure 4 – even with selectivity of greater than tenfold, substantial inhibition of COX-2 can be associated with significant inhibition of COX-1. In similar studies, indomethacin 25 mg day^{-1} markedly reduced platelet aggregation, serum TXB_2 levels and urinary excretion of PGE_2, while these parameters were unaffected by both 7.5 and 15 mg meloxicam at steady state[71,72]. Conversely, despite meloxicam demonstrating tenfold selectivity *in vitro*, it has been noted that dosing with meloxicam 7.5 and 15 mg day^{-1} for 7 days resulted in 51% and 70% reductions in *ex vivo* COX-2 activity and 25% and 35% reductions in *ex vivo* COX-1 activity (whole-blood assay)[73]. From this it has been concluded that the biochemical selectivity of meloxicam *in vitro* was inadequate to separate clearly the effects of meloxicam on COX-1 and COX-2 after oral dosing due to inter-individual variations in steady-state plasma levels. Despite the conclusion of these researchers it is still clear from the whole-blood inhibitor curves (Figure 6) that if supratherapeutic dosing is avoided, meloxicam retains its COX-2 selectivity. For example, as the meloxi- cam dose was increased from 7.5 to 15 mg day^{-1}, COX-2 inhibition increased by 20%, while COX-1 inhibition increased by 10%. There are no human pharmacology studies investigating the effect of etodolac on serum TXB_2, platelet aggregation or urinary PGE_2. However, in patients with rheumatoid arthritis, 4 weeks of dosing with etodolac (300 mg b.i.d.) produced fewer gastric erosions, as assessed by endoscopy, than naproxen (500 mg b.i.d.). At the same time naproxen but not etodolac produced significant reductions in the production of PGE_2 and PGI_2 by the gastric mucosa. There was, however, no correlation between PGE_2/PGI_2 levels and GI damage in the individual patients[74]. However, clinical pharmacology studies comparing the effects over 7 days of aspirin 2600 mg day^{-1} and etodolac up to 1200 mg day^{-1} showed that while aspirin increased faecal blood loss – an index of GI microbleeding – etodolac produced no increased blood loss[75].

Celecoxib did not inhibit collagen-, ADP- or arachidonate-induced platelet aggregation, and also had no effect on TXB_2 levels, 2 and 4 h after the last administration of 600 mg twice daily for 6 days[76]. Similarly, more recent studies looking at the effects of 100, 200 and 800 mg – and even up to 1200 mg – celecoxib, in comparison with 800 mg ibuprofen or 1000 mg naproxen, have shown that the traditional NSAIDs, but not celecoxib, inhibited *ex vivo* platelet aggregation induced by agonists such as collagen. Also, while naproxen but not celecoxib depressed circulating TXA_2 levels, both ibuprofen and celecoxib inhibited lipopolysaccharide-induced COX-2 expression *ex vivo*[77]. Interestingly, however, the plasma TXB_2 concentration, a more sensitive measure of COX-1 inhibition than platelet aggregation (see above), was significantly reduced by approximately 30% after a single administration of the supratherapeutic dose of 800 mg celecoxib[78]. In the same studies, both ibuprofen and celecoxib were found to inhibit urinary excretion of the PGI_2 metabolite 2,3-dinor-6-keto-$PGF_{1\alpha}$[78]. This may indicate that COX-2 is responsible for the formation of PGI_2 in the circulation. Indeed, further studies with rofecoxib have shown that like its comparator indomethacin, this COX-2-selective inhibitor also reduces the urinary excretion of the PGI_2 metabolite 2,3-dinor-6-keto-$PGF_{1\alpha}$[79]. At the same time even supratherapeutic doses of rofecoxib of up to 375 mg for 14 days produce no inhibition of COX-1 activity *ex vivo*, as assessed by TXB_2 generation in clotting blood, whereas there is profound inhibition of *ex vivo* COX-2 activity[80]. In shorter term studies doses of rofecoxib even as high as 1 g day^{-1} have similarly been found to be without effect on platelet TXB_2 production[81]. It may well be that such high doses of rofecoxib are not absorbed and are simply excreted. Effective concentrations may therefore not be as high as assumed.

Interestingly, although there has been much focus on the potential effects of COX-2-selective agents as anti-inflammatory drugs with reduced GI side effects, less attention has been paid to the ability of these new agents to promote renal toxicity. Clinical pharmacology has, however, provided some indications. In one study comparing celecoxib with naproxen in salt-depleted subjects it was noted that celecoxib caused increases in sodium and potassium retention, as did naproxen, suggesting that an increased selectivity for COX-2 does not spare the kidney[82]. It is not entirely clear presently whether or not glomerular filtration rate is also affected by COX-2-selective agents in a similar fashion to non-selective inhibitors. One study over 10 days has reported that celecoxib (up to 400 mg b.i.d.) produced less effect on glomerular filtration rate than naproxen (500 mg b.i.d.)[83], whereas another has reported that rofecoxib (25 mg day^{-1}) and indomethacin (50 mg t.i.d.) produced similar small reductions in glomerular filtration rate[84]. With drugs such as etodolac and meloxicam there is further clinical data. Thus, tests in small groups of patients have shown that etodolac produces transient effects on renal function, notably reductions in urinary sodium and chloride excretion and falls in urinary 6-keto-$PGF_{1\alpha}$[85]. However, studies in larger groups of patients, including those with mild to moderate renal impairment, have not shown etodolac to exacerbate renal insufficiencies[86]. Similar observations of renal tolerance have been made with meloxicam in renally impaired patients[87]. Taken together, however, we must probably conclude currently that COX-2 selective agents may affect renal function and renal PG formation and that similar caution should be exercised with these as with traditional NSAIDs[88].

CONCLUSIONS

Many *in vitro* assays have been developed to estimate the COX-1 and COX-2 selectivity of NSAIDs. Although there are notable variations, there are some consistent traits[1–3,7]. Clearly many of the older NSAIDs most closely associated with the production of side effects, such as GI disturbances, demonstrate selectivity towards COX-1, while newer compounds such as meloxicam, etodolac, nimesulide, celecoxib and rofecoxib demonstrate varying degrees of selectivity towards COX-2 and have been readily demonstrated to produce less GI disturbances and side effects.

Despite these broad conclusions one must be careful when drawing clinical conclusions from these *in vitro* systems. It is important to remember that the level of inhibition of COX-1 and COX-2 *in vivo*, at a given dose, cannot be predicted from *in vitro* data alone. The pharmacokinetic properties of each compound, including plasma levels, distribution and binding to plasma proteins, have to be taken into account. Despite these reservations it is becoming clear that compounds shown to be selective towards the inhibition of COX-2 demonstrate efficacy with less of the typical NSAID-induced side effects. As more experience is obtained with these drugs it will become clear whether or not these compounds will deliver on their promise of efficacy with safety. On a positive note, it has been recently observed from a meta-analysis of randomized controlled trials that meloxicam produces fewer adverse GI events than standard, non-selective NSAIDs[89]. Furthermore, in a prospective observational study, it was found that despite meloxicam being prescribed preferentially to patients with histories suggesting a higher risk of developing NSAID-induced GI toxicity, these patients still had lower rates of reported GI adverse drug reactions than those receiving standard NSAIDs[90]. The very latest reports of controlled trials with both celecoxib and rofecoxib also show that at therapeutic doses both of these drugs produce fewer severe GI side effects than standard comparators[91,92]. From this it would appear that the safety associated with COX-2 selectivity (i.e. as established in *in vitro* tests) seen in individual controlled trials is maintained both through meta-analysis and when drugs are used under normal prescribing conditions. This gives much hope for the future benefits of COX-2-selective drugs.

Address all correspondence to: Timothy D. Warner, Department of Cardiac, Vascular and Inflammation Research, The William Harvey Research Institute, St. Bartholomew's and the Royal London School of Medicine and Dentistry, Charterhouse Square, London EC1M 6BQ, UK. t.d.warner@mds.qmw.ac.uk

REFERENCES

1. Vane JR, Bakhle YS, Botting RM. Cyclo-oxygenase-1 and -2. *Annu Rev Pharmacol.* 1998;38:97–120.
2. Mitchell JA, Warner TD. Cyclo-oxygenase-2: pharmacology, physiology, biochemistry and relevance to NSAID therapy. *Br J Pharmacol.* 1999;128:1121–32.
3. Pairet M, Engelhardt G. Distinct isoforms (COX-1 and COX-2) of cyclooxygenase: possible physiological and therapeutic implications. *Fundam Clin Pharmacol.* 1996;10:1–15.
4. Fu JY, Masferrer JL, Seibert K, Raz A, Needleman P. The induction and suppression of prostaglandin H_2 synthase (cyclooxygenase) in human monocytes. *J Biol Chem.* 1990;265:16737–40.
5. Xie W, Chipman JG, Robertson DL, Erikson RL, Simmons DL. Expression of a mitogen-responsive gene encoding prostaglandin synthase is regulated by mRNA splicing. *Proc Natl Acad Sci USA.* 1991;88:1692–6.
6. Mitchell JA, Akarasereenont P, Thiemermann C, Flower RJ, Vane JR. Selectivity of nonsteroidal antiinflammatory drugs as inhibitors of constitutive and inducible cyclooxygenase. *Proc Natl Acad Sci USA.* 1993;90:11693–7.
7. Pairet M, Van Ryn J. Experimental models used to investigate the differential inhibition of cyclooxygenase-1 and cyclooxygenase-2 by non-steroidal anti-inflammatory drugs. *Inflamm Res.* 1998;47(Suppl 2):S93–101.
8. Futaki N, Takahashi S, Yokoyama M, Arai I, Higuchi S, Otomo S. NS-398, a new anti-inflammatory agent, selectively inhibits prostaglandin G/H synthase/cyclooxygenase (COX-2) activity *in vitro*. *Prostaglandins.* 1994;47:55–9.
9. Klein T, Nüsing RM, Pfeilschifter J, Ullrich V. Selective inhibition of cyclooxygenase 2. *Biochem Pharmacol.* 1994;48:1605–10.
10. Engelhardt G, Bogel R, Schnitzler C, Utzmann R. Meloxicam: influence on arachidonic acid metabolism: part 1. *In vitro* findings. *Biochem Pharmacol.* 1996;51:21–8.
11. Meade EA, Smith WL, DeWitt DL. Differential inhibition of prostaglandin endoperoxide synthase (cyclooxygenase) isozymes by aspirin and other non-steroidal anti-inflammatory drugs. *J Biol Chem.* 1993;268:6610–4.
12. Prasit P, Black WC, Chan CC, Ford-Hutchinson AW, Gauthier JY, Gordon R et al. L-745,337: a selective cyclooxygenase-2 inhibitor. *Med Chem Res.* 1995;5:364–74.
13. Barnett J, Chow J, Ives D, Chiou M, Mackenzie R, Osen E et al. Purification,

characterization and selective inhibition of human prostaglandin G/H synthase 1 and 2 expressed in the baculovirus system. *Biochim Biophys Acta.* 1994;1209:130–9.

14. Copeland RA, Williams JM, Giannaras J, Nurnberg S, Covington M, Pinto D et al. Mechanism of selective inhibition of the inducible form of prostaglandin G/H synthase. *Proc Natl Acad Sci USA.* 1994;91:11202–6.

15. Laneuville O, Breuer DK, Dewitt DL, Hla T, Funk CD, Smith WD. Differential inhibition of human prostaglandin endoperoxide H synthases-1 and -2 by non-steroidal anti-inflammatory drugs. *J Pharmacol Exp Ther.* 1994;271:927–34.

16. O'Neill GP, Mancini JA, Kargman S, Yergey J, Kwan MY, Falgueyret JP et al. Overexpression of human prostaglandin G/H synthase-1 and -2 by recombinant vaccinia virus: inhibition by nonsteroidal anti-inflammatory drugs and biosynthesis of 15-hydroxyeicosatetraenoic acid. *Mol Pharmacol.* 1994;45:245–54.

17. Glaser K, Sung ML, O'Neill K, Belfast M, Hartman D, Carlson R et al. Etodolac selectively inhibits human prostaglandin G/H synthase 2 (PGHS-2) versus human PGHS-1. *Eur J Pharmacol.* 1995;281:107–11.

18. Gierse JK, Hauser SD, Creely DP, Koboldt C, Rangwala SH, Isakson PC et al. Expression and selective inhibition of the constitutive and inducible forms of human cyclo-oxygenase. *Biochem J.* 1995;305:479–84.

19. Churchill L, Graham AG, Shih CK, Pauletti D, Farina PR, Grob PM. Selective inhibition of human cyclo-oxygenase-2 by meloxicam. *Inflammopharmacology.* 1996;4:125–35.

20. Cromlish WA, Kennedy BP. Selective inhibition of cyclooxygenase-1 and -2 using intact insect cell assays. *Biochem Pharmacol.* 1996;52:1777–85.

21. Kargman S, Wong E, Greig GM, Falgueyret JP, Cromlish W, Ethier D et al. Mechanism of selective inhibition of human prostaglandin G/H synthase-1 and -2 in intact cells. *Biochem Pharmacol.* 1996;52:1113–25.

22. Riendeau D, Percival MD, Boyce S, Brideau C, Charleson S, Cromlish W et al. Biochemical and pharmacological profile of a tetrasubstituted furanone as a highly selective COX-2 inhibitor. *Br J Pharmacol.* 1997;121:105–17.

23. Patrignani P, Panara MR, Greco A, Fusco O, Natoli C, Iacobelli S et al. Biochemical and pharmacological characterization of the cyclooxygenase activity of human blood prostaglandin endoperoxide synthases. *J Pharmacol Exp Ther.* 1994;271:1705–10.

24. Patrignani P, Panara MR, Santini G, Sciulli MG, Padovano R, Cipollone F et al. Differential inhibition of cyclooxygenase activity of prostaglandin endoperoxide synthase isozymes *in vitro* and *ex vivo* in man. *Prostagland Leukot Essent Fatty Acids.* 1996;55(Suppl I):PI 15.

25. Young JM, Panah S, Satchawatcharaphong C, Cheung PS. Human whole blood assays for inhibition of prostaglandin G/H synthases-1 and -2 using A23187 and lipopolysaccharide stimulation of thromboxane B_2 production. *Inflamm Res.* 1996;45:24653.

26. Brideau C, Kargman S, Liu S, Daflob AL, Ehrich EW, Rodger IW et al. A human whole blood assay for clinical evaluation of biochemical efficacy of cyclooxygenase inhibitors. *Inflamm Res.* 1996;45:68–74.

27. Prasit P. New highly selective COX-2 inhibitors. In: *Proceedings of the William Harvey Research Conference: Selective COX-2 Inhibitors.* Phuket, Sept. 17–19, 1997.

28. Warner TD, Giuliano F, Vojnovic I, Bukasa A, Mitchell JA, Vane JR. Nonsteroid drug selectivities for cyclo-oxygenase-1 rather than cyclo-oxygenase-2 are associated with human gastrointestinal toxicity: a full *in vitro* analysis. *Proc Natl Acad Sci USA.* 1999;96:7563–8.

29. Tavares IA, Bishai PM, Bennett A. Activity of nimesulide on constitutive and inducible cyclooxygenases. *Arzneimittel-Forschung/Drug Res.* 1995;45:1093–5.
30. Blanco F, Guitian R, Moreno 1, Hernandez A, Freire M, Atanes A et al. NSAIDs effects on COX-1 and COX-2 activity in human articular chondrocytes [abstract]. *Arthritis Rheum.* 1997;40 (Suppl 9):347.
31. Vergne P, Bertin P, Liagre B, Bonnet C, Pairet M, Rigaud M et al. Differential inhibition of COX- 1 and COX-2 by nonsteroidal anti-inflammatory drugs in cultured synovial cells [abstract]. *Arthritis Rheum.* 1997;40(Suppl 9):375.
32. Kawai S, Nishida S, Kato M, Furumaya Y, Okamoto R, Koshino T et al. Comparison of cyclooxygenase-1 and -2 inhibitory activities of various nonsteroidal anti-inflammatory drugs using human platelets and synovial cells. *Eur J Pharmacol.* 1998;347:87–94.
33. Kawai S. Cyclooxygenase selectivity and the risk of gastro-intestinal complications of various non-steroidal anti-inflammatory drugs: a clinical consideration. *Inflamm Res.* 1998;47(Suppl 2):S102–6.
34. Tavares IA. The effects of meloxicam, indomethacin or NS-398 on eicosanoid synthesis by fresh human gastric mucosa. *Aliment Pharmacol Ther.* 2000;14:795–9.
35. Gierse JK, Koboldt CM, Walker MC, Seibert K, Isakson PC. Kinetic basis for selective inhibition of cyclo-oxygenases. *Biochem J.* 1999;339:607–14.
36. Lanzo CA, Sutin J, Rowlinson S, Talley J, Marnett LJ. Fluorescence quenching analysis of the association and dissociation of a diarylheterocycle to cyclooxygenase-1 and cyclooxygenase-2: dynamic basis of cyclooxygenase-2 selectivity. *Biochemistry.* 2000;39:6228–34.
37. Berg J, Fellier H, Christoph T, Kremminger P, Hartmann M, Blaschke H et al. Pharmacology of a selective cyclooxygenase-2 inhibitor, HN-56249: a novel compound exhibiting a marked preference for the human enzyme in intact cells. *Naunyn-Schmiederbergs Arch Pharmacol.* 2000;361:363–72.
38. Riendeau D, Charleson S, Cromlish W, Mancini JA, Wong E, Guay J. Comparison of the cyclooxygenase-1 inhibitory properties of nonsteroidal anti-inflammatory drugs (NSAIDs) and selective COX-2 inhibitors, using sensitive microsomal and platelet assays. *Can J Physiol Pharmacol.* 1997;75:1088–95.
39. Chan CC, Boyce S, Brideau C, Charleson S, Cromlish W, Ethier D et al. Rofecoxib [Vioxx, MK-0966; 4-(4′-methylsulfonylphenyl)-3-phenyl-2-(5H)-furanone]: a potent and orally active cyclooxygenase-2 inhibitor. Pharmacological and biochemical profiles. *J Pharmacol Exp Ther.* 1999;290:551–60.
40. Davies NM, Anderson KE. Clinical pharmacokinetics of diclofenac. Therapeutic insights and pitfalls. *Clin Pharmacokinet.* 1997;33:184–213.
41. Brocks DR, Jamali F. Etodolac clinical pharmacokinetics. *Clin Pharmacokinet.* 1994;26:259–74.
42. Rainsford KD, Velo GP. *New Developments in Antirheumatic Therapy.* Dordrecht, Netherlands: Kluwer; 1989.
43. Insell PA. In: Hardman JG, Limbird LE, editors. *Goodman and Gilman's The Pharmacological Basis of Therapeutics,* 9th edition. New York: McGraw-Hill Companies Inc.; 1996:617–657.
44. Davies NM. Clinical pharmacokinetics of flurbiprofen and its enantiomers. *Clin Pharmacokinet.* 1995;28:100–14.
45. Buckley MM-T, Brogden RN. Ketorolac. A review of its pharmacodynamic and pharmacokinetic properties, and therapeutic potential. *Drugs* 1990;39:86–109.
46. Noble S, Balfour JA. Meloxicam. *Drugs* 1996;51:424–30.

47. Davies NM, Anderson KE. Clinical pharmacokinetics of naproxen. *Clin Pharmacokinet.* 1997;32:268–93.
48. Davis R, Brogden, RN. Nimesulide. An update of its pharmacodynamic and pharmacokinetic properties, and therapeutic efficacy. *Drugs* 1994;48:431–54.
49. Olkkola KT, Brunetto AV, Mattila MJ. Pharmacokinetics of oxicam nonsteroidal anti-inflammatory agents. *Clin Pharmacokinet.* 1994;26:107–20.
50. Davies NM, Watson, MS. Clinical pharmacokinetics of sulindac. A dynamic old drug. *Clin Pharmacokinet.* 1997;32:437–59.
51. Garcia-Rodriguez LA, Cattaruzzi C, Grazia-Troncon M, Agostinis L. Risk of hospitalization for upper gastrointestinal tract bleeding associated with ketorolac, other nonsteroidal anti-inflammatory drugs, calcium antagonists and other anti-hypertensive drugs. *Arch Intern Med.* 1998;158:33–39.
52. Henry DH, Lim LL-Y, Garcia-Rodriguez LA, Perez Gutthan S, Carson JL, Griffith M et al. Variability in risk of gastrointestinal complications with individual non-steroidal anti-inflammatory drugs: results of a collaborative meta-analysis. *Br Med J.* 1996;312:1563–6.
53. Henry D, Dobson A, Turner C. Variability in the risk of major gastrointestinal complications from nonaspirin nonsteroidal anti-inflammatory drugs. *Gastroenterol.* 1993;105:1078–88.
54. Blanco FJ, Guitian R, Moreno J, de Toro FJ, Galdo F. Effect of antiinflammatory drugs on COX-1 and COX-2 activity in human articular chondrocytes. *J Rheumatol.* 1999;26:1366–73.
55. Cryer B, Feldman M. Cyclooxygenase-1 and cyclooxygenase-2 selectivity of widely used nonsteroidal anti-inflammatory drugs. *Am J Med.* 1998;104:413–21.
56. Fenner H. New classification of aspirin like drugs. In: Vane J, Botting J, editors. *Selective Cyclooxygenase-2 Inhibitors: Pharmacology, Clinical Effects and Therapeutic Potential.* Dordrecht, The Netherlands: Kluwer Academic; London: William Harvey Press; 1998:109–16.
57. Day RO, Francis H, Vial J, Geisslinger G, Williams KM. Naproxen concentrations in plasma and synovial fluid and effects on prostanoid concentrations. *J Rheumatol.* 1995;22:2295–303.
58. Faust TW, Redfern JS, Podolsky I, Lee E, Grundy SM, Feldman M. Effects of aspirin on gastric mucosal prostaglandin E_2 and F_2 content and on gastric mucosal injury in humans receiving fish oil or olive oil. *Gastroenterology.* 1990;98:586–91.
59. Taha AS, McLaughlin S, Holland PJ, Kelly RW, Sturrock RD, Russell RI. Effect on gastric and duodenal mucosal prostaglandins of repeated intake of therapeutic doses of naproxen and etodolac in rheumatoid arthritis. *Ann Rheum Dis.* 1990;49:354–8.
60. Hudson N, Balsitis M, Filipowicz F, Hawkey C. Effect of *Helicobacter pylori* colonisation on gastric mucosal eicosanoid synthesis in patients taking non-steroidal anti-inflammatory drugs. *Gut.* 1993;34:748–51.
61. Bertin P, Lapicque F, Payan E, Rigaud M, Bailleul F, Jaeger S et al. Sodium naproxen: Concentration and effect on inflammatory response mediators in human rheumatoid synovial fluid. *Clin Pharmacol.* 1994;46:3–7.
62. Reilly IA, FitzGerald GA. Inhibition of thromboxane formation *in vivo* and *ex vivo*: implications for therapy with platelet inhibitory drugs. *Blood.* 1987;69:180–6.
63. Rane A, Oelz O, Frölich JC, Seyberth HW, Sweetman BJ, Watson J et al. Relationship between plasma concentrations of indomethacin and its effect on

prostaglandin synthesis and platelet aggregation in man. *Clin Pharmacol Ther.* 1978;23:658–68.

64. Cronberg S, Wallmark E, Sodeberg I. Effect on platelet aggregation of oral adminis-tration of 10 non-steroidal analgesics to humans. *Scand J Haematol.* 1984;33:155–9.

65. Vinge E. Arachidonic acid-induced platelet aggregation and prostanoid formation in whole blood in relation to plasma concentration of indomethacin. *Eur J Clin Pharmacol.* 1985;28:163–9.

66. Cox SR, Vanderlugt JT, Gumbleton TJ, Smith RB. Relationships between throm-boxane production, platelet aggregability, and serum concentrations of ibuprofen and flurbiprofen. *Clin Pharmacol Ther.* 1987;41:510–21.

67. Schafer AI. Effects of nonsteroidal antiinflammatory drugs on platelet function and systemic hemostasis. *J Clin Pharmacol.* 1995;35:209–19.

68. Cullen L, Kelly L, Coyle D, Forde R, Fitzgerald D. Selective suppression of COX-2 during chronic administration of nimesulide in man. In: *Proceedings of the William Harvey Research Conference: Selective COX-2 Inhibitors; Pharmacology, Clinical Effects and Therapeutic Potential*, Cannes, France, March 20–21, 1997, abstract P3.

69. Steinhauslin F, Munajo A, Buclin T, Macciochi A, Biollaz J. Renal effects of nime-sulide in furosemide-treated subjects. *Drugs.* 1993;46(Suppl 1):257–62.

70. Panara MR, Padovano R, Sciulli MG, Santini G, Renda G, Rotondo MT et al. Effects of nimesulide on constitutive and inducible prostanoid biosynthesis in human beings. *Clin Pharmacol Ther.* 1998;63:672–81.

71. Stichtenoth DO, Wagner B, Frolich JC. Effects of meloxicam and indomethacin on cyclooxygenase pathways in healthy volunteers. *J Invest Med.* 1997;45:44–49.

72. de Meijer A, Vollaard H, de Metz M, Verbruggen B, Thomas C, Novakova I. Meloxicam, 15 mg/day, spares platelet function in healthy volunteers. *Clin Pharmacol Ther.* 1999;66:425–30.

73. Panara MR, Renda G, Sciulli MG, Santini G, Di Giamberardino M, Rotondo MT et al. Dose-dependent inhibition of platelet cyclooxygenase-1 and monocyte cyclooxygenase-2 by meloxicam in healthy subjects. *J Pharmacol Exp Ther.* 1999;290:276–80.

74. Russell RI. Endoscopic evaluation of etodolac and naproxen and their relative effects on gastric and duodenal prostaglandins. *Rheum Int.* 1990;10:17–21.

75. Arnold JD, Mullane JF, Hayden DM, March L, Hart K, Perdomo CA et al. Etodolac, aspirin, and gastrointestinal microbleeding. *Clin Pharmacol Ther.* 1984;35:716–21.

76. Mengle-Gaw L, Hubbard R, Karim A, Yu S, Talwalker S, Isakson P. A study of the platelet effects of SC-58635, a novel COX-2 selective inhibitor [abstract]. *Arthritis Rheum.* 1997;40(Suppl 9):374.

77. Leese PT, Hubbard RC, Karim A, Isakson PC, Yu SS, Geiss GS. Effects of celecoxib, a novel cyclooxygenase-2 inhibitor, on platelet function in healthy adults: a randomised, controlled trial. *J Clin Pharmacol.* 2000;40:124–32.

78. McAdam BF, Catella-Lawson F, Mardini IA, Kapoor S, Lawson JA, FitzGerald GA. Systemic biosynthesis of prostacyclin by cyclooxygenase (COX)-2: the human pharmacology of a selective inhibitor of COX-2. *Proc Natl Acad Sci USA.* 1999;96:272–7.

79. Catella-Lawson F, McAdam B, Morrison BW, Kapoor S, Kujubu D, Antes L et al. Effects of specific inhibition of cyclooxygenase-2 on sodium balance, hemo-dynamics, and vasoactive eicosanoids. *J Pharmacol Exp Ther.* 1999;289:735–41.

80. Depre M, Ehrich E, Van Hecken A, De Lepeleire, I, Dallob A, Wong P et al. Pharmacokinetics, COX-2 specificity, and tolerability of supratherapeutic doses of rofecoxib in humans. *Eur J Clin Pharmacol.* 2000;56:167–74.

81. Ehrich E, Dallob A, Van Hecken A, Depre M, DeLepeleire I, Brideau C et al. Demonstration of selective COX-2 inhibition by MK-966 in humans [abstract]. *Arthritis Rheum.* 1996;39(Suppl 9):328.

82. Rossat J, Maillard M, Nussberger J, Brunner HR, Burnier M. Renal effects of selective cyclooxygenase-2 inhibition in normotensive salt-depleted subjects. *Clin Pharmacol Ther.* 1999;66:76–84.

83. Whelton A, Schulman G, Wallemark C, Drower EJ, Isakson PC, Verburg KM et al. Effects of celecoxib and naproxen on renal function in the elderly. *Arch Intern Med.* 2000;160:1465–70.

84. Swan SK, Rudy DW, Lasseter KC, Ryan CF, Buechel KL, Lambrecht LJ et al. Effect of cyclooxygenase-2 inhibition on renal function in elderly persons receiving a low salt diet. A randomized, controlled trial. *Ann Intern Med.* 2000;133:1–9.

85. Brater DC, Brown-Cartwright D, Anderson SA, Uaamnuichai M. Effect of high-dose etodolac on renal function. *Clin Pharmacol Ther.* 1987;42:283–9.

86. Brater DC. Evaluation of etodolac in subjects with renal impairment. *Eur J Rheumatol Inflamm.* 1990;10:44–55.

87. Boulton-Jones JM, Geddes CG, Heinzel G, Turck D, Nehmiz G, Bevis PJ. Meloxicam pharmacokinetics in renal impairment. *Br J Clin Pharmacol.* 1997;43:35–40.

88. Brater DC. Effects of nonsteroidal anti-inflammatory drugs on renal function: focus on cyclooxygenase-2-selective inhibition. *Am J Med.* 1999;107:65S–70S.

89. Schoenfeld P. Gastrointestinal safety profile of meloxicam: a meta-analysis and systematic review of randomized controlled trials. *Am J Med.* 1999;107:48S–54S.

90. Degner F, Sigmund R, Zeidler H. Efficacy and tolerability of meloxicam in an observational, controlled cohort study in patients with rheumatic disease. *Clin Ther.* 2000;22:400–10.

91. Silverstein FE, Faich G, Goldstein JL, Simon LS, Pinus T, Whelton A et al. Gastrointestinal toxicity with celecoxib versus nonsteroidal anti-inflammatory drugs for osteoarthritis and rheumatoid arthritis. *J Am Med Assoc.* 2000;284:1247–53.

92. Langman MJ, Jensen DM, Watson DJ, Harper SE, Zhao PL, Quan H et al. Adverse upper gastrointestinal effects of rofecoxib compared with NSAIDs. *J Am Med Assoc.* 1999;282:1929–33.

5 | Cyclooxygenase-2 in experimental models of inflammation

DEREK WILLOUGHBY, TOBY LAWRENCE
AND PAUL COLVILLE-NASH
*Department of Experimental Pathology, William Harvey
Research Institute, St Bartholomew's and Royal London School
of Medicine and Dentistry, Charterhouse Square, London
EC1M 6BQ, UK.*

THE INFLAMMATORY RESPONSE

Inflammation is a complex and dynamic process initiated by the body in response to tissue injury or infection. There is a sequential release of mediators which leads to vasodilation and increased blood flow, increased vascular permeability producing the accumulation of a fluid exudate, and activation of neurosensory pain fibres giving rise to the classical signs of acute inflammation of *calor* (heat), *rubor* (redness), *tumor* (swelling) and *dolor* (pain) first described by Celsus nearly 2000 years ago. In association with these events, cellular trafficking into the affected tissue is enhanced by the stimulation of the expression of endothelial and inflammatory cell adhesion molecules, coupled with the production of chemoattractants. Inflammatory cell influx also occurs in a sequential fashion such that there is initially a predominance of polymorphonuclear leukocytes (PMN) migrating into the tissue in the acute phases of inflammation, which are gradually replaced by increasing numbers of mononuclear cells (MN; mainly monocytes which transform into macrophages following migration, but also lymphocytes and eosinophils, etc.) as inflammation progresses into the stages of resolution. Ultimately, there is clearance of the injurious stimuli and restoration of normal tissue structure and function. Depending upon the ability of the host to clear the initiating stimulus, a number of inflammatory reactions have a delayed progression into the resolution phase giving rise to a MN-dominated phase of chronic inflammation. Coupled with this latter phase, there may be initiation of wound healing in an attempt to replace and/or restore damaged tissues.

It is well beyond the scope of this chapter to try to expound further upon the processes involved in the above events. However, it is important to appreciate that the descriptions of events in acute and chronic inflammation and wound healing are different facets of an ever changing continuum and frequently coexist. Certainly in the case of many chronic inflammatory diseases of man, such as rheumatoid arthritis (RA) and multiple sclerosis (MS), the presence of an underlying immune-driven chronic inflammatory reaction (perhaps in response to the presence of endogenous antigens, such as, for example, collagen II in the case of a proportion of RA sufferers) is superimposed with attempts by the host to remodel and repair lost or damaged tissue during periods of disease remission and overlying this may be further periods of acute inflammation when the disease relapses. It is the recognition of this dynamic nature which is the key to reaching an understanding of the mechanisms controlling an inflammatory reaction and the therapeutic implications of the vast amount of information available.

THE ROLE OF PROSTAGLANDINS

This topic has been elegantly reviewed by Vane and Botting[1,28], and only the briefest description of some of the more important facets of the activities of prostaglandins with regard to inflammation will be mentioned here. The term 'prostaglandin' (PG) was coined by von Euler in 1934[2] to describe a lipid soluble acid from seminal fluid with the ability to contract smooth muscle. Subsequently shown to consist of a large number of structurally related compounds, it was in 1964 that Bergstrom[3] and Van Dorp[4] independently showed that PGE_2 could be synthesized by tissue homogenates of sheep seminal vesicles from arachidonic acid. It is now known that the PGs are only one of the families of lipid mediators which can be produced from the enzymic conversion of arachidonic acid, the other major families including the thromboxanes and the leukotrienes.

Prostaglandins are amongst the earliest mediators which are released in an inflammatory reaction[5], much interest focusing on PGE_2 which is the major prostanoid released during the initiation of the inflammatory response. PGE_2 is a potent vasodilator[6], along with prostacyclin (PGI_2), and whilst it does not induce increases in vascular permeability directly, it will synergize potently with other mediators such as bradykinin or histamine[7], probably due to its vasodilator action. PGE_2 is also important in the pain pathways, where it is one of the mediators responsible for the hyperalgesia associated with inflammation[8], and also induces pyrexia[9]. PGE_2 can therefore be seen to contribute to all the classical signs of acute inflammation described above. However, it has been apparent for a long time that PGs can also have anti-inflammatory activities. Thus most of the effects of PGE_2 in the immune system suggest an immunosuppressive effect, this being evident both *in vivo* following antigen challenge to sensitized animals[10] and also *in vitro*, where PGE_2 can suppress lymphocyte proliferation[11], migration[12], cell mediated cytotoxicity[13] and secretion of cytokines such as interleukin-2 (IL-2) and interferon γ (IFNγ)[14]. In macrophages, PGE_2 also can suppress proinflammatory functions such as the secretion of interleukin-1 (IL-1) and TNF[15]. Indeed, in the cancer field, the elevated production of PGE_2 by some tumours and subsequent local immunosuppression has been suggested to be one of the reasons for the ability of tumours to survive attack by host defences[16]. Non-steroid anti-inflammatory drugs (NSAID) have been used as adjunctive therapeutic agents to treat some tumours[17] and recently there has been interest in the role of cyclooxygenase-2 (COX-2) in the pathogenesis of colon cancer and the ability of COX-2-selective inhibitors to prevent the development of this important group of carcinomas. This work is covered in detail by DuBois[18] and thus presents yet another apparent contradiction in the actions of prostaglandins.

Whilst PGE_2 has been extensively investigated, much less work has addressed the role of the other PGs in inflammation. However in a series of papers in the early 1970s by Willoughby's group[19-21], it was noted that there was an early rise in PGE_2 levels, which correlated with the onset of inflammation in a variety of non-immune and immune inflammatory models, and a fall during resolution (Figure 1). This was subsequently followed by a rise in levels of $PGF_{2\alpha}$ as inflammation waned, which Willoughby[22,23] had previously shown could inhibit the increased vascular permeability induced by other mediators such as histamine and serotonin. Thus it was suggested that there was a change in PG synthesis pathways during the resolution of inflammation, thus altering the PG profile. Whilst COX-2 was as yet undiscovered, it will become apparent later in this chapter that this enzyme may in fact be the source of the $PGF_{2\alpha}$ measured in these experiments.

In addition to the role of the PGs in inflammatory reactions, it is important to recognize that these substances play a role in routine physiological processes. The importance of this is highlighted by the various side effects of NSAID treatment, principally that on the gastrointestinal tract leading to gastric ulceration. This is excellently reviewed elsewhere in this volume (Harris[24], Whittle[25], Hawkey[26] and Rodriguez[27]) and will not be described further here.

PROSTAGLANDIN PRODUCTION BY CYCLOOXYGENASE – THE ADVENT OF COX-2

The enzyme responsible for the synthesis of the PGs is cyclooxygenase (COX), also called prostaglandin H synthase˙ and prostaglandin endoperoxidase (see review by Vane and Botting[28]). It was the demonstration by Vane in 1971[29] that the anti-inflammatory effects of aspirin-like non-steroid anti-

Figure 1 Distributions of prostaglandin E_2 and prostaglandin $F_{2\alpha}$ in pleural reactions of various aetiologies: (a) Arthus pleurisy; (b) delayed-type hypersensitivity, cell-mediated immune pleurisy. For carrageenan pleurisy, please see Figure 3b. (Figures modified from Capasso et al[21].)

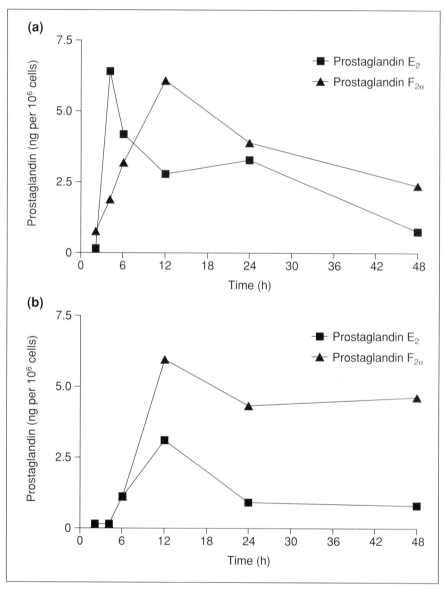

inflammatory drugs (NSAID) was via the prevention of PG biosynthesis by inhibition of this enzyme that provided the key breakthrough into the mode of action of this group of therapeutic agents. The discovery that COX exists in more than one isoform[30] was another huge leap in our understanding of the function of the prostanoid pathways. COX-1 is constitutively expressed in most tissues where it synthesizes low levels of PGs which help to maintain physiological processes. COX-2, in contrast, was shown to be highly inducible in response to proinflammatory stimuli, cytokines and mitogens, resulting in exaggerated PG release. This separation of function suggested that it might be possible to develop more selective NSAIDs which would target only the inducible isoform and spare COX-1, thus eliminating the major side effects of conventional NSAIDs which were either more selective for COX-1 (such as aspirin) or non-selective inhibitors of both isoforms[31]. Amongst the earliest COX-2 selective drugs to be described were DuP 697[32] and NS-398[33]. Whilst these were initially chosen on the basis of their gastrointestinal sparing therapeutic profile, they were subsequently shown to be effective COX-2 selective compounds[34]. DuP 697 is the parent compound for the diarylheterocyclic family of COX-2 selective inhibitors which include SC-58635 (celecoxib[35]) and MK-0966 (rofecoxib[36]), both of which were designed as COX-2 inhibitors using the enzyme protein.

As well as advancing the use of NSAIDs as anti-inflammatory agents, the further development of this group of drugs has also provided a useful means of investigating the roles of PGs and the contributions of COX-1 and COX-2 to inflammatory processes. Recently, their use in a number of experimental models has bought to light new concerns regarding a possible role for COX-2 in both wound healing, particularly in gastric ulcers[37-39], and in the resolution phase of inflammation[40]. It is the purpose of this chapter to describe the relative contributions of COX-1 and COX-2 in a variety of inflammatory models of differing aetiology. These are presented in an order which reflects, to some extent, the evolution of our understanding of the role of COX-2 in inflammation. Thus some of the initial findings in chronic inflammation and disease models of arthritis will be described first, followed by immune driven acute inflammatory models and finally acute inflammatory models driven by carrageenan, a non-specific inflammatory stimulus. Although these acute methods have been used since the conception of the COX-2 story, the investigations in these models have now produced evidence for a role for COX-2 in the resolution of inflammation. These will therefore be described towards the end of this chapter along with the potential mechanisms underlying this role and hence the therapeutic implications of manipulation of the COX system in inflammatory disease.

CYCLOOXYGENASE IN CHRONIC INFLAMMATION

The murine chronic granulomatous air pouch

Artificially induced subcutaneous air-filled cavities in rodents were originally used by Selye (1953)[41] to study chronic inflammatory reactions and later became widely used. The air pouch, prior to the application of irritants, develops into a structure which bears many similarities to that of the normal synovium, and following injection of an appropriate stimulus, the changes that occur, and the granulomatous tissue that develops, resemble those that are seen in an arthritic joint in diseases such as RA[42]. Indeed, the air pouch lining cells behave in a similar fashion to synovium in adjuvant arthritis, undergoing hyperplasia and exhibiting similar changes in their metabolism[43]. Subsequently, various forms of the model have been used to assess the impact of many anti-arthritic drugs[44] and they are amongst the best characterized of all inflammatory models. The murine chronic granulomatous air pouch has been used to study the processes involved in wound healing and in particular the development of new blood vessels – angiogenesis[45]. The model consists of a subcutaneous air pouch formed on the dorsum of mice by the injection of 3 ml air, followed 24 h later by 0.5 ml Freund's complete adjuvant supplemented with 0.1% vol/vol croton oil, resulting in an immune-driven chronic inflammatory reaction[46]. This results in an acute inflammatory response characterized by the influx of PMNs into the dermis and the periphery of the air pouch lining. By day 3, the air pouch lining has increased in thickness and the inflammatory cell population in the reaction is now dominated by macrophages. In addition to these cells, fibroblasts migrate into the tissue along with endothelial cells, and the beginning of a new vascular network to support the developing chronically inflamed tissue can be seen. Due to the persistence of the stimulus in the cavity of the air pouch, a zoned appearance develops in the pouch lining over time such that, adjacent to the cavity, a tissue similar to the early inflamed tissue described above can be seen. Underlying this, there is a zone consisting of macrophages with fibroblasts and newly formed capillaries, and deeper to this layer there is a more mature granulation tissue where wound healing has progressed further. This is highly vascular, with active deposition of collagen, and is densely populated with macrophages. From day 21 onwards, this tissue is replaced by a more mature fibrotic, less vascular tissue characteristic of scar formation. During these later stages, the irritant in the pouch is gradually being cleared and the lesion resolves by maturation of the chronically inflamed tissue into this fibrous tissue which contracts and remodels over a period of several weeks.

Due to the presence of the adjuvant and croton oil in the air pouch it is not possible to measure the levels of prostanoid mediators in the exudate; however, it is possible to measure the ability of the tissue to produce prostanoids by using tissue homogenates in an *ex vivo* biochemical assay, with exogenously added co-factors, and arachidonic acid to measure the activity of cyclooxygenase to produce PGE_2[47]. This technique revealed that COX activity rose during the first 24 h of inflammation, before falling slightly during the period of maximal increases in inflammatory tissue mass (day 3 to 5). Following this, a second delayed peak in COX activity was evident at day 14. As this assay cannot distinguish between COX-1 or COX-2, Western blotting was performed on the tissue homogenates. This revealed that COX-1 expression did not change during the inflammation, but the changes in PGE_2 production in the assay were mirrored by changes in the expression of COX-2 protein, suggesting this was the isoform responsible for the changes in prostaglandin synthesis. Immunohistochemical analysis of the distribution of COX-2 in this model[48] revealed that the predominant inflammatory cell expressing COX-2 was the macrophage at all times. However, by day 7, fibroblasts were also strongly immunopositive, and COX-2 was also evident in the capillaries of the tissue by day 14. At this time, COX-2 staining was strongly associated with the areas of active fibrogenesis in the mid-region of the granulomatous tissue. It was thus concluded from this study that COX-2 was the isoform responsible for the production of PGE_2 in this model in both the acute and chronic stages, and that its inhibition would be therapeutically desirable. However, it was also noted that there was a possibility that the function of COX-2 may change in the later stages of the model as inflammation begins to resolve. Whilst the earlier expression of COX-2 coincided with the highest levels of two key proinflammatory cytokines, interleukin-1 (IL-1) and tumour necrosis factor (TNF-α)[46], which are known inducers of COX-2 in a variety of cells including monocytes, the levels of these cytokines fall during the second peak in COX-2 expression at 14 days. However, at this time, there is increased expression of TGF-β. Considered to be generally an anti-inflammatory cytokine, TGF-β has been shown to induce COX-2 expression in fibroblasts[49] as well as promoting wound healing by increasing fibroblast collagen synthesis, for example[50]. This therefore suggests that COX-2 at this later stage may in fact aid the resolution of an inflammatory reaction. Thus COX-2 may promote resolution by regulating the immune component of this reaction by the immunosuppressive activities of some PGs and may also contribute to the control of extracellular matrix deposition induced by TGF-β, PGE_2 having been shown to antagonize the effects of TGF-β on fibroblast matrix deposition[51].

Further insight into the roles of COX-1 and COX-2 in this model have been gained by examining the effect of application of various NSAIDs with differing selectivity towards COX-1 and COX-2[52]. Such studies revealed that those inhibitors with selectivity towards COX-1 were more effective than COX-2 selective drugs. Thus treating animals with aspirin resulted in significant anti-inflammatory effects, inhibiting granuloma weight gain, vascularity and COX-activity. This suggests that despite not being induced, COX-1 appears to contribute significantly to PG production in inflammation. In contrast to the effect of aspirin, NS-398, a COX-2 selective inhibitor, had no effect on granuloma weight gain, tissue vascularity or COX activity when used at doses shown to be anti-inflammatory in other models of inflammation. Nimesulide, another NSAID with selectivity towards COX-2, again showed no anti-inflammatory effect and did in fact cause a significant increase in COX activity early in the model, which was followed by a subsequent increase in tissue vascularity by day 7, and an increase in the weight of the granulomas after 14 days of treatment was also noted. The induction of PGE_2 production by nimesulide has been reported from *in vitro* studies[53,54], one possible mechanism being the enhancement of COX-1 activity by enhancing the conversion of PGG_2 to PGH_2 by a radical scavenging mechanism[55]. Alternatively, a range of NSAIDs have been shown to induce the expression of mRNA for COX-1 and COX-2 in chick fibroblasts[54] and thus potentiate COX activity. However, analysis of the expression of COX-1 and COX-2 protein in this model showed no differences in expression following drug treatment and it thus appears likely that the effects of these drugs reflect either changes in enzyme activity or other effects such as changes in substrate availability. Certainly, there is evidence that PGE_2 can induce an angiogenic response *in vivo*[56] and also induce the expression of potent angiogenic growth factors such as vascular endothelial growth factor (VEGF) from various cells *in vitro* including rheumatoid synovial fibroblasts[57]. The link between angiogenesis and vascular growth has been demonstrated in the pouch model using angiostatic steroids[45], and thus the increase in vascularity may be responsible for the increased granuloma mass at day 14. Finally, in the above studies using the murine chronic granulomatous air pouch, the NSAIDs were applied not from the start of the model but from day 3 onwards, in an attempt to mimic therapeutic application, where inflammation in chronic diseases such as RA is often long-standing before treatment begins. In many studies, treatment is initiated at the time of application of the inflammatory stimulus; it is not known what effect this latter approach would have in the murine model; however, this is an important point to consider when examining papers investigating the effects of NSAIDs in chronic models because an effect on the acute stages of the inflammatory response are likely to change the subsequent dynamics of the chronic inflammatory response and thus different effects may be seen.

MANIPULATION OF CYCLOOXYGENASE IN ANIMAL MODELS OF ARTHRITIS

The above observations in a chronic inflammatory model, and the hypothesis for a role for COX-2 bringing about the onset of the inflammatory reaction as well as playing a role in the resolution of inflammation, suggested that the distribution of COX isoforms, and the efficacy of the various NSAIDs in chronic models of human inflammatory diseases, should be studied. These studies arguably give the closest idea of the therapeutic usefulness of an approach such as manipulation of COX-2 by novel NSAIDs before they are used clinically. Such information available in two of these models, adjuvant arthritis and monoarticular arthritis, will now be described.

Adjuvant arthritis

Adjuvant arthritis is induced by the sensitization of susceptible rats (usually the Lewis strain as many other strains of rat are not susceptible to this arthritis) to *Mycobacterium tuberculosis* in a light mineral oil (Freund's complete adjuvant). This causes a chronic arthritis affecting the hind limbs initially, progressing onto the forelimbs. It can also give rise to other manifestations of cartilage damage, for example an auricular chondritis[58]. Regulation of COX expression has long been reported in models of arthritis in rodents[59,60]. Early studies with non-isoform selective antibodies for COX showed elevations in expression of COX protein in synovium of animals with either adjuvant or streptococcal cell wall induced arthritis[59]. This was absent in normal tissues and the presence of this immunoreactivity paralleled the onset of clinical signs in these models. This elevated expression of COX protein was inhibited by dexamethasone, suggesting that the COX isoform being seen was inducible COX-2. More powerful studies[60] examined the expression of COX-2 using RNAse protection assays for COX-2 mRNA and COX-2 protein expression by ELISA with a specific antibody; these showed that paw oedema was concomitant with an increase in the expression of COX-2 and this was mirrored by elevations in the levels of PGE_2 in the paw tissue. Histological assessment showed that in arthritic paws, there was considerable infiltration of the joints with inflammatory cells by day 14, although little damage to cartilage or bone was evident at this time. By day 25, there was extensive infiltration by inflammatory leukocytes in the soft tissue but also into the hard tissues (bone and cartilage) of the joints with consequent cartilage and bone destruction. The effects of SC-58125[60], a COX-2 selective inhibitor, was examined using therapeutic doses in the presence of existing arthritis and this showed that the NSAID rapidly reversed the oedema present in the paws of arthritic rats, as did indomethacin (a non-selective inhibitor) and dexamethasone. This was associated with a fall in paw tissue PGE_2 levels. Curiously, treatment with the NSAIDs also reduced the production of mRNA for COX-2 in the tissues. Similarly, treatment with SC-58125 and indomethacin reduced the inflammatory changes evident in the joints as shown by histology. Cartilage integrity was maintained although there was still persistent inflammatory cell influx. Adjuvant arthritis is not, however, a very close model of the disease seen in human RA[58]. It is not a resolving and relapsing condition and whilst it does eventually resolve, joint destruction is progressive and resolution is by ankylosis. It therefore probably reflects the situation seen clinically during the onset of arthritis and during the periods of relapse in the disease.

Monoarticular arthritis

In this model, *Mycobacterium tuberculosis* is injected directly into the knee joints of CFHB Wistar rats (again this is a strain selective response) where it induces an acute inflammatory reaction leading to synovial hyperplasia and invasion of the joint with granulomatous tissue[61]. The model is useful in that it allows the quantitation of patella glycosaminoglycan loss, a measure of cartilage damage and bone loss, and therefore provides a convenient measure of joint destruction. The expression and modulation of COX-2 have also been described in this model[62]. Six hours after the injection of *Mycobacterium tuberculosis*, small clusters of inflammatory cells immunopositive for COX-2 are evident, which become widespread by 24 h. By four days, PMNs, macrophages and also fibroblasts in the synovium labelled positively for COX-2 protein expression. Nimesulide and piroxicam exacerbated patella glycosaminoglycan loss, though the more selective inhibitor for COX-2, NS-398, did not. Neither NS-398 nor nimesulide affected patella bone loss, though this was reduced by piroxicam. All of these drugs significantly reduced joint swelling assessed by joint diameter. These data are important as there is a large amount of information which suggests that traditional NSAIDs have an adverse effect on cartilage structure and chondrocyte function both *in vitro* and *in vivo*. The COX-2 selective drugs used in this study appear to have a better profile for sparing cartilage in arthritic joints than piroxicam and other NSAIDs such as naproxen and indomethacin that behave similarly. Thus, whilst they do not protect against bone loss, they do not exacerbate it and do protect cartilage, and the loss of cartilage is perhaps the key problem leading to failure of joint function in arthritic conditions.

CYCLOOXYGENASE ACTIVITY IN ACUTE INFLAMMATION

The majority of the work in the inflammation field, however, has utilized the acute phases of inflammatory models to examine the role of COX-2 and the effects of dual COX-1/COX-2 or selective COX-2 inhibitors.

Of the many acute inflammatory models that have been used, most information has been derived using non-specific inflammatory stimuli, mainly carrageenan (a seaweed extract). Therefore, despite the underlying immune nature of many human chronic inflammatory diseases, there is relatively little information regarding COX-2 expression and function from acute models with an immune component such as the Arthus (immediate-type hypersensitivity) or delayed-type hypersensitivity reactions, and thus effects of new generation NSAIDs with selectivity towards COX-2 have also not been reported in these models. Because of the sparse nature of information available, these immune driven models will be described first, followed by those induced by carrageenan.

Arthus (immediate-type hypersensitivity) reactions

The Arthus reaction is initiated by the deposition in tissues of a complex of antigen and antibody, resulting in the activation of complement. Rats are sensitized to bovine serum albumen (BSA) by a single injection of BSA 10 mg ml^{-1} in Freund's incomplete adjuvant followed 12 days later by intrapleural challenge with 0.1 ml BSA 10 mg ml^{-1} in saline[63]. This causes an acute allergic inflammatory reaction which peaks at 6 h and resolves at approximately 24 h post-application of antigen. The reaction is dominated by PMNs until resolution. Little work has been carried out on this model but COX activity peaks at 2 h and falls thereafter, this being mirrored by the expression of COX-2 protein assessed by Western blotting[64]. Immunocytochemistry identified the cell expressing COX-2 to be the PMN throughout the time course. There was, however, a slight increase in COX activity, assessed by PGE$_2$ production, at 24 h (50% greater than that seen at 6 h). Unfortunately, whilst it is known that the model is sensitive to inhibition by many older generation NSAIDs given prophylactically, the effects of COX-2 selective inhibitors have not been investigated, nor have the effects of treatment with NSAIDs once inflammation has been established. However, the role of traditional NSAIDs has been extensively investigated in a variety of other allergic reactions, particularly in the hamster allergic cheek pouch model[65]. In this model, indomethacin and diclofenac, which are non-selective inhibitors of COX-1 and COX-2, both significantly increased the release of histamine, plasma leakage and leukocyte accumulation. These effects were all reversed by the application of PGE$_2$ and this suggests a protective role for this COX product in these reactions.

In contrast, in the allergic pleurisy induced by sensitization to ovalbumin, aspirin and indomethacin failed to affect the exudation, cell accumulation or histamine release following challenge[66]. In this study, the authors also examined the role of the prostanoid pathway in the reductions in allergic inflammation which can be induced by the augmentation of eosinophil influx using platelet activating factor (PAF). Again, this PAF-induced hyporesponsiveness was associated with elevations in the levels of PGE$_2$ recoverable in the exudates. This protection was also lost following NSAID treatment with indomethacin or aspirin. In this case, the additional PGE$_2$ production induced by PAF treatment is thought to be caused by the newly arriving eosinophils, these having been shown to produce enough PGE$_2$ to inhibit histamine release induced by appropriate antigens *in vitro*. Unfortunately these experiments were not designed to examine specifically the role of COX-1 or COX-2 in the response and it is unclear as to the contribution of COX-1 or COX-2 to the production of PGE$_2$. However, the dose of aspirin used was very high (200 mg kg^{-1}) and given systemically rather than orally, and it is therefore likely that at these doses aspirin also inhibited COX-2. If the data correlate with those seen with the use of BSA as an antigen above, then these studies would suggest that the production of PGE$_2$ by COX-2 is protective in some phases of these models.

Cell mediated immune (delayed-type) hypersensitivity reactions

The substitution of methylated BSA for BSA in the sensitization and challenge protocol for the Arthus reaction described above gives rise to a delayed-type hypersensitivity reaction. Animals are sensitized by the injection of methylated BSA in Freund's incomplete adjuvant into the base of the tail, followed 12 days later by the intrapleural administration of the same antigen in saline. In contrast to the immediate hypersensitivity reaction of the Arthus, this model manifests a delayed response, with a modest initial acute response in inflammatory exudate formation and cell influx over the first 12 h, followed by a second, much greater, delayed reaction at 24 h. Whilst the early phase is dominated by PMN, the delayed phase consists almost entirely of macrophages. This reaction wanes over the next 24 h to be essentially resolved by 48 h[67]. COX activity in this model (as estimated by PG production) showed a steady increase as inflammation rose, particularly increasing as inflammation peaked (D. Gilroy, unpublished observations). However, after this time, COX activity was maintained during resolution and it was here that the highest levels of activity were measurable. Analysis of COX-2 protein expression showed a similar profile, with a clear increase in level of COX-2 protein at 24 h, which was further raised at 48 h, the COX-2 being associated with the macrophages dominating the exudate and in contrast to the expression of COX-2 in the immediate hypersensitivity models. As of yet, no manipulation of this model has been reported with NSAIDs, and the relevance of the differences in expression of COX-2 in resolution in PMNs in one model, but in macrophages in another, is intriguing but unknown.

However, in another model of delayed-type hypersensitivity, initiated by secondary antigen challenge in a rat air pouch model of allergic inflammation induced by sensitization and challenge with azobenzenecarsonate-conjugated BSA, the effects of COX-2 selective NSAID treatment has been reported[68]. This model manifests a slow progressive rise in exudate volume, leukocyte accumulation and mass of air pouch granulomatous tissue up to 48 h. Histological examination of the pouch fluid shows that whilst the percentage of macrophages and PMNs was roughly the same at the time of challenge, the secondary reaction was dominated by PMNs up to the time points measured (72 h). This suggests that this model has a slower rate of development compared with the methylated BSA model described previously and may not have developed fully into a delayed-type hypersensitivity reaction. Measurement of PGE_2 in the exudate showed a rapid accumulation which peaked at 6 h and was then maintained. Similar to the findings above, COX-1 expression was unchanged, whilst COX-2 was induced rapidly, peaking at 6 h, the profile subsequently reflecting the PGE_2 levels up to 48 h. Administration of the non-isoform selective NSAID, indomethacin, and the COX-2 selective inhibitor NS-398 immediately after the second antigen challenge and then subsequently daily, i.e. a prophylactic approach, inhibited the accumulation of fluid exudate, cell influx and granuloma development. However, it was noted that the reduction in cell number was accounted for by a reduction in PMN influx alone. These treatments both resulted in reduced levels of PGE_2 in the pouch fluid. The model was not taken beyond this point and the effects of inhibition of COX during resolution is therefore unknown, as are further details as to the expression of COX-1 and COX-2 during this period.

CARRAGEENAN-INDUCED INFLAMMATORY REACTIONS

Inflammatory reactions in response to carrageenan form a major part of the testing of NSAID efficacy *in vivo*. A number of variants of these exist, including: the rat carrageenan paw oedema test; the rat and murine carrageenan air pouch; and carrageenan pleurisy in the rat.

The rat carrageenan paw oedema test

Following the injection of 0.1 ml of 1% carrageenan solution in saline into the hind paw of a rat, there is a biphasic rise in oedema in the paw measured by a change in paw volume using a plethysmometer. There is an initial rapid phase of oedema formation for the first 30 min, followed by a slower but more sustained rate of oedema formation up to 5 h. After this time, inflammation begins to resolve. The carrageenan paw oedema model was developed by Winter, Risley and Nuss[69] to investigate the anti-inflammatory effects of indomethacin. Thirty years on, this model was also one of the first used to describe the efficacy of novel COX-2 selective NSAIDs, initially SC-58125[70]. Analysis of the expression of COX-1 and COX-2 within this model was by an RNAse protection assay. This showed no changes in the levels of mRNA for COX-1 but, in contrast, COX-2 mRNA was significantly induced, being evident from 60 min and maximal by 3 h. This correlated both with the formation of prostanoids in the paw tissue and oedema formation. Treatment with indomethacin or SC-58125 suppressed inflammation, oedema formation and hyperalgesia, being associated with suppression of paw tissue PG synthesis. However, PG production was assessed at 3 h, this time being chosen as it was the time of peak COX-2 mRNA expression over the time course (5 h) investigated. The distribution of COX isoforms and the effects of the COX inhibitors on the resolution of the model were not reported in this study and have yet to be determined. Other COX-2 selective NSAIDs have also been tested in this model (L-745,337[71], rofecoxib[72] and DFU[34]) but, again, a time point of 1 h or 3 h was used and the effects of administration later in the model was not investigated. However, the findings with the COX-2 selective drugs in this model have been questioned. Wallace et al. [73] showed that

NS-398, nimesulide and DuP 697 all required concentrations that were inhibiting not only COX-2 but also COX-1 to obtain a significant anti-inflammatory effect. Indeed, in Seibert's paper[70], the dose of SC-58125 required to inhibit oedema in the rat paw model was 1000 times that required to inhibit the synthesis of prostanoids in the paw tissue. This has been interpreted to suggest that COX-1 is important in this model despite its lack of inducibility. In the arachidonic acid-induced ear swelling test, deletion of the COX-1 gene effectively reduces the early phase of this inflammatory reaction[74]. Similarly, in mice with the COX-2 gene deleted, paw swelling and lymphocyte infiltration were similar to that seen in wild-type control mice[75]. However, a highly effective COX-1 inhibitor SC-560 failed to have any anti-inflammatory effect in the rat carrageenan paw model[76] at doses which inhibited COX-1 *in vivo*, although it did reduce the levels of prostanoids in the paws to the same degree as celecoxib, a selective COX-2 inhibitor that was shown to be anti-inflammatory. A key point was also raised in this paper – whilst prophylactic dosing with celecoxib was able to suppress inflammation, dosing when oedema was established (3 h) was without effect, confirming other reports using this treatment regime, although hyperalgesia associated with the inflammatory response was reduced.

The rat and murine carrageenan air pouch model

The usefulness of the rodent air pouch has been described briefly above. The injection of carrageenan into the rat air pouch 6 days after injection of air induces an acute inflammatory reaction, with influx of predominantly PMNs and macrophages, the latter only comprising 15% of the exudate cells at 24 h[77]. Carrageenan injection caused a time dependent increase in PGE_2 and prostacyclin levels in the exudates, though both of these peaked at 6 h and fell thereafter. This was parallelled by expression of COX-2 demonstrated by RNAse protection assay as well as by immunoprecipitation. However, despite the preponderance of PMNs, immunohistochemistry revealed that the cells expressing this COX-2 were the macrophages only. Examination of the pouch lining cells showed that COX-2 was also expressed in the superficial cells of the lining in both fibroblasts and macrophages. NS-398 given 6 h after the injection of carrageenan reduced exudate accumulation, cellular infiltration and PG content of the pouch exudate at 24 h post-injection of carrageenan. Previously, prophylactic dosing with NS-398[33] had shown similar beneficial effects of inhibition of COX-2. However, these studies have been only concerned with the acute phase of inflammation in the carrageenan air pouch, dominated by the PMN. If the time course of this model is extended, a chronic phase is seen, dominated by macrophages and with much larger exudative responses and leukocyte influx[78]. This does not reach resolution until approximately 4 weeks. It could be argued that this part of the time course is perhaps a better target for experimental investigations examining the role of various endogenous factors and drugs which are destined for use in chronic inflammatory diseases such as RA. Unfortunately no similar data exist for the resolution phase and it is largely ignored.

The time course of changes in the murine carrageenan air pouch is very different from that in the rat. In the mouse, the injection of carrageenan into a 6-day air pouch induces an acute inflammatory reaction in which exudation is maximal at 24 h and wanes thereafter. Unlike the rat model, a larger chronic phase is not seen, and the model gradually resolves over the next month[79]. Cellular influx peaks at 48 h, but by 72 h exudate volumes fall by 80% and cell numbers are halved. Initially dominated by PMNs, which form more than 99% of the cells at 6 h, these are gradually replaced by macrophages, which comprise 70% of the cells in the exudate at 72 h. Western blot analysis of the expression of COX-2 in the inflammatory cells showed that COX-2 was evident by 6 h in these cells (T. Lawrence, unpublished observations), but the amount of COX-2 protein subsequently continued to increase up to a peak at 48 h, which was maintained at 72 h during the resolution phase. Densitometry showed that COX-2 expression at this time was 3–4 times that seen during the acute phase of the reaction. Assessment of the inflammatory cell prostaglandin synthesis *ex vivo* showed that PGE_2 synthesis was maximal at 6 h, but this fell by 80% at 18 h and then remained low despite the continuing elevation of COX-2 protein expression. However, further analysis of the supernatants from these activity assays revealed that PGD_2 synthesis, which was detectable at 6 h, fell at 18 h as inflammation developed, and then gradually increased over the next 72 h, reflecting the raised expression of COX-2 protein. This poses the question as to the role of the COX-2 that is expressed during this resolution phase and what the effects of targeting this enzyme will be on the outcome of the inflammatory reaction. In the carrageenan air pouch in mice, these effects are currently being investigated and the effects of aspirin have been examined (T. Lawrence, unpublished observations). This drug at 100 mg kg^{-1} was anti-inflammatory if the model was terminated at 24 h post-injection of the carrageenan, but at 72 h, treatment with this dose of aspirin caused an exacerbation of both exudate volume and cellular influx. It is unclear from the limited preliminary data available in this model what role COX-1 has in its development and it cannot yet be determined whether this effect of aspirin is via an effect on COX-1 or COX-2 or both. Preliminary findings (T. Lawrence, unpublished observations) with a single oral dose of NS-398 at 10 mg kg^{-1} suggest that treatment with a COX-2 selective NSAID from the time of the peak in inflammation can retard the resolution of the inflammation (Figure 2), but the above concerns remain to be addressed and the effects of this treatment on prostaglandin synthesis during resolution is unknown at present. Although there is still much investigation required to establish more firmly the role of COX-2 in the resolution of the carrageenan inflammation in the air pouch in mice, similar

Figure 2 Influence of NS-398 on the resolution of inflammation in the murine carrageenan air pouch. Open symbols: vehicle treated animals; closed symbols: 10 mg kg⁻¹ p.o. q.i.d. from peak of inflammation. □■, exudate volume; ○●, cell numbers in pouch exudate. ($n = 10$ in all cases.)

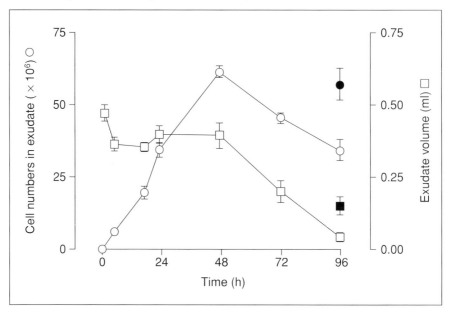

studies have been performed in rat carrageenan pleurisy where some of these problems have been addressed – these findings are described below.

The rat carrageenan pleurisy model

Carrageenan-induced pleurisy in the rat is a model of acute inflammation mediated by the activation of the complement system by the alternative pathway. The model has been used extensively to examine the sequential release of mediators in the acute inflammatory response[5]. Using a variety of inhibitors, this early work showed that initially histamine was released, followed by 5-hydroxytryptamine, kinins and subsequently PGs, initially PGE_2 but followed later by $PGF_{2\alpha}$ production. The inflammatory response is induced by the injection of 0.15 ml 1% carrageenan solution in saline. At various times post-injection of the irritant, the pleural exudates are harvested and can be assayed for a variety of mediators, and the cells within the exudate separated out for histological analysis, biochemical assay and Western blotting. The model is again very well characterized and extensively used for testing therapeutic agents. The peak in the inflammatory reaction, measured by exudate volume and cell influx, is at 24 h, inflammation then waning to be largely resolved by 48 h. Initially, PMNs dominate the reaction (up to 12 h). There is then a shift towards the mononuclear cells, with inwardly migrating monocytes that differentiate into macrophages which form the predominant cell type up to resolution at 48 h.

Examination of the profile of PGE_2 levels in the exudate revealed a peak at 2 h, which fell rapidly to near baseline values by 6 h and remained at these levels through to resolution[80]. Similarly, using the *ex vivo* biochemical assay for PGE_2 synthesis, this was also shown to peak at 2 h and similarly fell away rapidly. Western blotting for COX-1 and COX-2 revealed that whilst the expression of COX-1 was unchanged throughout the time course, the expression of COX-2 reflected these changes in PGE_2 up to 24 h. Immunohistochemistry revealed that the majority of PMNs and macrophages (more than 80%) contained COX-2. Later at 24 h, whilst the majority of PMNs present in the pleural cavity were still labelled for COX-2, only a small proportion of the macrophages (15%) were so labelled. This suggested that COX-2 protein expression in these cells is downregulated during the time at which exudate and cellular accumulation is still increasing to the peak of inflammation at 24 h. The above data were therefore highly suggestive of a role for COX-2 in the initial induction of this acute inflammatory response.

Prophylactic treatment with NSAIDs was initiated and the effects measured at 6 h, which is the most commonly used time point in this model for the assessment of this class of anti-inflammatory drugs[81]. The non-selective COX drugs, aspirin and piroxicam, suppressed exudate volume significantly and cell accumulation at 6 h, associated with a decrease in the levels of PGE_2. In contrast to these NSAIDs, those selective for COX-2 failed to show any anti-inflammatory effect on exudate volume and cell influx, although NS-398 did reduce the PGE_2 content of the exudate. Subsequently these experiments were repeated using an earlier time-point for the assessment of the response (3 h), this being closer to the peak of COX-2 expression. Using this time-point, but keeping the previous dosing regimes, both nimesulide and NS-398 inhibited exudation, cell influx and PGE_2 accumulation in the exudate. These drugs did not affect platelet thromboxane synthesis (dependent on COX-1) – this indicates that these effects at 3 h are due to COX-2 inhibition. However, even at 3 h, the non-selective NSAIDs were still much more potent inhibitors of inflammation. Further investigation of the apparent loss of the inhibitory activity of the COX-2-selective NSAIDs in this model revealed that at 6 h treatment caused a significant increase in leukotriene B_4 (LTB_4) production, whilst the COX-1-selective NSAIDs did not cause this. A similar effect has been noted in guinea pig anaphylaxis following indomethacin[82] and in the murine carrageenan air pouch using COX-2 knock-out mice, where the levels of LTB_4 in the pouch exudate were also elevated[83].

These findings highlight another crucial point for consideration – the time at which experimental models of inflammation are assessed. In many studies, single time-points are chosen and, as has been demonstrated, one obtains variable results if time-points are chosen with just a few hours difference. Thus, there are many studies which show the effectiveness of COX-2 inhibitors on the acute phase. The necessity of examining time courses which encompass the major phases of the inflammatory reaction through to resolution is clear, though seldom performed. This can also be seen in the case of the delayed-type hypersensitivity reactions described above. This loss of potentially important information can obviously have implications for the transposition of the data obtained to the clinical situation and data from these models in the literature therefore require careful scrutiny.

As part of this series of experiments, the effects of these COX inhibitors were examined in the same model but using the Lewis strain of rat, rather than the Wistar, which had been used in studies which showed an anti-inflammatory effect of NS-398 in the rat carrageenan air pouch. Lewis rats are in-bred and have low levels of circulating glucocorticoids and thus an exaggerated response to inflammatory stimuli, due to a poor glucocorticoid response following inflammatory stimuli. Using these rats, it was shown that both non-selective and COX-2-selective NSAIDs inhibited PGE_2 production and exudate accumulation at the 6 h time-point, though again the non-selective drugs were more effective (D. Gilroy, unpublished observations). It is of interest that cellular influx was still unaffected at this time, and again LTB_4 levels were raised only by the treatment with COX-2-selective drugs. It should be noted that the time course of changes in the gross parameters of inflammation were unaffected by the substitution of Lewis rats. It is possible that the lower levels of glucocorticoids produced in these animals may have resulted in elevated levels of COX-2 protein expression at 6 h, compared with that seen in Wistar rats, because COX-2 expression is inhibited by glucocorticoids, though this possibility has not been examined. However, it does highlight the differences that animal strain can have on the efficacy of a drug. This problem of strain differences becomes more important when one considers comparing data across species from rat to mouse models and, ultimately, translating concepts and findings into patients.

As has been emphasized, it is desirable to examine the role of COX isoforms throughout the different phases of inflammation rather than concentrating on the initial onset of an acute inflammatory reaction. This has been extensively investigated in the rat carrageenan pleurisy model[40], extending the observations made in the murine carrageenan air pouch model. There were two phases of COX-2 protein expression. Firstly, there was an early peak which was associated with the onset of inflammation, PMN influx and PGE_2 production *in vivo* and COX activity *ex vivo* (Figure 3a and b). This phase of the inflammatory response was inhibited by non-selective and COX-2-selective inhibitors. However, 48 h post-injection of irritant, a second much greater peak in COX-2 protein expression was seen, associated with later influx of mononuclear cells and the resolution of the inflammation. As in the carrageenan air pouch in mice previously described, this was at a time with-

Figure 3 Role of COX-2 in carrageenan pleurisy. (a) Inflammatory cell influx, exudate formation and COX-2 protein expression by Western blotting in the untreated model. (b) Profile of prostaglandin E_2, prostaglandin D_2 and prostaglandin 15-deoxy$\Delta^{12\text{-}14}$PGJ$_2$ in carrageenan pleurisy. (c) The effect of NS-398 (10 mg kg^{-1} p.o. q.i.d. from peak of inflammation) on cell number and exudate volume and concomitant replacement of prostaglandin D_2 and prostaglandin 15-deoxy$\Delta^{12\text{-}14}$PGJ$_2$. +++;*** $P < 0.001$, $n = 10$, in all cases. (From Gilroy[40].)

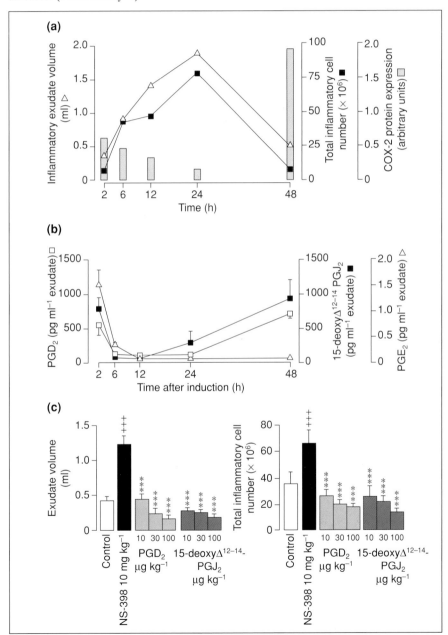

out the presence of detectable PGE_2 in the exudate or PGE_2 production *ex vivo* (Figure 3b). Treatment with the COX-2 selective inhibitors from 24 h to 48 h post-injection of irritant, i.e. during resolution, resulted in a prolongation of the inflammatory response. As it was considered that a prostanoid product of COX-2 was the most likely candidate responsible for this effect, we assayed the levels of PGD_2 and 15-deoxy$\Delta^{12-14}PGJ_2$ in the exudates, the latter PG being associated with anti-inflammatory functions in macrophages. Whilst the levels of these were initially raised, their levels fell during the onset and development of the inflammatory response but then rose again during resolution (Figure 3b). Furthermore, after treatment with the COX-2 inhibitors, their levels fell dramatically and, finally, replacement with exogenous PGD_2 and 15-deoxy$\Delta^{12-14}PGJ_2$ reversed the exacerbation of inflammation caused by these NSAIDs (Figure 3c). As a result of these findings, it may be hypothesized that COX-2 is proinflammatory during the early stages of the inflammatory response but contributes to the resolution of the inflammation by generating an alternative set of anti-inflammatory prostaglandins such as 15-deoxy$\Delta^{12-14}PGJ_2$ and other cyclopentenones. The mechanism behind this switch in prostaglandin profile is the subject of current research – perhaps it involves a switch in the prostaglandin synthases which act on PGH_2 (i.e. the reverse of the switch to PGE_2 synthesis seen in macrophages treated with TNF-α).

ANTI-INFLAMMATORY MECHANISMS AND A ROLE FOR COX-2 AND ITS PRODUCTS IN THE RESOLUTION OF INFLAMMATION

As described above in models of inflammation there is a change in PG profile during resolution, from PGE_2 at the onset of inflammation to a dominance of PGD_2 and the PGJs (which are spontaneously formed from PGD_2 in aqueous media in the presence of albumen[84]) produced via COX-2[40]. It is known that the cyclopentenone prostaglandin PGJ_2 and its metabolites are naturally occurring endogenous ligands for the peroxisome proliferator-activated receptor γ (PPARγ)[85]. The PPARs are a family of nuclear receptors which regulate lipid metabolism, glucose and energy homeostasis (see Schoonjans et al.[86]) and are the target of some hypolipidaemic and antidiabetic drugs. Currently three subclasses of PPAR have been described, PPARα, PPARβ and PPARγ. The metabolic oxidation pathways activated by PPAR ligands will metabolize lipid mediators such as PGs and leukotrienes and this has provoked interest in PPAR ligands as possible anti-inflammatory agents through the enhanced breakdown of proinflammatory eicosanoids. Thus, initial studies showed PPARα knockout mice have an exacerbated inflammatory response to arachidonic acid in the murine ear swelling assay[87]. This is a predominantly leukotriene-mediated response in which PGs play a minimal role. However, the response to 12-tetradecanoylphorbol-13-acetate (TPA) in the same model was unchanged in PPARα knockout mice; this reaction is PG mediated and involves the activation of NF-κB. In addition to these early studies *in vivo*, PPARγ ligands inhibit the production of an array of inflammatory mediators including cytokines such as TNF-α and IL-1 and pro-inflammatory PGs such as PGE_2 by activated human monocytes *in vitro*[88,89]. The suggestion was made that PPARγ activation may antagonize the DNA binding activity of NF-κB and other transcription factors of the signal transducer of activated T cells (STAT) family and activator protein-1 (AP-1)[88], which play pivotal roles in immune and inflammatory responses. In addition, we have shown that PPARγ ligands inhibit expression of inducible nitric oxide synthase (iNOS) by activated murine macrophages *in vitro*, associated with changes in expression of heme oxygenase-1 (HO-1)[90], an inducible heat shock protein which has been previously shown to be a possible endogenous anti-inflammatory enzyme system[91]. The use of an inhibitor for HO-1 revealed that at least part, but not all, of the inhibition of iNOS activity was due to HO-1-derived products. The induction of HO-1 by cyclopentenone prostaglandins has been shown to be independent of PPAR response elements[92]. This and other recent data clearly indicate that cyclopentenone PGs may have important actions independent of PPAR activation.

Peroxisome proliferator-activated receptor independent properties of cyclopentenone prostaglandins

Many of the observed pharmacological effects of PPAR agonists occur at doses far in excess of those required for the activation of the PPAR receptor. Previous studies evaluating PPARγ-dependent inhibition of macrophage activation *in vitro* indicated that 15-deoxyΔ$^{12-14}$PGJ$_2$ was significantly more effective than synthetic PPARγ ligands despite its relatively low binding affinity for PPARγ[88]. In addition, experiments with PPARγ-negative cell lines demonstrate that PGD_2 and its PGJ metabolites have modulatory effects independent of PPARγ. Thus, recent work in the PPARγ-negative HeLa cell line showed that 15-deoxyΔ$^{12-14}$PGJ$_2$ inhibits multiple steps in the proinflammatory NF-κB pathway by both PPARγ-dependent and PPARγ-independent mechanisms[93]. Treatment with 15-deoxyΔ$^{12-14}$PGJ$_2$ inhibited TPA-stimulated NF-κB activation in Hela cells in the absence of PPARγ expression. However, transfection of HeLa cells with a PPARγ expression plasmid potentiated the inhibitory effects of 15-deoxyΔ$^{12-14}$PGJ$_2$. In contrast, the synthetic PPARγ agonist BRL49653 inhibited NF-κB activation only in the presence of PPARγ expression and was less effective than 15-deoxyΔ$^{12-14}$PGJ$_2$ in this situation, an effect that has also previously been reported in murine macrophages[88]. Although less potent, these inhibitory effects of PGD_2 metabolites on proinflammatory signalling pathways were also seen with the cyclopentenone PGA_2 derived from PGE_2 metabolism but not with PPARγ agonists such as troglitazone.

This is a further indication of PPAR-independent anti-inflammatory effects of cyclopentenone PGs.

The cyclopentenone PGs are characterized by the presence of a cyclopentenone ring containing a highly reactive electrophilic carbon atom in the α,β-unsaturated carbonyl group of the cyclopentane ring. This carbon atom can react with nucleophiles, such as the free sulphhydryl groups of glutathione (GSH) and cysteine residues which form disulphides in proteins, by Michael addition reactions. Conserved cysteine residues are found in both the *trans* acting DNA-binding proteins of the NF-κB pathway and elements of the upstream kinase complex via which NF-κB activation in response to proinflammatory stimuli occurs. It has been postulated that the PPAR independent effects of the cyclopentenone PGs on the NF-κB pathway may be through the covalent modification of cysteine residues essential to the DNA binding and *trans* activation properties of NF-κB dimers and the activity of kinases which result in NF-κB activation[94].

Cyclopentenone prostaglandins, the heat shock response and inhibition of inflammation

As mentioned, in addition to the possible direct effects of these cyclopentenone PGs that could mediate the anti-inflammatory effects of COX-2 in the resolution of inflammation, many reports have shown that the cyclopentenone PGs of the A and J series induce the heat shock response in a variety of mammalian and human cell lines (reviewed by Santoro[95]). The heat shock response is a highly conserved cellular response to environmental and physiological stress and is characterized by the rapid expression of heat shock proteins (HSP). There are at least five families of HSPs classified according to their molecular weight, the best characterized of which is HSP-72 of the HSP-70 kDa family. In mammalian cells synthesis of HSPs is mediated by the inducible transcription factor heat shock factor 1 (HSF-1). The formation of non-native disulphides is a potent stimulus for HSF-1 activation and thus the modification of cysteine residues in proteins through Michael addition reactions with cyclopentenone prostaglandins may mediate the induction of HSP expression via HSF-1.

Many of the HSPs function as protein chaperones regulating protein–protein interactions during folding, transport and translocation. In recent years it has become clear that the heat shock response can involve the induction of proteins not classically defined as HSPs. This has led to the increased use of the term 'stress proteins'. The expression of a 32 kDa protein in response to heat shock (HSP-32) was later described as HO-1, the inducible form of the rate limiting enzyme in the catabolism of haem[96]. Both PGA and PGJ cyclopentenone prostaglandins induce HSP-72 and HO-1 expression in various mammalian and human cell lines[97,98] Induction of HSP-72 and HO-1 expression by cyclopentenone PGs confers protection against cytotoxic stress, such as heat[99] and viral infection[100]. In addition, similar treatments with cyclopentenone PGs inhibit expression of proinflammatory mediators and the activation of pro-inflammatory signalling pathways in human monocytes[88,89] and murine macrophages *in vitro*[90]. The inhibition of NF-κB activation by PGA$_1$ is associated with a dose-dependent increase in HSF-1 activation and the inhibitory effect is cycloheximide-sensitive, suggesting this requires *de novo* protein synthesis[101]. These data indicate that the mechanism by which the cyclopentenone PGA$_1$ inhibits NF-κB may involve the induction of HSP synthesis. Furthermore, both the induction of HSP-72 and inhibition of NF-κB are thought to contribute to the antiviral activity of cyclopentenone PGs *in vivo*[102]. Given the key position occupied by NF-κB in inflammatory processes[103], the elevations in production of these cyclopentenone prostanoids during the resolution of inflammation via COX-2 activity provides a plausible mechanism for the endogenous induction of the stress response in the latter stages of an inflammatory reaction.

Our recent work has demonstrated the expression of HSP-72 and HO-1 in leukocytes during the resolution phase of several experimental models of both immune-driven and non-immune models of acute inflammation *in vivo*. Using the rat carrageenan pleurisy model, induction of HO-1 activity attenuated inflammation, while inhibition of HO-1 activity exacerbated it[91]. These studies have now been extended to a murine model of acute inflammation, the carrageenan air pouch (T. Lawrence, unpublished observations). The resolution of inflammation in these models coincides with the induction of HSP-72 and HO-1 expression in inflammatory cells and, again, induction of HSP-72 expression with sodium arsenite or HO-1 with iron or cobalt protoporphyrin is anti-inflammatory. Furthermore, induction of the heat shock response with sodium arsenite inhibits activation of NF-κB in macrophages *in vivo* and *in vitro*, associated with the induction of HSP-72 and HO-1 expression. Work is also currently underway to examine what effect this chemical manipulation of the stress response may have on the temporal expression of COX-2 and thus whether changes in the expression of this enzyme, and hence changes in production of prostanoids, may also account for some of the observed anti-inflammatory effects.

The anti-inflammatory effects of HSP-72 and HO-1 induction, and the temporal correlation of HO-1 and HSP-72 expression with the resolution of inflammatory models *in vivo*, suggests that the heat shock response may play a role as a pathway for the resolution of inflammation. The demonstration of a possible role for cyclopentenone PGs in the resolution of inflammation, and the ability of cyclopentenone PGs to induce the heat shock response, suggests that the anti-inflammatory action of cyclopentenone prostaglandins may be mediated, at least in part, through the induction the heat shock response. The cyclopentenone PGs may thus represent endogenous pharmacological inducers of the heat shock response and this may account for their anti-inflammatory action – and places COX-2 in a pivotal role in the resolution of inflammation (Figure 4).

CYCLOOXYGENASE INHIBITORS AND THE FUTURE TREATMENT OF CHRONIC INFLAMMATORY DISEASES

The literature on the role of COX-2 in inflammation thus poses an interesting dilemma for the future development of selective inhibitors of this enzyme system. On the one hand, there is abundant evidence in experimental models and from the clinic that NSAIDs which target COX-2 are effective anti-inflammatory agents and analgesics, ameliorating the signs of acute inflammation. They have a much improved side effect profile compared with the traditional NSAIDs, which were less selective, and they thus avoid the marked morbidity, such as gastric ulceration, associated with NSAID treatment in the

Figure 4 Involvement of cyclopentenone PGs in the resolution of inflammation showing possible PPAR-dependent and independent inhibition of proinflammatory transcription factors and subsequent production of inflammatory mediators.

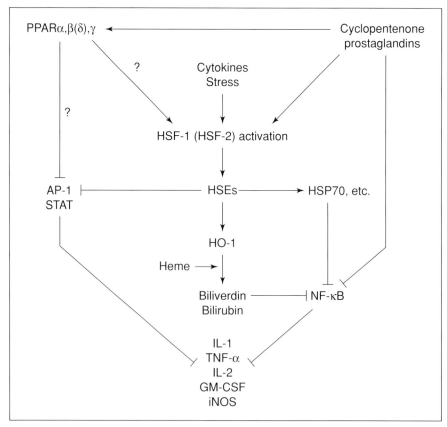

past. However, as can be seen from this review, there is evidence that COX-2 may play a role in the resolution of inflammation and that its inhibition during this phase of the inflammatory response may be less beneficial. A clue to the possible involvement of COX-2 in resolution arose from the development of COX-2 knockout mice, many of which develop spontaneous peritonitis (see Ballou[104] for overview of COX knockout mice). A number of postulates were proposed to explain this: COX-2 is not important in the generation of an inflammatory reaction; COX-2 has a role in immunity and prevention of infection; COX-2 may be important in the resolution of inflammation and tissue repair[105]. Evidence can also be found from models of gastrointestinal lesions that COX-2 may also be protective. For example in colitis models, use of the COX-2-selective L-745,337 markedly exacerbated mucosal damage, and long-term treatment was associated with death due to bowel perforation[106]. In models of gastric ulcer healing in rats, treatment of existing lesions with COX-2 inhibitors leads to a retardation of healing[37-39]. With chronic ulcers, epithelial proliferation, angiogenesis and granulation tissue development is retarded by use of COX-2 inhibitors. Whilst it is true that the non-selective inhibitors such as indomethacin share these problems, it is none the less apparent that there is room for further advances in the development of the NSAIDs.

The key to these advances may well be the nature of the COX isoform that is being expressed during the resolving stages of these model systems and whether it is actually COX-2 or another isoform entirely – a 'COX-3'[107]. Whilst not necessarily being used to denote a completely different protein, this term could perhaps be applied to this isoform responsible for the synthesis of anti-inflammatory PGs to denote its altered role compared with the enzyme responsible for prostanoid production in the acute phases of an inflammatory response (Figure 5).

There is evidence that a catalytic variant of COX-2 exists in transformed macrophages *in vitro* that have been exposed for long periods to high doses of NSAIDs[108]. Whilst this enzyme is recognized by an antibody raised against COX-2, it is far less sensitive to other NSAIDs than COX-2 induced by macrophages in response to LPS. This raises the question of demonstration and identification of proteins by antibodies. Antibodies are often raised against a relatively small epitope of the entire protein structure and it is possible that variants of that protein may share that epitope and thus be misidentified. Alternatively, the 'COX-2-like' or COX-3 protein seen during resolution may in fact be the same protein structure but have a completely different promoter system controlling its expression. This could be coupled with the change in expression of the associated synthases which govern the profile of prostanoids produced. This has been shown in macrophages following TNF-α treatment where the cells which constitutively produce PGD_2, switch to a PGE_2-producing phenotype following exposure to this cytokine, and can then be

Figure 5 A putative time course showing the involvement of COX-1, COX-2 and 'COX-3' in the generation and resolution of an inflammatory reaction. (Modified from Willoughby et al.[107].)

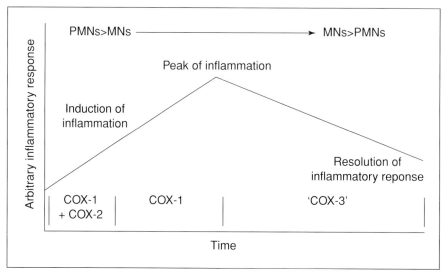

switched back[109]. Thus this could provide a simple mechanism for the findings in the carrageenan pleurisy and air pouch models, where a PGE_2-dominated acute inflammatory phase gives way to a PGD_2 dominated resolving phase has been demonstrated *in vivo*, leading to resolution. The changes in prostanoid profile during these inflammatory reactions supports such a hypothesis.

The findings presented in this chapter are from animal models, but they stress the urgent need to investigate whether these translate into the human. For example, the induction of such a system could be partly responsible for the initiation of remission which is seen in man in chronic inflammatory diseases such as RA. If this is in fact true, inhibition of this third inducible isoform by NSAIDs would not be desirable. On the contrary, a completely new form of therapy could be the induction of this isoform of COX-2 producing anti-inflammatory cyclopentenone PGs (see below). Thus, there would be a need to try to determine reliable markers of disease activity, such that when this isoform is functioning, i.e. in remission, alternative treatment modalities are used to avoid inhibiting an endogenous anti-inflammatory system. However, in the meantime, this could have a profound effect on prescribing habits for all classes of COX inhibitors, be they selective for COX-2 or non-selective inhibitors of both COX isoforms. Indeed, perhaps the reason for the failure of NSAIDs to affect disease progression in man significantly[110], unlike the situation in rodent models, may be the inhibition of resolution in periods of disease remission, because NSAIDs are traditionally in continuous use. The preliminary data from models of joint destruction in animals described above further indicate that COX-2 selective drugs may, in addition to their gastrointestinal sparing properties, also have a less damaging effect on cartilage. Thus the use of COX-2 selective NSAIDs, and improved targeting of these and even conventional therapy, may improve the clinical efficacy of this important family of anti-inflammatory agents in diseases such as RA, and other relapsing and remitting diseases such as MS.

The existence of such mechanisms, and perhaps of a COX-3 with an altered catalytic profile, suggests a number of potential avenues for therapeutic intervention. Perhaps the next generation of 'super-aspirins' may be able to differentiate further between COX-2 and COX-3? In addition, it may be possible to exploit the pathways behind the induction of this third COX iso-form and, if these isoforms are indeed the same protein, to induce a switch in the prostaglandin synthases to increase selectively the production of PGD_2 and its cyclopentenone derivatives. These products themselves may also offer opportunities for the development of novel anti-inflammatory agents in their own right. The answers to these questions and the exploration of the thera-peutic possibilities posed by current research into the role of the COX family of enzymes and its products are eagerly awaited.

Address all correspondence to: Derek Willoughby, Department of Experimental Pathology, William Harvey Research Institute, St Bartholomew's and Royal London School of Medicine and Dentistry, Charterhouse Square, London EC1M 6BQ, UK.

REFERENCES

1. Vane JR, Botting RM. The prostaglandins. In: Vane JR, Botting RM, editors. *Aspirin and Other Salicylates*. London: Chapman & Hall Medical. 1992;17–34.
2. Von Euler, US. Some aspects of the actions of prostaglandins. The First Hyemans Memorial Lecture. *Arch Int Pharmacodyn Ther.* 1973;202(Suppl):295–307.
3. Bergström S, Danielsson H, Sjövall J. The enzymatic formation of prostaglandin E_2 from arachidonic acid: prostaglandins and related factors. *Biochim Biophys Acta.* 1964;90:207–10.
4. Van Dorp DAA, Beerthuis RK, Nugteren DH, Vonkeman H. The biosynthesis of prostaglandins. *Biochim Biophys Acta.* 1964;90:204–7.
5. Di Rosa M, Giroud JP, Willoughby DA. Studies on the mediators of the acute inflammatory response induced in rats in different sites by carrageenan and turpentine. *J Path.* 1971;104:15–29.
6. Kaley G, Weiner R. Microcircultory studies with PGE_1. In: Ramwell PW, Shaw JE, editors. *Prostaglandin Symposium, Worcester Foundation for Experimental Biology.* New York: J. Wiley and Sons. 1968:321–28.
7. Williams TJ, Peck MJ. Role of prostaglandin-mediated vasodilatation in inflam-mation. *Nature.* 1977;270:530–32.
8. Ferreira SH. Prostaglandins, aspirin-like drugs and analgesia. *Nature New Biol.* 1972;240:200–3.

9. Milton AS, Wendlandt S. A possible role for PGE_1 as a modulator for temperature regulation in the central nervous system of the cat. *J Physiol.* 1970;207:76–7.

10. Webb DR, Osheroff PL. Antigen stimulation of prostaglandin synthesis and control of immune responses. *Proc Natl Acad Sci USA.* 1976;73:1300–4.

11. Goodwin JS, Messner RP, Peake GT. Prostaglandin suppression of mitogen-stimulated lymphocytes *in vitro.* Changes with mitogen dose and preincubation. *J Clin Invest.* 1978;62:753–60.

12. Van Epps DE. Suppression of human lymphocyte migration by PGE_2. *Inflammation.* 1981;5:81–7.

13. Meerpohl HG, Bauknecht T. Role of prostaglandins on the regulation of macrophage proliferation and cytotoxic functions. *Prostaglandins.* 1986;31:961–72.

14. Betz M, Fox BS. Prostaglandin E_2 inhibits production of Th1 lymphokines but not of Th2 lymphokines. *J Immunol.* 1991;146:108–13.

15. Kunkel SL, Spengler M, May MA, Spengler R, Larrick J, Remick D. Prostaglandin E_2 regulates macrophge-derived tumor necrosis factor gene expression. *J Biol Chem.* 1988;263:5380–4.

16. Goodwin JS, Ceuppens JL. Effect of non-steroidal anti-inflammatory drugs on immune function. *Semin Arthritis Rheum.* 1983;13:134–43.

17. Subbaramaiah K, Zakim D, Weksler BB, Dannenberg AJ. Inhibition of cyclooxygenase: novel approach to cancer prevention. *Proc Soc Exp Biol Med.* 1997;216:201–10.

18. DuBois RN. Cyclooxygenase-2: a target for prevention of colorectal cancer. In: Vane JR, Botting RM, editors. *Therapeutic roles of selective COX-2 inhibitors.* London: William Harvey Press. 2001;410–17.

19. Velo GP, Dunn CJ, Giroud JP, Timsit J, Willoughby DA. Distribution of prostaglandins in inflammatory exudate. *J Path.* 1973;111:149–58.

20. Capasso F, Dunn CJ, Yamamoto S, Willoughby DA, Giroud JP. Further studies on carrageenan-induced pleurisy in rats. *J Path.* 1975;116:117–24.

21. Capasso F, Dunn CJ, Yamamoto S, Deporter DA, Giroud JP, Willoughby DA. Pharmacological mediators of various immunological and non-immunological inflammatory reactions produced in the pleural cavity. *Agents Actions.* 1975;5:528–33.

22. Willoughby DA. Effects of prostaglandins $PGF_{2\alpha}$ and PGE_1 on vascular permeability. *J Path Bacteriol.* 1968;96:381–7.

23. Willoughby DA. The Heberden Oration, 1974. Human arthritis applied to animal models. Towards a better therapy. *Ann Rheum Dis.* 1975;34:471–8.

24. Harris R. Cyclooxygenase-2 in the kidney. In: Vane JR, Botting RM, editors. *Therapeutic roles of selective COX-2 inhibitors.* London: William Harvey Press. 2001;206–20.

25. Whittle BJR. Basis of gastrointestinal toxicity of non-steroid anti-inflammatory drugs. In: Vane JR, Botting RM, editors. *Therapeutic roles of selective COX-2 inhibitors.* London: William Harvey Press. 2001;329–54.

26. Hawkey CJ. Gastrointestinal toxicity of non-steroid anti-inflammatory drugs. In: Vane JR, Botting RM, editors. *Therapeutic roles of selective COX-2 inhibitors.* London: William Harvey Press. 2001;355–94.

27. Rodríguez LA García, Hernándex-Diáz S. Epidemiology of upper gastrointestinal side effects of non-steroid anti-inflammatory drugs. In: Vane JR, Botting RM, editors. *Therapeutic roles of selective COX-2 inhibitors.* London: William Harvey Press. 2001;394–409.

28. Vane JR, Botting RM. Formation and actions of prostaglandins and inhibition of their

synthesis. In: Vane JR, Botting RM, editors. *Therapeutic roles of selective COX-2 inhibitors.* London: William Harvey Press. 2001;1–47.

29. Vane JR. Inhibition of prostaglandin synthesis as a mechanism of action for aspirin-like drugs. *Nature New Biol.* 1971;231:232–5.

30. Xie W, Chipman JG, Robertson DL, Erikson RL, Simmons DL. Expression of a mitogen-responsive gene encoding prostaglandin synthase is regulated by mRNA splicing. *Proc Natl Acad Sci USA.* 1991;88:1692–6.

31. Vane JR. Towards a better aspirin. *Nature.* 1994;367:215–6.

32. Gans KR, Gailbraith W, Roman RJ, Haber SB, Kerr JS, Schmidt WK et al. Anti-inflammatory and safety profile of DuP697, a novel orally effective prostaglandin synthase inhibitor. *J Pharmacol Exp Ther.* 1990;254:180–7.

33. Futaki N, Yoshikawa K, Hamasaka Y, Arai I, Higuchi S, Iizuka H et al. NS-398, a novel non-steroidal anti-inflammatory drug with potent analgesic and anti-pyretic effects, which causes minimal stomach lesions. *Gen Pharmacol.* 1993;24:105–10.

34. Riendeau D, Percival MD, Boyce S, Brideau C, Charleson S, Cromlish W et al. *Br J Pharmacol.* 1997;121:105–17.

35. Lefkowith JB, Verburg KM, Geis GS. Clinical experience with celecoxib: a cyclooxygenase-2 specific inhibitor. In: Vane JR, Botting RM, editors. *Therapeutic roles of selective COX-2 inhibitors.* London: William Harvey Press. 2001;461–81.

36. Prasit P, Riendeau D, Chan CC. Discovery of Vioxx® (rofecoxib). In: Vane JR, Botting RM, editors. *Therapeutic roles of selective COX-2 inhibitors.* London: William Harvey Press. 2001;60–75.

37. Mizuno H, Sakamoto C, Matsuda K, Wada K, Uchida T, Noguchi H et al. Induction of cyclooxygenase 2 in gastric mucosal lesions and its inhibition by specific antagonist delays healing in mice. *Gastroenterology.* 1997;112:387–97.

38. Shigeta JI, Takahashi S, Okabe S. Role of cyclooxygenase 2 in the healing of gastric ulcers in rats. *J Pharmacol Exp Ther.* 1998;286:1383–90.

39. Schmassmann A, Peskar BM, Stettler C, Netzer P, Stroff T, Flogerzi B et al. Effects of inhibition of prostaglandin endoperoxide synthase-2 in chronic gastrointestinal ulcer models in rats. *Br J Pharmacol.* 1998;123:795–804.

40. Gilroy DW, Colville-Nash PR, Willis D, Chivers J, Paul-Clark MJ, Willoughby DA. Inducible cyclooxygenase may have anti-inflammatory properties. *Nature Med.* 1999;5:698–701.

41. Selye H. On the mechanism through which hydrocortisone affects the resistance of tissue to injury. *J Am Med Assoc.* 1953;152:1207–13.

42. Edwards JCW, Sedgwick AD, Willoughby DA. The formation of a structure with the features of synovial lining by subcutaneous injection of air: an *in vivo* tissue culture system. *J Path.* 1981;134:147–56.

43. Howat DW, Colville-Nash PR, Moore AR, Desa FM, Chander CL, Willoughby DA. A cytochemical study of the adjuvant inflamed air pouch in the rat. *Int J Tiss React.* 1989;11:219–23.

44. Bottomley KM, Griffiths RJ, Rising TJ, Steward A. A modified mouse air pouch model for evaluating the effects of compounds on granuloma induced cartilage degradation. *Br J Pharmacol.* 1988;93:627–35.

45. Colville-Nash PR, Alam CAS, Appleton I, Brown JR, Seed MP, Willoughby DA. The pharmacological modulation of angiogenesis in chronic granulomatous inflammation. *J Pharmacol Exp Ther.* 1995;274:1463–72.

46. Appleton I, Tomlinson A, Colville-Nash PR, Willoughby DA. Temporal and

spatial immunolocalisation of cytokines in murine chronic granulomatous tissue. *Lab Invest.* 1993;69:405–14.

47. Vane JR, Mitchell JA, Appleton I, Tomlinson A, Bishop-Bailey D, Croxtall J et al. Inducible isoforms of cyclooxygenase and nitric oxide synthase in inflammation. *Proc Natl Acad Sci USA.* 1994;91:2046–50.

48. Appleton I, Tomlinson A, Mitchell JA, Willoughby DA. Distribution of cyclooxygenase isoforms in murine chronic granulomatous inflammation. Implications for future anti-inflammatory therapy. *J Path.* 1995;176:413–20.

49. Herschmann HR, Gilbert RS, Xie W, Luner S, Reddy S. Regulation and role of TIS10/PGS2. *Adv Prost Thromb Leukot Res.* 1995;23:23–8.

50. Roberts AB, Sporn MB, Assoian RK, Smith JM, Roche NS, Wakefield LM, Transforming growth factor beta: rapid induction of fibrosis and angiogenesis *in vivo* and stimulation of collagen formation *in vitro. Proc Natl Acad Sci USA.* 1986;83:4167–71.

51. Barile F, Ripley-Rouzier C, Siddiqi ZE, Bienkowski, RS. Effects of PGE₁ on collagen production and degradation in human fetal lung fibroblasts. *Arch Biochim Biophys.* 1988;265;441–6.

52. Gilroy DW, Tomlinson A, Willoughby DA. Differential effects of inhibition of isoforms of cyclooxygenase (COX-1, COX-2) in chronic inflammation. *Inflamm Res.* 1998;47:79–85.

53. Tavares IA, Bishai PM, Bennett A. Activity of nimesulide on constitutive and inducible cyclooxygenases. *Arzneimittel-Forschung* 1995;45:1093–5.

54. Lu X, Xie W, Reed D, Bradshaw WS, Simmons DL. Non-steroidal anti- inflammatory drugs cause apoptosis and induce cyclooxygenases in chicken embryo fibroblasts. *Proc Natl Acad Sci USA.* 1995;92:7961–5.

55. Rufer C, Schillinger E, Bottcher I, Repenthim W, Hermann C. Non-steroidal anti-inflammatories. XII. Mode of action of anti-inflammatory methane sulphonilides. *Biochem Pharmacol.* 1982;31:3591–6.

56. Silverman KJ, Lund DP, Zetter BR, Lainey LL, Shahood JA, Freiman DG et al. Angiogenic activity of adipose tissue. *Biochem Biophys Res Commun.* 1988;153:347–52.

57. Ben-Av P, Crofford LJ, Wilder RL, Hla T. Induction of vascular endothelial growth factor expression in synovial fibroblasts by prostaglandin E and interleukin-1: a potential mechanism for inflammatory angiogenesis. *FEBS Letts.* 1995;372:83–7.

58. Billingham MEJ. Models of arthritis and the search for anti-rheumatic drugs. *J Pharmacol Ther.* 1983;21:389–428.

59. Sano H, Hla T, Maier JA, Crofford LJ, Case JP, Maciag T et al. *In vivo* cyclooxygenase expression in synovial tissues of patients with rheumatoid arthritis and osteoarthritis and rats with adjuvant and streptococcal cell wall arthritis. *J Clin Invest.* 1992;89:97–108.

60. Anderson GD, Hauser SD, McGarity KL, Bremer ME, Isakson PC, Gregory SA. Selective inhibition of cyclooxygenase (COX)-2 reverses inflammation and expression of COX-2 and interleukin 6 in rat adjuvant arthritis. *J Clin Invest.* 1996;97:2672–9.

61. Seed MP, Parker FL, Johns S, Curnock AP, Bowden A, Gardner CR. Mycobacterium tuberculosis-induced monoarticular arthritis in the rat, a new *in vivo* model for the assessment of anti-rheumatic drugs. *Clin Rheum.* 1991;10:461–2.

62. Gilroy DW, Tomlinson A, Greenslade K, Seed MP, Willoughby DA. The effects of cyclooxygenase 2 inhibitors on cartilage erosion and bone loss in a model of

mycobacterium tuberculosis-induced monoarticular arthritis in the rat. *Inflammation.* 1998;22:509–19.

63. Yamamoto S, Dunn CJ, Deporter DA, Capasso F, Willoughby DA, Huskisson EC. A model for the quantitative study of Arthus (immunologic) hypersensitivity in rats. *Agents Actions.* 1975;5:374–7.

64. Moore AR, Willis D, Gilroy D, Tomlinson A, Appleton I, Willoughby DA. Cyclooxygenase in rat pleural hypersensitivity reactions. *Adv Prost Thromb Leuk Res.* 1995;23:349–51.

65. Raud J, Dahlen SE, Sydbom A, Lindbom L, Hedqvist P. Prostaglandins modulation of mast cell-dependent inflammation. *Agents Actions.* 1989;26:42–4.

66. Bandeiro-Melo C, Singh Y, Cordeiro RB, e Silva PMR, Martins M. Involvement of prostaglandins in the down-regulation of allergic plasma leakage observed in rats undergoing pleural eosinophilia. *Br J Pharmacol.* 1996;118:2192–8.

67. Willis D, Moore AR, Willoughby DA. Heme oxygenase isoform expression in cellular and anti-body mediated models of acute inflammation in the rat. *J Path.* 2000;190:627–34.

68. Niki H, Tominga Y, Watanabe-Kobayashi M, Mue S, Ohuchi K. Possible participation of cyclooxygenase-2 in the recurrence of allergic inflammation in the rat. *Eur J Pharmacol.* 1997;320:193–200.

69. Winter CA, Risley EA, Nuss GW. Carrageenan induced edema in the hind paw of the rat as an assay for anti-inflammatory drugs. *Proc Soc Exp Biol Med.* 1962;111:544–52.

70. Seibert K, Zhang Y, Leahy K, Huser S, Masferrer J, Perkins W et al. Pharmacological and biochemical demonstration of the role of cyclooxygenase 2 in inflammation and pain. *Proc Natl Acad Sci USA.* 1994;91:12013–7.

71. Chan CC, Boyce S, Brideau C, Ford-Hutchinson AW, Gordon R, Guay D et al. Pharmacology of a selective cyclooxygenase-2 inhibitor, L-745,337: a novel non-steroidal anti-inflammatory agent with an ulcerogenic-sparing effect in rat and non-human primate stomach. *J Pharmacol Exp Ther.* 1995;274:1531–7.

72. Chan CC, Boyce S, Brideau C, Charleson S, Cromlish W, Ethier D et al. Rofecoxib [Vioxx, MK-0966; 4-(4(-methylsulfonylphenyl)-3-phenyl-2-(5H)-furanone]: a potent and orally active cyclooxygenase-2 inhibitor. Pharmacological and biochemical profiles. *J Pharmacol Exp Ther.* 1999;290:551–60.

73. Wallace JL, Bak A, McKnight W, Asfaha S, Sharkey K, MacNaughton WK. Cyclooxygenase 1 contributes to inflammatory responses in rats and mice: implications for gastrointestinal toxicity. *Gastroenterology.* 1998;115:101–9.

74. Langenbach R, Morham SG, Tiano HF, Loftin CD, Ghanayem BI, Chulada PC et al. Prostaglandin synthase 1 gene disruption in mice reduces arachidonic acid-induced inflammation and indomethacin-induced gastric ulceration. *Cell.* 1995;83;483–92.

75. Dinchuk JE, Car BD, Focht RJ, Johnston JJ, Jaffee BD, Covington MB et al. Renal abnormalities and an altered inflammatory response in mice lacking cyclooxygenase II. *Nature.* 1995;378:406–9

76. Smith CJ, Zhang Y, Koboldt CM, Muhammed J, Zweiffel BS, Shaffer A et al. Pharmacological analysis of cyclooxygenase 1 in inflammation. *Proc Natl Acad Sci USA.* 1998;95:13313–8.

77. Masferrer JL, Zweifel BS, Manning PT, Hauser SD, Leahy KM, Smith WG et al. Selective inhibition of inducible cyclooxygenase 2 *in vivo* is anti-inflammatory and nonulcerogenic. *Proc Natl Acad Sci USA.* 1994;91:3228–32.

78. Mackay AR, Sedgwick AD, Dunn CJ, Fleming WE, Willoughby DA. The transition from acute to chronic inflammation. *Br J Dermatol.* 1985;113(Suppl2):34–40.

79. Dawson J, Sedgwick AD, Edwards JCW, Lees P. A comparative study of the cellular, exudative and histological responses to carrageenan, dextran and zymosan in the mouse. *Int J Tiss Reac.* 1991;13:171–85.

80. Tomlinson A, Appleton I, Moore AR, Gilroy DW, Willis D, Mitchell JA et al. Cyclooxygenase and nitric oxide synthase isoforms in rat carrageenin-induced pleurisy. *Br J Pharmacol.* 1994;113:693–8.

81. Gilroy DW, Tomlinson A, Willoughby DA. Differential effects of inhibitors of cyclooxygenase (cyclooxygenase 1 and cyclooxygenase 2) in acute inflammation. *Eur J Pharmacol.* 1998;355:211–7.

82. Lee TH, Israel E, Drzen JM, Leitch G, Ravalese J, Corey EJ et al. Enhancement of plasma levels of biologically active leukotriene B compounds during anaphylaxis in guinea pigs pretreated by indomethacin or by a fish oil enriched diet. *J Immunol.* 1986;136:2575–82.

83. Langenbach R, Chulada PC, Lee C, Morham SG, Tino HF. Inflammatory responses in cyclooxygenase 1 and cyclooxygense 2 deficient mice. *J Leukocyte Biol.* 1996;(Suppl.15): Abs 11.

84. Mahmud I, Smith DL, Whyte MA, Nelson JT, Cho D, Tokes LG et al. On the identification and biological properties of prostaglandin J_2. *Prost Leuk Med.* 1984;16:131–46.

85. Forman BM, Tontonez P, Chen J, Brun RP, Spiegelman BM, Evans RM. 15-DeoxyΔ^{12-14}prostaglandinJ_2 is a ligand for the adipocyte determination factor PPARγ. *Cell.* 1995;83:803–12.

86. Schoonjans K Staels B, Auwerx J. The peroxisome proliferator-activated receptors (PPARs) and their effects on lipid metabolism and adipocyte differentiation. *Biochim Biophys Acta* 1996;1302:93–109.

87. Devchand PR, Keller H, Peters JM, Vazquez M, Gonalez FJ, Whli W. The PPARα-leukotriene pathway to inflammation control. *Nature.* 1996;384:39–42.

88. Ricote M, Li AC, Willson TM, Kelly CJ, Glass CK. The peroxisome proliferator activated receptor γ is a negative regulator of macrophage activation. *Nature.* 1998;391:79–82.

89. Jiang C, Ting AT, Seed B. PPAR γ agonists inhibit production of monocyte inflammatory cytokines. *Nature.* 1998;391:82–6.

90. Colville-Nash PR, Qureshi SS, Willis D, Willoughby DA. Inhibition of inducible nitric oxide synthase by peroxisome proliferator-activated receptor agonists: correlation with induction of heme oxygenase 1. *J Immunol.* 1998;161:978–84.

91. Willis D, Moore R, Frederick R, Willoughby DA. Heme oxygenase: a novel target for the modulation of the inflammatory response. *Nature Med.* 1996;2:87–90.

92. Koizumi T, Odani N, Okuyam T, Ichikaw A, Negishi M. Identification of a *cis*-regulatory element for Δ^{12}prostaglandin J_2-induced expression of the rat heme oxygenase gene. *J Biol Chem.* 1995;270:21779–84.

93. Straus DS, Pascual G, Li M, Welch JS, Ricote M, Hsiang C-H et al. 15-deoxy-Δ^{12-14}-prostaglandin J_2 inhibits multiple steps in the NFκB signalling pathway. *Proc Natl Acad Sci USA.* 2000;97:4844–9.

94. Rossi A, Kapahi P, Natoli G, Takahashi T, Chen Y, Karin M et al. Anti-inflammatory cyclopentenone prostaglandins are direct inhibitors of IκB kinase. *Nature.* 2000;403:103–8.

95. Santoro MG. Heat shock factors and the control of the stress response. *Biochem Pharmacol.* 2000;59:55–63.

96. Taketani S, Kohno H, Yoshinaga T, Tokunaga, R. Induction of heme oxygenase in rat hepatoma cells by exposure to heavy metals and hyperthermia. *Biochem Int.* 1988;17:665–72.

97. Elia G, Polla B, Rossi A, Santoro MG. Induction of ferritin and heat shock proteins by prostaglandin A_1 in human monocytes. Evidence for transcriptional and post-transcriptional regulation. *Eur J Biochem.* 1997;264:736–45.

98. Koizumi T, Yamauchi R, Irie A, Negishi M, Ichikawa A. Induction of a 31 000 dalton stress protein by prostaglandins D_2 and J_2 in porcine aortic endothelial cells. *Biochem Pharmacol.* 1991;42:777–85.

99. Amici C, Palmara AT, Santoro MG. Induction of thermotolerance by prostaglandin A in human cells. *Exp Cell Res.* 1993;207:230–4.

100. De Marco A, Carattoli A, Rozero C, Fortini D, Giorgi C, Belardo G et al. Induction of the heat shock response by antiviral prostaglandins in human cells infected with human immunodeficiency virus type 1. *Eur J Biochem.* 1998;256:334–41.

101. Rossi A, Elia G, Santoro MG. Inhibition of nuclear factor-κB by prostaglandin A_1: an effect associated with heat shock transcription factor activation. *Proc Natl Acad Sci USA.* 1997;94:746–50.

102. Santoro MG. Antiviral activity of cyclopentenone prostanoids. *Trends Microbiol.* 1997;5:276–81.

103. Barnes PJ, Karin M. Nuclear factor-kB: a pivotal transcription factor in chronic inflammatory diseases. *N Engl J Med.* 1997;336:1066–71.

104. Ballou LR, Blatteis CM, Ragow R. Elucidation of the pathophysiological functions of prostaglandins using cyclooxygenase gene deficient mice. In: Vane JR, Botting RM, editors. *Therapeutic roles of selective COX-2 inhibitors.* London: William Harvey Press. 2001;128–67.

105. De Witt D, Smith WL. Yes, but do they still get headaches? *Cell* 1995;83:473–82.

106. Reuter BK, Asfaha S, Buret A, Sharkey KA, Wallace JL. Exacerbation of inflammation-associated colonic injury in rat through inhibition of cyclooxygenase-2. *J Clin Invest.* 1996;98:2076–85.

107. Willoughby DA, Moore AR, Colville-Nash PR. COX-1, COX-2, and COX-3 and the future treatment of chronic inflammatory disease. *Lancet* 2000;355:646–48.

108. Simmons DL, Botting RM, Robertson PM, Madsen ML, Vane JR. Induction of an acetaminophen-sensitive cyclooxygenase with reduced sensitivity to non-steroid anti-inflammatory drugs. *Proc Natl Acad Sci USA.* 1999;96:3275–80.

109. Fournier T, Fadok V, Henson PM. Tumor necrosis factor-alpha inversely regulates prostaglandin D_2 and prostaglandin E_2 production in murine macrophages. *J Biol Chem.* 1997;272:31065–72.

110. Rashad S, Revell P, Hemingway A, Low F, Rainsford K, Walker F. Effect of non-steroidal anti-inflammatory drugs on the course of osteoarthritis. *Lancet* 1989;ii:519–22.

6 | Elucidation of the pathophysiological functions of prostaglandins using cyclooxygenase gene deficient mice

LESLIE R. BALLOU,[1,2,4] CLARK M. BLATTEIS[5] AND RAJENDRA RAGHOW[1,2,3]

[1]The Department of Veterans Affairs Medical Center, Memphis, TN 38104 and The Departments of [2]Medicine, [3]Pharmacology, [4]Molecular Sciences, [5]Physiology and Biophysics, The University of Tennessee Health Science Center, Memphis, TN 38163, USA.

The quest for developing optimal ways to study human diseases, and the burgeoning programmes aimed at testing experimental drugs *in vivo*, have created an unprecedented demand for laboratory animals that may be best suited for these purposes. As a result, the once lowly laboratory mouse, *Mus musculus*, has emerged as one of the most frequently used animals in contemporary biomedical research. The rise of the mouse as a pre-eminent experimental animal in biomedicine is due to a number of key attributes of its biology, as was recently described in a comprehensive review[1]. These include:

1. the availability of highly inbred, genetically defined strains;
2. a wealth of genetic data obtained via systematic breeding and selection, and information on the pedigrees of numerous well-defined mutants;
3. rapidly accumulating genomic sequences and their chromosomal organization;
4. superb fecundity; and
5. low cost of breeding and maintaining a mouse colony.

Above all, the mouse is endowed with another major advantage, resulting from our ability to alter precisely its genome during embryogenesis. Thus, a combination of methods of reverse genetics and embryo manipulation allow us to express or extinguish gene(s) in transgenic mice without the ethical concerns associated with similar experiments in humans. It is theoretically possible to alter any one of about 50 000 murine genes by transgenic technology and elucidate functional consequences of such changes *in vivo*. Since most of the murine genes have structural and functional homologues in the human genome, such experimental manipulations invariably reveal key insights into human pathophysiology[1].

Conversion of arachidonic acid (AA) to prostaglandin H_2 (PGH_2), the committed step in prostanoid biosynthesis, is mediated by two cyclooxygenase (COX) isoforms, COX-1 and COX-2, which are encoded by two unique genes, located on chromosomes 2 and 1, respectively[2,3]. Generally, while COX-1 is constitutively expressed, the expression of COX-2 is highly inducible[3,4]. Based on their respective modes of expression and selective inhibition of the two isozymes by drugs, 'constitutive' COX-1 was primarily thought to be involved in cellular homeostasis while 'inducible' COX-2 gene expression played a major role in inflammation and mitogenesis. However, prior to the availability of COX-1$^{-/-}$ and COX-2$^{-/-}$ mice, the precise contributions of the two COX genes to various pathophysiological processes had been difficult to assess. In this chapter, we will discuss the use of mice in which one or the other of the COX genes has been genetically ablated. Such genetically altered strains of mice have proved to be invaluable in deciphering the distinct biological roles of COX-1 and COX-2. The analysis of COX isozyme-deficient mice has uncovered specific roles for the prostaglandins (PGs) generated via the two COX isoforms in development, renal pathophysiology, reproduction, carcinogenesis, gastric ulceration, immune and inflammatory responses, the regulation of body temperature and nociception (Figure 1). There is mounting evidence to indicate that, in addition to the unique phenotypic consequences of COX-1 and COX-2-deficiency, COX gene ablation results in the compensatory upregulation of genes involved in eicosanoid biosynthesis and mobilization of AA[5,6]. Although we fully appreciate that the targeted ablation of many other genes (e.g. eicosanoid receptors, phospholipases and lipoxygenases) have enormously enhanced our understanding of eicosanoid biosynthesis and signalling pathways[7], a detailed discussion of these studies is beyond the scope of this chapter.

The data obtained from COX-deficient mice clearly indicate that the PGs produced by COX-1 or COX-2 can simultaneously elicit distinct as well as overlapping actions. These observations challenge the generally accepted concept that COX-1 is involved primarily in homeostatic/housekeeping functions while expression of COX-2 uniquely modulates inflammatory reactions. It appears more likely that both COX-1 and COX-2 are involved in homeostasis as well as in the inflammatory responses to specific stimuli. In fact, it could be argued that the basic effects of COX-1 and COX-2-deficiency on the

Figure 1 The phenotypic effects of COX deficiency. Based on experimental observations of COX isozyme-deficient mice, a number of unique as well as overlapping functions may be ascribed to COX-1 and COX-2. The tissue-restricted transcription and translation of the two COX isozymes, and the phospholipases that may be functionally coupled to COX-1 and COX-2, as well as signaling via specific cell-surface and nuclear (PPAR) receptors, play significant roles in regulating the functions of prostanoids.

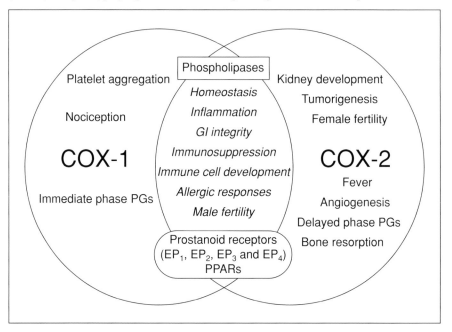

mouse phenotype might better support the opposite conclusion, since the ablation of the COX-2 gene manifests itself more profoundly than the ablation of the COX-1 gene.

PG biosynthesis is initiated by the phospholipase A_2 (PLA_2)-mediated release of membrane-associated arachidonic acid (AA) and subsequent conversion of AA to PGs by successive cyclooxygenase, hydroperoxidase and isomerase activities, respectively[3,4,8,9]. Although cytosolic phospholipase A_2 ($cPLA_2$) is primarily responsible for agonist-induced AA release from membrane phospholipids[10,11], secretory PLA_2 ($sPLA_2$) may also regulate AA availability via transcellular mechanisms[12]. PGs function as modulators of tissue homeostasis and their aberrant regulation can result in serious pathophysiological consequences[3,4,8]. The binding of PGs to either seven-transmembrane G-protein-coupled receptors or members of the nuclear peroxisomal proliferator-activated receptor (PPAR) family mediate their diverse actions[7].

The rate-limiting step in the biosynthesis of PGs, conversion of AA to PGH_2, is catalysed by COX-1 and COX-2. Although, historically, COX-1 is considered to be a constitutively expressed gene, recent evidence indicates that COX-1 can be induced under certain circumstances[13,14]. Furthermore, contrary to the generally accepted paradigm, COX-2 is constitutively expressed in the brain[15] and kidney[16]. Since, compared with COX-1-ablated mice, COX-2-deficient animals exhibit more serious abnormalities, the 'housekeeping' role attributed to COX-1 needs to be reconsidered[17-19].

Mechanistic interactions of PGs with their specific cellular targets are far from simple, however. In some cells the subcellular compartmentalization of the COX isoforms may play a critical role in determining their biological functions, as is the case for kidney and cells of the immune system[20-23]. On the other hand, in human umbilical vein endothelial cells (HUVECs) both COX-1 and COX-2 are equally distributed on the luminal surface of the endoplasmic reticulum (ER) but are freely diffusible among the ER and the inner and outer membranes of the nuclear envelope[24]. However, even in cells that show no discernible compartmentalization, the two COX isoforms still appear to function independently. The potential mechanisms may include the functional coupling of the COX isoforms to distinct phospholipase(s)[25-27] or differences in the kinetics of AA utilization by COX-1 and COX-2[24].

The non-steroid anti-inflammatory drugs (NSAIDs) act by inhibiting the cyclooxygenase activity of COX-1 and COX-2, thereby blocking their ability to convert AA to PGG_2[28,29]. In addition to their use as analgesics and for alleviation of acute and chronic inflammation, NSAIDs have proven effective in decreasing the frequency of heart attacks and strokes[28,30,31], and in reducing the incidence of colon cancer[32,33]. However, while the use of COX-1 or COX-2 selective NSAIDs has become widespread, some recent data suggest that NSAIDs have pharmacological activities independent of their abilities to inhibit COX activity[34].

A SYNOPSIS OF THE PHENOTYPIC MANIFESTATIONS OF CYCLOOXYGENASE DEFICIENCY IN MICE

In 1995, two groups independently ablated the genes encoding COX-1[35] and COX-2[36,37]. Homologous recombination techniques were used to produce mice that lacked the appropriately sized mRNA and corresponding COX-1 or COX-2 protein, while the heterozygotes expressed 50%-reduced levels of COX mRNA and protein compared with wild-type (WT) mice[35,36]. Even though these mice appeared generally normal, the heterozygous COX-deficient mice exhibited intermediate responses to some stimuli when compared with homozygous COX-deficient mice. Based upon the initial analysis it was reported that there was no apparent compensatory expression of the remaining COX isoform in COX-1- or COX-2-deficient mice. However, in the strictest sense, the ability of COX-deficient mice to overcome the effects of the missing COX isoform and to live relatively normal lives suggests compensatory PG biosynthesis (see below).

It is rather extraordinary that the phenotype of the COX-1$^{-/-}$ mouse is quite normal in the face of the complete absence of the 'housekeeping' PGs synthesized via the action of COX-1. Thus, the phenotype of the COX-1$^{-/-}$ mouse clearly calls in question the generally accepted 'housekeeping' role for COX-1. A complete absence of gastrointestinal and kidney pathology in COX-1$^{-/-}$ mice was particularly revealing, since COX-1-mediated PG biosynthesis has long been considered to be pivotal in the homeostasis of both of these organs[17–19,30,38,39].

As might be expected, platelet aggregation was found to be impaired in COX-1$^{-/-}$ mice[35]. While COX-1$^{-/-}$ males are fertile, COX-1$^{-/-}$ females exhibited parturition deficiency[40]. Surprisingly, however, COX-1$^{-/-}$ mice are born in normal numbers. The apparent normality of COX-1$^{-/-}$ animals derived from such matings is surprising, since the amount of PGs produced in most of their tissues is greatly reduced[35]. These findings indicate that the loss of constitutive PG production via COX-1 has little effect on normal murine physiology and requires that the notion that COX-1 mediates housekeeping functions needs to be revised. Clearly, compensatory pathways that can perform the necessary housekeeping functions of COX-1 maintain the normal phenotype, with a few notable exceptions (see below).

In contrast to the normal phenotype of mice lacking the COX-1 gene, mice lacking the COX-2 gene exhibit profound phenotypic consequences. Morham et al. originally reported that COX-2$^{-/-}$ mice of the 129 Ola/C57Bl/6 background are produced in normal ratios from heterozygous matings[36]. However, only 60% of the COX-2$^{-/-}$ pups survived to weaning; only three-quarters of the initial survivors lived for 1 year. Although the cause of death of the COX-2$^{-/-}$ pups prior to 3 weeks remained unknown, the older mice died mainly due to either peritonitis or kidney failure[36]. The renal phenotype of COX-2$^{-/-}$ mice was independently corroborated by Dinchuk et al., who demonstrated that these animals also frequently succumbed to cardiac fibrosis; COX-2-deficient females were invariably infertile[36,37].

The generally smaller kidneys of COX-2$^{-/-}$ mice were pale, had a reduced number of poorly developed glomeruli, and exhibited dilated and degenerating renal tubules[36]. The nephropathy associated with COX-2 deficiency was considered to be due to defective postnatal development, since the kidneys of newborn wild type and COX-2$^{+/-}$ mice were normal[36]. The renal pathology in COX-2$^{-/-}$ mice increased in severity with age, ultimately resulting in kidney failure[36].

The renal pathology seen in COX-2$^{-/-}$ mice prompted a comparison between the renal consequences of long-term use of NSAIDs and congenital COX-2 gene ablation. It appears that the kidney toxicity often associated with NSAID treatment in adult mice or humans appears to be quite distinct from the nephropathy exhibited in COX-2$^{-/-}$ mice[18,35,36]. This difference may be a function of the stage of renal development at which COX is actually inhibited. It was recently shown that the COX-2-selective inhibitor SC58236 given during pregnancy until weaning, impaired kidney development in both mice and rats in a manner that essentially mimicked the COX-2$^{-/-}$ mouse phenotype[16]. More precisely, treatment of newborn mice with the COX-2 inhibitor during the period between day 0 and day 21 severely reduced glomerular diameter, whereas treatment limited to the duration of pregnancy did not affect glomerular size. Since inhibition of COX-2 had no effect on glomerular volume in adult mice, there appears to be a rather narrow window of time during which COX-2 inhibition affects kidney development.

The peritonitis observed in COX-2 null mice involved multiple abdominal organs, with neutrophil infiltration and focal bacterial colonization[36]. Morham et al.[36] estimated that less than 5% of adult COX-2 null mice of the Ola 129/C57Bl/6 strain died of peritonitis. A strain of COX-2-deficient mouse bred in our laboratory, designated C57/DBA1, does not show an increased susceptibility or incidence of peritonitis. Thus, the precise phenotypic consequences of COX gene ablation may be greatly modified by the genetic background of a particular strain (see below).

Since the ablation of both COX-1 and COX-2 genes is embryonically lethal, primary fibroblast cell lines were derived from 'double' COX-deficient embryos, to investigate the roles of COX-1 and COX-2[34]. *In vitro*, cells lacking either COX-1, COX-2 or both genes could be transformed with oncogenes with equal efficiency. NSAIDs exerted antineoplastic effects on embryonic fibroblasts by enhancing apoptosis and suppressing colony formation in soft agar in the absence of either or both COX-1 and COX-2 genes. Thus, the antiproliferative and antineoplastic effects of NSAIDs occurred independently of the activity of either COX-1 or COX-2. Although the process of transformation remains unaffected in double COX knockout fibroblasts, these studies do not rule out roles for COX during subsequent stages of tumorigenesis.

The reproductive problems seen in the COX-2$^{-/-}$ C57Bl/6 mouse were ameliorated somewhat by developing a mixed 129 Ola/C57Bl/6 strain. We have also observed that the kidneys from C57/DBA1, COX-2$^{-/-}$ mice exhibited far less nephropathy (unpublished observation) than was reported in the COX-2$^{-/-}$, 129/j strain[36]. These data strongly indicate that additional genes can greatly modify the COX-deficient phenotype.

KIDNEY DEVELOPMENT IN THE CYCLOOXYGENASE-DEFICIENT MOUSE

In the adult kidney prostanoids are intimately involved in the regulation of renal pathophysiology[21]. Thus, mice with COX-1 gene ablation showed an altered inflammatory response to arachidonic acid[35] whereas COX-2$^{-/-}$ mice were born with severe renal pathology[36,37]. Normally, PGE$_2$, the main PG generated along the nephron and the collecting duct, exerts potent diuretic and natriuretic influences in the adult kidney[21]. Effects of PGE_2 on the kidney may be exactly opposite under some conditions; for instance, isolated perfused cortical collecting ducts exposed to PGE_2 generate more cyclic adenosine monophosphate (cAMP) and become more permeable to water. However, in vasopressin-treated collecting ducts, treatment with PGE_2 inhibited cAMP production and reduced water permeability[21]. Regulation of the haemodynamics of the renal vasculature and water and salt excretion in response to PGs involves two complementary processes. First, in response to pathophysiological signals (e.g. cytokines and hormones) there seems to be cell-specific and compartmentalized production of PGs *in vivo*. An additional level of complexity in the regulation of renal pathophysiology by PGs is achieved through preferential utilization of unique signalling receptors (EP_1 and EP_3 versus EP_2 and EP_4) with which various PGs may preferentially interact. The precise mechanistic interactions that govern localized, cell-specific expression of key enzymes involved in the production of PGs and the postreceptor signalling pathways are incompletely understood[21]. Experiments with mice containing targeted gene disruptions have greatly enhanced our appreciation of the intrinsic complexity of the varied, and sometimes paradoxical, actions of PGs in fetal and adult tissues[7,18,35–37,41].

Formation of PGs and their potential relationship to the expression of COX-1 or COX-2 genes has been investigated in the kidneys of several species, including humans[21,42]. These experiments have elucidated some interspecific differences in the patterns of expression of the two COX isozymes[42–46]. Immunolocalization and *in situ* hybridization experiments have demonstrated that COX-1 is abundantly expressed in the endothelial cells of renal blood vessels and collecting ducts, and in a subset of papillary interstitial cells in mice, rats, dogs, cynomolgus monkeys, and humans[46]. PGs, produced through the action of COX-1, are believed to regulate renal plasma flow and the rate of glomerular filtration, especially under conditions of angiotensin-stimulated vasoconstriction[21]. NSAIDs, such as aspirin, are believed to cause gastrointestinal and renal toxicity mainly by blocking the protective actions of PGs generated via COX-1[47,48]. However, it is well known that there is considerable variability among different species with regard to the susceptibility of kidneys to damage induced by NSAIDs. Such species-specific differences in the response of kidneys to NSAIDs may be due to variations in the tissue-specific expression of inducible and/or constitutive COXs, localized production of PGs, preferential modulation of prostanoid receptors and signalling mechanisms in different organisms[46].

The immunohistological staining of kidneys from mice, rabbits, rats and dogs with antibodies to COX-1 and COX-2 indicated that COX-2 protein is localized in the macula densa, the cells of the thick ascending limb (cTAL) of the loop of Henle and the papillary interstitial cells[44–46]. Basal expression of

COX-2 was also demonstrated in the glomerular podocytes and small blood vessels in the kidneys of monkeys and humans[45,46]. There was a noticeable absence of COX-2 gene expression in the arterioles and cells of the collecting ducts in both cortical and medullary regions of the adult kidney in all species. This finding is of considerable interest in order to assess a role of PGs as regulators of the vascular response of the kidney to chronic volume depletion. In the kidneys of chronically salt-deprived experimental animals, COX-2 gene expression was greatly increased in the macula densa and the adjoining cTAL cells in the renal cortex[43]. Similar brisk induction of expression of COX-2 mRNA and protein also occurred in cells of the macula densa and cTAL following subtotal renal ablation in rats. The relationship between the feedback regulation of the renal blood flow and rates of filtration by the renin–angiotensin system and COX-2 gene expression was explored by Cheng et al. in a recent study[49]. These investigators observed that treatment of mice with either an angiotensin-converting enzyme (ACE) inhibitor, captopril, or an angiotensin-II receptor antagonist, losartan, led to increased expression of COX-2 mRNA and protein in the macula densa. The enhanced COX-2 gene expression in the kidney under conditions of volume contraction, and in transgenic mice that lack both alleles of angiotensin-II receptors 1α and 1β (i.e. Agtr1α$^{-/-}$ and Agtr1β$^{-/-}$) was accompanied by elevated production of renin. Since simultaneous administration of SC58236 (a selective COX-2 inhibitor) could block renin production after partial renal ablation, these investigators postulated that induction of COX-2, and synthesis of PGs via the action of COX-2 enzyme, directly mediated augmented production of renin in response to decreased angiotensin-II levels or activity[49]. Based on the published literature, we may surmise that the actions of both COX-1 and COX-2 isoforms are uniquely involved in regulating renal pathophysiology.

An additional, and somewhat surprising, role of COX-2 gene expression (presumably via generation of PGs) during embryonic kidney development has come to be appreciated from gene ablation studies. It was noticed that mice lacking both alleles of COX-2 were born with severely underdeveloped kidneys[36,37]. The major manifestations of renal dysgenesis in COX-2$^{-/-}$ mice included hypoplastic glomeruli, the presence of fewer functional nephrons and an abundance of undifferentiated mesenchymal cells; the kidneys of COX-2$^{-/-}$ mice also contained numerous microcysts and medullary hyperplasia. Consistent with their abnormal renal histology, COX-2$^{-/-}$ mice were found to have elevated blood urea nitrogen and serum creatinine; as these animals aged, they developed renal hypertrophy, glomerular sclerosis and interstitial fibrosis, and ultimately died of renal failure[36,37]. Nephrogenesis in the developing embryo is carried out by co-operative interactions of many genes that include developmental morphogens, components of extracellular matrix (ECM) and transcription factors[50]. The multigenic nature of kidney development is consistent with the data showing that the severity of renal phenotype of COX-2[−/−] mice may depend on the genetic background of the strain of mice. For example, the renal complications of COX-2 deficiency are relatively mild in C57Bl/6 mice as compared to those seen in the 129/j strain (Laulederkind, Ballou and Raghow, unpublished). Strain-specific differences notwithstanding, the pathological manifestations seen in COX-2[−/−] mice greatly resemble the focal segmental glomerular sclerosis and chronic renal failure seen with human oligomeganephronia[51].

The question of how COX-2 gene expression and generation of PGs in the embryo relate mechanistically to the morphogenesis and perinatal maturation of the kidney remains unanswered. To elucidate this relationship, two plausible, although not mutually exclusive, scenarios need to be tested experimentally. First, the hypothesis that PGs, presumably generated via the action of COX-2, modulate a key step(s) involved in renal morphogenesis needs to be tested by rigorous experiments. Secondly, we need to investigate whether putative compensatory reactions elicited in the embryo, as a result of COX-2 gene ablation, modify a key signalling programme(s) that mediates developmental nephrogenesis. A recent study by Komhoff et al.[16] was directed towards investigating the first scenario proposed here. These investigators exposed mice to the COX-2 selective inhibitor, SC58236, *in utero* and demonstrated that prenatal inhibition of COX-2 activity in the embryo caused impaired glomerulogenesis and arrested cortical development. The overall pathology of kidneys from mice treated with SC58236 *in utero* appeared to be similar to that of COX-2[−/−] mice[36,37]. Furthermore, these investigators reported that selective inhibition of COX-2 between 0 and 21 days after birth also caused severe renal disease. The reduced glomerular diameter and associated renal pathology seen in mice treated with a COX-2 inhibitor during perinatal growth was similar to that seen in the kidneys of congenitally COX-2[−/−] mice[36,37].

REPRODUCTIVE ABNORMALITIES IN THE CYCLOOXYGENASE-DEFICIENT MOUSE

As potent vasoactive, mitogenic and differentiation-inducing agents, PGs regulate multiple steps of the normal ovarian cycle of the mammalian female. Although both COX-1 and COX-2 genes are known to be expressed in the uterus, the specific contribution of the two COX isozymes in regulating various uterine functions is far from clear. It has been appreciated for many years that PGs are critical to regulating the rhythmic contractions of uterus during parturition[52,53]. However, more recent observations indicate that prostanoids may play additional roles in the mechanisms of ovulation, fertilization, implantation and decidualization[6,40,54]. In the ovary, the pituitary gonadotrophins, follicle-stimulating hormone (FSH) and luteinizing hormone (LH), coordinate the development, maturation and rupture of the follicle to release the mature oocyte[52]. COX-2 gene expression in the uterus is induced immediately following the mid-cycle surge of LH and there is strong experimental data to suggest that PGs are required for normal follicular development and oocyte maturation[6,40,54]. The induction of extracellular matrix degrading proteinases in the uterine tissue, a phenomenon that is essential for the rupture of the antral follicles, is apparently regulated by prostanoids. Additional observations suggest that PGs, generated mainly via the enzymatic action of COX-1, and acting through the PGE_2 receptors, EP_1, EP_2 and EP_4, catalyse the physiological changes in the uterus needed for implantation of the embryo[40,53,55-58]. Characteristic changes in the vascular permeability of the endometrium that occur immediately after implantation of the blastocyst are also mediated by PGs but mainly through their interactions with the EP_2 receptors[59,60]. In light of these experimental observations, it is easy to appreciate the clinical data that show that regular consumption of NSAIDs is associated with reduced fertility[61,62]. Decreased rates of fertility, reduction in the number of implantation sites, with consequential reduction in the litter size, have also been observed in experimental animals. Late in pregnancy, an enhanced production of PGE_2, by uterine and fetal tissues, signals the ovary to undergo luteolysis. As fetal development comes to term, a sharp decline in the level of maternal progesterone and concomitant induction of oxytocin receptors occurs in the ovary; these cellular and molecular changes are responsible for the enhanced response of the myometrial tissue to oxytocin that is essential to initiate labour[63].

Based on their unique spatiotemporal patterns of expression in the uterus, it has been assumed *a priori* that the enzymatic actions of COX-1 and COX-2 regulate distinct uterine and ovarian functions during the normal menstrual cycle and pregnancy[64-67]. Nevertheless, the complex network of regulation in which PGs, generated via the action of either COX-1 or COX-2, became clear only recently, as a result of studies carried out with COX-deficient mice[6,40,54]. A number of careful studies have documented that COX-2$^{-/-}$ mice were unable to reproduce due to deficits of ovulation, inefficient fertilization, implantation and decidualization[37,40]. The anovulatory phenotype of COX-2$^{-/-}$ mice, attributed to impaired expansion of cumulus oophorum and stigmata formation, could be reversed by exogenous administration of PGE_2 or by injections of interleukin-1β, a potent inducer of PGE_2 biosynthesis[54].

In the preimplantation uterus, a consistent cell-specific expression of COX-1 (but not COX-2) in the uterine lumen is known to precede the characteristic vascular changes in WT mice. Elaboration of PGs, predominantly via the action of COX-1, is thought to modulate the normal physiological response of uterus before implantation. Therefore, a lack of overt reproductive deficiency in the COX-1-ablated mice was somewhat surprising. These studies suggested that activity of COX-2 adequately compensated for the lack of COX-1 in COX-1$^{-/-}$ mice and rescued these animals from reproductive failure. More detailed analysis of the cellular and biochemical changes in the uterus of COX-1$^{-/-}$ mice during oestrus and pregnancy by Reese et al.[6] have generally corroborated the concept of compensation. These authors reported that, compared with their WT counterpart, uteri of COX-1$^{-/-}$ mice exhibited significantly lower vascular permeability, reduced biosynthesis of PGs and smaller weight gain prior to implantation. Nevertheless, these blunted physiological responses could be adequately offset by the compensatory expression of COX-2 in the uterus of COX-1$^{-/-}$ mice. Thus, unlike what normally occurs in the WT mice, COX-1$^{-/-}$ uteri elicited a strong expression of COX-2 on the morning of day 4. Although these findings are consistent with the notion that PGs synthesized via the action of COX-2 rescued the deficiency of COX-1[6], the precise mechanisms that dictate tissue-specific compensatory regulation of COX-2 in COX-1$^{-/-}$ mice remain to be investigated. Furthermore, the published data do not provide an explanation as to why analogous compensatory mechanisms fail to be elicited in COX-2$^{-/-}$ animals.

CYCLOOXYGENASE AND THE GASTROINTESTINAL TRACT

A widespread clinical use of NSAIDs as anti-inflammatory agents has led to the recognition that these drugs invariably cause serious gastrointestinal (GI) distress due to GI bleeding, and gastric ulceration and perforation[68,69]. The activity of NSAIDs to inhibit biosynthesis and secretion of mucus and to promote acid secretion in the stomach, combined with their ability to abrogate platelet function, causes the known GI complications[70-72]. The generally accepted mechanism that the untoward effects of NSAIDs are caused by their ability to block the enzymatic activity of COX-1 is consistent with the observation that there is little constitutive expression of COX-2 in the normal gastric mucosal tissue and platelets. We believe, however, that the proposed mechanism to explain the GI complications that result from treatment with NSAIDs may be somewhat simplistic in light of some recent observations in COX-deficient mice. It is known that COX-1$^{-/-}$ mice do not develop gastric ulcers spontaneously, despite a greater than 90% reduction in the amount of PGs produced in their stomachs[7,18,35,36,41]. Furthermore, similar acute inflammatory responses of the GI tract to dextran sodium sulphate in COX-1$^{-/-}$ or COX-2$^{-/-}$ mice suggested that both isoforms of COX are equally effective in the defence of the intestinal mucosa under inflammatory conditions. The GI responses to inflammatory conditions are somewhat discordant with what occurs in the absence of injury and inflammation. Thus, under normal physiological conditions, neither COX isozyme appeared to be indispensable for maintaining the integrity of the gastric mucosa. The lack of spontaneous GI pathology in COX-1$^{-/-}$ mice is intriguing since a similar pharmacological block of COX-1 and consequent reduction of PGs by NSAIDs in normal mice consistently causes gastric ulceration and bleeding.

These dissimilar GI manifestations seen in WT mice treated with NSAIDs and in congenitally COX-1$^{-/-}$ or COX-2$^{-/-}$ mice suggest that the mechanisms by which the alternate isoform of COX regulates the homeostatic and post-inflammatory GI responses need to be examined in greater detail.

A number of recent observations suggests that induction of COX-2, and presumably PGs generated through its enzymatic action, may facilitate the process of postinflammatory tissue repair and regeneration after microbial infections[42,73]. A brisk induction of COX-2 gene expression during healing of experimentally induced acute ulceration, as well as in response to invasion of gut epithelium by *Salmonella* and other microorganisms has been documented[74,75]. PGs, elaborated in response to infection, may stimulate chloride and water secretion, thus facilitating expulsion of the bacteria from the GI tract. How the gut epithelial cells respond to bacterial infection in COX-2$^{-/-}$ mice compared with their normal littermates remains to be investigated.

TUMORIGENESIS/CARCINOGENESIS IN THE CYCLOOXYGENASE-DEFICIENT MOUSE

There are compelling epidemiological data to indicate that regular use of NSAIDs is associated with reduced morbidity and mortality caused by colorectal cancer. Since colorectal cancer is the second most common neoplasia in the developed world, these epidemiological findings have prompted extensive laboratory research on the potential relationship between PGs and the process of carcinogenesis[76–102].

Molecular bases of the chemopreventive effect of NSAIDs have been studied in a number of experimental systems. For example, sulindac and related NSAIDs have been shown to exert a potent inhibitory effect in a murine model of familial adenomatous polyposis (FAP)[101]. In a seminal study, Oshima et al.[103] combined the COX deficient phenotype with the mutation in adenomatous polyposis coli (*Apc*) gene, a mutation that invariably leads to the development of intestinal neoplasia. Using the COX-2$^{-/-}$/*Apc* mouse, they showed that COX-2 gene ablation dramatically reduced the induction of polyp formation. They also demonstrated that COX-2 selective inhibitors could reduce polyp formation in the *Apc* mouse. These observations clearly implicated COX-2 as an important early mediator of tumorigenesis referred to as 'self-promotion'[104]; COX-1$^{-/-}$/*Apc* mice were not studied.

Subsequently, Chulada et al.[105] used an alternative genetic approach to study tumorigenesis exploiting the COX-deficient mouse by making a COX$^{-/-}$/*Min* (multiple intestinal neoplasia) mouse[106–108]; the *Min* mouse is a model for FAP. Like the *Apc* mouse, the *Min* mouse invariably develops intestinal neoplasia resulting from a chemically-induced mutation of the *Apc* gene; however, the *Min* mouse does not develop nearly as many polyps as the

Apc deficient mouse. Using the COX$^{-/-}$/*Min* mouse, Chulada et al. found that the deficiency of either COX-1 or COX-2 significantly decreased intestinal polyp formation[105]. That both COX-1 and COX-2 appear to play significant roles in tumorigenesis in this model is not unexpected, given the fact that aspirin inhibits tumour formation *in vivo* and is a more effective inhibitor of COX-1 than COX-2. Similar results were obtained by the same group when COX-1$^{-/-}$ or COX-2$^{-/-}$ mice were examined for the development of skin papillomas; either COX-1 or COX-2 deficiency reduced tumour formation significantly and inhibitors of COX-1 or COX-2 similarly inhibited papilloma formation[109]. From these studies it is clear that both COX-1 and COX-2 are important in the tumorigenic process, but the potential effects of the COX isozymes in carcinogenesis are as yet less clear. Recently, however, Williams et al. found that tumour growth in COX-2$^{-/-}$ mice was greatly reduced compared with COX-1$^{-/-}$ and WT mice, demonstrating the importance of host COX-2 expression levels in regulating tumour growth; selective COX-2 inhibitors also inhibited tumour growth[110]. Mechanistically, COX-2 deficiency or treatment with COX-2 inhibitors reduced the ability of fibroblasts to produce the proangiogenic factor, VEGF, by over 90%, suggesting that this defect may play a significant role in modulating carcinoma growth[110]. While it appears that COX deficiency and the inhibition of COX activity have the same general inhibitory effects on tumorigenesis, there is little doubt that NSAIDs affect this process via mechanisms that may be independent of their ability to block COX.

A number of related observations suggest that the anti-neoplastic actions of NSAIDs may be attributed to their ability to inhibit cyclooxygenases and consequential suppression of biosynthesis of PGs[104,111,112]. Consistent with such a mechanism, it has been documented that enhanced COX-2 gene expression is invariably associated with a variety of tumours, especially of colorectal origin[112]. Additionally, experimental inactivation of COX-2 gene expression, either by homologous recombination or by treatment with selective inhibitors of COX-2 enzyme, reduces the rates of colorectal tumorigenesis in an experimental model of FAP[103].

Further support for COX-2 as a crucial mediator of the anti-neoplastic effect of NSAIDs was obtained with a COX-2 selective inhibitor, SC-58125. Sheng and coworkers demonstrated that experimental inhibition of COX-2 activity led to reduced rates of growth of tumours *in vivo*; additionally, treatment with SC-58125 induced apoptosis of cancer cells cultivated *in vitro*[113]. A number of additional observations have called in question the proposed cause and effect relationship between COXs (and PGs) and the process of carcinogenesis. First, NSAID derivatives, incapable of inhibiting cyclooxygenases, are potent suppressors of growth of colorectal tumours, both *in vivo* and *in vitro*[114–116]. Secondly, NSAIDs could inhibit the growth of colon cancer lines regardless of whether or not these cells contained detectable cyclooxygenase activity[117,118]. Finally, the most compelling evidence that COX activity may not be central to the process of neoplastic transformation was presented by Zhang et al.[34]. These investigators analysed primary embryonic fibroblasts from COX-1$^{-/-}$, COX-2$^{-/-}$ and double COX knockout mice for their ability to be transformed by Ha-*ras* and/or SV-40. These experiments revealed that regardless of whether embryonic fibroblasts lacked COX-1, COX-2 or both enzymes, they could be transformed with equal efficiency. Even more importantly, irrespective of the COX phenotype of the embryonic fibroblasts, treatment of H-*ras* transformed cells in culture with NSAIDs suppressed their rates of proliferation and colony formation in soft agar[34]. Thus, biosyntheses of PGs and COX expression were certainly not required for oncogenic transformation *in vitro*. However, these data do not rule out the possibility that PGs modulate a critical step in later stages of carcinogenesis. A number of additional observations corroborate and extend the concept that PGs may be only indirectly involved in the process of tumorigenesis. For example, while in the colorectal tumour in humans COX-2 gene expression is invariably elevated in the neoplastic epithelial cells[119,120], in murine intestinal cancer, enhanced COX-2 expression was restricted to non-cancerous stromal cells[103,121]. However, these critical differences in the cell-specific expression of COX-2 in the two species notwithstanding, NSAIDs exerted similar chemopreventive actions.

CYCLOOXYGENASE AND THE IMMUNE RESPONSE

COX-dependent production of PGs plays a central role in mediating the immune response; PGs appear to modulate both T cell development and activation[22,23]. PGE$_2$ alters the cytokine profiles of mature CD4$^+$T cells in both mice and humans by shifting the production of Th1-type cytokines to the production of Th2-type cytokines[122-126], and by inhibiting cytotoxic T lymphocyte function[127]; PG biosynthesis is associated with a variety of immunological disorders[128-130].

The immunological ramifications of COX deficiency are only beginning to be elucidated through the use of COX$^{-/-}$ mice. Recently, Rocca et al.[22,23] showed that both COX-1 and COX-2 were necessary for normal thymic T cell maturation in the fetal mouse; each isoform apparently plays a distinct role in T cell maturation and signals via particular PG receptors. While both COX-1 and COX-2 are expressed in the fetal thymus, their relative levels of expression vary significantly with respect to developmental stage. For example, while immature thymocytes expressed predominantly COX-1, COX-2 was highly expressed in the mature thymus. In the developing thymus COX-2 expression becomes localized to the medulla, unlike COX-1 which appears to be restricted to cortical thymic epithelial cells. Functionally, COX-1-mediated PGE$_2$ biosynthesis is thought to promote the transition of

$CD4^-CD8^-$ thymocytes to $CD4^+CD8^+$ cells, acting via the EP_2 receptor subtype. In mice lacking recombinase-activating gene-1 ($RAG\text{-}1^{-/-}$) that exhibit arrested thymocyte development at the $CD4^-CD8^-$ stage *in vivo* due to an inability to mediate T cell receptor rearrangements, COX-1 activity was essential for the development of $CD4^+CD8^+$ thymocyte populations[23]. Conversely, COX-2-mediated PGE_2 biosynthesis and utilization of EP_1 receptors favour the selection and maturation of $CD4^+$ lymphocytes.

Interestingly, COX-1 inhibitors are more effective than COX-1 gene ablation in preventing the transition of lymphocytes from $CD4^-CD8^-$ to $CD4^+CD8^+$, suggesting that COX-2 may compensate for the lack of COX-1 in genetically deficient mice or that non-COX related effects of these drugs can affect T cell maturation. However, higher COX-2 protein levels in the $COX\text{-}1^{-/-}$ thymus and a concordant increase in $CD4^+$ thymocytes is consistent with a compensatory mechanism. The compensatory expression of the alternate COX isoform in COX-deficient cells in culture[5] and *in vivo* (L. Ballou, unpublished observation) has been demonstrated[6].

Recently, in humans, increased COX-2 expression has been associated with a high risk for diabetes[131]. The enhanced expression of COX-2 in monocytes of subjects with insulin-dependent diabetes mellitus (IDDM) appears to correlate with risk for diabetes. Mechanistically, COX-2 elaborated products are thought to interact with diabetes-associated MHC class II antigens and thereby inhibit T cell activation. Thus, a COX-2 regulatory defect in an antigen-processing cell such as the monocyte results in an altered immune response that can be assessed directly as a risk factor for IDDM.

We are currently examining the immunological and inflammatory ramifications of COX-1 or COX-2 gene deletion, utilizing a murine model of autoimmune rheumatoid arthritis (RA), collagen-induced arthritis (CIA). The pathology observed in CIA closely resembles human RA[132]. To study CIA, COX-1 and COX-2 deficiency was bred into a DBA/1 strain, a mouse bearing the appropriate MHC class II molecules required to confer susceptibility to autoimmune arthritis[132]. This was accomplished by backcrossing the original C57/Bl6, $COX\text{-}2^{-/-}$ strain (that lacks MHC susceptibility genes for CIA) onto the DBA/1, bearing MHC ($I\text{-}A^q$).

Even though RA is classified as an autoimmune disease, the essence of its pathology is severe and chronic inflammation, making it difficult to separate the processes associated with immunity from those associated with inflammation. The COX pathway is critical to the pathogenesis of RA, and selective inhibition of COX by NSAIDs is the mainstay of RA therapy. However, since COX/PGs modulate immune, as well as inflammatory responses, the relative contribution of the two processes to the pathogenesis of RA remains to be elucidated. The importance of the immune system in the pathogenesis of RA is strongly supported by the presence of T cells in arthritic lesions and the association of this disease with MHC class II molecules. Histopathological and ultrastructural studies of rheumatoid synovial tissues show synovial lining cell hyperplasia along with chronic inflammatory infiltrates containing T and B lymphocytes, and macrophages characteristic of delayed-type hypersensitivity reactions[132]. The majority of the cells in the synovial tissues are activated T cells expressing MHC class II molecules[132]. It is postulated that the presumably antigen-specific T cells preferentially expand in the synovium and produce potent lymphokines that initiate inflammation. These cytokines stimulate B cells to produce antibodies that form immune complexes, which in turn activate the complement cascade, generating a cascade of complement proteins (e.g. C3a and C5a) that further amplify the inflammatory reaction. Phagocytosis of immune complexes by polymorphonuclear leukocytes, macrophages and synovial lining triggers the release of lysosomal enzymes, reactive oxygen species (ROS), AA metabolites, and matrix metalloproteinases (MMPs) that degrade the cartilage matrix. In parallel, mediators derived from activated macrophages and synovial fibroblast-like cells (e.g. IL-1, TNF-α, IL-6, GM-CSF, PGs, other AA metabolites and oxygen free-radicals) drive the process of inflammation. Concomitant release of MMPs leads to the degradation of the extracellular matrix of joint tissues. Thus, complex interactions of cells and mediators are involved in the chronic inflammation and destruction of cartilage, bone and surrounding connective tissues in RA.

An important approach to studying the role of the potential antigens in RA has been the establishment of animal models of experimental autoimmune arthritis[133]. Since RA is an autoimmune disease of articular joints, experimental animals immunized with constituents of cartilage, e.g. gp39, proteoglycan (aggrecan), or type II collagen (CII) invariably develop a polyarticular autoimmune arthritis. The susceptibility to CIA is linked to the expression of specific class II molecules of the murine MHC. As an aetiological autoantigen of RA, CII has received considerable attention for a number of reasons. First, CIA can be elicited in several species including mouse[134], rat[135] and monkey[136]. Secondly, the existence of T cell[137] or B cell[138–141] immunity to CII in RA patients, and anti-CII antibodies have been seen in the joint cartilage of RA patients[142]. The autoimmune response of mice in CIA is typified by both strong T cell and B cell responses, capable of recognizing the autoantigen, murine CII[143]. Like the studies in RA[142], antibody specific for homologous CII can be detected readily in the arthritic joints of mice. Based on experiments of passive transfer of disease with sera or CII-specific monoclonal antibodies[144–146], it appears that the pathogenesis in the CIA model is largely antibody-driven. Although for obvious ethical reasons it is yet to be demonstrated that the CII-specific antibody found in RA patients is pathogenic in humans, passive transfer of such antibodies into mice can induce a destructive arthritis[147].

Given the central role of COX in inflammation and the ability of COX to modulate the immune response, we studied CIA in the COX$^{-/-}$ mouse to gain insights into the precise roles of COX-1 and COX-2 in the pathogenesis of RA. To assess directly the roles of PGs produced uniquely via COX-1 or COX-2 in the pathogenesis of arthritis, we bred COX-1 and COX-2 deficiency onto a background expressing the MHC susceptibility gene (I-A^q) conferring susceptibility to CIA[148]. We examined the roles of COX-1 and COX-2 in the cascade of immune and inflammatory events mediating the pathogenesis of CIA in these mice. We found that COX-1$^{-/-}$ mice were susceptible to arthritis when immunized with CII, with onset and severity comparable with WT mice, while COX-2$^{-/-}$ mice exhibited a very low incidence of arthritis, with significantly delayed onset and greatly reduced severity. Conceivably, the inhibition of CIA in COX-2$^{-/-}$ mice may result from: (1) their inability to produce antibodies to CII, and (2) lack of appropriate quantity and/or quality of PGs. Intravenous infusion of anti-CII monoclonal antibodies caused CIA in 100% of the WT and COX-1$^{-/-}$ mice, while none of the COX-2-deficient mice developed disease. Therefore, simply bypassing the requirement for antibody production to CII via passive transfer is not sufficient to induce arthritis in COX-2$^{-/-}$ mice and suggests that production of inflammatory PGs via COX-2 may be more critical in the pathogenesis of CIA than mounting antibody responses to CII. Although the superficial inflammatory responses of COX-2$^{-/-}$ mice elicited by phorbol ester (TPA) or AA were reported to be normal[36], the immune-mediated, systemic inflammatory response associated with CIA was clearly compromised by the lack of COX-2. Further work using COX$^{-/-}$ mice in the CIA model will help to clarify the mechanism(s) by which COX-2 activity is related to autoimmune arthritis.

CYCLOOXYGENASE DEFICIENCY AND THE INFLAMMATORY RESPONSE

The process of inflammation involves the activation and migration of neutrophils and macrophages to sites of tissue damage, and is facilitated by increased blood flow and vascular permeability. The activation and migration of inflammatory cells is controlled by many inflammatory mediators, including the PGs. Inflammatory reactions often accompany an immune response but can also be completely separate, as in an acute physical injury. The inhibition of PG production by NSAIDs is therefore mainly responsible for the anti-inflammatory actions of the latter.

In the original studies with COX-1$^{-/-}$ and COX-2$^{-/-}$ mice, the ear oedema model of inflammation was used to assess the effects of COX isozyme deficiency on the inflammatory response. Either AA or phorbol ester (TPA) was applied to the ear and swelling was measured as an indicator of inflammation. It was somewhat surprising that AA-induced inflammation was significantly blunted in COX-1$^{-/-}$ mice, whereas the COX-2$^{-/-}$ and WT mice responded with a robust swelling of the ear. On the other hand, TPA induced an equivalent inflammatory response in both COX-1$^{-/-}$ and COX-2$^{-/-}$ and in WT mice. The apparent discrepancy between the AA and TPA results may be explained by the fact that COX-1 (highly expressed in skin) is able to utilize exogenously added AA more effectively than COX-2. Since TPA-induced ear inflammation was similar in COX-1$^{-/-}$ and COX-2$^{-/-}$ mice, it was concluded that the remaining COX isoform produced sufficient levels and types of PGs to elicit an inflammatory response. However, in light of the data from the CIA model, the respective roles of COX-1 and COX-2 may be different in different tissues and may be dependent on the type of inflammatory stimuli.

Recently, Wallace et al.[149] showed that COX-2$^{-/-}$ and WT mice both developed carageenan-induced inflammation, and that indomethacin, but not NS-398 (a COX-2 selective inhibitor), inhibited the inflammatory response. This result clearly implicates COX-1 in the inflammatory process, since indomethacin was used at a concentration that likely had an inhibitory effect on COX-1 activity. However, during the latter stages of the inflammatory response, the resolution phase, it appears that COX-2 may play a more significant role, because cellular infiltration and oedema are present for longer periods of time in COX-2$^{-/-}$ than in WT mice. Differential COX isozyme activation patterns during 'immediate' and 'delayed' phases of PG synthesis in macrophages further corroborate a role for both COX-1 and COX-2 in the inflammatory process[150,151]. Macrophages lacking COX-1 produced less PGs after stimulation, whereas COX-2$^{-/-}$ macrophages produced normal PG levels, indicating a role for COX-1 in the immediate phase of PG production[151]. The dependence of immediate and delayed PG biosynthesis on COX-1 and COX-2 was also demonstrated in mast cells derived from COX-deficient mice[150].

To test the role of PGs in bone resorption, Okada et al.[152] used cultured cells obtained from COX-deficient mice to show that PGE$_2$ production in bone marrow cultures from COX-2$^{-/-}$ mice was greatly reduced, compared with WT and COX-1$^{-/-}$ cultures. Fewer osteoclasts were formed by COX-2$^{-/-}$ marrow cells[152] and treatment of normal marrow cells with NSAIDs similarly reduced osteoclastogenesis. The reduced osteoclastogenesis in COX-2$^{-/-}$ marrow cells appeared to be correlated with reduced expression in osteoblasts of receptor activator of NF-κB ligand (RANKL), a protein essential for resorption. Consistent with this was the finding that exogenously added RANKL inhibited osteoclast formation in COX-2$^{-/-}$ spleen cell cultures but not in COX-1$^{-/-}$ or WT cultures. In vivo, the injection of parathyroid hormone (PTH) above the calvaria caused hypercalcaemia in WT but not COX-2$^{-/-}$ mice. Thus, in this bone resorption model, although COX-2 may not play an essential role in normal bone turnover, AA metabolites elaborated via the action of COX-2 may be involved in modulating bone resorption in response to inflammatory mediators.

Recently, Gavett et al.[153] investigated the roles of COX-1 and COX-2 in allergic lung responses in COX$^{-/-}$ mice immunized and then challenged with ovalbumin. In non-immunized mice PGE$_2$ levels in bronchoalveolar lavage (BAL) fluid of COX-1$^{-/-}$ mice were lower compared with normal and COX-2$^{-/-}$ mice; there were no obvious differences in lung function or lung pathology among the three groups. However, when immunized and then challenged with ovalbumin, both COX-1$^{-/-}$ and COX-2$^{-/-}$ mice mounted a more aggressive inflammatory response when compared with WT mice. A number of parameters, including measurement of lung function, the infiltration of inflammatory cells and the production of IgE, substantiated this conclusion. Both COX-1$^{-/-}$ and COX-2$^{-/-}$ mice exhibited reduced allergic lung function. But only allergic COX-1$^{-/-}$, not COX-2$^{-/-}$ mice, exhibited an increase in baseline resistance and responsiveness to methacholine. Based upon these data it was concluded that COX-1 is responsible for PGE$_2$ production in the normal mouse lung, whereas both COX-1 and COX-2 are involved in reducing allergic lung inflammation.

Angiogenesis is often associated with post-inflammatory tissue repair and regeneration, and PGs are known to modulate neovascularization. Based on studies with COX-selective inhibitors, it has been concluded previously that both COX-1 and COX-2 isozymes are involved in the mechanism of angiogenesis, especially during colorectal tumorigenesis. Recent experiments with Lewis lung carcinoma (LLC) transplanted in different strains of mice suggested that the rate of growth of LLC tumours was significantly lower in the COX-2$^{-/-}$ animals compared with either in COX-1$^{-/-}$ or WT mice. The slower rate of LLC tumour growth in COX-2$^{-/-}$ mice was correlated with weaker angiogenic response, as judged by the lower vascular density of these tumours. Thus PGs of the host, generated via the action of COX-2, modulate angiogenesis and growth of tumour models of xenotransplantation. We examined the neovacularization response in the corneas of COX-1$^{-/-}$ and COX-2$^{-/-}$ mice following silver nitrate injury. As shown in Figure 2, neovasculogenesis in the COX-2$^{-/-}$ mice was found to be much more vigorous than in either COX-1$^{-/-}$ or WT animals. The rate of angiogenesis in the COX-1$^{-/-}$ animals was also significantly lower than that seen in WT mice. These data suggest that the contribution of PGs to neovascularization occurs through complex interactions between COX-1 or COX-2, and the mechanistic bases of these interactions need to be examined more rigorously, using COX-1$^{-/-}$ and COX-2$^{-/-}$ mice.

CYCLOOXYGENASE AND FEVER

Fever is the most manifest of the body's acute phase reactions to an infectious challenge. It is elicited, prototypically, by the entry into the body of infectious microorganisms, e.g. bacteria, or their products, such as lipopolysaccharides

Figure 2 Neovascularization in COX-deficient mice. Silver nitrate was applied to the corneas of wild-type (top panel), COX-1$^{-/-}$ (middle panel) and COX-2$^{-/-}$ (bottom panel) mice, and eyes were examined for the newly formed blood vessels 7 days after corneal injury. In the wild type mouse cornea, neovascularization is evident in about 50% of the area (double arrows) between the limbus and burn (black line). The newly formed vessels in the cornea of the COX-1$^{-/-}$ mice occupy about 30% of the space (double arrows) between the limbus and the burn. The area covered by newly sprouted vessels in the COX-2$^{-/-}$ corneas (double arrows) encompasses about 75% of the corneal surface between the limbus and the silver nitrate burn.

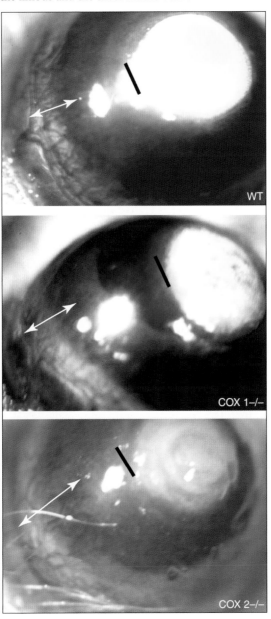

(LPSs) ('exogenous pyrogens'), that then induce the generation, chiefly by mononuclear phagocytes, of various pyrogenic cytokines ('endogenous pyrogens'), in particular, TNF-α, IL-1 and IL-6. These, in turn, by means that are not yet fully understood, alter the activity of thermoregulatory neurons in the anterior hypothalamic preoptic area (POA, the primary brain region in which body core temperature [T_c] is regulated), such that co-ordinated thermoeffector responses are initiated that result in a regulated rise in T_c (reviewed in ref. 154). Since the febrile response thus induced can be suppressed by the administration of drugs that interfere with the production of PGE_2 or with its binding to its receptors, it is thought that PGE_2 is an intermediate, more proximal substance that is released in the POA subsequent to the cytokines and that it drives the observed febrile response. Since the first step in the synthesis of PGE_2 is the conversion of AA into the PG endoperoxides, PGG_2 and PGH_2, by COX and its associated hydroperoxidase, respectively, it follows that COX, too, should have a major regulatory role in fever production.

PROSTAGLANDIN E$_2$ AS A PUTATIVE FEVER MEDIATOR

Milton and Wendlandt were the first to suggest that PGE_2 may be a central mediator of fever[155]. Much evidence since then has consolidated its position in fever genesis. Thus, it is now well established that PGE_2 occurs naturally in the brain, including the POA, and that it is febrigenic when administered intracerebroventricularly (i.c.v.) or directly into the POA (iPO). Moreover, its levels rise and fall in the cerebrospinal fluid (CSF) and preoptic extracellular fluid after peripheral exogenous or endogenous pyrogen administration, in parallel with the febrile course. Both exogenous and endogenous pyrogens enhance PGE_2 synthesis by POA tissue *in vitro*, and, as already mentioned, prostaglandin synthesis inhibitors and PGE_2 receptor antagonists abolish LPS-induced fever in parallel with the reversal of PGE_2 activity (reviewed in ref. 156). This notwithstanding, the mode of action of PGE_2 in fever induction is still unclear. Thus, PGE_2 has been implicated in various models of peripheral cytokine-to-brain signalling (reviewed in refs 157, 158).

CYCLOOXYGENASE-MEDIATED MODULATION OF FEVER

It is now well documented that exogenous (e.g. LPS) and endogenous (e.g. IL-1β) pyrogens activate COX-2 *in vivo*. For example, in recent studies, COX-2-like immunoreactivity[159] and COX-2 mRNA[160–162] were found to be expressed in rat cerebral endothelial cells of capillaries and venules approximately 1.5 h after intraperitoneal (i.p.) LPS administration, and in perivascular microglia and meningeal macrophages approximately 2.5 h after intravenous (i.v.) LPS or IL-1β administration. The different latencies of appearance of COX-2 in the two cell groups may be due to the different routes of LPS administration, i.e. endothelial and phagocytic cells exhibit differential sensitivities to LPS depending on the stimulation or 'priming' conditions[163]. In contrast, COX-1 expression was not affected anywhere in the brain by the peripheral administration of pyrogens. Moreover, the i.p. pre-administration of a COX-1-selective inhibitor, SC560, did not affect the febrile response of guinea pigs to i.v. injected LPS (unpublished observations), whereas treatment with specific inhibitors of COX-2 (NS-398, L-745, 337, DFU, celexoxib, nimesulide) orally after i.v. LPS[164], i.p. before i.p. LPS[160,165,166], i.p. before i.v. or i.c.v. LPS, or i.c.v. before i.v. or i.c.v. LPS (unpublished observations), dose-dependently attenuated the febrile response, but did not affect basal T_c. These antipyretic effects were not different from those produced by conventional NSAIDs, which inhibit both COX-1 and COX-2. Finally, we[167] found that COX-2 gene-deleted heterozygous (COX-2$^{+/-}$) and homozygous (COX-2$^{-/-}$) mice were unable to develop a febrile response to i.p. LPS, whereas their COX-1-deficient littermates produced fevers not different than their WT counterparts. Thus, our data were the first to show that WT, C57BL/6J, COX-1$^{+/-}$ and COX-1$^{-/-}$ mice responded similarly to LPS (*E. coli*, 1 μg animal^{-1}; i.p.) with a 1°C rise in T_c within 1 h after pyrogen administration; the fever abated gradually over the following 3 h. By contrast, COX-2$^{+/-}$ and COX-2$^{-/-}$ mice displayed no T_c rise after LPS. Pyrogen-free saline (PFS) did not affect the T_c of any animal. We concluded from these data that COX-2 is critically important for LPS-induced fever production. This study also served to demonstrate the suitability of such gene knockout mice as conscious animal models for investigating the roles of COX and PGE$_2$ in fever production. These latter findings have meanwhile been extended to show the equally critical dependence on COX-2, but not on COX-1, of the febrile responses of mice to i.v. and i.c.v. LPS and to i.p. and i.c.v. IL-1 (unpublished observations). The febrigenic response to i.c.v. PGE$_2$, on the other hand, is not affected by either COX-1 or COX-2 gene ablation (unpublished observations).

Taken together, these studies confirm the essential role of COX-2 in PGE$_2$, and hence fever, production by various pyrogens delivered by different routes into diverse species. As expected, COX-2 seems to be particularly crucial to the development of the late rather than the early phase of i.v. LPS fever, and its delayed appearance may account for the slow onset latency of i.c.v. LPS fever. It is noteworthy in this context that, compared with their WT counterparts, COX-1$^{-/-}$ and COX-2$^{-/-}$ cells overexpress the alternate functional COX isozyme as well as both basal and IL-1 induced cytosolic phospholipase A$_2$ (cPLA$_2$) and, consequently, exhibit elevated PGE$_2$ biosynthesis[5]. Taken together, therefore, these data provide compelling support for the critical importance of COX-2 in fever genesis.

These data notwithstanding, there are still many unanswered questions. For example, 2 h or more are required for new gene expression and translation of COX-2[168]. By contrast, T_c rises within 8–15 min after i.v. LPS or IL-1β administration[169,170], and preoptic PGE_2 levels are significantly elevated within 30 min[171]. This temporal incongruence between COX-2 induction and fever onset implies, therefore, that the prompt, pyrogen-induced elevation of PGE_2 cannot be accounted for by the inducible form of this enzyme, but rather by its constitutive form, which occurs both in neurons[172] and in cerebro-microvascular endothelial cells[207]. Hence, it may be hypothesized that the regulation of PGE_2 synthesis may be determined by two mechanisms, i.e. an early one involving stimulus-induced activation of the pre-existing enzyme, and a later one requiring *de novo* protein synthesis. The responses of the gene knockout mice in our studies would indicate that the enzyme implicated in LPS-induced fever may indeed be, first, 'constitutive' neuronal or endothelial cell COX-2, then 'inducible' COX-2 in, presumably, the barrier cells, but possibly also in neurons, e.g. refs 173–175. Thus, according to this notion, PGE_2 production after addition of exogenous or endogenous pyrogens may occur in the POA region at two distinct time intervals, viz. an initial release within 20 min and a second, more protracted one, over 2–4 h; the first increase in PGE_2 levels being COX-2 synthesis-independent and the second mediated by *de novo* synthesis of COX-2. However, this requires verification. It is probable that the secondary increased production of PGE_2 also involves the upregulation of $cPLA_2$[176,177]. Very recently, lipid body like structures have been found in cultured, quiescent neurons[178]. These organelles, which contain COX-2, are rapidly inducible in leukocytes at sites of inflammation[179]; as a ready source of AA, they are postulated to be a means of quickly upregulating PGE_2 production[151,180]. They are not seen in quiescent, non-neural cells or in COX-1 labelled cells[151]. The initiating afferent signal, if neurally mediated, could be provided by noradrenaline (NE)[181–183], or simply by synaptic excitation[184–186]; nitric oxide (NO) may also be involved[181,187,188]. Alternatively, if the initiating afferent signal were endothelial cell-mediated, blood-borne LPS could itself be the triggering stimulus. Hence, the regulation of POA PGE_2 synthesis for LPS-induced fever production may be determined by two successive mechanisms, i.e. an early one associated with the first febrile rise, involving, for example, NE- or LPS-induced activation of the pre-existing COX-2 isozyme in neurons or in endothelial cells, respectively, and a later one associated with the second febrile rise, requiring *de novo* COX-2 synthesis by macrophages and/or endothelial cells. It should be noted, importantly, that the secondary increased production of PGE_2 is not associated with elevated preoptic NE levels; these decrease to control levels in parallel with the decline of the first febrile rise[182]. But a role for COX-1 cannot yet be discounted completely. Indeed, selective inhibition of COX-2 only partially reduces the levels of PGs at sites of either acute or chronic inflammation, in comparison with non-selective NSAIDs, which reduce PGs to undetectable levels[189–191], and new data suggest that COX-1 expression may be upregulated under certain inflammatory conditions[192].

Thus, as already emphasized, the observed increase in the plasma levels of PGE_2 simultaneously with the onset of fever after i.v. pyrogen administration occurs too rapidly to be accounted for by the induction of COX-2 in peripheral phagocytic and/or endothelial cells; i.e. the latency of fever onset is too short under these conditions for *de novo* COX-2 induction. Hence, the observed, quick augmentation of circulating PGE_2 would have to be mediated by the activation of COX-1 constitutively expressed in these cells. However, as stated earlier, COX-1 is not normally activated by pyrogenic factors, nor does its congenital absence or pharmacological blockade alter the febrile response. But be that as it may, the available data would nevertheless support the notion that central rather than peripheral PGE_2 is the indispensable mediator in fever genesis. Indeed, we and many others have shown that peripheral LPS causes marked increases in AV3V/POA PGE_2 levels that are sensitive to NSAID inhibition[160,162,193,194]. However, it is not yet established whether LPS-enhanced preoptic PGE_2 is differentially sensitive to selective COX-1 or COX-2 inhibition, and, if so, which, and when after LPS administration.

A different set of events may occur when an infectious noxa originates within the brain or, for experimental purposes, pyrogens are injected i.c.v. In such instances, the febrile response has a long latency of onset and develops gradually[170,195,196]. Originally, this paradoxically slow time-course was ascribed to poor accessibility of the organum vasculosum laminae terminalis (OVLT) to agents originating within the brain and the consequently less coordinated attendant activation of the mechanism(s), whether neural or humoral, mediating the response to blood-borne pyrogens (reviewed in ref. 157); or, alternatively, to the expression by brain tissue of IL-1 receptor antagonist (IL-1ra)[197,198] or of some other antipyretic agent (e.g. arginine vasopressin[199]) upon direct exposure to pyrogens. Such modulatory processes, however, can hardly account for the slow course of fever after iPO injection of pyrogens, including IL-1β[196], and the observation that pyrogens produce a faster fever by intra-OVLT than iPO microinjection[200]. It is conceivable that the stimulated release of PGE_2 by pyrogens acting directly inside the blood–brain barrier (BBB) proceeds only through the activation of inducible, and not constitutive, COX-2. If correct, it may be further speculated that the second febrile rise after i.v. LPS is mediated by IL-1β synthesized meanwhile in the brain[201,202]. However, this too must be verified experimentally.

While the available data generally concur in indicating that the fever-mediating PGE_2 is synthesized in brain via COX-2, the relative roles of constitutive (neurons, endothelial cells) and inducible (microglia, macrophages, endothelial cells) COX-2 are unknown. Their respective involvement may depend on the time elapsed since, and the route and dose of, pyrogen administration; even the pyrogen type may be a factor. An intermediary agent, NE, may be involved. Thus, our hypothesis is that the release of PGE_2 in the POA proceeds in two steps, an early one triggered by NE and mediated by constitutive COX-2 in neurons, and a later one activated by IL-1 and mediated by inducible COX-2 in non-neural cells. A role for COX-1 seems unlikely.

CYCLOOXYGENASE AND NOCICEPTION

PGs formed by COX-1 or COX-2 mediate hyperalgesia in sensory nerve endings. Recently, we[203] assessed the respective roles of COX-1 and COX-2 in pain processing by comparing nociception[204] in WT mice with that in animals lacking either COX-1 or COX-2. There were no differences in gross parameters of behaviour between the different groups of male COX-deficient mice. There was significantly less nociception in COX-1$^{-/-}$ and COX-1$^{+/-}$ (heterozygotes) compared with COX-2$^{-/-}$, COX-2$^{+/-}$ and WT (Figure 3). While the writhing response was somewhat reduced in COX-2$^{-/-}$ and heterozygous animals, compared with WT mice, this difference was not statistically significant.

Figure 3 Nociception in COX-deficient mice. Writhing responses in COX-1 or COX-2-deficient male mice. The number of writhing responses in 15 min in the stretching test for COX-1$^{-/-}$ mice injected i.p. with 1.2% acetic acid (0.1 ml 10 g^{-1}) was less than the number of responses by wild-type (WT) or COX-2$^{-/-}$ animals, which indicates a decrease in nociception in these mice. Histograms represent means for 4–6 animals SEM. *$P < 0.05$.

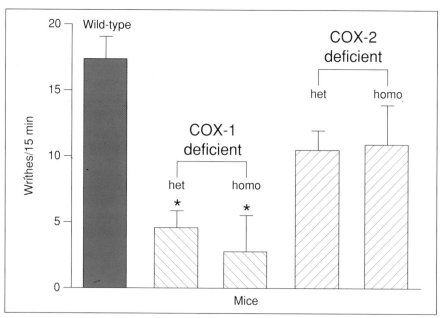

Measurements of mRNA levels by reverse transcriptase polymerase chain reaction (RT-PCR) demonstrated a compensatory increase of COX-1 mRNA in spinal cords of COX-2$^{-/-}$ mice. There was no compensatory COX-2 expression in the spinal cords of COX-1$^{-/-}$ mice. Reduction in the number of writhes of COX-1$^{-/-}$ animals may be due to the absence of COX-1 at the site of stimulation with acetic acid. Thus, PGs made by COX-1 are mainly involved in pain transmission in the stretching test in these animals[203]. Eguchi et al. recently showed that PGD$_2$ plays an essential role in the transmission of tactile pain in mice in a PGD$_2$ synthase deficient model[205].

COMPENSATORY CYCLOOXYGENASE EXPRESSION

Compensatory COX expression may, at least in part, explain why COX-deficient mice are able to function as well as they do, and may also explain some of the surprising phenotypic traits, such as the lack of development of spontaneous ulcers in COX-1$^{-/-}$ mice. The diversity of the COX-1$^{-/-}$ or COX-2$^{-/-}$ phenotype and the apparent overlap between the functions of COX-1 and COX-2 have prompted a re-examination of the question of compensatory regulation of these enzymes *in vitro* and *in vivo*. Interestingly, both COX-1$^{-/-}$ and COX-2$^{-/-}$ cells produced six- to tenfold higher amounts of PGE$_2$ compared with WT cells. Interleukin-1β further enhanced PGE$_2$ output of the WT and COX-1$^{-/-}$ cells but not COX-2$^{-/-}$ cells[5,206].

The dramatic differences we observed in basal PGE$_2$ biosynthesis among WT and COX-1$^{-/-}$ or COX-2$^{-/-}$ cells prompted us to compare the expression of COX-1, COX-2 and cPLA$_2$ genes, encoding three key enzymes that regulate PGE$_2$ biosynthesis. The constitutive levels of COX-2 protein were significantly greater ($\approx$2.4-fold) in unstimulated COX-1$^{-/-}$ cells, consistent with the higher basal PGE$_2$ levels in COX-1$^{-/-}$ cells. IL-1β treatment dramatically increased COX-2 protein levels in COX-1$^{-/-}$ cells[5]. COX-1 protein levels in unstimulated COX-2$^{-/-}$ cells were also much greater ($\approx$14 fold) than in WT cells, likely accounting for the higher basal PGE$_2$ levels. However, IL-1 had no stimulatory effect on COX-1 protein levels in COX-2$^{-/-}$ cells. Whether PGE$_2$ synthase expression may also be altered in COX-deficient cells and play a role in the compensatory synthesis of PGE$_2$ in these cells remains to be examined.

We also discovered that the constitutive levels of cPLA$_2$ protein in COX-1$^{-/-}$ or COX-2$^{-/-}$ embryonic fibroblasts was much higher than in WT cells. Therefore, the enhanced expression of cPLA$_2$ could contribute directly to higher PGE$_2$ levels in both types of COX-deficient cells by generating greater AA substrate for PGE$_2$ biosynthesis. Stimulation of COX-1$^{-/-}$ or COX-2$^{-/-}$ cells with IL-1 resulted in a further increase in the amount of cPLA$_2$ protein. In contrast, WT cells showed little change in the levels of cPLA$_2$ protein after treatment with IL-1. Taken together, these data support the hypothesis that long-term COX isoenzyme deficiency leads to the co-ordinated upregulation of the key enzymes involved in arachidonic acid metabolism[5,206]. We are currently assessing our WT and COX-deficient mice for levels of COX-1 and COX-2 mRNA in a variety of tissues, using competitive RT-PCR. The preliminary data, summarized in Table 1, indicate that compensation may be a tissue-specific phenomenon. Together, these observations suggest that there may be an intricate network involving cross-talk among those enzymes involved in regulating the metabolism of AA. The mechanisms by which tissue-specific compensatory responses 'normalize' prostanoid biosynthesis remain to be elucidated.

INSIGHTS GAINED FROM CYCLOOXYGENASE-DEFICIENT MICE

Based on the phenotypes of COX-1- and COX-2-deficient mice, we may conclude that COX-deficient mice have significantly extended earlier observations that the COX isozymes mediate distinct as well as overlapping functions *in vivo* (Figure 1). However, these studies also provide compelling evidence that ascribing COX-1 and COX-2 exclusive housekeeping or inflammatory functions, respectively, is somewhat simplistic. Since the congenital deficiency of COX-2 is more detrimental than that of COX-1, it may be argued that COX-2 is indeed an important mediator of 'housekeeping' functions. Conversely, COX-1 clearly plays a more important role in certain inflammatory reactions than was previously appreciated.

The use of congenitally COX-deficient mice has enabled us to assess the precise contributions of each COX isozyme to various pathophysiological processes more accurately than was possible through the use of selective COX-1 or COX-2 inhibitors. Although some of the phenotypic effects of COX deficiency can certainly be mimicked by the use of COX-selective inhibitors, these genetically deficient animals have given us a portal with which to view the complexity of regulatory pathways that mediate the homeostatic and inducible functions of the COXs. A number of obvious avenues of research

Table 1 Compensatory COX expression in COX-deficient mouse tissues

	Brain	Heart	Kidney	Liver	Lung	Spinal cord	Spleen	Stomach
COX-1 mRNA in COX-2$^{-/-}$ mice	++	+	−	+	−	++++++	−	−
COX-2 mRNA in COX-1$^{-/-}$ mice	++	−	++	ND	−	−	ND	++

+; increase in mRNA level relative to WT.
−; no change in mRNA level relative to WT.
ND; mRNA below a detectable level.

have been opened by these studies. The two rather surprising phenotypic manifestations, the lack of GI pathology in COX-1$^{-/-}$ mice and the aberrant kidney development of COX-2$^{-/-}$ mice deserve more detailed mechanistic studies. We need to gain a greater understanding of how different tissues are able to differentiate between, and respond differently to, COX-1 or COX-2-derived metabolites. Does differential cellular localization of COX-1, COX-2 and phospholipases modulate tissue-specific responses? We need to elucidate whether COX-1- and COX-2-derived products are functionally linked to distinct cell-surface and nuclear receptors to differentiate between the paracrine, autocrine and intracrine effects of PGs derived from each isozyme. Whether qualitatively different metabolites of AA are expressed in the tissues of COX-deficient versus WT animals remains to be established. The nuclear mechanisms of compensation for the absence of COX isozyme expression and how this phenomenon affects specific pathophysiological processes remain to be studied. The development of conditional mutants in which tissue-specific and temporal expression of the COX isoforms may be precisely regulated and analyses of tissue-specific gene expression using genome wide cDNA micro-arrays will be invaluable in answering these vexing questions.

ACKNOWLEDGEMENTS

The observations from the authors' laboratories included in this review were supported by the Office of Research and Development (R&D), Medical Research Service, Department of Veterans Affairs (DVA), the National Arthritis Foundation and NIH grants AR-43589, AR-45987 and NS 34857. R.R. is a Senior Research Career Scientist of the DVA.

Address all correspondence to: Leslie R. Ballou, Ph.D., Research Chemist, Department of Veterans Affairs Medical Center, Research 151, 1030 Jefferson Avenue, Memphis, TN 38104, USA.

REFERENCES

1. Malakoff D. The rise of the mouse, biomedicine's model mammal. *Science.* 2000;288:248–53.
2. Wen P, Wardern C, Fletcher B, Kujubu D, Herschman H, Lusis A. Chromosomal organization of the inducible and constitutive prostaglandin synthase/cyclooxygenase genes in mouse. *Genomics.* 1993;15:458–60.
3. Smith WL, Garavito RM, DeWitt DL. Prostaglandin endoperoxide H synthase (cyclooxygenases)-1 and -2. *J Biol Chem.* 1996;271:33157–60.
4. Herschman H. Prostaglandin synthase 2. *Biochim Biophys Acta.* 1996;1299:125–40.
5. Kirtikara K, Morham SG, Raghow R, Laulederkind SJ, Kanekura T, Goorha S, Ballou LR. Compensatory prostaglandin E$_2$ biosynthesis in cyclooxygenase 1 or 2 null cells. *J Exp Med.* 1998;187:517–23.

6. Reese J, Brown N, Paria BC, Morrow J, Dey SK. COX-2 compensation in the uterus of COX-1 deficient mice during the pre-implantation period. *Mol Cell Endocrinol.* 1999;150:23–31.

7. Austin SC, Funk CD. Insight into prostaglandin, leukotriene, and other eicosanoid functions using mice with targeted gene disruptions. *Prostaglandins Lipid Mediat.* 1999;58:231–52.

8. Goetzl EJ, An S, Smith WL. Specificity of expression and effects of eicosanoid mediators in normal physiology and human diseases. *FASEB J.* 1995;9:1051–8.

9. Herschman HR, Gilbert RS, Xie W, Luner S, Reddy ST. The regulation and role of TIS10 prostaglandin synthase-2. *Adv Prostaglandin Thromboxane Leukot Res.* 1995;23:23–8.

10. Lin LL, Lin AY, Knopf JL. Cytosolic phospholipase A2 is coupled to hormonally regulated release of arachidonic acid. *Proc Natl Acad Sci USA.* 1992;89:6147–51.

11. Clark JD, Lin LL, Kriz RW, Ramesha CS, Sultzman LA, Lin AY et al. A novel arachidonic acid-selective cytosolic PLA_2 contains a $Ca^{(2+)}$-dependent translocation domain with homology to PKC and GAP. *Cell.* 1991;65:1043–51.

12. Reddy ST, Herschman HR. Transcellular prostaglandin production following mast cell activation is mediated by proximal secretory phospholipase A_2 and distal prostaglandin synthase-1. *J Biol Chem.* 1996;271:186–91.

13. Murakami M, Matsumoto R, Urade Y, Austen KF, Arm JP. c-kit ligand mediates increased expression of cytosolic phospholipase A_2, prostaglandin endoperoxide synthase-1, and hematopoietic prostaglandin D_2 synthase and increased IgE-dependent prostaglandin D_2 generation in immature mouse mast cells. *J Biol Chem.* 1995;270:3239–46.

14. Murakami M, Bingham CO, Matsumoto R, Austen KF, Arm JP. IgE-dependent activation of cytokine-primed mouse cultured mast cells induces a delayed phase of prostaglandin D_2 generation via prostaglandin endoperoxide synthase-2. *J Immunol.* 1995;155:4445–53.

15. Maslinska D, Kaliszek A, Opertowska J, Toborowicz J, Deregowski K, Szukiewicz D. Constitutive expression of cyclooxygenase-2 (COX-2) in developing brain. A. Choroid plexus in human fetuses. *Folia Neuropathol.* 1999;37:287–91.

16. Komhoff M, Wang JL, Cheng HF, Langenbach R, McKanna JA, Harris RC, Breyer MD. Cyclooxygenase-2-selective inhibitors impair glomerulogenesis and renal cortical development. *Kidney Int.* 2000;57:414–22.

17. Langenbach R, Morham SG, Tiano HF, Loftin CD, Ghanayem BI, Chulada PC et al. Disruption of the mouse cyclooxygenase 1 gene. Characteristics of the mutant and areas of future study. *Adv Exp Med Biol.* 1997;407:87–92.

18. Langenbach R, Loftin C, Lee C, Tiano H. Cyclooxygenase knockout mice: models for elucidating isoform-specific functions. *Biochem Pharmacol.* 1999;58:1237–46.

19. Langenbach R, Loftin CD, Lee C, Tiano H. Cyclooxygenase-deficient mice. A summary of their characteristics and susceptibilities to inflammation and carcinogenesis. *Ann N Y Acad Sci.* 1999;889:52–61

20. Breyer MD, Jacobson HR, Breyer RM. Functional and molecular aspects of renal prostaglandin receptors. *J Am Soc Nephrol.* 1996;7:8–17.

21. Breyer M, Bader K. Arachidonic acid metabolites and the kidney. In: Brenner M, editor. *The Kidney*, vol. 1. Philidelphia: W. B. Sanders; 1996:754–88.

22. Rocca B, Spain LM, Ciabattoni G, Patrono C, FitzGerald GA. Differential expression and regulation of cyclooxygenase isozymes in thymic stromal cells. *J Immunol.* 1999;162:4589–97.

23. Rocca B, Spain LM, Pure E, Langenbach R, Patrono C, FitzGerald GA. Distinct roles of prostaglandin H synthases 1 and 2 in T-cell development. *J Clin Invest.* 1999;103:1469–77.

24. Spencer AG, Woods JW, Arakawa T, Singer, Smith WL. Subcellular localization of prostaglandin endoperoxide H synthases-1 and -2 by immunoelectron microscopy. *J Biol Chem.* 1998;273:9886–93.

25. Murakami M, Kambe T, Shimbara S, Higashino K, Hanasaki K, Arita H et al. Different functional aspects of the group II subfamily (Types IIA and V) and type X secretory phospholipase A_2s in regulating arachidonic acid release and prostaglandin generation. Implications of cyclooxygenase-2 induction and phospholipid scramblase-mediated cellular membrane perturbation. *J Biol Chem.* 1999;274:31435–44.

26. Murakami M, Kambe T, Shimbara S, Yamamoto S, Kuwata H, Kudo I. Functional association of type IIA secretory phospholipase A_2 with the glycosylphosphatidylinositol-anchored heparan sulfate proteoglycan in the cyclooxygenase-2-mediated delayed prostanoid-biosynthetic pathway. *J Biol Chem.* 1999;274:29927–36.

27. Balsinde J, Balboa MA, Dennis EA. Functional coupling between secretory phospholipase A_2 and cyclooxygenase-2 and its regulation by cytosolic group IV phospholipase A_2. *Proc Natl Acad Sci USA.* 1998;95:7951–6.

28. Vane JR, Botting RM. A better understanding of anti-inflammatory drugs based on isoforms of cyclooxygenase (COX-1 and COX-2). *Adv Prostaglandin Thromboxane Leukot Res.* 1995;23:41–8.

29. DeWitt DL, Meade EA, Smith WL. PGH synthase isozyme selectivity: potential safer nonsteroidal antiinflammatory drugs. *Am J Med.* 1993;95:40s–4s.

30. Vane JR, Botting RM. Regulatory mechanisms of the vascular endothelium: an update. *Pol J Pharmacol.* 1994;46:499–21.

31. Vane JR, Botting RM. New insights into the mode of action of anti-inflammatory drugs. *Inflamm Res.* 1995;44:1–10.

32. Kargman SL, O'Neill GP, Vickers PJ, Evans JF, Mancini JA, Jothy S. Expression of prostaglandin G/H synthase-1 and -2 protein in human colon cancer. *Cancer Res.* 1995;55:2556–9.

33. Rigas B, Goldman IS, Levine L. Altered eicosanoid levels in human colon cancer. *J Lab Clin Med.* 1993;122:518–23.

34. Zhang X, Morham SG, Langenbach R, Young DA. Malignant transformation and antineoplastic actions of nonsteroidal antiinflammatory drugs (NSAIDs) on cyclooxygenase-null embryo fibroblasts. *J Exp Med.* 1999;190:451–9.

35. Langenbach R, Morham SG, Tiano HF, Loftin CD, Ghanayem BI, Chulada PC et al. Prostaglandin synthase 1 gene disruption in mice reduces arachidonic acid-induced inflammation and indomethacin-induced gastric ulceration. *Cell.* 1995;83:483–92.

36. Morham SG, Langenbach R, Loftin CD, Tiano HF, Vouloumanos N, Jennette JC et al. Prostaglandin synthase 2 gene disruption causes severe renal pathology in the mouse. *Cell.* 1995;83:473–82.

37. Dinchuk JE, Car BD, Focht RJ, Johnston JJ, Jaffee BD, Covington MB et al. Renal abnormalities and an altered inflammatory response in mice lacking cyclooxygenase II. *Nature.* 1995;378:406–9.

38. Vane JR. NSAIDs, Cox-2 inhibitors, and the gut. *Lancet.* 1995;346:1105–6.

39. Mahler JF, Davis BJ, Morham SG, Langenbach R. Disruption of cyclooxygenase genes in mice. *Toxicol Pathol.* 1996;24:717–19.

40. Lim H, Paria BC, Das SK, Dinchuk JE, Langenbach R, Trzaskos JM et al. Multiple female reproductive failures in cyclooxygenase 2-deficient mice. *Cell.* 1997;91:197–208.
41. Lipsky PE, Brooks P, Crofford LJ, DuBois R, Graham D, Simon LS et al. Unresolved issues in the role of cyclooxygenase-2 in normal physiologic processes and disease. *Arch Intern Med.* 2000;160:913–20.
42. Dubois RN, Abramson SB, Crofford L, Gupta RA, Simon LS, Van De Putte LB et al. Cyclooxygenase in biology and disease. *FASEB J.* 1998;12:1063–73.
43. Harris RC, McKanna JA, Akai Y, Jacobson HR, Dubois RN, Breyer MD. Cyclooxygenase-2 is associated with the macula densa of rat kidney and increases with salt restriction. *J Clin Invest.* 1994;94:2504–10.
44. Guan Y, Chang M, Cho W, Zhang Y, Redha R, Davis L et al. Cloning, expression, and regulation of rabbit cyclooxygenase-2 in renal medullary interstitial cells. *Am J Physiol.* 1997;273:F18–26.
45. Komhoff M, Grone HJ, Klein T, Seyberth HW, Nusing RM. Localization of cyclooxygenase-1 and -2 in adult and fetal human kidney: implication for renal function. *Am J Physiol.* 1997;272:F460–8.
46. Khan KN, Venturini CM, Bunch RT, Brassard JA, Koki AT, Morris DL et al. Interspecies differences in renal localization of cyclooxygenase isoforms: implications in nonsteroidal antiinflammatory drug-related nephrotoxicity. *Toxicol Pathol.* 1998;26:612–20.
47. Zambraski EJ. The effects of nonsteroidal anti-inflammatory drugs on renal function: experimental studies in animals. *Semin Nephrol.* 1995;15:205–13.
48. Palmer BF, Henrich WL. Clinical acute renal failure with nonsteroidal anti-inflammatory drugs. *Semin Nephrol.* 1995;15:214–27.
49. Cheng HF, Wang JL, Zhang MZ, Miyazaki Y, Ichikawa I, McKanna JA et al. Angiotensin II attenuates renal cortical cyclooxygenase-2 expression. *J Clin Invest.* 1999;103:953–61.
50. Stuart RO, Nigam S. Developmental biology of the kidney. In: Brenner BM, editor. *The Kidney*, vol. 1, 6th edn. Philadelphia: W. B. Sanders; 2000:68–92.
51. Anderson CE, Wallerstein R, Zamerowski ST, Witzleben C, Hoyer JR, Gibas L et al. Ring chromosome 4 mosaicism coincidence of oligomeganephronia and signs of Seckel syndrome. *Am J Med Genet.* 1997;72:281–5.
52. Richards JS, Fitzpatrick SL, Clemens JW, Morris JK, Alliston T, Sirois J. Ovarian cell differentiation: a cascade of multiple hormones, cellular signals, and regulated genes. *Recent Prog Horm Res.* 1995;50:223–54.
53. Sugimoto Y, Yamasaki A, Segi E, Tsuboi K, Aze Y, Nishimura T et al. Failure of parturition in mice lacking the prostaglandin F receptor. *Science.* 1997;277:681–3.
54. Davis BJ, Lennard DE, Lee CA, Tiano HF, Morham SG, Wetsel WC et al. Anovulation in cyclooxygenase-2-deficient mice is restored by prostaglandin E_2 and interleukin-1. *Endocrinology.* 1999;140:2685–95.
55. Yang ZM, Das SK, Wang J, Sugimoto Y, Ichikawa A, Dey SK. Potential sites of prostaglandin actions in the periimplantation mouse uterus: differential expression and regulation of prostaglandin receptor genes. *Biol Reprod.* 1997;56:368–79.
56. Katsuyama M, Sugimoto Y, Morimoto K, Hasumoto K, Fukumoto M, Negishi et al. 'Distinct cellular localization' of the messenger ribonucleic acid for prostaglandin E receptor subtypes in the mouse uterus during pseudopregnancy. *Endocrinology.* 1997;138:344–50.
57. Murata T, Ushikubi F, Matsuoka T, Hirata M, Yamasaki A, Sugimoto Y et al.

Altered pain perception and inflammatory response in mice lacking prostacyclin receptor. *Nature.* 1997;388:678–82.

58. Nguyen M, Camenisch T, Snouwaert JN, Hicks E, Coffman TM, Anderson PA et al. The prostaglandin receptor EP_4 triggers remodelling of the cardiovascular system at birth. *Nature.* 1997;390:78–81.

59. Austin S, FitzGerald GA. Not a mouse stirring: deletion of the EP_2 and love's labor's lost. *J Clin Invest.* 1999;103:1481–2.

60. Tilley SL, Audoly LP, Hicks EH, Kim HS, Flannery PJ, Coffman TM et al. Reproductive failure and reduced blood pressure in mice lacking the EP_2 prostaglandin E_2 receptor. *J Clin Invest.* 1999;103:1539–45.

61. Akil M, Amos RS, Stewart P. Infertility may sometimes be associated with NSAID consumption. *Br J Rheumatol.* 1996;35:76–8.

62. Athanasiou S, Bourne TH, Khalid A, Okokon EV, Crayford TJ, Hagstrom HG et al. Effects of indomethacin on follicular structure, vascularity, and function over the periovulatory period in women. *Fertil Steril.* 1996;65:556–60.

63. Gross L. The role of viruses in the etiology of cancer and leukemia in animals and in humans. *Proc Natl Acad Sci USA.* 1997;94:4237–8.

64. Chakraborty I, Das SK, Wang J, Dey SK. Developmental expression of the cyclooxygenase-1 and cyclooxygenase-2 genes in the peri-implantation mouse uterus and their differential regulation by the blastocyst and ovarian steroids. *J Mol Endocrinol.* 1996;16:107–22.

65. Bany BM, Kennedy TG. Regulation of cyclooxygenase gene expression in rat endometrial stromal cells: the role of epidermal growth factor. *Dev Genet.* 1997;21:109–15.

66. Kim JJ, Wang J, Bambra C, Das SK, Dey SK, Fazleabas AT. Expression of cyclooxygenase-1 and -2 in the baboon endometrium during the menstrual cycle and pregnancy. *Endocrinology.* 1999;140:2672–8.

67. Song JH, Sirois J, Houde A, Murphy BD. Cloning, developmental expression, and immunohistochemistry of cyclooxygenase 2 in the endometrium during embryo implantation and gestation in the mink (*Mustela vison*). *Endocrinology.* 1998;139:3629–36.

68. Langman MJ, Weil J, Wainwright P, Lawson DH, Rawlins MD, Logan RF et al. Risks of bleeding peptic ulcer associated with individual non-steroidal anti-inflammatory drugs. *Lancet.* 1994;343:1075–8.

69. Kargman S, Charleson S, Cartwright M, Frank J, Riendeau D, Mancini J et al. Characterization of prostaglandin G/H synthase 1 and 2 in rat, dog, monkey, and human gastrointestinal tracts. *Gastroenterology.* 1996;111:445–54.

70. Schafer AI. Effects of nonsteroidal antiinflammatory drugs on platelet function and systemic hemostasis. *J Clin Pharmacol.* 1995;35:209–19.

71. Patrono C. Aspirin as an antiplatelet drug. *N Engl J Med.* 1994;330:1287–94.

72. Vane JR, Botting RM. Mechanism of action of aspirin-like drugs. *Semin Arthritis Rheum.* 1997;26 (suppl 1):2–10.

73. Cirino G. Multiple controls in inflammation. Extracellular and intracellular phospholipase A_2, inducible and constitutive cyclooxygenase, and inducible nitric oxide synthase. *Biochem Pharmacol.* 1998;55:105–11.

74. Mizuno H, Sakamoto C, Matsuda K, Wada K, Uchida T, Noguchi H et al. Induction of cyclooxygenase 2 in gastric mucosal lesions and its inhibition by the specific antagonist delays healing in mice. *Gastroenterology.* 1997;112:387–97.

75. Eckmann L, Stenson WF, Savidge TC, Lowe DC, Barrett KE, Fierer J et al. Role

of intestinal epithelial cells in the host secretory response to infection by invasive bacteria. Bacterial entry induces epithelial prostaglandin H synthase-2 expression and prostaglandin E_2 and $F_{2\alpha}$ production. *J Clin Invest.* 1997;100:296–309.

76. Bak AW, McKnight W, Li P, Del Soldato P, Calignano A, Cirino G et al. Cyclooxygenase-independent chemoprevention with an aspirin derivative in a rat model of colonic adenocarcinoma. *Life Sci.* 1998;62:367–73.

77. Bamba H, Ota S, Kato A, Adachi A, Itoyama S, Matsuzaki F. High expression of cyclooxygenase-2 in macrophages of human colonic adenoma. *Int J Cancer.* 1999;83:470–5.

78. Fischer SM, Lo HH, Gordon GB, Seibert K, Kelloff G, Lubet RA et al. Chemopreventive activity of celecoxib, a specific cyclooxygenase-2 inhibitor, and indomethacin against ultraviolet light-induced skin carcinogenesis. *Mol Carcinog.* 1999;25:231–40.

79. Fukuda K, Hibiya Y, Mutoh M, Koshiji M, Akao S, Fujiwara H. Inhibition by berberine of cyclooxygenase-2 transcriptional activity in human colon cancer cells. *J Ethnopharmacol.* 1999;66:227–33.

80. Hwang D, Scollard D, Byrne J, Levine E. Expression of cyclooxygenase-1 and cyclooxygenase-2 in human breast cancer. *J Natl Cancer Inst.* 1998;90:455–60.

81. Kalgutkar AS, Kozak KR, Crews BC, Hochgesang GP, Marnett LJ. Covalent modification of cyclooxygenase-2 (COX-2) by 2-acetoxyphenyl alkyl sulfides, a new class of selective COX-2 inactivators. *J Med Chem.* 1998;41:4800–18.

82. Kalgutkar AS, Crews BC, Rowlinson SW, Garner C, Seibert K, Marnett LJ. Aspirin-like molecules that covalently inactivate cyclooxygenase-2. *Science.* 1998;280:1268–70.

83. Kawamori T, Rao CV, Seibert K, Reddy BS. Chemopreventive activity of celecoxib, a specific cyclooxygenase-2 inhibitor, against colon carcinogenesis. *Cancer Res.* 1998;58:409–12.

84. Langenbach N, Kroiss MM, Ruschoff J, Schlegel J, Landthaler M, Stolz W. Assessment of microsatellite instability and loss of heterozygosity in sporadic kerato-acanthomas. *Arch Dermatol Res.* 1999;291:1–5.

85. Lim HY, Joo HJ, Choi JH, Yi JW, Yang MS, Cho DY et al. Increased expression of cyclooxygenase-2 protein in human gastric carcinoma. *Clin Cancer Res.* 2000;6:519–25.

86. Lipsky PE. The clinical potential of cyclooxygenase-2-specific inhibitors. *Am J Med.* 1999;106 (5B):51S–57S.

87. Lipsky PE. Role of cyclooxygenase-1 and -2 in health and disease. *Am J Orthop.* 1999;28 (suppl):8–12.

88. Nakajima T, Hamanaka K, Fukuda T, Oyama T, Kashiwabara K, Sano T. Why is cyclooxygenase-2 expressed in neuroendocrine cells of the human alimentary tract? *Pathol Int.* 1997;47:889–91.

89. Nakatsugi S, Fukutake M, Takahashi M, Fukuda K, Isoi T, Taniguchi Y et al. Suppression of intestinal polyp development by nimesulide, a selective cyclo-oxygenase-2 inhibitor, in Min mice. *Jpn J Cancer Res.* 1997;88:1117–20.

90. Narko K, Ristimaki A, MacPhee M, Smith E, Haudenschild CC, Hla T. Tumorigenic transformation of immortalized ECV endothelial cells by cyclo-oxygenase-1 overexpression. *J Biol Chem.* 1997;272:21455–60.

91. Reddy BS, Hirose Y, Lubet R, Steele V, Kelloff G, Paulson S et al. Chemoprevention of colon cancer by specific cyclooxygenase-2 inhibitor, celecoxib, administered during different stages of carcinogenesis. *Cancer Res.* 2000;60:293–7.

92. Shao J, Sheng H, Aramandla R, Pereira MA, Lubet RA, Hawk E et al. Coordinate

regulation of cyclooxygenase-2 and TGF-β1 in replication error-positive colon cancer and azoxymethane-induced rat colonic tumors. *Carcinogenesis*. 1999;20:185–91.

93. Sheng H, Shao J, Kirkland SC, Isakson P, Coffey RJ, Morrow J et al. Inhibition of human colon cancer cell growth by selective inhibition of cyclooxygenase-2. *J Clin Invest*. 1997;99:2254–9.

94. Shiota G, Okubo M, Noumi T, Noguchi N, Oyama K, Takano Y et al. Cyclooxygenase-2 expression in hepatocellular carcinoma. *Hepato-gastroenterology*. 1999;46:407–12.

95. Singh J, Hamid R, Reddy BS. Dietary fat and colon cancer: modulation of cyclo-oxygenase-2 by types and amount of dietary fat during the postinitiation stage of colon carcinogenesis. *Cancer Res*. 1997;57:3465–70.

96. Tsujii M, Kawano S, Tsuji S, Sawaoka H, Hori M, DuBois RN. Cyclooxygenase regulates angiogenesis induced by colon cancer cells. *Cell*. 1998;5:705–16.

97. Uefuji K, Ichikura T, Mochizuki H, Shinomiya N. Expression of cyclooxygenase-2 protein in gastric adenocarcinoma. *J Surg Oncol*. 1998;69:168–72.

98. Hursting SD. Experimental models of gene–environment interaction for cancer chemoprevention studies. *Curr Opin Oncol*. 1997;9:487–91.

99. Majerus PW. Prostaglandins: critical roles in pregnancy and colon cancer. *Curr Biol*. 1998;8:R87–9.

100. Oshima M, Taketo MM. Colon cancer and cyclooxygenase. *Nippon Shokakibyo Gakkai Zasshi*. 1998;95:1327–32.

101. Taketo MM. COX-2 and colon cancer. *Inflamm Res*. 1998;47 (suppl 2):S112–6.

102. Watanabe K, Kawamori T, Nakatsugi S, Ohta T, Ohuchida S, Yamamoto H et al. Role of the prostaglandin E receptor subtype EP$_1$ in colon carcinogenesis. *Cancer Res*. 1999;59:5093–6.

103. Oshima M, Dinchuk JE, Kargman SL, Oshima H, Hancock B, Kwong E et al. Suppression of intestinal polyposis in *Apc δ716* knockout mice by inhibition of cyclooxygenase 2 (COX-2). *Cell*. 1996;87:803–9.

104. Prescott SM, White RL. Self-promotion? Intimate connections between APC and prostaglandin H synthase-2. *Cell*. 1996;87:783–6.

105. Chulada PC, Doyle C, Gaul B, Tiano HF, Mahler JF, Lee CA et al. Cyclooxygenase-1 and -2 deficiency decrease spontaneous intestinal adenomas in the *Min* mouse. *Proc Am Assoc Cancer Res*. 1998;39:195.

106. Shoemaker AR, Gould KA, Luongo C, Moser AR, Dove WF. Studies of neoplasia in the *Min* mouse. *Biochim Biophys Acta*. 1997;1332:F25–48.

107. Shoemaker AR, Luongo C, Moser AR, Marton LJ, Dove WF. Somatic mutational mechanisms involved in intestinal tumor formation in Min mice. *Cancer Res*. 1997;57:1999–2006.

108. Moser AR, Luongo C, Gould KA, McNeley MK, Shoemaker AR, Dove WF. *ApcMin*: a mouse model for intestinal and mammary tumorigenesis. *Eur J Cancer*. 1995;31A:1061–4.

109. Tiano HF, Chulada PC, Spalding J, Lee CA, Loftin CD, Mahler JF et al. Effects of cyclooxygenase deficiency on inflammation and papilloma formation in mouse skin. *Proc Am Assoc Cancer Res*. 1998;38:257.

110. Williams C, Tsujii M, Reese J, Dey S, DuBois R. Host cyclooxygenase-2 modulates carcinoma growth. *J Clin Invest*. 2000;105:1589–94.

111. Smalley WE, DuBois RN. Colorectal cancer and nonsteroidal anti-inflammatory drugs. *Adv Pharmacol*. 1997;39:1–20.

112. Shiff SJ, Rigas B. The role of cyclooxygenase inhibition in the antineoplastic effects of nonsteroidal antiinflammatory drugs (NSAIDs). *J Exp Med.* 1999;190:445–50.

113. Sheng GG, Shao J, Sheng H, Hooton EB, Isakson PC, Morrow JD et al. A selective cyclooxygenase 2 inhibitor suppresses the growth of H-*ras*-transformed rat intestinal epithelial cells. *Gastroenterology.* 1997;113:1883–91.

114. Piazza GA, Rahm AL, Krutzsch M, Sperl G, Paranka NS, Gross PH et al. Antineoplastic drugs sulindac sulfide and sulfone inhibit cell growth by inducing apoptosis. *Cancer Res.* 1995;55:3110–16.

115. Mahmoud NN, Boolbol SK, Dannenberg AJ, Mestre JR, Bilinski RT, Martucci C et al. The sulfide metabolite of sulindac prevents tumors and restores enterocyte apoptosis in a murine model of familial adenomatous polyposis. *Carcinogenesis.* 1998;19:87–91.

116. Reddy BS, Kawamori T, Lubet RA, Steele VE, Kelloff GJ, Rao CV. Chemopreventive efficacy of sulindac sulfone against colon cancer depends on time of administration during carcinogenic process. *Cancer Res.* 1999;59:3387–91.

117. Hanif R, Pittas A, Feng Y, Koutsos MI, Qiao L, Staiano-Coico L et al. Effects of nonsteroidal anti-inflammatory drugs on proliferation and on induction of apoptosis in colon cancer cells by a prostaglandin-independent pathway. *Biochem Pharmacol.* 1996;52:237–45.

118. Elder DJ, Halton DE, Hague A, Paraskeva C. Induction of apoptotic cell death in human colorectal carcinoma cell lines by a cyclooxygenase-2 (COX-2)-selective nonsteroidal anti- inflammatory drug: independence from COX-2 protein expression. *Clin Cancer Res.* 1997;3:1679–83.

119. Eberhart CE, Coffey RJ, Radhika A, Giardiello FM, Ferrenbach S, DuBois RN. Up-regulation of cyclooxygenase 2 gene expression in human colorectal adenomas and adenocarcinomas. *Gastroenterology.* 1994;107:1183–8.

120. Sano H, Kawahito Y, Wilder RL, Hashiramoto A, Mukai S, Asai K et al. Expression of cyclooxygenase-1 and -2 in human colorectal cancer. *Cancer Res.* 1995;55:3785–9.

121. Shattuck-Brandt RL, Lamps LW, Heppner Goss KJ, DuBois RN, Matrisian LM. Differential expression of matrilysin and cyclooxygenase-2 in intestinal and colorectal neoplasms. *Mol Carcinog.* 1999;24:177–87.

122. Betz M, Fox BS. Prostaglandin E_2 inhibits production of Th1 lymphokines but not of Th2 lymphokines. *J Immunol.* 1991;146:108–13.

123. Anastassiou ED, Paliogianni F, Balow JP, Yamada H, Boumpas DT. Prostaglandin E_2 and other cAMP-elevating agents modulate IL-2 and IL-2R alpha gene expression at multiple levels. *J Immunol.* 1992;148:2845–52.

124. Paliogianni F, Kincaid RL, Boumpas DT. Prostaglandin E_2 and other cAMP elevating agents inhibit interleukin 2 gene transcription by counteracting calcineurin-dependent pathways. *J Exp Med.* 1993;178:1813–17.

125. Hilkens CM, Vermeulen H, van Neerven RJ, Snijdewint FG, Wierenga EA, Kapsenberg ML. Differential modulation of T helper type 1 (Th1) and T helper type 2 (Th2) cytokine secretion by prostaglandin E_2 critically depends on interleukin-2. *Eur J Immunol.* 1995;25:59–63.

126. van der Pouw Kraan TC, Boeije LC, Smeenk RJ, Wijdenes J, Aarden LA. Prostaglandin E_2 is a potent inhibitor of human interleukin-12 production. *J Exp Med.* 1995;181:775–9.

127. Valitutti S, Dessing M, Lanzavecchia A. Role of cAMP in regulating cytotoxic T lymphocyte adhesion and motility. *Eur J Immunol.* 1993;23:790–5.

128. Mastino A, Grelli S, Piacentini M, Oliverio S, Favalli C, Perno CF et al.

Correlation between induction of lymphocyte apoptosis and prostaglandin E$_2$ production by macrophages infected with HIV. *Cell Immunol.* 1993;152:120–30.

129. Cayeux SJ, Beverley PC, Schulz R, Dorken B. Elevated plasma prostaglandin E$_2$ levels found in 14 patients undergoing autologous bone marrow or stem cell transplantation. *Bone Marrow Transplant.* 1993;12:603–8.

130. Leung DY. Atopic dermatitis: the skin as a window into the pathogenesis of chronic allergic diseases. *J Allergy Clin Immunol.* 1995;96:302–18.

131. Litherland SA, Xie XT, Hutson AD, Wasserfall C, Whittaker DS, She JX et al. Aberrant prostaglandin synthase 2 expression defines an antigen-presenting cell defect for insulin-dependent diabetes mellitus. *J Clin Invest.* 1999;104:515–23.

132. Rosloneic E, Ballou LR, Raghow R, Hasty K, Kang AH. Molecular biology of autoimmune arthritis. In: Serhan CN, Ward PA editors. *Molecular and Cellular Basis of Inflammation.* Totowa, NJ: Humana Press; 1999:289–307.

133. Brahn E. Animal models of rheumatoid arthritis. Clues to etiology and treatment. *Clin Orthop.* 1991;265:42–53.

134. Courtenay JS, Dallman MJ, Dayan AD, Martin A, Mosedale B. Immunization against heterologous type II collagen induces arthritis in mice. *Nature.* 1980;283:666–8.

135. Trentham DE, Townes AS, Kang AH. Autoimmunity to type II collagen: An experimental model of arthritis. *J Exp Med.* 1977;146:857–68.

136. Terato K, Arai H, Shimozuru Y, Fukuda T, Tanaka H, Watanabe H et al. Sex-linked differences in susceptibility of cynomolgus monkeys to type II collagen-induced arthritis: Evidence that epitope-specific immune suppression is involved in the regulation of type II collagen autoantibody formation. *Arthritis Rheum.* 1989;6:748–58.

137. Londei M, Savill CM, Verhoef A, Brennan F, Leech ZA, Duance V et al. Persistence of collagen type II-specific T-cell clones in the synovial membrane of a patient with rheumatoid arthritis. *Proc Natl Acad Sci USA.* 1989;86:636–40.

138. Jasin HE. Autoantibody specificities of immune complexes sequestered in articular cartilage of patients with rheumatoid arthritis and osteoarthritis. *Arthritis Rheum.* 1985;28:241–8.

139. Watson W, Cremer M, Wooley P, Townes A. Assessment of the potential pathogenicity of type II collagen autoantibodies in patients with rheumatoid arthritis. *Arth Rheum.* 1986;29:1316–21.

140. Terato K, Shimozuru Y, Katayama K, Takemitsu Y, Yamashita I, Miyatsu M et al. Specificity of antibodies to type II collagen in rheumatoid arthritis. *Arthritis Rheum.* 1990;33:1493–500.

141. Stuart JM, Huffstutter EH, Townes AS, Kang AH. Incidence and specificity of antibodies to type I, II, III, IV, and V collagen in rheumatoid arthiritis and other rheumatic diseases as measured by ^{125}I-radioimmunoassay. *Arthritis Rheum.* 1983;26:832–40.

142. Watson WC, Tooms RE, Carnesale PG, Dutkowsky JP. A case of germinal center formation by CD45RO T and CD20 B lymphocytes in rheumatoid arthritic subchondral bone: Proposal for a two-compartment model of immune-mediated disease with implications for immunotherapeutic strategies. *Clin Immunol Immunopath.* 1994;73:27–37.

143. Brand DD, Marion TN, Myers LK, Rosloniec EF, Watson WC, Stuart JM et al. Autoantibodies to murine type II collagen in collagen induced arthritis: A comparison of susceptible and non susceptible strains. *J Immunol.* 1996;157:5178–84.

144. Terato K, Hasty KA, Reife RA, Cremer MA, Kang AH, Stuart JM. Induction of arthritis with monoclonal antibodies to collagen. *J Immunol.* 1992;148:2103–8.

145. Stuart JM, Tomoda K, Townes AS, Kang AH. Serum transfer of collagen induced arthritis. II. Identification and localization of autoantibody to type II collagen in donor and recipient rats. *Arthritis Rheum.* 1983;26:1237–44.

146. Stuart JM, Dixon FJ. Serum transfer of collagen induced arthritis in mice. *J Exp Med.* 1983;158:378–92.

147. Wooley PH, Luthra, S. H, Singh S, Huse A, Stuart JM, David CS. Passive transfer of arthritis in mice by human anti-type II collagen antibody. *Mayo Clinic Proc.* 1984;59:737–43.

148. Myers L, Rosloneic E, Cremer M, Kang AH. Collagen-induced arthritis: an animal model of autoimmunity. *Life Sci.* 1997;61:1861–78.

149. Wallace JL, Bak A, McKnight W, Asfaha S, Sharkey KA, MacNaughton WK. Cyclooxygenase 1 contributes to inflammatory responses in rats and mice: implications for gastrointestinal toxicity. *Gastroenterology.* 1998;115:101–9.

150. Reddy ST, Tiano HF, Langenbach R, Morham SG, Herschman HR. Genetic evidence for distinct roles of COX-1 and COX-2 in the immediate and delayed phases of prostaglandin synthesis in mast cells. *Biochem Biophys Res Commun.* 1999;265:205–10.

151. Bozza PT, Payne JL, Morham SG, Langenbach R, Smithies O, Weller PF. Leukocyte lipid body formation and eicosanoid generation: cyclooxygenase-independent inhibition by aspirin. *Proc Natl Acad Sci USA.* 1996;93:11091–6.

152. Okada Y, Lorenzo JA, Freeman AM, Tomita M, Morham SG, Raisz LG et al. Prostaglandin G/H synthase-2 is required for maximal formation of osteoclast-like cells in culture. *J Clin Invest.* 2000;105:823–32.

153. Gavett SH, Madison SL, Chulada PC, Scarborough PE, Qu W, Boyle JE et al. Allergic lung responses are increased in prostaglandin H synthase-deficient mice. *J Clin Invest.* 1999;104:721–32.

154. Blatteis CM. Fever. In: Blatteis CM, editor. *Physiology and Pathophysiology of Temperature Regulation.* Singapore: World Scientific; 1998:177–92.

155. Milton AS, Wendlandt S. A possible role for prostaglandin E_2 as a modulator for temperature regulation in the central nervous system of the cat. *J Physiol (Lond).* 1970;207:76P–77P.

156. Blatteis CM, Sehic E. Prostaglandin E_2: a putative fever mediator. In: Mackowiak P, editor. *Basic Mechanisms and Management,* 2nd edn. New York: Raven–Lippincott; 1997:117–48.

157. Blatteis C, Sehic E. Fever: how many circulating pyrogens signal the brain? *News Physiol Sci.* 1997;12:1–9.

158. Coceani F, Akarsu ES. Prostaglandin E_2 in the pathogenesis of fever. An update. *Ann N Y Acad Sci.* 1998;856:76–82.

159. Matsumura K, Cao C, Ozaki M, Morii H, Nakadate K, Watanabe Y. Brain endothelial cells express cyclooxygenase-2 during lipopolysaccharide-induced fever: light and electron microscopic immunocytochemical studies. *J Neurosci.* 1998;18:6279–89.

160. Cao C, Matsumura K, Yamagata K, Watanabe Y. Involvement of cyclooxygenase-2 in LPS-induced fever and regulation of its mRNA by LPS in the rat brain. *Am J Physiol.* 1997;272:R1712–R25.

161. Quan N, Whiteside M, Herkenham M. Cyclooxygenase 2 mRNA expression in rat brain after peripheral injection of lipopolysaccharide. *Brain Res.* 1998;802:189–97.

162. Elmquist JK, Breder CD, Sherin JE, Scammell TE, Hickey WF, Dewitt D et al. Intravenous lipopolysaccharide induces cyclooxygenase 2-like immunoreactivity in rat brain perivascular microglia and meningeal macrophages. *J Comp Neurol.* 1997;381:119–29.

163. Koll S, Goppelt-Struebe M, Hauser I, Goerig M. Monocytic–endothelial cell interaction: regulation of prostanoid synthesis in human coculture. *J Leukoc Biol.* 1997;61:679–88.

164. Futaki N, Takahashi S, Yokoyama M, Arai I, Higuchi S, Otomo S. NS-398, a new anti-inflammatory agent, selectively inhibits prostaglandin G/H synthase/cyclooxygenase (COX-2) activity *in vitro. Prostaglandins.* 1994;47:55–9.

165. Taniguchi Y, Yokoyama K, Inui K, Deguchi Y, Furukawa K, Noda K. Inhibition of brain cyclooxygenase-2 activity and the antipyretic action of nimesulide. *Eur J Pharmacol.* 1997;330:221–9.

166. Chan CC, Boyce S, Brideau C, Ford-Hutchinson AW, Gordon R, Guay D et al. Pharmacology of a selective cyclooxygenase-2 inhibitor, L-745,337: a novel nonsteroidal anti-inflammatory agent with an ulcerogenic sparing effect in rat and nonhuman primate stomach. *J Pharmacol Exp Ther.* 1995;274:1531–7.

167. Li S, Wang Y, Matsumura K, Ballou LR, Morham SG, Blatteis CM. The febrile response to lipopolysaccharide is blocked in cyclooxygenase-2$^{(-/-)}$, but not in cyclooxygenase-1$^{(-/-)}$ mice. *Brain Res.* 1999;825:86–94

168. Masferrer JL, Seibert K, Zweifel B, Needleman P. Endogenous glucocorticoids regulate an inducible cyclooxygenase enzyme. *Proc Natl Acad Sci USA.* 1992;89:3917–21.

169. Blatteis CM. Influence of body weight and temperature on the pyrogenic effect of endotoxin in guinea pigs. *Toxicol Appl Pharmacol.* 1974;29:249–58.

170. Stitt JT, Bernheim HA. Differences in endogenous pyrogen fevers induced by iv and icv routes in rabbits. *J Appl Physiol.* 1985;59:342–7.

171. Sehic E, Szekely M, Ungar AL, Oladehin A, Blatteis CM. Hypothalamic prostaglandin E$_2$ during lipopolysaccharide-induced fever in guinea pigs. *Brain Res Bull.* 1996;39:391–9.

172. Norton JL, Adamson SL, Bocking AD, Han VK. Prostaglandin-H synthase-1 (PGHS-1) gene is expressed in specific neurons of the brain of the late gestation ovine fetus. *Brain Res Dev Brain Res.* 1996;95:79–96.

173. Breder CD, Dewitt D, Kraig RP. Characterization of inducible cyclooxygenase in rat brain. *J Comp Neurol.* 1995;355:296–315.

174. Lacroix S, Rivest S. Effect of acute systemic inflammatory response and cytokines on the transcription of the genes encoding cyclooxygenase enzymes (COX-1 and COX-2) in the rat brain. *J Neurochem.* 1998;70:452–66.

175. Smith CJ, Zhang Y, Koboldt CM, Muhammad J, Zweifel BS, Shaffer A et al. Pharmacological analysis of cyclooxygenase-1 in inflammation. *Proc Natl Acad Sci USA.* 1998;95:13313–8.

176. Lin LL, Lin AY, DeWitt DL. Interleukin-1α induces the accumulation of cytosolic phospholipase A$_2$ and the release of prostaglandin E$_2$ in human fibroblasts. *J Biol Chem.* 1992;267:23451–4.

177. Hoeck WG, Ramesha CS, Chang DJ, Fan N, Heller RA. Cytoplasmic phospholipase A$_2$ activity and gene expression are stimulated by tumor necrosis factor: dexamethasone blocks the induced synthesis. *Proc Natl Acad Sci USA.* 1993;90:4475–9.

178. Thore CR, Beasley TC, Busija DW. *In vitro* and *in vivo* localization of prostaglandin H synthase in fetal sheep neurons. *Neurosci Lett.* 1998;242:29–32.

179. Dvorak AM, Weller PF, Harvey VS, Morgan ES, Dvorak HF. Ultrastructural localization of prostaglandin endoperoxide synthase (cyclooxygenase) to isolated, purified fractions of guinea pig peritoneal macrophage and line 10 hepatocarcinoma cell lipid bodies. *Int Arch Allergy Immunol.* 1993;101:136–42.

180. Weller PF, Dvorak AM. Lipid bodies: intracellular sites for eicosanoid formation. *J Allergy Clin Immunol.* 1994;94:1151–6.

181. Rettori V, Gimeno M, Lyson K, McCann SM. Nitric oxide mediates norepinephrine-induced prostaglandin E_2 release from the hypothalamus. *Proc Natl Acad Sci USA.* 1992;89:11543–6.

182. Linthorst AC, Flachskamm C, Holsboer F, Reul JM. Intraperitoneal administration of bacterial endotoxin enhances noradrenergic neurotransmission in the rat preoptic area: relationship with body temperature and hypothalamic–pituitary–adrenocortical axis activity. *Eur J Neurosci.* 1995;7:2418–30.

183. Sehic E, Ungar AL, Blatteis CM. Interaction between norepinephrine and prostaglandin E_2 in the preoptic area of guinea pigs. *Am J Physiol.* 1996;271:R528–36.

184. Kaufmann WE, Worley PF, Pegg J, Bremer M, Isakson P. COX-2, a synaptically induced enzyme, is expressed by excitatory neurons at postsynaptic sites in rat cerebral cortex. *Proc Natl Acad Sci USA.* 1996;93:2317–21.

185. Yamagata K, Andreasson KI, Kaufmann WE, Barnes CA, Worley PF. Expression of a mitogen-inducible cyclooxygenase in brain neurons: regulation by synaptic activity and glucocorticoids. *Neuron.* 1993;11:371–86.

186. Adams J, Collaco-Moraes Y, de Belleroche J. Cyclooxygenase-2 induction in cerebral cortex: an intracellular response to synaptic excitation. *J Neurochem.* 1996;66:6–13.

187. Salvemini D, Misko TP, Masferrer JL, Seibert K, Currie MG, Needleman P. Nitric oxide activates cyclooxygenase enzymes. *Proc Natl Acad Sci USA.* 1993;90:7240–4.

188. Salvemini D, Settle SL, Masferrer JL, Seibert K, Currie MG, Needleman P. Regulation of prostaglandin production by nitric oxide; an *in vivo* analysis. *Br J Pharmacol.* 1995;114:1171–8.

189. Seibert K, Zhang Y, Leahy K, Hauser S, Masferrer J, Perkins W et al. Pharmacological and biochemical demonstration of the role of cyclooxygenase 2 in inflammation and pain. *Proc Natl Acad Sci USA.* 1994;91:12013–17.

190. Portanova JP, Zhang Y, Anderson GD, Hauser SD, Masferrer JL, Seibert K et al. Selective neutralization of prostaglandin E_2 blocks inflammation, hyperalgesia, and interleukin 6 production *in vivo*. *J Exp Med.* 1996;184:883–91.

191. Anderson GD, Hauser SD, McGarity KL, Bremer ME, Isakson PC, Gregory SA. Selective inhibition of cyclooxygenase (COX)-2 reverses inflammation and expression of COX-2 and interleukin 6 in rat adjuvant arthritis. *J Clin Invest.* 1996;97:2672–9.

192. Murakami M, Matsumoto R, Austen KF, Arm JP. Prostaglandin endoperoxide synthase-1 and -2 couple to different transmembrane stimuli to generate prostaglandin D_2 in mouse bone marrow- derived mast cells. *J Biol Chem.* 1994;269:22269–75.

193. Matsumura K, Watanabe Y, Onoe H, Hayaishi O. High density of prostaglandin E_2 binding sites in the anterior wall of the 3rd ventricle: a possible site of its hyperthermic action. *Brain Res.* 1990;533:147–51.

194. Scammell TE, Griffin JD, Elmquist JK, Saper CB. Microinjection of a cyclooxygenase inhibitor into the anteroventral preoptic region attenuates LPS fever. *Am J Physiol.* 1998;274:R783–9.

195. Coceani F, Bishai I, Dinarello CA, Fitzpatrick FA. Prostaglandin E$_2$ and thromboxane B$_2$ in cerebrospinal fluid of the afebrile and febrile cat. *Am J Physiol.* 1983;244:R785–93.

196. Sirko S, Bishai I, Coceani F. Prostaglandin formation in the hypothalamus *in vivo*: effect of pyrogens. *Am J Physiol.* 1989;256:R616–24.

197. Licinio J, Wong ML, Gold PW. Localization of interleukin-1 receptor antagonist mRNA in rat brain. *Endocrinology.* 1991;129:562–4.

198. Xin L, Blatteis CM. Blockade by interleukin-1 receptor antagonist of IL-1 beta-induced neuronal activity in guinea pig preoptic area slices. *Brain Res.* 1992;569:348–52.

199. Cooper K. *Fever and Antipyresis: the Role of the Nervous System.* Cambridge: Cambridge University Press; 1995:1–182.

200. Stitt JT. Differential sensitivity in the sites of fever production by prostaglandin E$_1$ within the hypothalamus of the rat. *J Physiol (Lond).* 1991;432:99–110.

201. Ban E, Haour F, Lenstra R. Brain interleukin-1 gene expression induced by peripheral lipopolysaccharide administration. *Cytokine.* 1992;4:48–54.

202. Konsman JP, Kelley K, Dantzer R. Temporal and spatial relationships between lipopolysaccharide-induced expression of *Fos*, interleukin-1 and inducible nitric oxide synthase in rat brain. *Neuroscience.* 1999;89:535–48.

203. Ballou LR, Botting R, Goorha S, Zhang J, Vane JR. Nociception in cyclooxygenase isozyme-deficient mice. *Proc Natl Acad Sci USA* 2000;97:10272–6.

204. Collier HO, Dinneen LC, Johnson CA, Schneider C. The abdominal constriction response and its suppression by analgesic drugs in the mouse. *Br J Pharmacol.* 1968;32:295–310.

205. Eguchi N, Minami T, Shirafuji N, Kanaoka Y, Tanaka T, Nagata A et al. Lack of tactile pain (allodynia) in lipocalin-type prostaglandin D synthase-deficient mice. *Proc Natl Acad Sci USA.* 1999;96:726–30.

206. Ballou L. The regulation of cyclooxygenase-1 and -2 in knockout cells and cyclooxygenase and fever in knockout mice. In: Serhan C, Perez H, editors. *Advances in Eicosanoid Research*, vol. 31. Berlin: Springer; 2000:97–124.

207. Parfenova H, Eidson TH, Leffler CW. Upregulation of COX-2 in cerebral microvascular endothelial cells by smooth muscle signals. *Am J Physiol.* 1997;273:C277–88.

7 | Role of spinal cyclooxygenases in nociceptive processing

Tony L. Yaksh and Camilla Svensson

Department of Anesthesiology, University of California, San Diego, 9500 Gilman Drive, La Jolla, CA 92093-0818, USA.

Local tissue injury and inflammation results in ongoing pain and an enhanced response to subsequent noxious stimuli, i.e. a local hyperalgesia[1]. Hyperalgesia is operationally defined as a reduction in the magnitude of the stimulus required to evoke an escape response or a decrease in the latency of the escape response evoked by a given stimulus. In humans, such an exaggerated response is considered to be an important psychophysical component of post-tissue injury pain (surgery, trauma or inflammation)[2]. In animals, studies have consistently demonstrated that the systemic delivery of aspirin and its congeners has little or no effect on the normal nociceptive response threshold or latency, but instead they reverse, in a dose-dependent manner, the hyperalgesic component which occurs secondary to tissue injury and inflammation (see Table 1). This observation was considered to be a defining characteristic of agents that were classified as non-steroid anti-inflammatory drugs (NSAIDs). This functional selectivity stands in contrast to agents such as opiates which also suppress the response in acute pain models in normal rats (e.g. thermal escape latency test, mechanical pressure) and represents one of the defining functional characteristics of this class of agents (see Figure 1).

PERIPHERAL MECHANISMS OF HYPERALGESIA AND NSAID ACTION

Peripheral mechanisms

Interpretation of the mechanisms of the antihyperalgesic action of NSAIDs was initially based on the hypothesis of the effects of NSAIDs on peripheral mechanisms of post-tissue injury hyperalgesia. This linkage was predicated

Table 1 Relative effect of intrathecal NSAIDs or μ-opioid receptor agonists on different pain models (for details see refs 1 and 113)

Assay (rat)	Stimulus	NSAID	μ-opioid
Hot plate test	thermal stimulus	0	+ +
Tail flick test	thermal stimulus	0	+ +
Writhing test	chemical irritation	+ +	+ +
Formalin phase 1	acute chemical stimulus	+	+ +
Formalin phase 2	prolonged chemical stimulus	+ +	+ +
Normal paw	mechanical pressure	0	+ +
Inflamed paw	mechanical pressure	+ +	+ +
Nerve constriction	thermal hyperesthesia	0	+
Spinal strychnine	tactile allodynia	0	+

Figure 1 Dose–response curves for systemic (intraperitoneal) morphine (MOR) and acetylsalicylic acid (ASA) in rats showing the effects of these agents on the threshold pressure in grams required to produce a withdrawal of the hindpaw in a normal paw and in a paw inflamed previously with the local injection of carrageenan. As indicated, the carrageenan-injected paw shows a lower threshold than the normal paw (vehicle = VEH) or a hyperalgesia. Morphine elevates the threshold to maximum (400 g) in both paws (though it takes more in the inflamed paw) while ASA only elevates the threshold of the inflamed paw (but not the normal paw) and the effect of ASA is limited to reversing the hyperalgesic component.

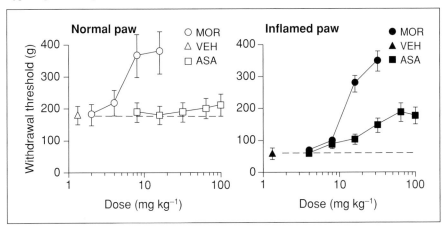

on three observations: (i) injury and inflammation led to spontaneous activity and produced a leftward shift in the stimulus–response relationship in sensory afferents; (ii) the effects of injury could be mimicked by the direct subcutaneous delivery of products known to be present in the inflammatory milieu, including the lipidic acid prostaglandins (PGs). These PGs, locally elaborated following tissue injury, served to sensitize peripheral nerve endings and facilitate pain behaviour in animal models[3]; (iii) the non-narcotic, non-steroid antipyretic agents, in spite of their structural variations, were shown to share the ability to inhibit cyclooxygenase (COX)-mediated synthesis of PGs[4,5]. These properties were consistent with the unifying hypothesis that NSAIDs acted in models of peripheral inflammation where the hallmark of nociception was a 'hyperalgesic state'[6,7]. In this manner, it has been widely appreciated that NSAIDs, by inhibiting the biosynthesis of PGs, do not, strictly speaking, produce analgesia but rather inhibit the hyperalgesic state resulting from the sensitization of the peripheral afferent nerve terminals. Under such conditions, it would be anticipated that these agents would only be effective when the *peripheral* afferent terminal reactivity had been sensitized by the local release of PGs.

Dissociation of the anti-hyperalgesic from the anti-inflammatory actions of NSAIDs

In spite of this emphasis on peripheral action, several lines of evidence indicate that the actions of NSAIDs extend beyond these peripheral mechanisms:

1. Persistent electrical stimulation of small primary afferents will evoke facilitated activity in dorsal horn and thalamic neurons. This central activation occurs in the absence of any peripheral inflammation. Nevertheless, this facilitated state is diminished by systemically administered NSAIDs[8–11].
2. NSAIDs delivered spinally have been shown to have little effect upon acute afferent-evoked spinal excitation, but will diminish the 'wind up' responses of spinal neurones evoked by electrical stimulation of the sural nerve at C-fibre strength[12–15].
3. The behavioural relevance of these central effects is indicated by the observation that the delivery of NSAIDs into the neuraxis produces a significant attenuation in the nocifensive activity of the animal evoked by certain chemical stimuli. Thus, Ferreira[16,17] reported that intracerebroventricular administration of NSAIDs will inhibit the carrageenan-evoked hyperalgesia in the rat paw, and Yaksh[18] observed that intrathecal NSAIDs would diminish the writhing response in rats at doses that were without systemic activity.
4. This activity observed in animal models is mirrored by comparable activity in man. In normal humans, the nociceptive reflex evoked by electrical sural nerve stimulation is diminished by systemically delivered ketoprofen,

diflunisal, indomethacin, acetylsalicylic acid or paracetamol[19–21]. A comparable reflex evoked in the orbicularis oculi muscle by electrical stimulation is inhibited by piroxicam[22].

In summary, these observations suggest that NSAIDs may express their anti-hyperalgesic actions in human and animal models by a central action that reflects mechanisms that are independent of a peripheral anti-inflammatory action. Importantly, systematic comparison of the clinical anti-hyperalgesic activity and the anti-inflammatory activity of a wide variety of NSAIDs has indeed indicated that there is a significant dissociation between the anti-inflammatory potency and the anti-hyperalgesic action of several agents[23,24].

SPINAL MECHANISMS OF HYPERALGESIA AND NSAID ACTION

An important advance in our understanding of the biology of nociception is that persistent small afferent input (as generated by tissue injury and inflammation) evokes a spinal sensitization such that spinal neurons will display an enhanced responsiveness and an increase in the size of the peripheral receptive field of the neuron. Iontophoretic delivery of substance P (SP) or excitatory amino acid (EAA) agonists evokes background firing and enhances the response of spinal dorsal horn neurons to subsequent thermal and mechanical stimuli[25]. The 'wind up' generated by persistent afferent input and the effects of the iontophoretically delivered transmitters are reversed by the spinal delivery of neurokinin 1 (NK1), N-methyl-D-aspartate (NMDA) and 2-amino-3,3-hydroxy-5-methyl-isoxasol-4-yl propionic acid (AMPA) receptor antagonists, respectively, while the intrathecal delivery of these agonists will evoke a brief thermal and mechanical hyperalgesia, which is reversed by their respective antagonists[26]. Activation of these receptors thus initiates a complex spinal cascade, which involves increased intracellular calcium ($[Ca^{2+}]_i$) levels and activation of spinal kinases, phospholipases and synthases. A variety of kinases phosphorylate membrane channels (calcium) and receptors (NMDA) and enhance their function[27]. Cytosolic ($cPLA_2$) and secretory ($sPLA_2$) phospholipases release arachidonic acid (AA) from cellular membranes through hydrolysis of phospholipids[28,29]. AA is converted by COX to PGH_2, which is then isomerized to yield biologically active prostanoid products. As will be reviewed below, prostanoids frequently serve to augment transmitter release and spinal excitability. Increases in $[Ca^{2+}]_i$ by glutamate will also activate synthesis of NO, shown in several preparations to activate PG synthesis itself[30,31]. These findings are thus consistent with a central sensitization by which afferent activation induced by peripheral injury and inflammation initiates a cascade of events that leads to a facilitated state of processing.

Spinal actions of NSAIDs

Further work on the elucidation of the events following persistent afferent activation led to the consideration of the effects of NSAIDs given spinally. The appreciation that neuronal systems could release prostanoids yielded the speculative hypothesis that spinal COX might play a role in the facilitated (hyperalgesic) state initiated by tissue injury. In these studies, it was shown that lumbar intrathecal (i.t.) injection of structurally diverse NSAIDs has no effect upon acute escape behaviour but resulted in a dose-dependent suppression of the pain behaviour evoked by: (i) peripheral injury caused by dilute formalin injection into the rat paw[32] (see Figure 2); (ii) acetic acid in the peritoneal cavity[18]; (iii) inflammation in the paw as produced by the local injection of an irritant such as carrageenan[33]; and (iv) the thermal hyperalgesia induced by intrathecal SP and NMDA in rats[34] (see Figure 3). The last example is of particular importance as it emphasizes that the anti-hyperalgesic effects of the spinal agent are observed independently of any peripheral injury or inflammation.

The effects of i.t. NSAIDs have several functionally distinctive properties[32,35]:

1. The anti-hyperalgesic effects occur at doses that have no effect upon motor function or upon acute thermal or mechanical nociception.
2. This effect reflects a spinal effect and is not secondary to a systemic redistribution. The spinal action is indicated by the observation that systemic NSAIDs are also able to produce a dose-dependent reduction of the behaviours in the carrageenan-induced hyperalgesia and formalin tests, but the doses required to produce an equal anti-nociception are 100–300 times more than those required after spinal delivery.
3. Both the systemic and spinal NSAIDs produce a similar reduction of carrageenan- and formalin-evoked behaviours. This reduction displayed a clear and comparable plateau effect independent of the route of delivery (see Figure 2). The similarity in plateau effects observed by the two routes of delivery and the low dose required after spinal injection raises the possibility that the action of the systemic NSAID may be mediated centrally.

Consistent with a role for spinal COX products, PGE antagonists given i.t. diminish formalin-induced hyperalgesia[36] while prostanoids given i.t., including PGE_2, $PGF_{2\alpha}$, TXA_2 and PGI_2, produce a thermal and mechanical hyperalgesia[37–39] and enhance the formalin response[40]. These results suggest a protracted afferent input through the release of glutamate and SP, which through the activation of spinal NK1/NMDA/AMPA receptors evokes the release of COX products. These spinal prostanoids act through one or more PG receptors (see below) to facilitate afferent-evoked excitation and sustain a hyperalgesic state.

Figure 2 Time–effect curve of the effects of intrathecal S(+)-ibuprofen (top = 2.7–80 nmol) and R(−)-ibuprofen (bottom = 27–270 nmol) or vehicles administered 2 min before the intraplantar injection of formalin (0.5%; 50 µl). The number of flinches per min is plotted versus the time after the formalin injection into the dorsal surface of the right hind paw. The line representing the control group includes 20 animals, otherwise each line represents the mean and SEM of 4–6 animals. Note that S(+)-ibuprofen produced a dose-dependent reduction in phase two down to a plateau at the 27 nmol dose, whereas R(−)-ibuprofen had no effect even at ten times the S(+) plateau dose (adapted from ref. 32; i.t. = intrathecal).

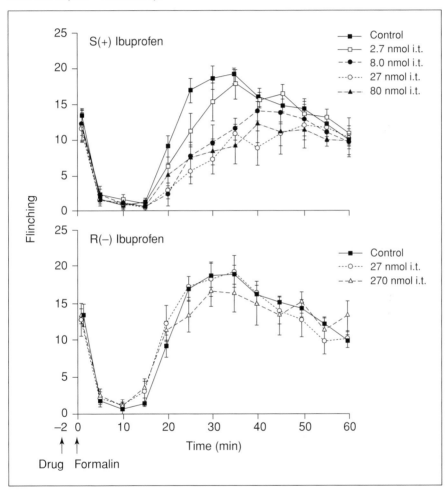

Spinal pharmacology of cyclooxygenase inhibitors

The effects of a spinally delivered drug may reflect upon a number of actions. To define the site of action requires consideration of its pharmacology.

Figure 3. Time–effect curve for formalin-evoked behaviour (top), and spinal release of PGE$_2$ (middle) or glutamate (Glu) (bottom), following intrathecal (i.t.) S(+)-ibuprofen (1 or 10 µg) or vehicle 25 min before the formalin test. The behavioural data are presented as the mean (± SEM) number of flinches versus the time after formalin injection. Spinal release of PGE$_2$ or Glu are presented as mean (± SEM) of the percentage change from baseline release versus time after formalin injection. The asterisks indicate significantly decreased release compared with saline control (Kruskal–Wallis followed by Dunn's multiple comparisons test; $*$ = $P < 0.05$; $**$ = $P < 0.01$; $***$ = $P < 0.001$; ns not significant). In addition to these results, it was shown that intraperitoneal S(+)-ibuprofen (10 mg kg^{-1}) had the same effect and that intrathecal R(−)-ibuprofen (10 µg) was without effect (data from ref. 50).

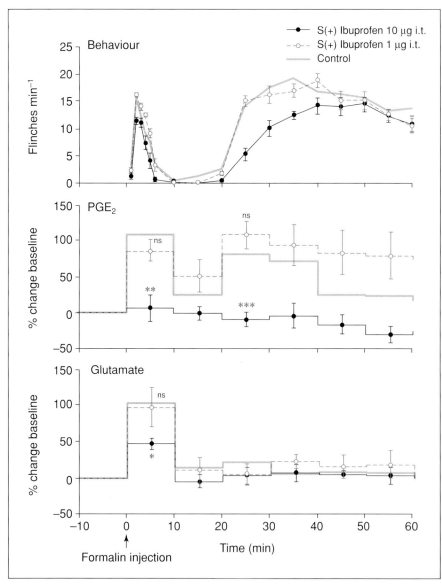

(I) STRUCTURE ACTIVITY RELATIONSHIP

In studies examining the anti-hyperalgesic effects of intrathecal NSAIDs, all agents produced comparable maximum reductions in effect, but they varied by over 100-fold in apparent potency in several tests. Thus, in the writhing test, the rank order of potency was: zomepirac sodium > aspirin[18]. In the formalin test, the rank order of potency was: indomethacin > flurbiprofen > ketorolac > zomepirac > S(+)-ibuprofen > ibuprofen > aspirin > paracetamol > R(−)-ibuprofen = 0[35]. For the carrageenan-evoked thermal hyperalgesia, the rank order of potency was: ketorolac > zomepirac > S(+)-ibuprofen > ibuprofen > aspirin > R(−)-ibuprofen = 0[33]. For the thermal hyperalgesia induced by SP given i.t., the rank order of potency was: ketorolac > S(+)-ibuprofen > aspirin > R(−)-ibuprofen = 0[26]. This order of potency approximates to that for blocking the activity of COX isozymes (see below).

(II) STEREOSPECIFICITY

In the formalin test, the effect was stereospecific in that the S-enantiomer of ibuprofen, which is active as an inhibitor of COX[41], produced anti-nociception, while the R-enantiomer, which has no COX inhibitory activity, was inactive. This further supports the notion that the spinal anti-nociceptive effect is related to inhibition of COX.

(III) COX-1 VERSUS COX-2 PHARMACOLOGY

The discovery of the two COX isozymes (see below) leads to the query as to whether one or the other, if not both, contribute to the spinal anti-hyperalgesic actions of the non-selective COX inhibitors. COX-2, but not COX-1, inhibitors given i.t. suppress the thermal hyperalgesia observed with an inflamed paw, with the order of activity paralleling their respective potency for COX-2 inhibition[33]. The thermal hyperalgesia induced by the spinal delivery of SP or NMDA is reversed by COX-2, but not COX-1, inhibitors delivered systemically or intrathecally [42,43]. These observations are of particular significance as they emphasize that the COX-2 inhibitors are: (i) acting at a time when there could have been no induction of the target isozyme, i.e. through a constitutively expressed isozyme; (ii) that systemically administered inhibitors, at doses which have no effect upon normal thermal escape latencies, are able to reduce the centrally-evoked thermal hyperalgesia at doses that are considered to be effective in models of inflammatory pain. These observations emphasize that the COX-2 agents at systemic doses are altering central processing.

Spinal prostaglandin release

An important corollary of the anti-hyperalgesic activity of spinal COX inhibition is the likelihood that prostanoids are released by the corresponding stimuli. Early work by Ramwell[44] demonstrated that stimulation of the sciatic nerve would lead to an increase in the levels of bioassayable prostanoid activity in the perfusate from the spinal cord of the frog. Yaksh demonstrated an increase of PGE from spinal superfusates of the rat *in vivo* evoked by potassium[18]. Subsequent work emphasized that there was a close correspondence between manipulations that induce a hyperalgesic state and the spinal release of COX products. Thus, *in vivo* spinal microdialysis in rats shows increases in spinal extracellular concentrations of prostanoids (PGE_2, PGI_2) induced by: (i) acute activation of small afferents with intraplantar formalin[45] and thermal stimulation[46]; (ii) persistent inflammation (carrageenan in knee joint)[47]; and (iii) SP or kainate given i.t.[48,49]. This spinal PG release is blocked by i.t. or i.p. doses of COX inhibitors which indeed reverse the respective hyperalgesia[50] (see Figure 4).

Figure 4. Time–effect curve for thermal escape latency observed following the intrathecal injection at time 0 of substance P (SP; 20 nmol) in animals pretreated 15 min before with vehicle, S(+)-ibuprofen (S(+) Ibu 80 nmol: non-selective COX inhibitor), R(−)-ibuprofen (R(−) Ibu 80 nmol: inactive isomer), SC-58125 (50 nmol: COX-2 inhibitor) or SC-560 (840 nmol: COX-1 inhibitor). Each point represents the mean ± SEM of 6–8 rats. BL = basal level. (Data from ref. 42).

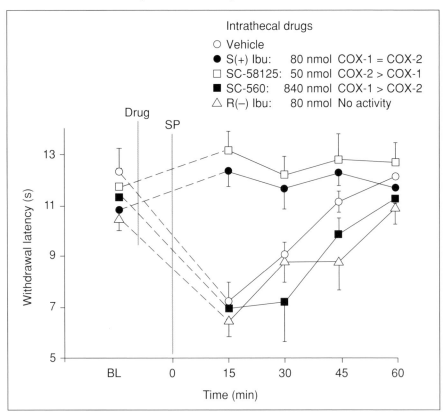

Role of spinal prostanoids and receptors in facilitated processing and hyperalgesic behaviour

The ability of spinal COX inhibitors to alter the injury-evoked hyperalgesic state argues for an important role of prostanoids at the spinal level in altering afferent-evoked excitation. Prostanoids bind at five classes of receptors (DP, EP, FP, IP and TP), defined by their primary binding ligand. Most endogenous ligands display significant cross-reactivity. While there is no space to review the extensive literature on the effects of PG receptor activation, cloned receptor sequences predict seven transmembrane domains coupled to a regulatory G protein[51–53]. Accordingly, the actions of these several classes of receptors include: stimulation of inositol triphosphate[54]; activation of PLC[55]; stimulation of adenylate cyclase[56]; and increases in $[Ca^{2+}]_i$[57]. Conversely, inhibitory effects on cAMP production inhibited by a pertussis toxin-sensitive mechanism have also been reported[58,59]. Thus, PGE_2: (i) increases calcium influx in cultured spinal oligodendrocytes[60] and avian sensory neurons[61]; (ii) decreases an outward potassium current[62]; and (iii) increases tetrodotoxin-resistant sodium influx in rat sensory neurons[63]. Depolarization-evoked increases in $[Ca^{2+}]_i$ and the correlated release of SP from dorsal root ganglia (DRG) is enhanced by prostanoids[61] and this may account for the enhanced release of spinal SP observed in arthritic rats[64]. The increase in glutamate release *in vivo* evoked by capsaicin and NMDA given i.t. is significantly, but incompletely, attenuated by prior i.t. delivery of COX inhibitors[50,65], suggesting that spinal terminals from which glutamate is released are sensitized by COX products. In this regard, the highest density of PGE_2 binding sites are found in laminae I and II of the dorsal horn[66]. The mRNA of a PGE_2 receptor mediating increase in intracellular calcium has also been found to be highly expressed in dorsal root ganglion cells and in neurons of the brain[67]. Therefore, it appears possible that PGE_2 synthesized and released within the spinal cord may act on presynaptic terminals to enhance neurotransmitter release.

At the behavioural level and consistent with the above observations, the spinal injection of a variety of prostanoids, including PGE_2 and thromboxane B_2 (TXB_2), result in thermal and mechanical hyperalgesic states[37–39]. Conversely, as noted above, EP_1 receptor antagonists given i.t. can reduce hyperalgesia produced by tissue injury.

Spinal cyclooxygenase isozymes

After release of AA, the essential enzyme for PG synthesis is COX. There are two COX isozymes, COX-1 and COX-2, encoded by distinct single copy genes (>22 kb pairs and 8–9 kb pairs in length), residing on chromosomes 2 and 1 (murine), respectively[68]. Both COX-1 and COX-2 have been cloned[69,70] and the crystal structures of both the original COX-1[71] as well as COX-2[72] have now been determined. In the periphery, COX-1 is constitutively expressed. COX-2 is thought to be inducible, although constitutive expression of COX-2 has been demonstrated in testis, macula densa and brain (see below). COX-2 expression is induced in peripheral cell line cultures by growth factors and cytokines, and *in vivo* by carrageenan-mediated tissue injury and inflammation, thus suggesting differential pharmacological targets for the management of PG synthesis in post-injury pain states.

Importantly, commonly available NSAIDs (ibuprofen, indomethacin) inhibit both COX-1 and COX-2 with varying selectivities[73], whereas recently developed compounds have been reported to be selective for COX-2 without inhibition of COX-1[74]. This potential difference in inhibitor specificity between COX-1 and COX-2 has been proposed to depend on one amino acid difference between COX-1 and COX-2 within the hydrophobic active site. COX-2 has a valine in a position where COX-1 has an isoleucine[75]. This differential activity has been of great interest due the observations that gastric mucosa cells express primarily COX-1, and specific COX-2 inhibitors are effective anti-inflammatory/analgesic agents without the gastric side effects that are known to be the major dose-limiting side effect for NSAIDs in the clinic[76].

The COX-1 gene is consistent with it being constitutively expressed as a 'housekeeping gene'[77], i.e. it does not have a TATA-box which is typical for developmentally regulated housekeeping genes. In contrast to COX-1, COX-2 is subject to rapid regulation at the transcription/translation level. COX-2 mRNA displays consensus sequences for nuclear transcription factors including NF-κB, providing potent mechanisms for induction. The gene also displays repeated motifs in the untranslated regions (ATTTA) which renders the mRNA less stable[68]. These properties resemble those of an immediate early gene (e.g. *cFOS*) and show that COX-2 allows a dynamic regulation of the PG-mediated cascade. A notable feature of COX is that it undergoes suicide inactivation during catalysis.

In spite of their co-localization and constitutive presence in spinal cells, the differential effects of COX-1 and COX-2 inhibitors on pain behaviour and PG release noted above indicate that these enzymes do not play equivalent roles. Differential effects have been noted *in vitro* in cells co-transfected with combinations of phospholipases and COX isozymes[78]. Based on electron micrograph studies, the differences do not appear to result from differential localization[79,80]. Two possibilities may be that: (i) COX-1 requires higher AA concentrations than COX-2[51]; or (ii) differential coupling to cytosolic, secretory and non-calcium-dependent phospholipases[78,79,81,82].

Location of spinal COX isozymes

In normal rats, COX-1 mRNA and protein are expressed constitutively in dorsal horn neurons, in the ventral horns of the spinal cord and in DRG as shown by *in situ* hybridization[81] (see also ref. 82), Northern blotting[83–86], immunohistochemistry[14,84] and Western blot techniques[14,42,84,87]. There is at present controversy as to whether the cells within which the spinal COX-1 and COX-2 are constitutively expressed. There is little doubt that at least a portion of the COX-2 isozymes are found within stimulated microglia and astrocytes[88,89]. While it is less certain that such activity is expressed by spinal neurons under untreated conditions, COX-1 is constitutively expressed in dorsal horn neurons and in DRG[81]. In DRG primary cell cultures, we have observed COX-1 and COX-2 immunoreactivity in SP-expressing cells (I. Khan, C. Svensson and T. Yaksh, unpublished observations). In this regard, it is interesting to note that interleukin-1β (IL-1β) induces SP release from primary afferent neurons and this effect is blocked by COX-2 inhibition[90].

Regulation of spinal COX isozymes

With few exceptions, COX-1 expression is relatively fixed, whereas increases in central COX-2 expression often occur after tissue injury and inflammation.

(I) TISSUE INJURY AND COX UPREGULATION

Tissue injury and inflammation increases COX-2 but not COX-1 expression in the spinal cord. Intraplantar injection of zymosan in mice, or Freund's adjuvant arthritis, results in an increase in mRNA and COX-2 expression in neurons ipsilaterally, with increases also observed in contralateral dorsal horn neurons[91]. Intraplantar carrageenan results in bilateral increases in COX-2 expression in dorsal (but not ventral) horn cells over an interval of 4–24 h[86,92]. The increase is paralleled by an increase in basal and SP- or NMDA-evoked release of spinal PGE_2[93]. The increase in COX-2 may occur in non-neuronal or neuronal elements, e.g. around 6 h after unilateral hind paw injection of carrageenan, COX-2-mRNA is bilaterally expressed in non-neuronal cells in the spinal grey and white matter and along leptomeninges and blood vessels[82].

What is the 'stimulus' that initiates this upregulation? As noted above, tissue injury leads to afferent activation *and* to an increase in circulating factors. To the degree that upregulation reflects activity in primary afferents, we anticipate that increased COX-2 expression will be in populations of neurons receiving that input (e.g. ipsilateral lumbar after unilateral hindpaw injury). As noted, spinal COX-2 was increased bilaterally after unilateral inflammation, suggesting a contribution by circulating factors.

(II) NEURAL ACTIVATION

In brain, neuronal expression of COX-2 is rapidly and transiently induced by NMDA-dependent synaptic activity[94,95].

The above observations, taken together, make it seem likely that both neuronal activation and circulating inflammatory products can initiate upregulation of COX-2 in CNS. Since upregulation reflects activity in primary afferents it can be anticipated that increased COX-2 expression will be in populations of neurons receiving that input (e.g. ipsilateral lumbar after unilateral hindpaw injury). Thus, *cFOS*, also an immediate early gene like COX-2, displays an increase in *ipsilateral* lumbar expression within hours after intraplantar injection of formalin. Importantly, the enhanced *cFOS* expression is prevented by spinal lignocaine, and systemic morphine, ketamine, propofol, alphaxalone and NK1-receptor antagonists, but not barbiturate[96-99]. This anatomical specificity associated with intraplantar formalin injection is consistent with single unit activity that emphasizes local activation of small afferents[100] and the comparative lack of swelling or inflammation observed several hours after formalin injection, in contrast to models employing agents leading to systemic inflammation (carrageenan, Freund's adjuvant). As noted, spinal COX-2 was increased bilaterally after unilateral inflammation, suggesting a contribution by circulating factors.

(III) CIRCULATING FACTORS

After tissue injury there are increases in a variety of circulating factors, including TNF-α and IL-1β[101]. Following systemic delivery of lipopolysaccharide (LPS), IL-1β and TNF-α, constitutive levels of COX-2 mRNA in brain neurons appear to be unaltered. In contrast, COX-2 mRNA expression in cells throughout the brain in proximity to the microvasculature and leptomeninges was observed to peak at 2 h and to subside by 24 h[102-104]. Co-activation of IL-1β and TNF-α serves to enhance synergistically: (i) release of AA; and (ii) the expression of COX-2 mRNA and the release of PGs[105].

In summary, we suggest that the net spinal COX-2 upregulation and the PG-mediated hyperalgesia will reflect synergy between effects produced by: (i) segmental input; and (ii) from an action upon the entire neuraxis secondary to the circulatory distribution of inflammatory products. The increase will thus reflect the contribution of a heterogeneous population of neurons and non-neuronal elements.

CENTRAL ACTIONS OF NSAIDS IN HUMANS

Preclinical approaches indicate that NSAIDs can have a central action even when administered peripherally. The developing appreciation of the CNS effects produced by NSAIDs has provided an important insight into an additional element explaining the surprisingly potent action of these agents and provides a rationale as to why the analgesic action may exceed that anticipated given their moderate anti-inflammatory activities. Comparable lines of investigation also exist which support a central anti-algesic action in humans.

1. Electrically-evoked nociceptive reflexes can be caused by direct electrical activation of peripheral sensory nerves. The nociceptive response of the biceps femoris flexion reflex evoked by sural nerve stimulation can be diminished by systemically delivered ketoprofen, diflunisal, indomethacin, acetylsalicylic acid or paracetamol[19-21]. A comparable reflex, evoked in the orbicularis oculi muscle by electrical stimulation, is blocked by piroxicam[22]. These results, reflecting the direct activation of small afferent nerve input, support a central antinociceptive action of these agents.

2. In human cancer patients, i.t. delivery of lysine acetylsalicylate produced significant pain relief[106-108]. These several lines of observations provide evidence for a direct spinal interaction in animal models and in humans.

3. In clinical studies, COX-2-selective inhibitors have been shown to have significant anti-hyperalgesic activity in post-surgical pain states[109]. In models of third molar extraction, the onset of pain occurs in less than a few hours after surgery and COX-2 inhibitors have been shown to have a rapid onset of action. Given that COX-2 is not constitutively expressed in the periphery, rapid onset of COX sensitivity suggests that these agents must be exerting their action at a site where the COX-2 is constitutively expressed. Thus, though indirect, these observations argue for a site within the central nervous system where this isozyme is constitutively expressed.

SUMMARY

The information outlined in this chapter suggests that the hyperalgesic state induced by tissue injury is at least in part the consequence of a complex spinal cascade which serves to increase PG synthesis and release through a constitutive spinal COX-2 pathway. These prostanoids are part of the cascade that results in a spinal state of facilitated processing. The elements of this pathway are summarized below and presented schematically in Figure 5.

1. Persistent small afferent input (as generated by tissue injury and inflammation) evokes the release of EAAs (e.g. glutamate) and peptides (e.g. substance P).

2. The effects of injury are mimicked by the spinal delivery of SP or EAA agonists, which serve to enhance the response of spinal dorsal horn neurons to subsequent noxious stimuli and produce hyperalgesia.

3. The peptide and EAA receptors initiate a complex local cascade, one component of which is the activation of phospholipases to form AA, which is acted upon by spinal COX to yield PGs.

4. Prostanoids, by an action on local receptors, serve to augment transmitter release and spinal excitability. These results are thus consistent with a central sensitization by which afferent activation induced by peripheral

Figure 5. Schematic illustration of the dorsal horn presenting potential structures from which prostaglandins (PGs) may derive and mechanisms whereby cyclooxygenase (COX) products may alter spinal nociceptive processing. C fibre activation yields the release of a variety of excitatory neurotransmitters, including substance P (SP) and glutamate. This results in increased intracellular calcium ($[Ca^{2+}]_i$) which in turn results in the activation of a number of intracellular enzymes, including phospholipase A_2 (PLA_2). This causes an increase in free arachidonic acid (AA) which then enters the cyclooxygenase (COX) cascade leading to the formation of a variety of PGs that gain access to the extracellular space. Several of these prostanoids have been shown to increase intracellular calcium in sensory afferents and thus would serve to facilitate afferent transmitter release. Though it is suggested that the spinal prostanoids are acting only on the sensory C fibre, it is suspected that many terminals in the dorsal horn will be similarly affected. COX-1 and possibly COX-2 are believed to be present in dorsal root ganglion cells and hence sensory afferent terminals. The evidence that COX-2 is found in second order neurons is not consistent. This system is, however, quite dynamic Thus, there is an enhanced expression of mRNA and protein for COX-2 that is initiated by persistent afferent input generated by peripheral tissue injury and inflammation. It is important to note that several structures within the dorsal horn may account for the expression of COX-2, including non-neuronal elements that may be activated secondary to activity in adjacent synaptically-coupled systems (e.g. via glutamate) as well as by circulating cytokines. The net result is an increase in extravascular, extracellular prostanoids which can act upon local receptor populations to enhance transmitter release, perhaps by augmenting the opening of voltage-sensitive calcium channels (see text for further comments).

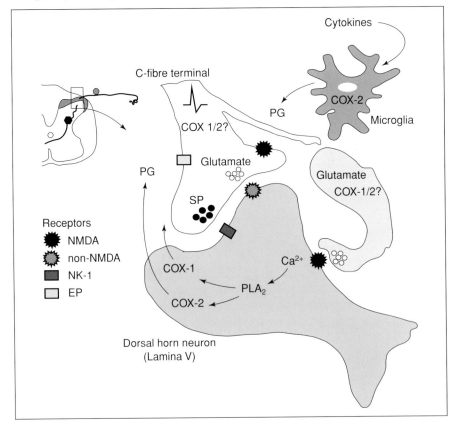

injury and inflammation initiates a cascade of events that lead to a facilitated state of processing (see Figure 2).

5. Though the evidence is controversial, both COX-1 and COX-2 appear to be constitutively present in the dorsal horn and in the dorsal root ganglion.

6. The pharmacology of systemic and i.t. delivered COX inhibitors indicates that the sensitization evoked by peripheral tissue injury (formalin), or the direct activation of spinal neurokinin 1 or glutamatergic receptors, is mediated by spinal COX-2 and not by COX-1 isozyme

7. A variety of neurogenic (e.g. NMDA-receptor activation) and circulating factors (IL-1β, TNF-α and LPS) can serve to upregulate the expression of COX-2, particularly in microglia and astrocytes. *In vitro* work has indicated that these cells can release prostanoids. Accordingly, these non-neuronal cells found within the CNS may contribute to the facilitated state associated with tissue injury and inflammation, which, by its pharmacology, may be mediated in part by spinal prostanoids acting upon spinal prostanoid receptors.

In conclusion, Flower et al.[110] in their chapter in the sixth edition of Goodman and Gilman's *The Pharmacological Basis of Therapeutics* noted that whereas "… the analgesic actions of morphine occur centrally, aspirin works peripherally … preventing the synthesis and release of prostaglandins in inflammation …". In the eighth edition, it was emphasized that the aspirin-like drugs are particularly effective in "… settings in which inflammation has caused sensitization of pain receptors to normally painless mechanical or chemical stimuli"[111]. It is interesting to note that we have now come full circle. Woodbury in his chapter in the third edition of Goodman and Gilman[112] noted that "… the salicylates are capable of alleviating certain types of pain by virtue of a selective depressant effect on the CNS, the mechanism of which has not been elucidated. A sub-cortical site is suggested by the fact that analgesic doses do not cause mental disturbances, hypnosis or changes in the modality of sensations other than pain".

Address all correspondence to: Tony L. Yaksh, Department of Anesthesiology, University of California, San Diego, 9500 Gilman Drive, La Jolla, CA 92093-0818, USA.

REFERENCES

1. Yaksh TL. Preclinical models of nociception. In: Yaksh TL, Lynch III C, Zapol WM, Maze M, Biebuyck JF, Saidman LJ, editors. *Anesthesia: Biologic Foundations.* Philadelphia: Lippincott-Raven Publishers; 1997;685–718.

2. Price DD. Psychophysical measurement of normal and abnormal pain states and

analgesia. In: Yaksh TL, Lynch III C, Zapol WM, Maze M, Biebuyck JF, Saidman LJ, editors. *Anesthesia: Biologic Foundations.* Philadelphia: Lippincott-Raven; 1997;719–33.

3. Lim RK. Pain. *Annu Rev Physiol.* 1970;32:269–88.

4. Smith JB, Willis AL. Aspirin selectively inhibits prostaglandin production in human platelets. *Nature.* 1971;231:235–7.

5. Vane JR. Inhibition of prostaglandin synthesis as a mechanism of action for aspirin-like drugs. *Nature New Biol.* 1971;231:232–5.

6. Ferreira SH. Prostaglandins, aspirin-like drugs and analgesia. *Nature New Biol.* 1972;240:200–3.

7. Moncada S, Ferreira SH, Vane JR. Inhibition of prostaglandin biosynthesis as the mechanism of analgesia of aspirin-like drugs in the dog knee joint. *Eur J Pharmacol.* 1975;31:250–60.

8. Attal N, Kayser V, Eschalier A, Benoist JM, Guilbaud G. Behavioural and electro-physiological evidence for an analgesic effect of a non-steroidal anti-inflammatory agent, sodium diclofenac. *Pain.* 1988;35:341–8.

9. Carlsson KH, Monzel W, Jurna I. Depression by morphine and the non-opioid analgesic agents, metamizol (dipyrone), lysine acetylsalicylate, and paracetamol, of activity in rat thalamus neurones evoked by electrical stimulation of nociceptive afferents. *Pain.* 1988;32:313–26.

10. Groppetti A, Braga PC, Biella G, Parenti M, Rusconi L, Mantegazza P. Effect of aspirin on serotonin and met-enkephalin in brain: correlation with the antinoci-ceptive activity of the drug. *Neuropharmacology.* 1988;27:499–505.

11. Jurna I, Brune K. Central effect of the non-steroid anti-inflammatory agents, indomethacin, ibuprofen, and diclofenac, determined by C fibre-evoked activity in single neurones of the rat thalamus. *Pain.* 1990;41:71–80.

12. Herrero JF, Parrado A, Cervero F. Central and peripheral actions of the NSAID ketoprofen on spinal cord nociceptive reflexes. *Neuropharmacology.* 1997;36:1425–31.

13. Mazario J, Rozqa C, Herrero JF. The NSAID dexketoprofen, trometamol is as potent as mu-opioids in the depression of wind-up and spinal cord nociceptive reflexes in normal rats. *Brain Res.* 1999;816;512–7.

14. Willingale HL, Gardiner NJ, McLymont N, Giblett S, Grubb BD. Prostanoids synthesized by cyclo-oxygenase isoforms in rat spinal cord and their contribution to the development of neuronal hyperexcitability. *Br J Pharmacol.* 1997;122:1593–604.

15. Pitcher GM, Henry JL. NSAID-induced cyclooxygenase inhibition differentially depresses long-lasting versus brief synaptically-elicited responses of rat spinal dorsal horn neurons in vivo. *Pain.* 1999;82:173–86.

16. Ferreira SH, Lorenzetti BB, Corrêa FM. Central and peripheral antialgesic action of aspirin-like drugs. *Eur Pharmacol.* 1978;53:39–48.

17. Ferreira SH, Lorenzetti BB, Corrêa FM. Blockade of central and peripheral generation of prostaglandins explain the antialgic effect of aspirin like drugs. *Pol J Pharmacol Pharm.* 1978;30:133–40.

18. Yaksh TL. Central and peripheral mechanisms for the antialgesic action of acetyl-salicyclic acid. In: Barnet JM, Hirsh J, Mustard JF, editors. *Acetylsalicyclic Acid: New Uses for an Old Drug.* New York: Raven Press; 1982;137–52.

19. Willer JC, De Broucker T, Bussel B, Roby-Brami A, Harrewyn JM. Central anal-gesic effect of ketoprofen in humans: electrophysiological evidence for a supraspinal mechanism in a double-blind and cross-over study. *Pain.* 1989;38:1–7.

20. Piletta P, Porchett HC, Dayer P. Central analgesic effect of acetaminophen but not of aspirin. *Clin Pharmacol Ther*. 1991;49:350–4.
21. Guieu R, Blin O, Pouget J, Serratrice G. Analgesic effect of indomethacin shown using the nociceptive flexion reflex in humans. *Ann Rheum Dis*. 1992;51:391–3.
22. Fabbri A, Cruccu G, Sperti P, Ridolfi M, Ciampani T, Leardi MG et al. Piroxicam-induced analgesia: evidence for a central component which is not opioid mediated. *Experientia*. 1992;48:1139–42.
23. Mehlisch DR. Review of the comparative analgesic efficacy of salicylates, acetaminophen, and pyrazolones. *Am J Med*. 1983;75:47–52.
24. McCormack K, Brune K. Dissociation between the antinociceptive and anti-inflammatory effects of the nonsteroidal anti-inflammatory drugs. A survey of their analgesic efficacy. *Drugs*. 1991;41:533–47.
25. Dougherty PM, Willis WD. Enhanced responses of spinothalamic tract neurons to excitatory amino acids accompany capsaicin-induced sensitization in the monkey. *J Neurosci*. 1992;12:883–94.
26. Malmberg AB, Yaksh TL. Hyperalgesia mediated by spinal glutamate or substance P receptor blocked by spinal cyclooxygenase inhibition. *Science*. 1992;257:1276–9.
27. Yaksh TL, Hua XY, Kalcheva I, Nozaki-Taguchi N, Marsala M. The spinal biology in humans and animals of pain states generated by persistent small afferent input. *Proc Natl Acad Sci USA*. 1999;96:7680–6.
28. Bingham III CO, Austen KF. Phospholipase A_2 enzymes in eicosanoid generation. *Proc Assoc Am Physicians*. 1999;111:516–24.
29. Farooqui AA, Yang HC, Rosenberger TA, Horrocks LA. Phospholipase A_2 and its role in brain tissue. *J Neurochem*. 1997;69:889–901.
30. Salvemini D, Misko TP, Masferrer JL, Seibert K, Currie MG, Needleman P. Nitric oxide activates cyclooxygenase enzymes. *Proc Natl Acad Sci USA*. 1993;90:7240–4.
31. Swierkosz TA, Mitchell JA, Warner TD, Botting RM, Vane JR. Co-induction of nitric oxide synthase and cyclo-oxygenase: interactions between nitric oxide and prostanoids. *Br J Pharmacol*. 1995;114:1335–42.
32. Malmberg AB, Yaksh TL. Pharmacology of the spinal action of ketorolac, morphine, ST-91, U50488H, and L-PIA on the formalin test and an isobolographic analysis of the NSAID interaction. *Anesthesiology*. 1993;79:270–81.
33. Dirig DM, Isakson PC, Yaksh TL. Effect of COX-1 and COX-2 inhibition on induction and maintenance of carrageenan-evoked thermal hyperalgesia in rats. *J Pharmacol Exp Ther*. 1998;285:1031–8.
34. Björkman R, Hallman KM, Hedner J, Hedner T, Henning M. Nonsteroidal anti-inflammatory drug modulation of behavioral responses to intrathecal N-methyl-D-aspartate, but not to substance P and amino-methyl-isoxazole-propionic acid in the rat. *J Clin Pharmacol*. 1996;36:20S–26S.
35. Malmberg AB, Yaksh TL. Antinociceptive actions of spinal nonsteroidal anti-inflammatory agents on the formalin test in the rat. *J Pharmacol Exp Ther*. 1992;263:136–46.
36. Malmberg AB, Rafferty MF, Yaksh TL. Antinociceptive effect of spinally delivered prostaglandin E receptor antagonists in the formalin test on the rat. *Neurosci Lett*. 1994;173:193–6.
37. Minami T, Uda R, Horiguchi S, Ito S, Hyodo M, Hayaishi O. Allodynia evoked by intrathecal administration of prostaglandin E_2 to conscious mice. *Pain*. 1994;57:217–23.
38. Minami T, Uda R, Horiguchi S, Ito S, Hyodo M, Hayaishi O. Allodynia evoked by

intrathecal administration of prostaglandin F$_2$ alpha to conscious mice. *Pain.* 1992;50:223–9.

39. Uda R, Horiguchi S, Ito S, Hyodo M, Hayaishi O. Nociceptive effects induced by intrathecal administration of prostaglandin D$_2$, E$_2$ or F$_2$ alpha to conscious mice. *Brain Res.* 1990;510:26–32.

40. Takano Y, Kuno Y, Sato E, Takano M, Sato I. The enhancement of formalin induced agitation behavior by intrathecal administration of prostaglandin E. *Masui.* 1999;48:841–6.

41. Adams SS, Bresloff P, Mason CG. Pharmacological differences between the optical isomers of ibuprofen: evidence for metabolic inversion of the (−)-isomer. *J Pharm Pharmacol.* 1976;28:256–7.

42. Yaksh TL, Dirig DM, Conway CM, Svensson C, Luo D, Isakson PC. The acute antihyperalgesic action of NSAIDs and release of spinal PGE$_2$ is mediated by inhibition of constitutive spinal COX-2, but not COX-1. *J Neurosci.* 2001; in press.

43. Yamamoto T, Sakashita, Y. COX-2 inhibitor prevents the development of hyperalgesia induced by intrathecal NMDA or AMPA. *Neuroreport.* 1998;9:3869–73.

44. Ramwell PW, Shaw JE, Jessup R. Spontaneous and evoked release of prostaglandins from frog spinal cord. *Am J Physiol.* 1966;211:998–1004.

45. Scheuren N, Neupert W, Ionac M, Neuhuber W, Brune K, Geisslinger G. Peripheral noxious stimulation releases spinal PGE$_2$ during the first phase in the formalin assay of the rat. *Life Sci.* 1997;60:L295–300.

46. Coderre TJ, Gonzales R, Goldyne ME, West J, Levine JD. Noxious stimulus-induced increase in spinal prostaglandin E$_2$ is noradrenergic terminal-dependent. *Neurosci Lett.* 1990;115:253–8.

47. Yang LC, Marsala M, Yaksh TL. Characterization of time course of spinal amino acids, citrulline and PGE$_2$ release after carrageenan/kaolin-induced knee joint inflammation: a chronic microdialysis study. *Pain.* 1996;67:345–54.

48. Hua XY, Chen P, Marsala M, Yaksh TL. Intrathecal substance P-induced thermal hyperalgesia and spinal release of prostaglandin E$_2$ and amino acids. *Neuroscience.* 1999;89:525–34.

49. Yang LC, Marsala M, Yaksh TL. Effect of spinal kainic acid receptor activation on spinal amino acid and prostaglandin E$_2$ release in rat. *Neuroscience.* 1996;75:453–61.

50. Malmberg AB, Yaksh TL. Cyclooxygenase inhibition and the spinal release of prostaglandin E$_2$ and amino acids evoked by paw formalin injection: a microdialysis study in unanesthetized rats. *J Neurosci.* 1995;15:2768–76.

51. Versteeg HH, van Bergen en Henegouwen PM, van Deventer SJ, Peppelenbosch MP. Cyclooxygenase-dependent signalling: molecular events and consequences. *FEBS Lett.* 1999;445:1–5.

52. Armstrong RA, Wilson NH. Aspects of the thromboxane receptor system. *Gen Pharmacol.* 1995;26:463–72.

53. Negishi M, Sugimoto Y, Ichikawa A. Molecular mechanisms of diverse actions of prostanoid receptors. *Biochim Biophys Acta.* 1995;1259:109–19.

54. Yousufzai SY, Chen AL, Abdel-Latif AA. Species differences in the effects of prostaglandins on inositol triphosphate accumulation, phosphatidic acid formation, myosin light chain phosphorylation and contraction in iris sphincter of the mammalian eye: interaction with the cyclic AMP sytem. *J Pharmacol Exp Ther.* 1988;247:1064–72.

55. Birnbaumer L, Abramowitz J, Brown AM. Receptor-effector coupling by G proteins. *Biochim Biophys Acta.* 1990;1031:163–224.

56. Samuelsson B, Goldyne M, Granström E, Hamberg M, Hammarström S, Malmsten C. Prostaglandins and thromboxanes. *Annu Rev Biochem.* 1978;47:997–1029.

57. Woodward DF, Fairbairn CE, Goodrum DD, Krauss AH, Ralston TL, Williams LS. Ca²⁺ transients evoked by prostanoids in Swiss 3T3 cells suggest an FP-receptor mediated response. *Adv Prostaglandin Thromboxane Leukotriene Res.* 1991;21A:367–70.

58. Melien O, Winsnes R, Refsnes M, Gladhaug IP, Christoffersen T. Pertussis toxin abolishes the inhibitory effects of prostaglandins E_1, E_2, I_2 and F_2 alpha on hormone-induced cAMP accumulation in cultured hepatocytes. *Eur J Biochem.* 1988;172:293–7.

59. Negishi M, Ito S, Hayaishi O. Prostaglandin E receptors in bovine adrenal medulla are coupled to adenylate cyclase via Gi and to phosphoinositide metabolism in a pertussis toxin-insensitive manner. *J Biol Chem.* 1989;264:3916–23.

60. Soliven B, Takeda M, Shandy T, Nelson DJ. Arachidonic acid and its metabolites increase $[Ca^{2+}]_i$ in cultured rat oligodendrocytes. *Am J Physiol.* 1993;264:C632–40.

61. Nicol GD, Klingberg DK, Vasko MR. Prostaglandin E_2 increases calcium conductance and stimulates release of substance P in avian sensory neurons. *J Neurosci.* 1992;12:1917–27.

62. Nicol GD, Vasko MR, Evans AR. Prostaglandins suppress an outward potassium current in embryonic rat sensory neurons. *J Neurophys.* 1997;77:167–76.

63. Gold MS, Reichling DB, Shuster MJ, Levine JD. Hyperalgesic agents increase a tetrodotoxin-resistant Na⁺ current in nociceptors. *Proc Natl Acad Sci USA.* 1996;93:1108–12.

64. Oku R, Satoh M, Takagi H. Release of substance P from the spinal dorsal horn is enhanced in polyarthritic rats. *Neurosci Lett.* 1987;74:315–9.

65. Sorkin LS. Release of amino acids and PGE_2 into the spinal cord of lightly anesthetized rats during development of an experimental arthritis: enhancement of C-fiber evoked release. *Soc Neurosci Abstr.* 1992;18:429.10.

66. Matsumura K, Watanabe Y, Imai-Matsumura K, Connolly M, Koyama Y, Onoe H et al. Mapping of prostaglandin E_2 binding sites in rat brain using quantitative autoradiography. *Brain Res.* 1992;581:292–8.

67. Coleman RA, Smith WL, Narumiya S. International Union of Pharmacology VIII. Classification of Prostanoid receptors: properties, distribution and structure of the receptors and their subtypes. *Pharmacol Rev.* 1994;46:205–29.

68. Vane JR, Bakhle YS, Botting RM. Cyclooxygenases 1 and 2. *Annu Rev Pharmacol Toxicol.* 1998;38:97–120.

69. DeWitt DL, Smith WL. Cloning of sheep and mouse prostaglandin endoperoxide synthases. *Methods Enzymol.* 1990;187:469–79.

70. Xie W, Chipman JG, Robertson DL, Erikson RL, Simmonds DL. Expression of a mitogen-responsive gene encoding prostaglandin synthase is regulated by mRNA splicing. *Proc Natl Acad Sci USA.* 1991;88:2692–6.

71. Picot D, Loll PJ, Garavito RM. The X-ray crystal structure of the membrane protein prostaglandin H_2 synthase-1. *Nature.* 1994;367;243–9.

72. Kurumbail RG, Stevens AM, Gierse JK, McDonald JJ, Stegeman RA, Pak JY et al. Structural basis for selective inhibition of cyclooxygenase-2 by anti-inflammatory agents. *Nature.* 1996;384:644–8. (Published erratum appears in *Nature.* 1997;385:555.)

73. Meade EA, Smith WL, DeWitt DL. Differential inhibition of prostaglandin endoperoxide synthase (cyclooxygenase) isozymes by aspirin and other non-steroidal anti-inflammatory drugs. *J Biol Chem.* 1993;268:6610–4.

74. Seibert K, Zhang Y, Leahy K, Hauser S, Masferrer J, Perkins W et al. Pharmacological and biochemical demonstration of the role of cyclooxygenase 2 in inflammation and pain. *Proc Natl Acad Sci USA.* 1994;91:12013–7.

75. Gierse JK, McDonald JJ, Hauser SD, Rangwala SH, Koboldt CM, Seibert K. A single amino acid difference between cyclooxygenase-1 (COX-1) and -2 (COX-2) reverses the selectivity of COX-2 specific inhibitors. *J Biol Chem.* 1996;271:15810–4.

76. Masferrer JL, Zweifel BS, Manning PT, Hauser SD, Leahy KM, Smith WG et al. Selective inhibition of inducible cyclooxygenase 2 in vivo is antiinflammatory and nonulcerogenic. *Proc Natl Acad Sci USA.* 1994;91:3228–32.

77. Herschman HR. Prostaglandin synthase 2. *Biochim Biophys Acta.* 1996;1299:125–40.

78. Murakami M, Kambe T, Shimbara S, Kudo I. Functional coupling between various phospholipase A_2s and cyclooxygenases in immediate and delayed prostanoid biosynthetic pathways. *J Biol Chem.* 1999;274:3103–15.

79. Leslie CC. Properties and regulation of cytosolic phospholipase A_2. *J Biol Chem.* 1997;272:16709–12.

80. Spencer AG, Woods JW, Arakawa T, Singer II, Smith WL. Subcellular localization of prostaglandin endoperoxide H synthases-1 and -2 by immunoelectron microscopy. *J Biol Chem.* 1998;273:9886–93.

81. Chopra B, Giblett S, Little JG, Donaldson LF, Tate S, Evans RJ et al. Cyclooxygenase-1 is a marker for a subpopulation of putative nociceptive neurons in rat dorsal root ganglia. *Eur J Neurosci.* 2000;12:911–20.

82. Ichitani Y, Shi T, Haeggstrom JZ, Samuelsson B, Hökfelt, T. Increased levels of cyclooxygenase-2 mRNA in the rat spinal cord after peripheral inflammation: an *in situ* hybridization study. *Neuroreport.* 1997;8:2949–52.

83. Beiche F, Scheuerer S, Brune K, Geisslinger G, Goppelt-Struebe M. Up-regulation of cyclooxygenase-2 mRNA in the rat spinal cord following peripheral inflammation. *FEBS Lett.* 1996;390:165–9.

84. Beiche F, Brune K, Geisslinger G, Goppelt-Struebe M. Expression of cyclo-oxygenase isoforms in the rat spinal cord and their regulation during adjuvant-induced arthritis. *Inflamm Res.* 1998;47:482–7.

85. Beiche F, Klein T, Nusing R, Neuhuber W, Goppelt-Struebe M. Localization of cyclooxygenase-2 and prostaglandin E_2 receptor EP_3 in the rat lumbar spinal cord. *J Neuroimmunol.* 1998;89:26–34.

86. Hay CH, de Belleroche JS. Dexamethasone prevents the induction of COX-2 mRNA and prostaglandins in the lumbar spinal cord following intraplantar FCA in parallel with inhibition of oedema. *Neuropharmacology.* 1998;37:739–44.

87. Ebersberger A, Grubb BD, Willingale HL, Gardiner NJ, Nebe J, Schaible HG. The intraspinal release of prostaglandin E_2 in a model of acute arthritis is accompanied by an up-regulation of cyclo-oxygenase-2 in the spinal cord. *Neuroscience.* 1999;93:775–81.

88. Bauer MK, Lieb K, Schulze-Osthoff K, Berger M, Gebicke-Haerter PJ, Bauer J et al. Expression and regulation of cyclooxygenase-2 in rat microglia. *Eur J Biochem.* 1997;243:726–31.

89. Petrova TV, Akama KT, Van Eldik LJ. Selective modulation of BV-2 microglial activation by prostaglandin E(2). Differential effects on endotoxin-stimulated cytokine induction. *J Biol Chem.* 1999;274:28823–7.

90. Inoue A, Ikoma K, Morioka N, Kumagai K, Hashimoto T, Hide I et al. Interleukin-

1 beta induces substance P release from primary afferent neurons through the cyclooxygenase-2 system. *J Neurochem.* 1999;73:2206–13.

91. Geisslinger G, Yaksh TL. Spinal actions of cyclooxygenase isozyme inhibitors. In: Devor M, Rowbotham MC, Wiesenfelld-Hallin Z, editors. *Proceedings of the 9th World Congress on Pain.* Seattle: IASP Press; 2000;771–85.

92. Hay C, de Belleroche J. Carrageenan-induced hyperalgesia is associated with increased cyclo-oxygenase-2 expression in spinal cord. *Neuroreport.* 1997;8:1249–51.

93. Dirig DM, Yaksh TL. *In vitro* prostanoid release from spinal cord following peripheral inflammation: effects of substance P, NMDA and capsaicin. *Br J Pharmacol.* 1999;126:1333–40.

94. Yamagata K, Andreasson KI, Kaufmann WE, Barnes CA, Worley PF. Expression of a mitogen-inducible cyclooxygenase in brain neurons: regulation by synaptic activity and glucocorticoids. *Neuron.* 1993;11:371–86.

95. Miettinen S, Fusco FR, Yrjänheikki J, Keinänen R, Hirvonen T, Roivainen R et al. Spreading depression and focal brain ischemia induces cyclooxygenase-2 in cortical neurons through N-methyl-D-aspartic acid-receptors and phospholipase A_2. *Proc Natl Acad Sci USA.* 1997;94:6500–5.

96. Gilron I, Quirion R, Coderre TJ. Pre- versus post-formalin effects of ketamine or large-dose alfentanil in the rat: discordance between pain behavior and spinal Fos-like immunoreactivity. *Anesth Analg.* 1999;89:128–35.

97. Gilron I, Quirion R, Coderre TJ. Pre-versus postinjury effects of intravenous GABAergic anesthetics on formalin-induced Fos immunoreactivity in the rat spinal cord. *Anesth Analg.* 1999;88:414–20.

98. Presley RW, Menétrey D, Levine JD, Basbaum AI. Systemic morphine suppresses noxious stimulus-evoked Fos protein-like immunoreactivity in the rat spinal cord. *J Neurosci.* 1990;10:323–35.

99. Yashpal K, Mason P, McKenna JE, Sharma SK, Henry JL, Coderre TJ. Comparison of the effects of treatment with intrathecal lidocaine given before and after formalin on both nociception and Fos expression in the spinal cord dorsal horn. *Anesthesiology.* 1998;88:157–64.

100. Puig S, Sorkin LS. Formalin-evoked activity in identified primary afferent fibers: systemic lidocaine suppresses phase-2 activity. *Pain.* 1996;64:345–55.

101. Watkins LR, Nguyen KT, Lee JE, Maier SF. Dynamic regulation of proinflammatory cytokines. *Adv Exp Med Biol.* 1999;461:153–78.

102. Quan N, Whiteside M, Herkenham M. Cyclooxygenase 2-mRNA expression in rat brain after peripheral injection of lipopolysaccharide. *Brain Res.* 1998;802:189–97.

103. Lacroix S, Rivest S. Effect of acute systemic inflammatory response and cytokines on the transcription of the genes encoding cyclooxygenase enzymes (COX-1 and COX-2) in the rat brain. *J Neurochem.* 1998;70:452–66.

104. Matsumura K, Cao C, Ozaki M, Morii H, Nakadate K, Watanabe Y. Brain endothelial cells express cyclooxygenase-2 during lipopolysaccharide-induced fever: light and electron microscopic immunocytochemical studies. *J Neurosci.* 1998;18:6279–89.

105. Yucel-Lindberg T, Nilsson S, Modéer T. Signal transduction pathways involved in the synergistic stimulation of prostaglandin production by interleukin-1beta and tumor necrosis factor alpha in human gingival fibroblasts. *J Dent Res.* 1999;78:61–8.

106. Devoghel JC. Small intrathecal doses of lysine-acetylsalicylate relieve intractable pain in man. *J Int Med Res.* 1983;11:90–1.

107. Devoghel JC. Intrathecal injection of lysine-acetylsalicylate in man with intractable cancer pain. In: Juma I, Yaksh TL, editors. *Progress in Pharmacology and Clinical Pharmacology.* Gustav Fischer Verlag. 1993:111–8.

108. Pellerin M, Hardy F, Abergel A, Boule D, Palacci JH, Babinet P et al. [Chronic refractory pain in cancer patients. Value of the spinal injection of lysine acetylsal-icylate. 60 cases]. *Presse Med.* 1987;16:1465–8.

109. Malmstrom K, Daniels S, Kotey P, Seidenberg BC, Desjardins PJ. Comparison of rofecoxib and celecoxib, two cyclooxygenase-2 inhibitors, in postoperative dental pain: a randomized, placebo- and active-comparator-controlled clinical trial. *Clin Ther.* 1999;21:1653–63.

110. Flower RJ, Moncada S, Vane JR. Analgesic-antipyretics and anti-inflammatory agents; drugs employed in the treatment of gout. In: Gilman AG, Goodman LS, Gilman A, editors. *The Pharmacological Basis of Therapeutics,* 6th Edition. New York: Macmillan; 1980:682–728.

111. Insel PA. Analgesic-antipyretics and anti-inflammatory agents; drugs employed in the treatment of rheumatoid arthritis and gout. In: Gilman AG, Rall TW, Nies AW, Taylor P, editors. *The Pharmacological Basis of Therapeutics,* 8th Edition. New York: Macmillan. 1999:640–681.

112. Woodbury DM. Analgesics and antipyretics. In: Goodman LS, Gilman A, editors. *The Pharmacological Basis of Therapeutics,* 3rd Edition. New York: Macmillan. 1965:312–44.

113. Yaksh TL, Dirig DM, Malmberg AB. Mechanism of action of nonsteroidal anti-inflammatory drugs. *Cancer Invest.* 1998;16:509–27.

8 | Cyclooxygenase and inflammation in the clinical progression of Alzheimer's disease dementia

Giulio Maria Pasinetti

Neuroinflammation Research Center, Department of Psychiatry, Mount Sinai Medical Center, One Gustave L. Levy Place, New York, NY 10029, USA.

THE INFLAMMATORY HYPOTHESIS OF ALZHEIMER'S DISEASE

In the past few years, a large number of epidemiological studies have addressed the possible protective effect of the use of anti-inflammatory drugs with regard to Alzheimer's disease (AD)[1]. Perhaps the most convincing of these studies – the Baltimore Longitudinal Study of Aging – utilized data collected prospectively, thereby minimizing recall bias issues. As corroborated by related studies, their results indicated a protective effect from the use of non-steroid anti-inflammatory drugs (NSAIDs)[2]. One small controlled trial of indomethacin suggested that the drug slowed cognitive deterioration[3]. More recently, a small controlled trial of the NSAID diclofenac showed similar results (though not statistically significant because of a high drop-out rate)[4].

However, in spite of the prior research on this hypothesis, whether the inflammatory mechanisms actually cause damage in AD, or are merely present to remove the debris of the neurodegenerative events, is still uncertain. Although clinical features of inflammation are absent, on a molecular level inflammatory responses appear to accompany the neuropathological features of AD[5,6]. Amyloid plaques are surrounded by reactive microglia (as well as astrocytes) which have the characteristics of antigen-presenting tissue macrophages, including HLA-DR surface markers. In addition, there is clear evidence of an acute phase response[7], with upregulation of inflammatory cytokines such as IL-1, IL-6 and tumour necrosis factor (TNF)-α, accompanied by an increase in acute phase proteins such as α1-antichymotrypsin (ACT) and α2-macroglobulin (α2-MAC). Further, there is an active complement system in the AD brain[8] with generation of the lytic membrane attack complex[9] and, presumably, with release of anaphylatoxins. Our previous findings show that complement peptides potentiate amyloid neurotoxicity *in vitro*[10], which is consistent with the evidence showing that overexpression of the inflammatory cytokine IL-6 in the brain leads to neurodegeneration[11]. Finally, upregulation of cyclooxygenase(COX)-2 but not COX-1 in AD neurons suggests that inflammatory lipids may also be involved in the pathogenesis of the disease[12].

The elucidation of the role of inflammatory processes has provided an impetus to the development of anti-inflammatory therapy for AD[13]. Yet there remains a critical need both to improve the diagnosis of patients who are in the very earliest stage of AD, and to identify very early neurobiological inflammatory abnormalities, so that effective treatment can be developed.

INFLAMMATION AND THE CLINICAL PROGRESSION OF ALZHEIMER'S DISEASE DEMENTIA

Recent evidence suggests that different indices of classical inflammatory cascades may have distinct associations with different phases of the clinical progression of AD, as reflected in the clinical dementia rating (CDR)[14]. For example, it appears that COX-2 (but not COX-1) expression in the neurons of the hippocampal formation, a brain region at risk for AD neurodegeneration, may be a predictor of progression of very early AD before neurodegeneration occurs[15]. Surprisingly, in contrast to COX-2, other classical markers of inflammatory neurodegeneration, such as cytokine expression[16], microglial reactivity and complement component gene expression (unpublished observation) showed increased expression, but only at later stages of AD dementia (Figure 1). The evidence showing induction of neuronal COX-2 early in AD dementia is very interesting and suggests that independent segments of the inflammatory cascade may play important and possibly independent roles in separate phases of the disease, to influence the progression of AD dementia (Figure 1). Given these findings, selection of anti-inflammatory drugs for studies of AD patients at a particular clinical stage should be based on their activity against the inflammatory processes most pronounced at that stage, e.g COX-2 inhibitors in the early phase of AD. Thus, the identification of specific early markers involved in destructive brain inflammation would provide critically important selection criteria, and/or possible covariance, for clinical trials of anti-inflammatory drugs. Below, I will outline recent evidence implicating COX-2, microglia, cytokines and the complement system in AD neurodegeneration.

Figure 1 Inflammatory markers and clinical progression of Alzheimer's disease dementia.

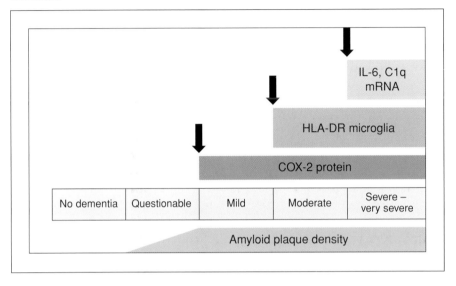

CYCLOOXYGENASE AND ALZHEIMER'S DISEASE

While the mechanism of action of NSAIDs is not entirely clear, it is generally assumed that their effects are mediated by competitive inhibition of COX catalytic activity, reducing the production of inflammatory prostaglandins (PGs) from membrane-derived arachidonate. The apparent protective effect of NSAIDs suggests that COX might be involved in neurodegenerative mechanisms. In view of the great interest in clinical trials of NSAIDs in AD, we have investigated the role of COX in neurodegeneration[17].

In recent years it has been established that COX exists in two isoforms, coded by distinct genes on different chromosomes[18–20]. The two isoforms show about 60% homology and have similar catalytic activity, but are physiologically distinct. COX-2 is inducible in inflammatory cells in response to inflammatory signals such as cytokines and lipopolysaccharide, and is down-regulated by glucocorticoids. In contrast, COX-1 is generally constitutive. It thus appears that COX-2 mediates inflammatory activity, while COX-1 has housekeeping functions, including gastric cytoprotection and platelet aggregation. Traditional NSAIDs are non-selective COX inhibitors; their beneficial effects derive from inhibiting COX-2 activity. COX-1 inhibition, however, is more likely to cause gastrointestinal and renal toxicity and inhibit platelet aggregation. Thus, the use of newly developed, highly selective COX-2 inhibitors holds promise for maintained efficacy with vastly reduced toxicity[21,22].

To clarify the neuroprotective mechanisms of NSAIDs, we have studied the role of COX-1 and COX-2 in the developing brain and in experimental models of neurodegeneration. We found that in the rat brain, COX-2 is expressed primarily in limbic structures and is developmentally regulated[24]. We next examined COX-2 and COX-1 expression in an excitotoxic model of neurodegeneration: apoptosis induced by systemic injection of kainic acid. The results showed that neuronal COX-2, but not COX-1, was induced in response to kainic acid injection[23]. Moreover, COX-2, but not COX-1, induction is elevated during the response leading to apoptotic neuron death[24]. A related study shows that glutamate excitotoxicity is potentiated in primary neuron cultures derived from transgenic mice with neuronal overexpression of human COX-2[25]. Interestingly, COX-2-specific inhibitors may also protect against glutamate neurotoxicity[26].

The discovery that in brain COX-2 is expressed in neurons[23,27–29] and not in glia, suggests some important implications for the treatment of neuro-degenerative disorders. We hypothesized that while COX-2 is involved in neuronal death mechanisms, it may not necessarily be linked to the classical inflammatory cascades[17]. For example, recent studies in our laboratories indicated that COX-2 overexpression in neurons may influence genes involved in the cell cycle and cell differentiation[30], suggesting alternative roles for COX-2 in brain.

Major efforts are now under way to determine whether COX inhibitors can help control the destructive progression of AD. Large National Institutes of Health (NIH)-supported clinical trials are evaluating whether selective COX-2 inhibitors, or low dose non-selective NSAIDs, can delay the diagnosis of AD. Industry-sponsored trials of selective COX-2 inhibitors currently target individuals with mild cognitive impairment. Additional trials are in the planning stages as new COX-2 inhibitors continue to be developed. Further elucidation of the role of COX-2 (and COX-1) in various clinical stages of AD, defined by CDR, will clearly aid the clinical design of such trials. As discussed earlier, the elevation of neuronal COX-2 expression during the early phase (mild dementia) of the clinical progression of AD dementia might set favourable circumstances for later inflammatory neurodegenerative conditions. This would be consistent with the apparent early upregulation of COX-2 in AD brain, prior to an increase in microglial activity (unpublished observation) and elevation of cytokine (e.g. IL-6, transforming growth factor (TGF)-β1) expression[14].

MICROGLIA AS AN INFLAMMATORY CELL COMPONENT INVOLVED IN THE CLINICAL PROGRESSION OF ALZHEIMER'S DISEASE

Microglia represent the main cellular component of the inflammatory response in the AD brain[31]. They carry HLA-DR surface antigens, and therefore may act as antigen processing and presenting cells. The activated microglia may also secrete neurotoxins that contribute to neuronal loss in AD[32,33]. It is unclear, however, whether these processes represent a reaction to the neurodegeneration in AD.

Microglia may participate in complement-mediated mechanisms in the AD brain. The HLA-DR+ microglia (with class II antigen presentation capability) also express leucocyte common antigen and FcRI or FcRII receptors that promote phagocytosis[34]. Such reactive microglial cells are often found within or intimately associated with senile plaques[35], where they express complement receptors CR3 and CR4. These receptors bind to IC3b, a potent opsonin (a cell-associated tag for phagocytosis) on target cell surfaces[36]. Moreover, the local degenerative environment of the AD brain, which contains an abundance of β-amyloid (Aβ), neurofibrillary tangles, dystrophic neurites, neurophil threads and possibly injured neurons, may be favourable for complement system activation. We hypothesized that complement fragments released during activation of the cascade might have important roles in chemo-attraction of the microglia and astrocytes frequently observed in the tissue surrounding AD plaques[37]. Thus microglia may play a role in complement-mediated phagocytosis in the brain.

Independent of the potential chemotactic role of microglia, the relation-ship of microglia to Aβ plaque evolution is still controversial. One possibility is that microglia play a direct role through synthesis, processing or catabolism of amyloid precursor protein (APP) or Aβ. Of these alternatives, primary synthesis of APP leading to Aβ deposition is the least clear. On the one hand, cultured microglia can secrete Aβ and metabolize APP in a manner that might favour Aβ deposition[38]. Neurons, by virtue of their high expression of APP, have been postulated as the primary source of Aβ[39]. Another potential role for microglia in plaque formation may involve processing of APP and Aβ derived from other cellular sources; there is evidence suggesting that microglia aggregate much more around amyloid-containing neuritic plaques than diffuse plaques, both in AD and normal ageing[40]. This suggests that microglia may be involved in the conversion of non-fibrillar Aβ into amyloid fibrils, a role similar to that ascribed to peripheral macrophages in systemic amyloidosis[41].

Activated microglia are also capable of producing a variety of pro-inflammatory mediators[42] and potentially neurotoxic substances[43] that could contribute to localized or more widespread brain injury. These include complement, cytokines, reactive oxygen intermediates and nitric oxide, among others[44,45]. Moreover, conditions in the AD brain may enhance constitutive production of inflammation-related molecules. Aβ, for example, is a particularly potent stimulator of the microglial production of IL-6, IL-1, TNF-α, nitric oxide and superoxide free radicals[44,46]. Consistent with these observations *in vitro*, immunohistochemical and *in situ* hybridization studies of AD and control cortical samples have revealed plaque-associated microglia expressing IL-6[47], IL-1 and TNF-α[48].

We hypothesized that microglia-mediated responses at later stages of the clinical progression of AD dementia may play an important role in fuelling a cycle of inflammatory cascades leading to accelerated AD neuropathology, possibly through elevation of microglia-derived cytokines. The precise identification of the clinical stage at which pro-inflammatory molecules become available for microglia activation will facilitate the development of anti-inflammatory strategies aimed at slowing the clinical progression of AD.

CYTOKINE EXPRESSION AND ALZHEIMER'S DISEASE DEMENTIA

Among other inflammatory mediators, cytokines presumably subserve inter- and intracellular signalling processes in the brain, similar to their responses to inflammatory cascades in the periphery. However, some mechanisms may be unique to their role in the brain. The expression of several cytokines has been investigated in the AD brain, and many of them, including IL-6, TGF-β1 and IL-1, showed upregulation in neuropathologically defined AD brain[49]. For example IL-6 appears to be highly involved in AD neuropathology. In the AD brain, the cortical elevation of IL-6 mRNA expression coincides with the elevation of acute phase proteins such as C-reactive protein and α2-MAC expression[50]. Moreover, there is immunocytochemical evidence showing that in the AD brain, IL-6 is preferentially associated with diffuse, but not neuritic, AD plaques[51]. Thus, IL-6 may play an important role in the maturational process of AD plaques, leading to neuritic degeneration.

Like IL-6, TGF-β1 is a cytokine apparently playing a major role in brain tissue injury and repair[52]. The expression of TGF-β1 is elevated in AD plaques and its expression is especially prominent along cerebrovascular vessels that exhibit Aβ deposition (congophilic angiopathy)[52]. While TGF-β1 expression correlates with the extent of amyloidosis in the AD brain[46], overexpression of TGF-β1 in a mouse brain results in exacerbation of AD neuropathology[53].

Unlike IL-6 and TGF-β1, the potential role of TNF-α in AD is highly controversial, given the almost universal acceptance of this cytokine as a potent pro-inflammatory, cytotoxic polypeptide in disorders such as brain trauma and Parkinson's disease[54]. Excess TNF-α is reported to destroy human cortical neurons. However, TNF-α has also been reported to be trophic to rat hippocampal neurons[55] and to protect against glutamate, free-radical and Aβ toxicity in enriched cultures of primary neurons[54]. Pharmacological inhibition of TNF-α release or activity ameliorates tissue damage in ischaemia models, but genetic ablation of TNF receptors has been suggested to worsen excitotoxic damage[56].

As discussed above, it appears that the elevation of cytokine expression

Figure 2 Potential role of COX-2 in the progression of Alzheimer's disease dementia.

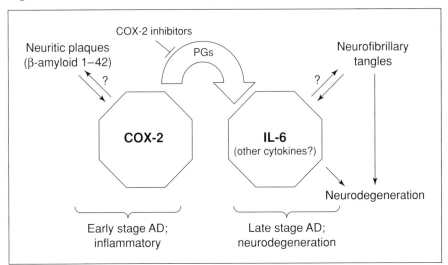

during AD becomes evident only at late stages of the clinical dementia[14] (Figure 1), when it may be too late for preventive measures. Thus, it might be possible to view the elevation of cytokines in brain of AD as a consequence, rather than a cause, of neurodegeneration. Because of the evidence showing that COX-2-generated prostaglandins (PGs) may influence cytokine gene expression[57], the finding tentatively suggests that treatment of early AD with a specific COX-2 inhibitor may be an appropriate therapeutic intervention for preventing cytokine-mediated neurodegeneration at later AD clinical stages, as illustrated in Figure 2.

THE COMPLEX ROLE OF THE COMPLEMENT SYSTEM IN ALZHEIMER'S DISEASE

Demonstration of complement activation in the AD brain has caused much speculation about the role of this inflammatory cascade in neurodegenerative mechanisms[39]. There is evidence that complement proteins can augment aspects of Aβ toxicity. Recent studies suggest that the interaction of C1q (the first component of the complement cascade) with Aβ peptides increases the aggregability and toxicity of Aβ and initiates the complement cascade[58,59] and generation of the membrane attack complex[9]. These potentially destructive roles for complement proteins suggest that drugs inhibiting complement activation may be useful in the treatment of AD[60]. As shown for IL-6, C1q was also found elevated only at the late stage of AD clinical dementia (unpublished observation) (Figure 1).

However, recent studies from our laboratory indicate that the situation may be more complex. While activation of the complement cascade in the brain may be destructive, activation of selective complement components such as C5 may lead to the generation of the anaphylatoxin, C5a, that we found to be highly neuroprotective[61]. While little is known about the generation of C5a in the brain, we found that C5a is expressed locally in the mouse brain[62], where it can be generated proteolytically from C5 even in the absence of classical complement activation[63]. It is possible then that C5a might contribute to neuronal and glial functions in a normal brain even in the absence of classical complement activation. This suggests that the complement system in the brain may have unexpected roles in neuronal homeostasis; specifically, release of anaphylatoxins during complement activation may increase the resistance of neurons to toxic stress. If complement activation has a dual role during AD, general suppression of the complement system may have unpredictable results. For this reason, developing drugs that target specific complement peptides or receptors may hold greater promise.

Recent studies suggest that the broad anti-inflammatory activity of glucocorticoids may have actually contributed to the failure of the attempt of the prednisone study to slow the clinical progression of AD dementia (see below). As discussed above, there is evidence that some inflammatory mediators, such as the C5-derived anaphylatoxin C5a[61,62] and TNF-α[64], are actually neuroprotective. The finding that low dose prednisone suppresses anaphylatoxin levels in AD[65] may suggest a deleterious effect on the disease process. Based in part on this evidence, the Alzheimer's Disease Cooperative Study (ADCS) is now beginning a second set of trials of anti-inflammatory therapies. The complications found in the aforementioned studies eliminated the ADCS's consideration of another glucocorticoid regimen in selecting drug regimens for these trials. Next, potential implications regarding the recent evidence showing the failure of the prednisone clinical trial in AD[66] and ongoing interventional studies designed to control inflammatory neurodegeneration in Alzheimer's disease will be discussed.

STATUS OF ANTI-INFLAMMATORY DRUG TRIALS IN ALZHEIMER'S DISEASE

The most effective drugs for the suppression of COX-2 and other inflammatory mediators have been glucocorticoids, a class of drugs that has also been found to downregulate COX-2 (among other inflammatory mediators)[65]. A multi-centre placebo-controlled trial of the synthetic glucocorticoid prednisone has been conducted by the ADCS, a consortium funded by the National Institute on Aging. The study enrolled 138 subjects, randomized to receive a regimen of prednisone (initial dose 20 mg, tapered to a maintenance dose of 10 mg) or matching placebo. The primary outcome measures were the Alzheimer's Disease Assessment Scale (ADAS-cog)[66], and the CDR scores[67]. The primary, intent-to-treat, analysis of the one-year change in the ADAS-cog showed no significant difference between treatment groups. Secondary analyses, including completers-only analyses, similarly showed no significant effect of the intervention on cognitive function or clinical stage of disease as assessed by the CDR[68].

Several explanations have been suggested for the failure of the prednisone regimen to slow the rate of cognitive decline[66]. First, the dose may have been too low; much higher doses are used routinely to treat inflammatory diseases of brain, such as lupus cerebritis. However, data from the study suggests that higher doses among this population are not feasible. The low dose regimen also caused some decline in lumbar spine bone density, despite calcium and vitamin D supplementation, and a few asymptomatic vertebral fractures were detected in the prednisone group. There were also a number of subjects with significant hyperglycaemia. Finally, the prednisone treatment group showed significant behavioural decline, as assessed by the Brief Psychiatric Rating Scale[69], compared with the placebo group.

This adverse effect on behaviour may have contributed to the failure to favourably influence cognitive function. It is possible that glucocorticoid therapy has an adverse effect on hippocampal function (demonstrated in rodents) that may negate any beneficial effect on AD brain pathology. However, a recent study suggests that the hippocampal neurodegeneration seen in rodents does not occur in primates with long-term exogenous glucocorticoid exposure[70].

On the other hand, the characterization of inflammatory processes in the AD brain has led to efforts to develop anti-inflammatory treatment strategies to slow the rate of disease progression. These strategies target one or more of the processes discussed above: COX-2 , cytokines, complement cascade and microglial accumulation and activation. The recent elucidation of the respective physiological roles of COX-1 and COX-2 has resulted in great interest by the pharmaceutical industry in the development of selective inhibitors of COX-2[22]. These agents may be equally effective in suppressing inflammation in diseases such as rheumatoid arthritis, but with reduced gastrointestinal toxicity. Selective COX-2 inhibitors may be excellent candidates for therapeutic trials in AD because of their improved safety and because they target the COX isoform that may be involved in AD neurodegeneration. Two pharmaceutical companies are now conducting large-scale trials of selective COX-2 inhibitors to slow the progression of AD; one of these trials using rofecoxib (Vioxx®) targets the earliest stage of the disease (i.e. slowing the progression from questionable to mild dementia).

FUTURE DIRECTIONS IN ANTI-INFLAMMATORY STUDIES IN ALZHEIMER'S DISEASE

Toxicity remains a major block to a study of the anti-inflammatory dosage of a traditional NSAID. One way to reduce NSAID toxicity is to add a cytoprotective agent to the treatment regimen. Misoprostol is a synthetic prostaglandin proven to reduce the incidence of NSAID gastropathy. However, a recent report of a trial of diclofenac plus misoprostol in AD patients indicated that this combination was not tolerated any better than indomethacin; the drop-out rate in this 25-week trial was 50% in the active drug group, rendering the results of the study inconclusive[71]. It is unlikely that a study of a treatment regimen that is tolerated (over the course of a year) by a minority of subjects will yield definitive results. The ADCS has opted to study two NSAID-type regimens that are expected to have substantially less toxicity than the reported indomethacin and diclofenac regimens. The first is the new selective COX-2 inhibitor, rofecoxib. As discussed above, COX-2 may be the target of action of NSAIDs in the AD brain, and since COX-2 inhibitors appear to carry a much reduced risk of serious gastrointestinal toxicity, rofecoxib may be effective.

The second active drug regimen in the new ADCS trial is low dose naproxen (200 mg twice daily). Naproxen is a non-selective COX inhibitor, and therefore carries the risk of toxicity at full dose, similar to indomethacin and diclofenac. However, if in fact COX-1 is an important target for NSAID action in AD, naproxen may be more effective than a selective COX-2 inhibitor. It is important to note that 200 mg is the over-the-counter analgesic dose, which is substantially less than a full anti-inflammatory dose. Nevertheless, studies suggest that this regimen is reasonably well tolerated in the elderly[72,73], although there are few data on long-term treatment. In rodents, it has been found that systemic administration of naproxen suppresses COX activity in the brain[74,75], indicating effective brain penetration. But will the low dose tested in the ADCS trial be sufficient to alter the AD process? The epidemiological studies suggest that casual use of NSAIDs obtained over-the-counter may be neuroprotective, supporting further study of a low dose regimen.

ACKNOWLEDGEMENTS

This work was supported by AG13799, AG14239, and AG16743 to GMP. We thank Christian M. Kolarz for editorial assistance.

Address all correspondence to: Giulio Maria Pasinetti, M.D., Ph.D., Neuroinflammation Research Center, Department of Psychiatry, The Mount Sinai School of Medicine, One Gustave L. Levy Place, New York, NY 10029, USA.

REFERENCES

1. McGeer PL, Schulzer M, McGeer EG. Arthritis and anti-inflammatory agents as possible protective factors for Alzheimer's disease: A review of 17 epidemiologic studies. *Neurology*. 1996;47:425–32.

2. Stewart WF, Kawas C, Corrada M, Metter EJ. Risk of Alzheimer's disease and duration of NSAID use. *Neurology*. 1997;48:626–32.

3. Rogers J, Kirby LC, Hempelman SR, Berry DL, McGeer PL, Kaszniak AW et al. Clinical trial of indomethacin in Alzheimer's disease. *Neurology*. 1993;43:1609–11.

4. Scharf S, Mander A, Ugoni A, Vajda F, Christophidis N. A double-blind, placebo-controlled trial of diclofenac/misoprostol in Alzheimer's disease. *Neurology*. 1999;53:197–201.

5. Aisen PS. Inflammation and Alzheimer's disease: Mechanisms and therapeutic strategies. *Gerontology*. 1997;43:143–9.

6. Pasinetti GM. Cyclooxygenase and inflammation in Alzheimer's disease: experimental approaches and clinical interventions. *J Neurosci Res*. 1998;54:1–6.

7. Vandenabeele P, Fiers W. Is amyloidogenesis during Alzheimer's disease due to an IL-1/IL-6-mediated 'acute phase response' in the brain? *Immunol Today*. 1991;12:217–9.

8. Pasinetti GM. Inflammatory mechanisms in neurodegeneration and Alzheimer's disease: The role of the complement system. *Neurobiol Aging*. 1996;17:707–16.

9. Webster S, Lue LF, Brachova L, Tenner AJ, McGeer PL, Terai K et al. Molecular and cellular characterization of the membrane attack complex, C5b-9, in Alzheimer's disease. *Neurobiol Aging*. 1997;18:415–21.

10. Oda T, Lehrer-Graiwer J, Finch CE, Pasinetti GM. Complement and beta-amyloid neurotoxicity *in vitro*: a model for Alzheimer disease. *Alzheimer's Res*. 1995;1:29–34.

11. Campbell IL, Abraham CR, Masliah E, Kemper P, Inglis JD, Oldstone MB et al. Neurologic disease induced in transgenic mice by cerebral overexpression of interleukin 6. *Proc Natl Acad Sci USA*. 1993;90:10061–5.

12. Pasinetti GM, Aisen PS. Cyclooxygenase-2 expression is increased in frontal cortex of Alzheimer's disease brain. *Neuroscience*. 1998;87:319–24.

13. Aisen PS. Inflammation and Alzheimer's disease. Mechanisms and therapeutic strategies. *Gerontology*. 1997;43:143–9.

14. Pasinetti G. The role of inflammation in the clinical progression of Alzheimer's disease dementia. *Soc Neurosci Abstr*. 2001; in press.

15. Ho L, Purohit D, Haroutunian V, Luterman JD, Willis F, Naslund J et al. Neuronal cyclooxygenase 2 is a marker of progression of early Alzheimer's disease. *Arch Neurol*. 2001; in press.

16. Luterman JD, Haroutunian V, Yemul S, Ho L, Purohit D, Aisen PS et al. Cytokine gene expression as a function of the clinical progression of Alzheimer's disease dementia. *Arch Neurol*. 2001; in press.

17. Pasinetti GM. Cyclooxygenase and inflammation in Alzheimer's disease: experimental approaches and clinical interventions. *J Neurosci Res*. 1998;54:1–6.

18. Kujubu DA, Fletcher BS, Varnum BC, Lim RW, Herschman HR. TIS10, a phorbol ester tumor promoter-inducible mRNA from Swiss 3T3 cells, encodes a novel prostaglandin synthase/cyclooxygenase homologue. *J Biol Chem*. 1991;266:12866–72.

19. Cao C, Matsumura K, Yamagata K, Watanabe Y. Induction by lipopolysaccharide

of cyclooxygenase-2 mRNA in rat brain; its possible role in the febrile response. *Brain Res.* 1995;697:187–96.

20. O'Banion MK, Winn VD, Young DA. cDNA cloning and functional activity of a glucocorticoid-regulated inflammatory cyclooxygenase. *Proc Natl Acad Sci USA.* 1992;89:4888–92.

21. Vane JR, Botting RM. New insights into the mode of action of anti-inflammatory drugs. *Inflamm Res.* 1995;44:1–10.

22. Warner TD, Giuliano F, Vojnovic I, Bukasa A, Mitchell JA, Vane JR. Nonsteroid drug selectivities for cyclo-oxygenase-1 rather than cyclo-oxygenase-2 are associated with human gastrointestinal toxicity: a full *in vitro* analysis. *Proc Natl Acad Sci USA.* 1999; 96:563–8.

23. Tocco G, Freire MJ, Schreiber SS, Sakhi SH, Aisen PS, Pasinetti GM. Maturational regulation and regional induction of cyclooxygenase-2 in rat brain: implications for Alzheimer's disease. *Exp Neurol.* 1997;144:339–49.

24. Ho L, Osaka H, Aisen P, Pasinetti GM. Induction of cyclooxygenase (COX)-2 but not COX-1 gene expression in apoptotic cell death. *J Neuroimmunol.* 1998;89:142–9.

25. Kelley KA, Ho L, Winger D, Freire-Moar J, Borelli CB, Aisen PS et al. Potentiation of excitotoxicity in transgenic mice overexpressing neuronal cyclooxygenase-2. *Am J Pathol.* 1999;155:995–1004.

26. Hewett SA, Ulizsz TF, Vidwans AS, Hewett JA. Cyclooxygenase-2 contributes to N-methyl-D-aspartate-mediated neuronal cell death in primary cortical cell culture. *J Pharmacol Exp Therap.* 2000;293:417–25.

27. Adams J, Collazo-Moraes Y, de Belleroche J. Cyclooxygenase-2 induction in cerebral cortex: an intacellular response to synaptic excitation. *J Neurochem.* 1996;66:6–13.

28. Kaufmann WE, Worley PF, Pegg J, Bremer M, Isakson P. COX-2, a synaptically induced enzyme, is expressed by excitatory neurons at postsynaptic sites in rat cerebral cortex. *Proc Natl Acad Sci USA.* 1996;93:2317–21.

29. Yamagata K, Andreasson KI, Kaufmann WE, Barnes CA, Worley PF. Expression of a mitogen-inducible cyclooxygenase in brain neurons: regulation by synaptic activity and glucocorticoids. *Neuron.* 1993;11:371–86.

30. Mirjani M, Ho L, Yemul S, Pasinetti GM. Cyclooxygenase-2 dependent cell cycle activities in brain. Implications in the clinical progression of Alzheimer's disease dementia. *Soc Neurosci Abstr.* 2001; in press.

31. McGeer PL, Itagaki S, Tago H, McGeer EG. Reactive microglia in patients with senile dementia of the Alzheimer type are positive for the histocompatibility glycoprotein HLA-DR. *Neurosci Lett.* 1987;79:195–200.

32. Dzenko KA, Weltzien RB, Pachter JS. Suppression of amyloid beta-induced monocyte neurotoxicity by antiinflammatory compounds. *J Neuroimmunol.* 1997;80:6–12.

33. Giulian D, Li J, Leara B, Keenen C. Phagocytic microglia release cytokines and cytotoxins that regulate the survival of astrocytes and neurons in culture. *Neurochem Int.* 1994;25:227–33.

34. McGeer PL, Akiyama H, Itagaki S, McGeer EG. Immune system response in Alzheimer's disease. *Can J Neurol Sci.* 1989;16:516–27.

35. Styren SD, Civin WH, Rogers J. Molecular, cellular and pathologic characterization of HLA-DR immunoreactivity in normal elderly and Alzheimer's disease brain. *Exp Neurol.* 1990;110:93–104.

36. Rozemuller JM, Van der Valk P, Eikelenboom P. Activated microglia and cerebral amyloid deposits in Alzheimer's disease. *Res Immunol.* 1992;143:646–9.

37. Pasinetti GM. Inflammatory mechanisms in neurodegeneration and Alzheimer's disease: The role of the complement system. *Neurobiol Aging.* 1996;17:707–16.

38. Bauer J, Konig G, Strauss S, Jonas U, Ganter U, Weidemann A et al. In-vitro matured human macrophages express Alzheimer's beta A4-amyloid precursor protein indicating synthesis in microglial cells. *FEBS Lett.* 1991;282:335–40.

39. LeBlanc A. Increased production of 4 kDa amyloid beta-peptide in serum deprived human primary neuron cultures: possible involvement of apoptosis. *J Neurosci.* 1995;15:7837–46.

40. Itagaki S, McGeer PL, Akiyama H, Zhu S, Selkoe D. Relationship of microglia and astrocytes to amyloid deposits of Alzheimer disease. *J Neuroimmunol.* 1989;24:173–82.

41. Shirahama T, Miura K, Ju ST, Kisilevsky R, Gruys E, Cohen AS. Amyloid enhancing factor-loaded macrophages in amyloid fibril formation. *Lab Invest.* 1990;62:61–8.

42. Sawada M, Kondo N, Suzumura A, Marunouchi T. Production of tumor necrosis factor-• by microglia and astrocytes in culture. *Brain Res.* 1989;491:394–7.

43. Yoo AS, McLarnon JG, Xu RL, Lee YB, Krieger C, Kim SU. Effects of phorbol ester on intracellular Ca^{2+} and membrane currents in cultured human microglia. *Neurosci Lett.* 1996;218:37–40.

44. Colton CA, Gilbert DL. Production of superoxide anions by a CNS macrophage, the microglia. *FEBS Lett.* 1987;223:284–8.

45. Cotman CW, Tenner AJ, Cummings BJ. Beta amyloid converts an acute phase injury response to chronic injury responses. *Neurobiol Aging.* 1996;17:723–31.

46. Chao CC, Ala TA, Hu S, Crossley KB, Sherman RE, Peterson PK et al. Serum cytokine levels in patients with Alzheimer's disease. *Clin Diagn Lab Immunol.* 1994;1:433–6.

47. Griffin W, Sheng JG, Roberts GW, Mrak RE. Interleukin-1 expression in different plaque types in Alzheimer's disease: significance in plaque evolution. *J Neuropath. Exp Neurol.* 1995;54:276–81.

48. Dickson DW, Lee SC, Mattiace LA, Yen SH, Brosnan C. Microglia and cytokines in neurological disease, with special reference to AIDS and Alzheimer's disease. *Glia.* 1993;7:75–83.

49. Benveniste E. Cytokine actions in the central nervous system. *Cytokine Growth Factor Rev.* 1998;9:259–75.

50. Wood JA, Wood PL, Ryan R, Graff-Radford NR, Pilapil C, Robtaille Y et al. Cytokine indices in Alzheimer's temporal cortex: no changes in mature IL-1β or IL-1RA but increases in the associated acute phase proteins IL-6, α2-macroglobulin and C-reactive protein. *Brain Res.* 1993;629: 245–52.

51. Hull M, Strauss S, Berger M, Volk B, Bauer J. Inflammatory mechanisms in Alzheimer's disease. *Eur Arch Psych Clin Neurosci.* 1996;246:124–8.

52. Finch CE, Laping NJ, Morgan TE, Nichols NR, Pasinetti GM. TGF-beta 1 is an organizer of responses to neurodegeneration. *J Cell Biochem.* 1993;53:314–22.

53. Wyss-Coray T, Masliah E, Mallory M, McConlogue L, Johnson-Wood K, Lin C et al. Amyloidogenic role of cytokine TGF-beta1 in transgenic mice and in Alzheimer's disease. *Nature.* 1997;389:603–6.

54. Barger SW, Hörster D, Furukawa K, Goodman Y, Krieglestein J, Mattson MP. Tumor necrosis factors α and β protect neurons against amyloid β-peptide toxicity:

Evidence for involvement of a κB-binding factor and attenuation of peroxide and Ca^{2+} accumulation. *Proc Natl Acad Sci USA*, 1995;92:9328–32.

55. Feuerstein GZ, Liu T, Barone FC. Cytokines, inflammation, and brain injury: role of tumor necrosis factor-alpha. *Cerebr Brain Metab Rev.* 1994;6:341–60.

56. Bruce AJ, Boling W, Kindy MS, Peschon J, Kraemer PJ, Carpenter MK et al. Altered neuronal and microglial responses to excitotoxic and ischemic brain injury in mice lacking TNF receptors. *Nature Med.* 1996;2:788–94.

57. Fiebich BL, Hull M, Lieb K, Gyufko K, Berger M, Bauer J. Prostaglandin E$_2$ induces interleukin-6 synthesis in human astrocytoma cells. *J Neurochem.* 1997;68:704–9.

58. Jiang H, Burdick D, Glabe CG, Cotman CW, Tenner AJ. Beta-amyloid activates complement by binding to a specific region of the collagen-like domain of the C1q A chain. *J Immunol.* 1994;152:5050-9.

59. Velazquez P, Cribbs DH, Poulos TL, Tenner AJ. Aspartate residue seven in beta amyloid protein is critical for classical complement pathway activation: implications for Alzheimer's disease pathogenesis. *Nature Med.* 1997;3:77–9.

60. Rogers J, Civin WH, Styren SD, McGeer PL. Immune-related mechanism of Alzheimer's disease pathogenesis. In: Khachaturian ZS, Blass JB editors. *Alzheimer's disease: New Treatment Strategies*. New York: Marcel Dekker; 1992:147–63.

61. Osaka H, Mukherjee P, Aisen PS, Pasinetti GM. Complement-derived anaphyla-toxin C5a protects against glutamate-mediated neurotoxicity. *J Cell Biochem.* 1999;73:303–11.

62. Mukherjee P, Pasinetti GM. The role of complement anaphylatoxin C5a in neurodegeneration: implications in Alzheimer's disease. *J Neuroimmunol.* 2000;105:124–30.

63. Wingrove JA, DiScipio RG, Chen Z, Potempa J, Travis J, Hugli TE. Activation of complement components C3 and C5 by a cysteine proteinase (gingipain-1) from *Porphyromonas (Bacteroides) gingivalis*. *J Biol Chem.* 1992;267:18902–7.

64. Mattson MP, Barger SW, Furukawa K, Bruce AJ, Wyss-Coray T, Mark RJ et al. Cellular signaling roles of TGF-beta , TNF-alpha and beta-APP in brain injury responses and Alzheimer's disease. *Brain Res Rev.* 1997;23:47–61.

65. Fagarasan MO, Sevilla D, Baruch B, Santoro J, Marin D, Aisen PS. Plasma C3a levels in Alzheimer's disease. *Alzheimer's Res.* 1997;3:137–40.

66. Aisen PS, Davis KL, Berg JD, Campbell K, Thomas RG, Weiner MF et al. A randomized controlled trial of prednisone in Alzheimer's disease. Alzheimer's disease cooperative study. *Neurology* 2000;54:588–93.

67. Rosen WG, Mohs RC, Davis KL. A new rating scale for Alzheimer's disease. *Am J Psych.* 1984;141:1356–64.

68. Morris JC. The Clinical Dementia Rating (CDR): Current version and scoring rules. *Neurology.* 1993;43:2412–4.

69. Overall JE, Gorham DR. Brief Psychiatric Rating Scale. *Psychol Reports.* 1962;10:799–812.

70. Leverenz JB, Wilkinson CW, Wamble M, Corbin S, Grabber JE, Raskind MA et al. Effect of chronic high-dose exogenous cortisol on hippocampal neuronal number in aged nonhuman primates. *J Neurosci.* 1999;19:2356–61.

71. Scharf S, Mander A, Ugoni A, Vajda F, Christophidis N. A double-blind, placebo-controlled trial of diclofenac/misoprostol in Alzheimer's disease. *Neurology.* 1999;53:197–201.

72. DeArmond B, Francisco CA, Lin J-S, Huang FY, Halladay S, Bartziek RD et al. Safety profile of over-the-counter naproxen sodium. *Clin Ther.* 1995;17:587–601.

73. Gecsy M, Peltier L, Wolbach R. Naproxen tolerability in the elderly: A summary report. *J Rheumatol.* 1987;14:348–54.

74. Abdel-Halim MS, Sjoquist B, Anggard E. Inhibition of prostaglandin synthesis in rat brain. *Acta Pharmacol Toxicol.* 1978;43:266–72.

75. Ferrari RA, Ward SJ, Sobre CM, Van Liew DKP, Connell MJ, Haubrich DR. Estimation of the *in vivo* effect of cyclooxygenase inhibitors on prostaglandin E_2 levels in mouse brain. *Eur J Pharmacol.* 1990;179:25–34.

9 | Cyclooxygenase-2 in the kidney

RAYMOND C. HARRIS

Division of Nephrology, Department of Medicine, Vanderbilt University School of Medicine, Nashville, TN 37232, USA.

Prostaglandins (PG) are produced constitutively by many tissues in the body, including brain, gut and kidney, and their synthesis increases at sites of inflammation. Cyclooxygenase (COX), the enzyme responsible for the initial rate-limiting metabolism of arachidonic acid to PGG_2 and subsequently to PGH_2, was first purified from ram seminal vesicles and was cloned in 1988 by DeWitt and Smith[1]. This enzyme has been renamed cyclooxygenase-1 (COX-1) to indicate that it encodes the constitutive enzyme.

The seminal observation of Sir John Vane that COX was the target of aspirin[2] provided confirmation that PGs play myriad roles as local mediators of inflammation and as modulators of physiological functions, such as maintenance of gastric mucosal integrity and modulation of renal microvascular haemodynamics, renin release and tubular salt and water reabsorption[3]. The pharmaceutical industry subsequently developed a substantial number of non-steroid anti-inflammatory drugs (NSAIDs), whose mechanism of action involves competitive or non-competitive inhibition of COX activity. However, by the early 1990s, experimental studies began to suggest that COX-1 might not be the enzyme responsible for increased prostanoid production in inflammatory states. In cultured cells and tissues, COX activity increased rapidly in response to mitogens and cytokines[4-6], although COX-1 mRNA and immuno-reactive protein were not altered. Furthermore, glucocorticoid administration was shown to decrease the rise in COX activity in peritoneal macrophages following lipopolysaccharide (LPS)[7] but not to affect constitutive renal medullary COX activity. These results led Needleman and co-workers to postulate the existence of a second, inflammation-mediated pool of COX activity isoform.

Shortly after the Needleman hypothesis was formulated, Simmons and co-workers detected the presence of a second avian COX mRNA species[8], and

Herschman and co-workers identified a phorbol ester-activated immediate early murine gene (*TIS10*) that possesses similar COX activity but shares only ~66% homology in amino acid sequence[9]. This second COX isoform has subsequently been renamed COX-2, and a vast amount of research has identified it to be derived from an inducible glucocorticoid-sensitive gene that is highly expressed in many tissues in response to inflammatory stimuli. Expression of recombinant enzymes and determination of the crystal structure of COX-2 has provided insights into the observed physiological and pharmacological similarities to, and differences from, COX-1[10,11]. The identification of COX-2 has also led to the development and marketing of both relatively and highly selective COX-2 inhibitors for use as analgesics, antipyretics and anti-inflammatory agents. In addition to its central role in inflammation, aberrantly upregulated COX-2 expression is increasingly implicated in the pathogenesis of a number of epithelial cell carcinomas, including those of the colon, oesophagus, breast and skin and also in Alzheimer's disease and possibly other neurological conditions[12–14].

COX-2 EXPRESSION IN THE KIDNEY

It was initially postulated that the major GI and renal side effects of the original NSAIDs, termed 'non-selective' because of their inhibition of both COX-1 and COX-2, would be avoided by the development of COX-2 selective NSAIDs, since COX-1 was recognized to be abundantly expressed in gastric mucosa and in kidney. However, some COX-2 is expressed in the normal gastric mucosa, and there has now been definitive indication of localized and regulated COX-2 expression in the mammalian kidney. Identification of the pattern of distribution of COX-2 in the kidney has also begun to resolve previous conundrums concerning renal prostanoid physiology.

We initially determined that COX-2 mRNA was present at low but detectable levels in normal adult rat kidney and that immunoreactive COX-2 could be detected in microsomes from cortex and papilla[15]. *In situ* hybridization and immunolocalization demonstrated localized expression of COX-2 mRNA and immunoreactivity in the cells of the macula densa, and adjacent cortical thick ascending limb in adult rat kidney cortex. The immunoreactivity of stained cells was intense, but only one (and rarely two) COX-positive cells were observed per site (Figure 1a). The majority of identified glomeruli sectioned through the juxtaglomerular apparatus did not have COX-2 positive cells in the macula densa. No COX-2 immunoreactivity was detected in arterioles, glomeruli or cortical or medullary collecting ducts.

REGULATION OF COX-2 EXPRESSION IN KIDNEY

Role in renin release

In the mammalian kidney, the macula densa is involved in regulating renin release[16] by sensing alterations in luminal chloride via changes in the rate of $Na^+/K^+/2Cl^-$ cotransport[17]. Inhibition of $Na^+/K^+/2Cl^-$ cotransport with loop diuretics results in a decrease in chloride reabsorption by the macula densa and an increase in renin secretion[18]. It has long been recognized that NSAID administration can elicit a reduction in plasma renin levels, and studies using an isolated perfused juxtaglomerular preparation indicated that NSAID administration prevented the increases in renin release mediated by macula densa sensing of decreases in luminal NaCl[19]. Immunoreactive COX-1 cannot be detected in cortical thick limb or macula densa[15,20]. In our initial studies, we established a high renin level, induced by imposition of a salt deficient diet, and demonstrated that macula densa/cortical thick ascending limb of Henle (cTALH) COX-2 mRNA and immunoreactive protein increased significantly[15].

Harding et al. first demonstrated a direct role for macula densa COX-2 activity in mediating renin production and release by showing that NS398, a selective COX-2 inhibitor, inhibited increases in renal renin expression in response to a low salt diet[21]. Our group has subsequently demonstrated that increases in renin mRNA expression and renal renin activity in response to angiotensin converting enzyme (ACE) inhibition were also blunted by the highly selective COX-2 inhibitor, SC59236[22]. We have further shown that in experimental renovascular hypertension, in which macula densa COX-2 expression is increased (Figure 2)[23,24], COX-2 inhibition blunted increases in renin expression and lowered blood pressure[24]. In addition, our preliminary results have indicated that in COX-2 knockout mice, renal renin activity did not increase in

---

Figure 1 Localization of COX-2 in kidney sections from control and low salt rats. *In situ* hybridization of COX-2 mRNA (a–d). Darkfield photomicrographs demonstrating increased COX-2 message in specific foci within cortex of low salt kidney (b) compared with control (a). At higher magnification (c), the COX-2 mRNA signal in renal cortex of low salt animals can be seen to be concentrated in the region of the macula densa (arrow). Substantial COX-2 mRNA signal is also detectable in the papillary tip (d). Cortex and papilla (pap) are noted. COX-2 immunoreactive protein (e–h). Typical sections of renal cortex show paucity of COX-2 immunoreactivity in either control (e) or low salt (f) rats. Sparse populations of densely stained COX-2-positive cells (arrows) usually are singlets in control renal cortex (e) but are often grouped in low salt (f). At higher magnification (g), clusters of COX-2-positive cells are apparent within the macula densa (1), adjacent to the macula densa (2) and in the cortical thick ascending limb proximal to the macula densa (3). In the tip of the papilla (h), COX-2 is absent from collecting ducts (C) but is localized to cytoplasmic granules and the perinuclear cysternae of interstitial cells. Scale bar in g = 100 μm (reprinted with permission from ref. 15).

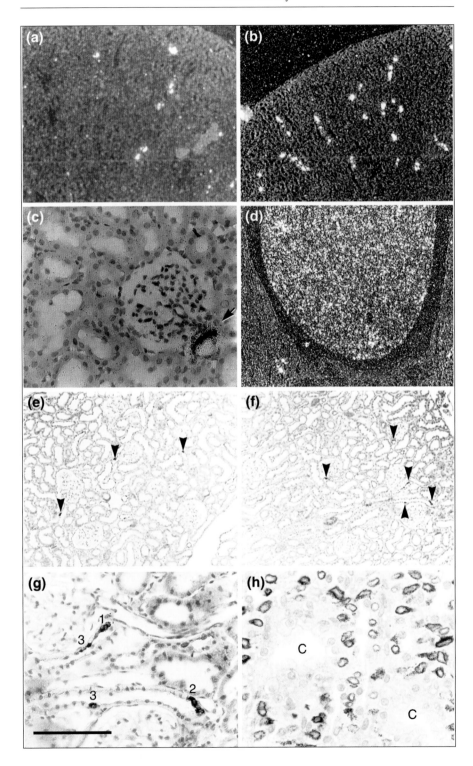

Figure 2 Cyclooxygenase-2 (COX-2) expression in renal cortex following one week of aortic coarctation. Representative experiments of COX-2 mRNA (a) and COX-2 immunoreactive protein (b) are presented. Lanes: 1. sham-operated control; 2. aortic coarctation, right kidney; 3. aortic coarctation, left kidney; 4. aortic coarctation + SC58236, right kidney; 5. aortic coarctation + SC58236, left kidney. In (a), relative expression of GAPDH mRNA expression is provided for comparison. (Reprinted from ref. 24 with permission.)

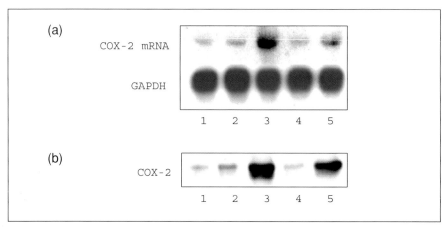

response to ACE inhibition[25]. Direct evidence of a role for COX-2 has recently been provided by Traynor et al., who determined that in an isolated perfused juxtaglomerular preparation, increased renin release in response to lowering the perfusate NaCl concentration was blocked by NS398[26].

Because COX-2 is involved in regulation of renin production and release, we have also examined whether components of the renin–angiotensin system might be involved in mediating expression of macula densa/cTALH COX-2 expression. Administration of either an ACE inhibitor or an angiotensin type 1 (AT_1) receptor antagonist to rats led to increases in cortical COX-2 expression *in vivo* (Figure 1b) and mice that are double nullizygotes for both angiotensin type 1a (AT_{1a}) and type 1b (AT_{1b}) also expressed high levels of COX-2 in the macula densa[25]. In addition, we determined that adrenalectomy increased macula densa/cTALH expression, which was reversed by administration of either glucocorticoids or mineralocorticoids[27]. Furthermore, not only the glucocorticoid receptor (GR) antagonist, RU486, but also the mineralocorticoid receptor (MR) antagonist, spironolactone, increased macula densa/cTALH COX-2, suggesting that MR as well as GR may inhibit basal COX-2 expression[27].

Interactions with the renin–angiotensin system

It is known that renal renin production is modulated by angiotensin II[28,29]. Increased renal tubule reabsorption, mediated directly by angiotensin II and indirectly by aldosterone, will re-establish intravascular volume homeostasis and thereby decrease the stimulus for renin release. In addition, angiotensin II directly inhibits renal renin production and release by a so-called 'short loop feedback inhibition'[29]. Administration of either ACE inhibitors or AT_1 receptor antagonists results in increases in juxtaglomerular renin expression, even in the absence of any detectable alteration in intravascular volume or renal haemodynamics[28,30,31].

It has traditionally been assumed that angiotensin II inhibits renin production by a direct action on the juxtaglomerular (JG) cells[32,33]. However, a recent study by Matsusaka et al. in chimeric mice carrying 'regional' null mutation of the AT_{1a} receptor, the AT_1 receptor subtype exclusively present in mouse JG cells, has questioned whether angiotensin II does act directly on JG cells[34]. In these studies, the JG apparatus (JGA) of $AT_{1a}^{(-/-)}$ receptor mice was markedly enlarged, with intense expression of renin mRNA and protein. In the chimeric mice, the changes in the JGA were proportional to the degree of chimerism, but the degree of JGA hypertrophy/hyperplasia and the expression of renin mRNA and protein were not different in $AT_{1a}^{(+/+)}$ receptor and $AT_{1a}^{(-/-)}$ receptor JG cells. Therefore, the presence or absence of AT_1 receptors on JG cells did not appear to be the determining factor of whether angiotensin II could regulate JGA renin synthesis.

The results of our studies of COX-2 expression suggest an alternative or additional mechanism by which angiotensin II may inhibit renin release. Angiotensin II may act to inhibit cTALH/macula densa COX-2 expression by a direct action and indirectly by increasing aldosterone production, thereby limiting the relative increases in COX-2 expression in response to volume depletion, and thus the ability of the macula densa to signal renin release (Figure 3).

Regulation by nitric oxide

Because of the localization of neuronal nitric oxide synthase (nNOS) to the same regions of the kidney as COX-2 (macula densa and inner medulla), we have examined whether nNOS activity might be involved in mediating increased renal COX-2 expression. Increases in cTALH/macula densa COX-2 expression induced by a low salt diet or low salt diet + ACE inhibition were significantly inhibited by simultaneous administration of the selective nNOS inhibitors, 7-NI or SMTC. In addition, increased papillary COX-2 expression induced by a high salt diet was significantly inhibited by simultaneous 7-NI administration[35].

In primary cultures of immunodissected rabbit cTALH cells, which express immunoreactive nNOS, administration of either cGMP or a nitric oxide (NO) donor increased COX-2 expression, while administration of either non-selective (L-N-methyl arginine methyl ester) or nNOS-selective (7-NI) nitric oxide synthase inhibitors decreased basal COX-2 expression. Basal renal cortical COX-2 was also decreased in response to nNOS inhibition[35]. Therefore, it is

Figure 3 Proposed interactions of COX-2, neuronal nitric oxide synthase (nNOS) and the renin–angiotensin system in macula densa regulation of renin secretion.

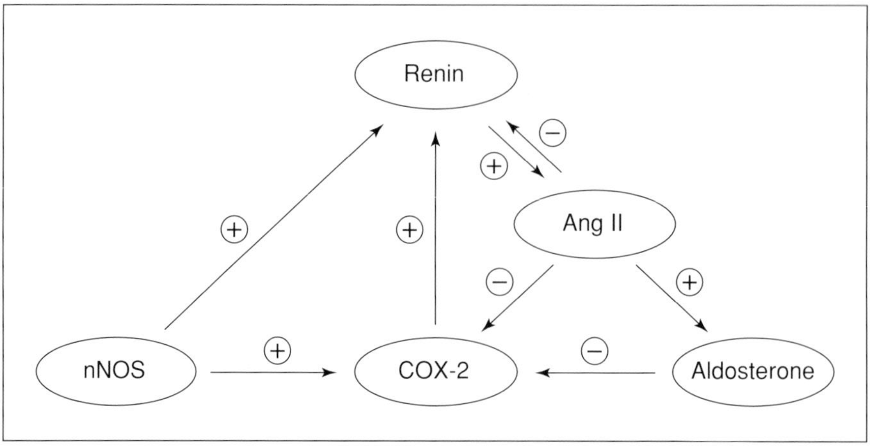

plausible to suggest that NO may be a positive regulator of COX-2 expression under both basal and stimulated conditions.

Although there is experimental evidence that macula densa-derived NO may counteract the vasoconstriction of tubuloglomerular (TG) feedback and also mediate renin release signalled by the macula densa, it has been argued that the short half-life of NO and the long (for NO) potential distance between macula densa cells and the glomerular vascular pole make it less likely that macula densa-derived NO acts directly on renin producing cells, especially in conditions that lead to recruitment of renin-producing cells. Rather, direct effects of NO on JG cells might be expected to be mediated by NO derived from vascular endothelial NOS[36]. Recent studies by Ichihara et al. have suggested that NO-mediated counteraction of TG feedback vasoconstriction is blocked by selective COX-2 specific inhibitors[37].

Regulation of medullary COX-2
In addition to cortical COX-2 expression, localized COX-2 expression was detected in the lipid-laden medullary interstitial cells in the tip of the papilla. The medullary collecting duct expresses abundant COX-1[15,20], and it has been proposed that papillary PGs mediate vasa recta dilatation to maintain medullary blood flow and antagonize vasopressin-mediated water and solute reabsorption[38]. However, in addition to the collecting duct, a subset of medullary interstitial cells has long been recognized to contain abundant arachidonic acid and to be a rich source of PGs[39], although COX-1 expression in these cells was sparse. Medullary COX-2 expression decreases significantly with salt depletion and increases with a high salt diet[40,41] and with water deprivation[42]. COX-2 in cultured medullary interstitial cells increases in response to

extracellular hyperosmolarity and appears to confer protection against hyperosmolarity-induced apoptosis[42,43].

In addition to the medullary interstitial cells, COX-2 has also been implicated in the functioning of the medullary thick ascending limb (MTAL), which metabolizes arachidonic acid (AA) via cytochrome P450- and COX-dependent pathways[44]. Tumour necrosis factor (TNF) and phorbol ester increased COX-2 expression in cultured MTAL cells, and COX-2 inhibitors blocked increases in PGE_2 production by these agents. Expression of COX-2 protein in unstimulated MTAL cells was attenuated by preincubation for 2 h with dexamethasone but did not affect COX-2 expression in cells challenged with either PMA or TNF. Furthermore, time-dependent inhibition of ^{86}Rb uptake by MTAL cells challenged with TNF was diminished if the cells were pretreated with a COX-2 inhibitor, suggesting that induction of COX-2 protein accounted for the lag-time required for this cytokine to inhibit ^{86}Rb uptake in MTAL cells[44].

ROLE OF COX-2 IN KIDNEY DEVELOPMENT

Fetal and early postnatal kidneys possess functional COX activity and are a rich source of PGs[45,46]. Our studies localized COX-2 mRNA and immunoreactive protein in the kidneys of normal rats beginning at E16 and determined that renal COX-2 expression is highly developmentally regulated. During kidney development, immunoreactive COX-2 is first observed in mid-gestation embryonic stages, notably in cells undergoing induction and/or morphogenesis; this form is found in subcapsular epithelial structures in the kidney for the duration of nephrogenesis (through postnatal week two in the rat). The mature intense form of immunoreactive COX-2 appears primarily in functional nephrons as they mature[47]. A similar pattern of COX-2 expression is seen in the developing mouse kidney[48]. In the postnatal kidney, COX-2 expression is relatively low at birth, increases in the first two postnatal weeks, and gradually declines to low levels in normal adult rats[47]. Increased postnatal COX-2 expression was the result of expression at high levels in specific epithelial cells in the cortical segment of Henle's TAL.

This expression pattern of COX-2 in the developing kidney is of interest because of the evidence that COX metabolites play important functional and developmental roles in the fetal kidney. Matson et al. administered the non-specific COX inhibitor, indomethacin, to fetal lambs during the third trimester of gestation. These lambs developed increased renal vascular resistance and decreased fetal renal blood flow, as well as increases in urinary sodium and chloride excretion and decreases in plasma renin activity[49]. In humans an increased incidence of oligohydramnios has been observed in women who chronically consumed significant amounts of aspirin or other COX inhibitors during the third trimester of pregnancy[50]. Since the fetal urine is the source of a significant amount of the amniotic fluid, these studies suggested that inhibition of COX led to the suppression of fetal renal function.

There also is evidence that COX metabolites may mediate normal renal development. Chronic administration of indomethacin to pregnant rhesus monkeys led to renal hypoplasia in the neonates, with kidney mass reduced by 15% compared with control animals[51]. The observed defect was specific for the kidney, since in the treated animals, development of other organs was not affected, except for hepatic hypertrophy. Chronic use of COX inhibitors during human pregnancy has also been related to fetal renal maldevelopment – kidneys from infants who came to term or died in the early postnatal period had few differentiated proximal tubules in the inner cortex and crowding of the glomeruli[52,53]. The outer cortex was more severely affected, with evidence of poorly differentiated glomeruli, undifferentiated tubule epithelia and tubular dilation. In addition, the medullary pyramids were crowded with small immature tubules.

Targeted disruption of murine COX-2 has indicated an important role for this enzyme in renal development[54,55]. At maturity in homozygous COX-2 null mice, the kidneys are small, with fewer developed nephrons than in wild-type kidneys. Undeveloped mesenchymal tissue, immature glomeruli, and dysplastic tubules were present in the outer cortex. Hypoplasia or atrophy of the medulla accompanied by microcystic lesions in the corticomedullary junction was also present in the knockout mice. No apparent developmental or functional abnormalities have been described in mice with targeted disruption of COX-1[56]. Of interest, maternal administration of a selective COX-2 inhibitor to wild-type mice and rats during the fetal and/or perinatal period led to renal lesions similar to those observed in the homozygous COX-2 null mice[48].

EXPRESSION OF COX-2 IN RENAL INJURY

COX metabolites have been implicated in functional and structural alterations in glomerular and tubulointerstitial inflammatory diseases[57-59]. Studies have suggested that prostanoids may also mediate altered renal function and glomerular damage following subtotal renal ablation, and glomerular PG production may be altered in such conditions[60-66]. Following subtotal renal ablation, there were selective increases in renal cortical COX-2 mRNA and immunoreactive protein expression, without significant alterations in COX-1 expression. This increased COX-2 expression was most prominent in the macula densa and surrounding cTALH, the site of expression of cortical COX-2 in the normal rat kidney[67]. In addition, there was detectable COX-2 immunoreactivity in some glomeruli from remnant kidneys, with increased expression in visceral epithelial cells and mesangial cells.

We have determined that administration of the COX-2 selective inhibitor, SC58236, decreased proteinuria and inhibited development of glomerular sclerosis in rats with reduced functioning renal mass. In addition, the COX-2 inhibitor decreased mRNA expression of TGF-β1 and of types III and IV collagen is consistent with an inhibition of thromboxane-mediated responses in the remnant kidney[68]. Whether the effects of COX-2 inhibition were the result of modulation of inflammatory stimuli that may mediate cell injury and alterations in matrix deposition or effects on glomerular haemodynamics will require further study. However, it is of interest that the same degree of hypertension was present in both vehicle-treated and SC58236-treated animals, indicating that the decreases in renal injury were not the result of alterations in systemic blood pressure. Decreases in proteinuria, and preservation of renal structural integrity in passive Heymann nephritis, have also been observed with administration of the relatively selective COX-2 inhibitor, flosulide[69,70]. Since renal COX-2 expression also increases in glomerulonephridities such as lupus nephritis[71], it is possible that COX-2 inhibitors may also alter the natural history of glomerular inflammatory lesions.

EXPRESSION OF COX-2 IN HUMAN KIDNEY

Although published studies have documented a similar pattern of COX-2 expression (macula densa/cTALH and medullary interstitial cells) in the kidney of the mouse, rat, rabbit and dog[15,48,72,73], it was previously controversial whether the human kidney demonstrated the same COX-2 localization. The initial studies of COX-2 localization in human kidney failed to detect COX-2 in either location and instead reported expression in podocytes and arteriolar smooth muscle cells[74]. However, a more recent study in humans > 60 years of age, was able to detect COX-2 in the macula densa and medullary interstitial cells[75] and a preliminary report has also detected increased macula densa COX-2 in patients with congestive heart failure and in Bartter's syndrome[76]. Therefore, it is likely that COX-2 may well play similar physiological roles in the human kidney as has been noted for other mammals.

In summary, COX-2 mRNA and immunoreactive protein are constitutively expressed at high levels in restricted locations in the mammalian kidney, the macula densa and surrounding cTALH, and the medullary interstitial cells. Regulation of expression during development and in a variety of physiological and pathophysiological conditions indicates potentially important roles for COX-2 metabolites in glomerulogenesis, regulation of renal haemodynamics and the renin–angiotensin system.

ACKNOWLEDGEMENTS

This work was supported by the Vanderbilt George O'Brien Kidney and Urologic Diseases Center (National Institutes of Health Grant DK 39261) and by funds from the Department of Veterans Affairs.

Address all correspondence to: R.C. Harris MD, Division of Nephrology, S 3223 MCN, Vanderbilt University School of Medicine, Nashville, TN 37232, USA.

REFERENCES

1. DeWitt DL, Smith WL. Primary structure of prostaglandin G/H synthase from sheep vesicular gland determined from the complementary DNA sequence. *Proc Natl Acad Sci USA.* 1988;85:1412–16.

2. Vane JR. Inhibition of prostaglandin synthesis as a mechanism of action for aspirin-like drugs. *Nat New Biol.* 1971;231:232–5.

3. Needleman P, Turk J, Jakschik BA, Morrison AR, Lefkowith JB. Arachidonic acid metabolism. *Annu Rev Biochem.* 1986;55:69–102.

4. Habenicht AJ, Goerig M, Grulich J, Rothe D, Gronwald R, Loth U et al. Human platelet-derived growth factor stimulates prostaglandin synthesis by activation and by rapid *de novo* synthesis of cyclooxygenase. *J Clin Invest.* 1985;75:1381–7.

5. Raz A, Wyche A, Siegel N, Needleman P. Regulation of fibroblast cyclooxygenase synthesis by interleukin-1. *J Biol Chem.* 1988;263:3022–8.

6. Harris RC, Badr KF. Recovery of prostaglandin synthesis in rat glomerular mesangial cells after aspirin inhibition: induction of cyclooxygenase activity by serum and epidermal growth factor. *Prostaglandins.* 1990;39:213–22.

7. Masferrer JL, Zweifel BS, Seibert K, Needleman P. Selective regulation of cellular cyclooxygenase by dexamethasone and endotoxin in mice. *J Clin Invest.* 1990;86:1375–9.

8. Xie W, Chipman, JG, Robertson DL, Erikson RL, Simmons DL. Expression of a mitogen-responsive gene encoding prostaglandin synthase is regulated by mRNA splicing. *Proc Natl Acad Sci USA.* 1991;88:2692–6.

9. Kujubu DA, Fletcher BS, Varnum BC, Lim RW, Herschman HR. TIS 10, a phorbol ester tumor promoter-inducible mRNA from Swiss 3T3 cells, encodes a novel prostaglandin synthase/cyclooxygenase homolog. *J Biol Chem.* 1991;266:12866–72.

10. Luong C, Miller A, Barnett J, Chow J, Ramesha C, Browner MF. Flexibility of the NSAID binding site in the structure of human cyclooxygenase-2. *Nat Struct Biol.* 1996;3:927–33.

11. Marnett LJ, Rowlinson SW, Goodwin DC, Kalgutkar AS, Lanzo CA. Arachidonic acid oxygenation by COX-1 and COX-2. Mechanisms of catalysis and inhibition. *J Biol Chem.* 1999;274:22903–6.

12. Fosslien E. Molecular pathology of cyclooxygenase-2 in neoplasia. *Ann Clin Lab Sci.* 2000;30:3–21.

13. Lipsky PE. Specific COX-2 inhibitors in arthritis, oncology, and beyond: where is the science headed? *J Rheumatol.* 1999;26(Suppl.56):25–30.

14. Smalley WE, DuBois RN. Colorectal cancer and nonsteroidal anti-inflammatory drugs. *Adv Pharmacol.* 1997;39:1–20.

15. Harris RC, McKanna JA, Akai Y, Jacobson HR, Dubois RN, Breyer MD. Cyclooxygenase-2 is associated with the macula densa of rat kidney and increases with salt restriction. *J Clin Invest.* 1994;94:2504–10.

16. Persson AEG, Salomonsson M, Westerlund P, Greger R, Schlatter E, Gonzalez E. Macula densa function. *Kidney Int.* 1991;32:S39–44.

17. Schlatter E, Salomonsson M, Persson AEG, Greger R. Macula densa cells sense

luminal NaCl concentration via furosemide sensitive $Na^+2Cl^-(K^+$ cotransport. *Pflügers Arch.* 1989;414:286–90.

18. Martinez-Maldonado M, Gely R, Tapia E, Benabe JE. Role of macula densa in diuretics-induced renin release. *Hypertension.* 1990;16:261–8.

19. Greenberg SG, Lorenz JN, He XR, Schnermann JB, Briggs JP. Effect of prostaglandin synthesis inhibition on macula densa-stimulated renin secretion. *Am J Physiol.* 1993;265:F578–83.

20. Smith WL, Bell TG. Immunohistochemical localization of the prostaglandin-forming cyclooxygenase in renal cortex. *Am J Physiol.* 1978;235:F451–7.

21. Harding P, Sigmon DH, Alfie ME, Huang PL, Fishman MC, Beierwaltes WH et al. Cyclooxygenase-2 mediates increased renal renin content induced by low-sodium diet. *Hypertension.* 1997;29:297–302.

22. Cheng HF, Wang JL, Zhang MZ, Miyazaki Y, Ichikawa I, McKanna JA et al. Angiotensin II attenuates renal cortical cyclooxygenase-2 expression. *J Clin Invest.* 1999;103:953–61.

23. Hartner A, Goppelt-Struebe M, Hilgers KF. Coordinate expression of cyclooxygenase-2 and renin in the rat kidney in renovascular hypertension. *Hypertension.* 1998;31:201–5.

24. Wang JL, Cheng HF, Harris RC. Cyclooxygenase-2 inhibition decreases renin content and lowers blood pressure in a model of renovascular hypertension. *Hypertension.* 1999;34:96–101.

25. Cheng H-F, Wang J-L, Wang S-W, McKanna JA, Harris RC. Angiotensin converting enzyme inhibitor-mediated increases in renal renin expression are not seen in cyclooxygenase-2 knockout mice. *J Am Soc Nephrol.* 1999;10:343A.

26. Traynor TR, Smart A, Briggs JP, Schnermann J. Inhibition of macula densa-stimulated renin secretion by pharmacological blockade of cyclooxygenase-2. *Am J Physiol.* 1999;277:F706–10.

27. Zhang MZ, Harris RC, McKanna JA. Regulation of cyclooxygenase-2 (COX-2) in rat renal cortex by adrenal glucocorticoids and mineralocorticoids. *Proc Natl Acad Sci USA.* 1999;96:15280–5.

28. Hackenthal E, Paul M, Ganten D, Taugner R. Morphology, physiology, and molecular biology of renin secretion. *Physiol Rev.* 1990;70:1067–116.

29. Shricker K, Holmer S, Kramer BK, Riegger GA, Kurtz A. The role of angiotensin II in the feedback control of renin gene expression. *Pflügers Archiv.* 1997;434:166–72.

30. Gomez RA, Chevalier RL, Everett AD, Elwood JP, Peach MJ, Lynch KR et al. Recruitment of renin gene-expressing cells in adult rat kidneys. *Am J Physiol.* 1990;259:F660–5.

31. Campbell DJ, Lawrence AC, Towrie A, Kladis A, Valentijn AJ. Differential regulation of angiotensin peptide levels in plasma and kidney of the rat. *Hypertension.* 1991;18:763–73.

32. Johns DW, Peach MJ, Gomez RA, Inagami T, Carey RM. Angiotensin II regulates renin gene expression. *Am J Physiol.* 1990;259:F882–7.

33. Inagami T, Mizuno K, Kawamura M, Okamura T, Clemens DL, Higashimori K. Localization of components of the renin–angiotensin system within the kidney and sustained release of angiotensins from isolated and perfused kidney. *Tohoku J Exper Med.* 1992;166:17–26.

34. Matsusaka T, Nishimura H, Utsunomiya H, Kakuchi J, Nümrua F, Imagami T et al. Chimeric mice carrying 'regional' targeted deletion of the angiotensin type 1A

receptor gene. Evidence against the role for local angiotensin in the *in vivo* feedback regulation of renin synthesis in juxtaglomerular cells. *J Clin Invest.* 1996;98:1867–77.

35. Cheng H-F, Wang J-L, Zhang MZ, McKanna JA, Harris RC. Nitric oxide upregulates cyclooxygenase-2 expression in cTALH. *Am J Physiol.* 2000;279:F122–9.

36. Kurtz A, Wagner C. Role of nitric oxide in the control of renin secretion. *Am J Physiol.* 1998;275:F849–62.

37. Ichihara A, Imig JD, Inscho EW, Navar LG. Cyclooxygenase-2 participates in tubular flow-dependent afferent arteriolar tone: interaction with neuronal NOS. *Am J Physiol.* 1998;275:F605–12.

38. Stokes JB. Integrated actions of renal medullary prostaglandins in the control of water excretion. *Am J Physiol.* 1981;240:F471–80.

39. Dunn MJ, Staley RS, Harrison M. Characterization of prostaglandin production in tissue culture of rat renal medullary cells. *Prostaglandins.* 1976;12:37–49.

40. Jensen BL, Kurtz A. Differential regulation of renal cyclooxygenase mRNA by dietary salt intake. *Kidney Int.* 1997;52:1242–9.

41. Yang T, Singh I, Pham H, Sun D, Smart A, Schnermann JB et al. Regulation of cyclooxygenase expression in the kidney by dietary salt intake. *Am J Physiol.* 1998;274:F481–9.

42. Yang T, Schnermann JB, Briggs JP. Regulation of cyclooxygenase-2 expression in renal medulla by tonicity *in vivo* and *in vitro*. *Am J Physiol.* 1999;277:F1–9.

43. Hao CM, Komhoff M, Guan Y, Redha R, Breyer MD. Selective targeting of cyclooxygenase-2 reveals its role in renal medullary interstitial cell survival. *Am J Physiol.* 1999;277:F352–9.

44. Ferreri NR, An SJ, McGiff JC. Cyclooxygenase-2 expression and function in the medullary thick ascending limb. *Am J Physiol.* 1999;277:F360–8.

45. Day NA, Attallah AA, Lee JB. Letter: Presence of prostaglandin A and F in fetal kidney. *Prostaglandins.* 1974;5:491–3.

46. Moel DI, Cohn RA, Penning J. Renal prostaglandin E2 synthesis and degradation in the developing rat. *Biol Neonate.* 1985;48:292–8.

47. Zhang MZ, Wang JL, Cheng HF, Harris RC, McKanna JA. Cyclooxygenase-2 in rat nephron development. *Am J Physiol.* 1997;273:F994–1002.

48. Komhoff M, Wang JL, Cheng HF, Langenbach R, McKanna JA, Harris RC et al. Cyclooxygenase-2-selective inhibitors impair glomerulogenesis and renal cortical development. *Kidney Int.* 2000;57:414–22.

49. Matson JR, Stokes JB, Robillard JE. Effects of inhibition of prostaglandin synthesis on fetal renal function. *Kidney Int.* 1981;20:621–7.

50. Schoenfeld A, Bar Y, Merlob P, Ovadia Y. NSAIDs: maternal and fetal considerations. *Am J Reprod Immunol.* 1992;28:141–7.

51. Novy MJ. Effects of indomethacin on labor, fetal oxygenation, and fetal development in rhesus monkeys. *Adv Prostaglandin Thromboxane Res.* 1978;4:285–300.

52. Kaplan BS, Restaino I, Raval DS, Gottlieb RP, Bernstein J. Renal failure in the neonate associated with *in utero* exposure to non-steroidal anti-inflammatory agents. *Pediatr Nephrol.* 1994;8:700–4.

53. Voyer LE, Drut R, Mendez JH. Fetal renal maldevelopment with oligohydramnios following maternal use of piroxicam. *Pediatr Nephrol.* 1994;8:592–4.

54. Morham SG, Langenbach R, Loftin CD, Tiano HF, Voloumaos N, Jennette JC et al. Prostaglandin synthase 2 gene disruption causes severe renal pathology in the mouse. *Cell.* 1995;83:473–82.

55. Dinchuk JE, Car BD, Focht RJ, Johnston JJ, Jaffee BD, Covington MB et al. Renal abnormalities and an altered inflammatory response in mice lacking cyclooxygenase II. *Nature.* 1995;378:406–9.

56. Langenbach R, Morham SG, Tiano HF, Loftin CD, Gharnayem BI, Chulada PC et al. Prostaglandin synthase 1 gene disruption in mice reduces arachidonic acid-induced inflammation and indomethacin-induced gastric ulceration. *Cell.* 1995;83:483–92.

57. Feng L, Sun W, Xia Y, Tang WW, Chanmugam P, Soyoola E et al. Cloning two isoforms of rat cyclooxygenase: differential regulation of their expression. *Arch Biochem Biophys.* 1993;307:361–8.

58. Klahr S, Morrissey JJ. The role of growth factors, cytokines, and vasoactive compounds in obstructive nephropathy. *Semin Nephrol.* 1998;18:622–32.

59. Takahashi K, Schreiner GF, Yamashita K, Christman BW, Blair I, Badr KF. Predominant functional roles for thromboxane A_2 and prostaglandin E2 during late nephrotoxic serum glomerulonephritis in the rat. J Clin Invest 1990;85:1974–82.

60. Don BR, Blake S, Hutchison FN, Kayson GA, Schambelan M. Dietary protein intake modulates glomerular eicosanoid production in the rat. *Am J Physiol.* 1989;252:F711–8.

61. Nath KA, Chmielewski DH, Hostetter TH. Regulatory role of prostanoids in glomerular microcirculation of remnant nephrons. *Am J Physiol.* 1987;252:F829–37.

62. Pelayo JC, Shanley PF. Glomerular and tubular adaptive responses to acute nephron loss in the rat. Effect of prostaglandin synthesis inhibition. *J Clin Invest.* 1990;85:1761–9.

63. Schmitz PG, Krupa SM, Lane PH, Reddington JC, Salinas-Madrigal L. Acquired essential fatty acid depletion in the remnant kidney: amelioration with U-63557A. *Kidney Int.* 1994;46:1184–91.

64. Stahl RAK, Kudelka S, Paravicini M, Schollmeyer P. Prostaglandin and thromboxane formation in glomeruli from rats with reduced renal mass. *Nephron.* 1986;42:242–57.

65. Stahl RAK, Kudelka S, Helmchen U. High protein intake stimulates glomerular prostaglandin formation in remnant kidneys. *Am J Physiol.* 1987;252:F1083–94.

66. Stahl RA, Thaiss F, Wenzel U, Schoeppe W, Helmchen U. A rat model of progressive chronic glomerular sclerosis: the role of thromboxane inhibition. *J Am Soc Nephrol.* 1992;2:1568–77.

67. Wang J-L, Cheng H-F, Zhang M-Z, McKanna JA, Harris RC. Selective increase of cyclooxygenase-2 expression in a model of renal ablation. *Am J Physiol.* 1998;275:F613–22.

68. Wang J-L, Cheng H-F, Shappell S, Harris RC. A selective cyclooxygenase-2 inhibitor, decreases proteinuria and retards progressive renal injury in rats. *Kidney Int.* 2000;57:2334–42.

69. Blume C, Heise G, Muhlfeld A, Bach D, Schror A, Gerhardz CD et al. Effect of flosulide, a selective cyclooxygenase 2 inhibitor, on passive Heymann nephritis in the rat. *Kidney Int.* 1999;56:1770–8.

70. Heise G, Grabensee B, Schror K, Heering P. Different actions of the cyclooxygenase 2 selective inhibitor flosulide in rats with passive Heymann nephritis. *Nephron.* 1998;80:220–6.

71. Tomasoni S, Noris M, Zappella S, Gotti E, Casiraghi F, Bonazzola S et al. Upregulation of renal and systemic cyclooxygenase-2 in patients with active lupus nephritis. *J Am Soc Nephrol.* 1998;9:1202–12.

72. Guan Y, Chang M, Cho W, Zhang Y, Redha R, Davis L et al. Cloning, expression, and regulation of rabbit cyclooxygenase-2 in renal medullary interstitial cells. *Am J Physiol.* 1997;273:F18–26.

73. Khan KN, Venturini CM, Bunch RT, Brassard JA, Koki AT, Morris DL et al. Interspecies differences in renal localization of cyclooxygenase isoforms: implications in nonsteroidal antiinflammatory drug-related nephrotoxicity. *Toxicol Pathol.* 1998;26:612–20.

74. Komhoff M, Grone HJ, Klein T, Seyberth HW, Nusing RM. Localization of cyclooxygenase-1 and -2 in adult and fetal human kidney: implication for renal function. *Am J Physiol.* 1997;272:F460–8.

75. Nantel F, Meadows E, Denis D, Connolly B, Metters KM, Giaid A. Immunolocalization of cyclooxygenase-2 in the macula densa of human elderly. *FEBS Lett.* 1999;457:475–7.

76. Komhoff M, Seyberth HW, Nusing RM, Breyer MD. Cyclooxygenase-2 expression is associated with the macula densa in kidneys from patients with Bartter like syndrome. *J Am Soc Nephrol.* 1999;10:437A.

10 | Apoptosis induced with non-steroid anti-inflammatory drugs

DANIEL L. SIMMONS AND JOEL E. WILSON

Department of Chemistry and Biochemistry, Brigham Young University, Provo, Utah, USA.

APOPTOSIS IN HOMEOSTASIS OF ANIMAL DEVELOPMENT

Apoptosis plays an important role both in development and in homeostasis of metazoans. Apoptosis is a form of cell death that removes infected, mutated, damaged or unneeded cells from an organism. During animal development, apoptosis plays a major role in removing unwanted cells. Apoptosis functions to: (1) control cell numbers by removing surplus cells; (2) sculpt structures by deleting unneeded cells; and (3) remove infected, mutated or damaged cells[1]. Apoptotic events include DNA fragmentation, chromatin condensation, membrane blebbing, cell shrinkage and disassembly into membrane-enclosed vesicles, known as apoptotic bodies.

In humans about 100 000 cells are produced every second by mitosis, and a similar number undergo apoptosis during the same time period[2]. Without these homeostatic mechanisms of apoptosis, organisms die early in development due to an excess of cells. For example, mice in which CPP3 (caspase-3) has been deleted by homologous recombination die within 1–3 weeks of birth, with a vast excess of cells in their central nervous system as a result of decreased apoptosis[3]. Developmentally, the formation of digits in higher vertebrates is an example of apoptosis serving to sculpt structures by removal of the unnecessary cells between developing digits. The tail of a tadpole is removed by apoptosis during frog development. In many organs, cells are over-produced and then selected through apoptosis. For example, in vertebrates, neurons are produced in excess, and up to half are eliminated by apoptosis. The neurons are thought to compete for survival signals secreted by their target cells, and those cells that do not receive enough signal undergo

221

apoptosis. This mechanism helps to match appropriately the number of neurons with the target cells they innervate, as well as to delete neurons that are inappropriately connected. Similar examples exist in other tissues to ensure that cells only survive when they are needed[1].

Cells that are non-functional or harmful are also removed by apoptosis. Damaged cells are removed by various mechanisms, including one mediated by the p53 tumour-suppressor protein (discussed below). Nuclear DNA is cleaved at the linker regions between nucleosomes, producing DNA fragments of 180–200 base pairs. The cleavage of DNA in the apoptotic process serves to protect the transfer of damaged DNA to nearby cells, which engulf the genetic material[4].

APOPTOSIS IN THE GASTROINTESTINAL TRACT

The epithelium of the gastrointestinal (GI) tract is an area of massive cellular proliferation and cycling, as the lining of the tract is replaced every 2–3 days in mammals. These tissues maintain homeostasis through apoptosis of both the epithelium and the immediate subepithelial fibroblast layer[5]. Apoptosis occurs in both proliferative and non-proliferative tissue layers of the mammalian GI tract. Apoptosis in the GI epithelium is not uniform and occurs with increasing frequency as cells migrate from the proliferative to non-proliferative zones of crypts[5]. The clearance of apoptotic bodies appears to be accomplished through engulfment by neighbouring epithelial cells, although macrophages may be involved at the subepithelial level.

The inhibition of apoptosis in the GI tract is a major component of the genesis of colorectal adenomas and carcinomas[6]. This inhibition may contribute to tumour growth, clonal evolution, and acquired resistance to chemotherapeutic agents. In normal colonic crypts, the expression of the anti-apoptotic *Bcl-2* is restricted to the proliferative zone at the base and lower third of the crypt epithelial column. *Bcl-2* expression is lost as cells differentiate and migrate toward the luminal surface, which contributes to the increasing frequency of apoptosis at the distal end of villi. In primary human colorectal tumours, *Bcl-2* expression is frequently dysregulated[6]. In addition, the tumour-suppressor protein p53 is commonly mutated in colorectal cancers.

APOPTOTIC SIGNALS

In vivo studies reveal that developing vertebrate tissues require signals from other cells to avoid apoptosis. These studies also suggest that many cell deaths result from specific cells not receiving necessary signals. Still, some cell deaths in animals are produced as a response to apoptosis-inducing signals, which can act systemically or locally and override the action of survival signals. An example of systematic induction is amphibian tadpoles at metamorphosis, where an increase in thyroid hormone in the blood induces cells in the tail to undergo apoptosis[1]. The great majority of cell deaths that occur in normal development probably result from a combination of apoptotic-inducing and apoptotic-suppressing signals.

Cell proliferation, differentiation and apoptosis must be properly balanced, for an imbalance in a cell's proliferative or apoptotic machinery results in cancer. For example, increased cell cycling because of c-*Myc* oncogene over-expression and reduced apoptosis expression because of inhibition of the *Bcl-2* oncogene leads to tumorigenesis in mammary glands[7].

The tumour suppressor protein p53 is a transcription factor normally expressed at low levels due to interaction with the Mdm-2 protein. DNA damage may induce phosphorylation of either p53 or Mdm-2. Phosphorylation of p53 or Mdm-2 inhibits the interaction of these proteins, thus increasing the levels of p53 inside the cell. p53 serves to: (1) promote cell cycle arrest at the G_1/S checkpoint; and (2) induce apoptosis. p53-dependent cell-cycle arrest occurs as a result of induction of the cyclin-dependent kinase (CDK) inhibitor p21[7]. For example, γ-irradiation activates p53 to turn on transcription of p21, which, in turn, inhibits CDKs. The inhibition of CDKs limits the phosphorylation of retinoblastoma protein (Rb) and prevents the release of E2F, inhibiting the transition from the G_1 to S phase.

The transcription of *bax*, which in turn promotes apoptosis through the activation of caspases, may also be activated by p53 (see below). Apoptosis can also be induced by p53 independently of transcriptional pathways[8]. Interestingly, p53 is frequently mutated in human cancers, such as human colorectal carcinomas[9]. The absence of functional p53 in these tissues leads to a partial lack of control of the pathways that control cell-cycle arrest and apoptosis, resulting in genomic instability and, consequently, tumour production.

c-*Myc* possesses both mitogenic and pro-apoptotic qualities. The expression of *Myc* is sufficient to drive cells into the cell cycle in the absence of external mitogens; however, *Myc* has also been shown to promote apoptosis in certain circumstances[9]. The precise mechanism by which *Myc* induces apoptosis is unclear, although *Myc* has been shown to trigger apoptosis indirectly through the activation of p53[10]. Dysregulated c-*Myc* expression is frequent in cancer.

The Bcl-2 protein family serves to regulate apoptosis. Anti-apoptotic proteins (Bcl-2, Bcl-X, Bcl-W, A1 and Mcl-1) function to inhibit apoptosis and are regulated by the pro-apoptotic members of the Bcl-2 family (Bax, Bid, Bad and Bim), which can actually stimulate apoptosis[11]. Bad expression is necessary for ceramide-induced apoptosis through a pathway involving kinase suppressor of Ras (KSR)/ceramide-activated protein kinase (CAPK), Ras, Raf-1 and MEK1[12]. Bcl-2-like proteins are present in the outer mitochondrial membrane and have pore-forming domains, allowing them to form ion channels in biological membranes. Bcl-2 is thought to inhibit the release of pro-apoptotic factors from the mitochondria, such as cytochrome c, thereby blocking caspase activation through Apaf-1 and the apoptotic process[13]. Overexpression of *Bcl-2* also prevents apoptosis by downregulating NF-κB activity[14]. NF-κB is a transcription factor whose target genes include: the Fas/Apo-1 ligand, c-*myc*, p53 and IL-1β converting enzyme (ICE).

In addition to the Bcl-2 family, inhibitor of apoptosis proteins (IAP) can regulate apoptosis. In humans, the IAP proteins – XIAP, cIAP1 and cIAP2, survivin, and NAIP – appear to inhibit apoptosis by specifically binding to and inactivating caspases[11].

CASPASE-MEDIATED PROTEIN CLEAVAGE IN APOPTOSIS

Apoptosis is mediated by a family of cysteine proteases termed caspases (cysteine aspartases). There are about a dozen mammalian caspases that exist in cells as inactive zymogens[2]. Caspases are specific, hydrolysing peptide bonds on the carboxyl side of an aspartate residue. When initiator caspases are cleaved, due to initial apoptotic signals, they become active and can activate other effector caspases, creating a proteolytic cascade. Effector caspases function in cell disassembly.

Caspases cause cell death by degrading critical cell structures such as lamins and gelsolin (a protein that severs actin filaments in a regulated manner). Caspases also cause cell death by activating latent enzymes through proteolysis of their inhibitors[7]. For example, caspase-mediated cleavage of ICAD (inhibitor of caspase-activated DNAase) leads to activation of CAD and, subsequently, degradation of the cell's DNA[2].

Two distinct pathways for activating effector caspases exist. One pathway for activating caspases is through death receptors, as in the CD-95 (Fas/Apo-1) system[11]. CD-95 is part of the tumour necrosis factor receptor (TNFR) family and functions to remove activated T cells following the immune response. The binding of the Fas ligand to the Fas receptor induces trimerization of the receptor. The cytoplasmic region of the trimerized Fas recruits the adapter molecule FADD (Fas-associating protein with death domain; also termed MORT1), which recruits pro-caspase-8 into a multimeric complex termed DISC (death-inducing signal complex). Caspase-8, an initiator caspase, then cleaves other zymogenic caspases, such as caspase-3. Caspase-8 also cleaves Bid, a pro-apoptotic member of the *Bcl-2* family, which amplifies the death signal by triggering cytochrome c release from the mitochondria[11].

Apaf-1 is another molecule that activates caspases in mammals. Apaf-1 can bind to the pro-domain of pro-caspase-9 and activate it in the presence of cytochrome c and dATP in a cell-free system[13]. As cytochrome c is usually located between the inner and outer membranes of the mito-chondria, it has been proposed that the release of cytochrome c from the mitochondria is a crucial step in the initiation of apoptosis. In contrast to the death-receptor-induced apoptosis mentioned above, members of the anti-apoptotic Bcl-2 family can inhibit Apaf-1-mediated activation of caspase-9 (ref. 7).

CHEMOTHERAPEUTIC AGENTS AND APOPTOSIS

Despite the vast array of anticancer drugs in use today, neoplastic cells often develop resistance to these chemotherapeutic agents and continue to prolif-erate, due to high mutation rates and genetic instability. Chemotherapeutic agents can cause tumour regression through induced apoptosis of the tumour cells themselves or through an anti-angiogenic mechanism. Conventional chemotherapy consists of administering high drug doses, followed by a re-covery period to permit the recovery of normal host cells. Chemotherapeutic agents such as 5-fluorouracil (5-FU) are commonly used to treat lung, breast and GI carcinomas. 5-FU, and other chemotherapeutic agents, induce apop-tosis in these cancerous cells by a variety of mechanisms, leading to the regres-sion of tumours. 5-FU is thought to induce expression of the p53 gene, which in turn, induces the expression of p21 and the proapoptotic gene *bax*, result-ing in the induction of apoptosis. Other drugs that operate through a p53-independent mechanism are used to induce apoptosis in p53-mutant tumours.

Folkman and his colleagues[15] have postulated that vascular endothelial cells in the tumour bed might also renew growth during the conventional recovery period. This new vasculature could support the regrowth of tumour cells and contribute to the emergence of drug-resistant tumour cells. Treatment of tumours on a more consistent, anti-angiogenic schedule, however, results in the regression of existing tumours. Folkman and his colleagues[15] demonstrated that the chemotherapeutic agent cyclophosphamide also has anti-angiogenic properties. Cyclophosphamide induced the apoptosis of endothelial cells within tumours, which preceded the apoptosis of the tumour cells themselves, even in previously demonstrated drug-resistant tumours. Folkman's results also suggest that the apoptosis of drug-resistant tumour cells most likely resulted from endothelial cell growth suppression and not direct killing of the cells. Tumour regrowth after 13 days, evident in conventional treatment, was prevented by treatment on a consistent, low-level cyclophosphamide schedule, which resulted in sustained inhibition of angiogenesis within the tumour bed. Moreover, combining cyclophosphamide with another angio-genesis inhibitor, TNP-470, resulted in the eradication of drug-resistant Lewis lung carcinomas. These results suggest that chemotherapeutic agents such as cyclophosphamide and other drugs, including NSAIDs, may be used to retard tumour growth and/or eradicate tumours by causing apoptosis in the developing vascular endothelial cells.

SULINDAC, AN NSAID INDUCER OF APOPTOSIS AND TUMOUR REGRESSION

Sulindac (*cis*-5-fluoro-2-methyl-1[*p*-(methylsulphinyl)benzylidene]indene-3-acetic acid) was first introduced as a potentially safe NSAID in 1973 under the brand name Clinoril[®16]. At that time, it was proposed that sulindac was safer than other NSAIDs, based on its property as a prodrug that required metabolic activation *in vivo* to its anti-inflammatory form. Unfortunately, like many NSAIDs introduced during this period, the increased safety hoped for was not fully realized because the active metabolite of sulindac, sulindac sulphide, inhibits both COX-1 and COX-2. In addition to its anti-inflammatory activity, sulindac has been shown to exhibit clear antineoplastic activity against polyps of the colon, where it also induces apoptosis. Sulindac constitutes the best-studied NSAID with regard to the reduction of tumours in humans, as well as with regard to the induction of apoptosis in tumour cells. Thus, sulindac is currently the best model compound for understanding the antineoplastic activity of NSAIDs.

CHEMICAL PROPERTIES OF SULINDAC AND ITS METABOLITES

Sulindac (Figure 1) is an amphipathic molecule of the indene class. It is given orally but can also be administered topically, intravenously and as a suppository. Its uptake is reported to be inhibited by food, but, otherwise, approximately 90% of the orally administered drug is absorbed[17]. Sulindac sulphide, the COX-inhibitory metabolite of sulindac, is significantly more lipophilic than sulindac and is 100 times less soluble in water[17]. Once systemically absorbed, sulindac binds avidly to blood serum albumin[17–19]. More than 95% of sulindac and its major metabolites sulindac sulphide and sulindac sulphone are protein-bound in the blood. However, sulindac sulphide binds with greater affinity to blood proteins than does sulindac[19]. Peak plasma concentrations in young, healthy adults given sulindac (400 mg once a day for 7 days) were 26 μM (sulindac), 17 μM (sulindac sulphide) and 6 μM (sulindac sulphone)[17]. Elderly patients may exhibit approximately twice the plasma concentrations of young adults[20]. Half-lives for sulindac and its metabolites have been reported as: 1.7–7 h (sulindac); 15.3–16.4 h (sulindac sulphide) and 16.6–19.6 h (sulindac sulphone)[17].

Bioactivation of sulindac requires reductive metabolism to sulindac sulphide by intestinal flora of the large bowel or by microsomal enzymes of the liver and kidney[21–23]. Both aerobic and anaerobic bacteria in the bowel

Figure 1 The metabolic fates of sulindac in mammals. Sulindac, a sulphoxide, is reduced to sulindac sulphide by flora in the large bowel, as well as by renal and hepatic enzymes. It is also oxidatively metabolized to sulindac sulphone by the same organs. The sulphide potently inhibits COX-1 and COX-2, whereas sulindac or sulindac sulphone are essentially inactive at inhibiting COX enzymes at physiological concentrations. IC$_{50}$ values are from Warner[24].

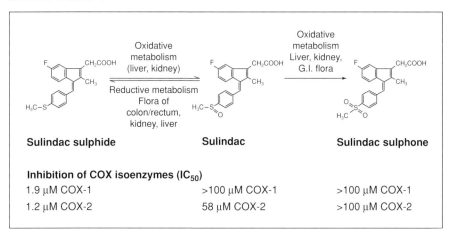

Oxidative metabolism (liver, kidney)

Reductive metabolism Flora of colon/rectum, kidney, liver

Oxidative metabolism Liver, kidney, G.I. flora

Sulindac sulphide   **Sulindac**   **Sulindac sulphone**

Inhibition of COX isoenzymes (IC$_{50}$)
1.9 µM COX-1   >100 µM COX-1   >100 µM COX-1
1.2 µM COX-2   58 µM COX-2   >100 µM COX-2

function in reducing the sulphoxide of sulindac to the sulphide (Figure 1). The importance of colon/rectum flora in the conversion of sulindac to sulindac sulphide in humans is underscored by the fact that patients who have experienced total colectomy have markedly reduced plasma levels of sulindac sulphide[23]. Hence, sulindac is in dynamic equilibrium with sulindac sulphide as intestinal flora and kidney/liver enzymes interconvert sulindac to sulindac sulphide and back again to the sulphoxide (Figure 1).

Sulindac sulphide is a potent inhibitor of COX-1 and COX-2[24] in humans and other organisms (Figure 1). By virtue of this activity, it is also a potent anti-inflammatory agent[25]. Sulindac, in contrast, inhibits COX-1 and COX-2 only at concentrations that are greater than 50 µM (Figure 1). In addition to sulindac's reductive metabolism to the sulphide, sulindac is also oxidatively metabolized to sulindac sulphone in the liver, colon, and kidney[26]. Like sulindac, sulindac sulphone inhibits COX-1 and COX-2, only at very high, non-physiological concentrations in the millimolar range.

From a chemical standpoint, sulphones are difficult to reduce. They can be chemically reduced in a test tube using potent reducing agents such as LiAlH$_4$, in which case the majority of sulphone molecules are reduced completely to the sulphide, rather than to the intermediate sulphoxide[27,28]. It is not known whether this difficult reduction can occur *in vivo*. Because of the known difficulty of reducing sulphones, the oxidation of sulindac to sulindac sulphone *in vivo* is generally thought to be an irreversible reaction (Figure 1).

SULINDAC AS AN ANTI-TUMORIGENIC AGENT

The prodrug property of sulindac does not eliminate the significant gastropathy typical of NSAIDs that inhibit both COX-1 and COX-2. Prodrugs still cause ulceration of the stomach and intestines through delivery of the drug via the vasculature, and not through topical exposure on the mucosal surface of the gut (see Whittle, Chapter 15). Nevertheless, the reported efficacy of sulindac as a potent anti-inflammatory agent with potentially lower side effects led Waddell and Loughry[29] in 1983 to administer sulindac chronically to four patients with Gardner's syndrome, a form of familial adenomatosis polyposis (FAP). Prior to treatment these patients exhibited colorectal polyps and one patient had dermal desmoid growths. The rationale for treatment with sulindac was that a beneficial effect of indomethacin had been observed in reducing desmoid growth. However, chronic sulindac treatment (150–300 mg day^{-1} for up to 2 years) produced the unexpected result of almost complete disappearance (70–100%) of the colorectal polyps in all patients treated[29]. Gastric polyps and ileal hyperplastic nodules were unaffected. Since this seminal observation, numerous investigators have reported success in both decreasing growth of colorectal polyps (chemoprevention) as well as inducing the disappearance of pre-existing polyps (tumour regression). Most of these studies have used FAP patients who have previously experienced colectomy and ileorectal anastomosis. The tumours arising in these patients occur primarily in the rectum and in the periampullary region of the small intestine. Chemoprevention and/or tumour regression has been observed frequently for rectal adenomas in FAP patients, but less frequently for periampullary tumours of the small intestine[30]. The reason for this regional effect may reflect greater exposure to drug, either through higher concentration or more prolonged contact, or to yet undefined regional cell/tissue differences that govern susceptibility to sulindac treatment. In addition to studies of FAP patients, a small number of studies have investigated the effect of sulindac on sporadic adenomas of the colon/rectum, with contradictory conclusions as to whether sulindac is efficacious in tumour regression and chemoprevention of sporadic tumours[31,32].

In one of the first double-blind, randomized, placebo-controlled studies of sulindac, Giardello[33] investigated 22 patients with FAP, including 18 without prior colectomy. Patients were given sulindac (300 mg day^{-1}) for 9 months and were endoscoped at 3, 6 and 9 months. A statistically significant reduction in colorectal polyps was observed by 3 months. After 9 months treated patients exhibited a 56% decrease in polyp number and a 65% decrease in polyp size relative to placebo controls. Following cessation of treatment, regrowth of polyps was observed. The finding of colorectal polyp reduction by 60–100% as a result of sulindac treatment is typical of the many small studies that have been performed on this drug since the initial study of Waddell and Loughry[29].

Present data also support the concept that the effect of sulindac is not permanent and that growth of tumours will recur upon removal of the drug.

THE CELLULAR EFFECTS OF SULINDAC

Nugent et al.[34] reported a randomized controlled trial of sulindac in 24 FAP patients in which bromodeoxyuridine labelling showed a statistically significant decrease in cell proliferation in the intestinal mucosa of sulindac-treated patients. However, similar experiments using tritiated thymidine labelling failed to show a difference in cell proliferation, as did ki67 (a proliferation-associated antigen) labelling[35,36]. Using cell cytometry to assess both changes in cell cycle distribution and apoptosis, Giardello and colleagues[37] failed to detect a significant change in cytokinetic variables or cell-cycle distribution in patients treated for 3 months with sulindac (150 mg day^{-1}). However, the sub-diploid apoptotic fraction was significantly increased from 10% to 31%, suggesting that induction of apoptosis was an important part of the anti-proliferative effect of sulindac.

Induction of apoptosis is consistent with the ability of sulindac to induce tumour regression, where, by definition, cell death and cell removal, the hallmarks of apoptosis, must occur. Current data are insufficient to support the claim that induction of apoptosis by NSAIDs is the sole mechanism by which tumour regression or chemoprevention occurs, since it is clear that changes in cyclooxygenase expression, both overexpression and inhibition, can dramatically influence the cell cycle in cells of various origin[38,39].

Numerous studies have now evaluated sulindac and its metabolites in rodents and in cell lines explanted from human tumours[40-45]. Sulindac is effective at inhibiting intestinal tumorigenesis in rodents treated with azoxymethane[43] or in mice heterozygous for a null mutation of the adenomatous polyposis coli (APC) gene[46-48]. In the latter murine model for intestinal polyposis, aggressive sulindac treatment (1.6 mg [in humans the equivalent of approximately 3 g on a weight : weight basis] day^{-1} for 11 weeks) produced up to a 96% decrease in polyp number.

When used in tissue culture, sulindac is a weak inducer of apoptosis and typically requires levels approaching millimolar concentrations to be effective. Thus, a metabolite of sulindac, rather than the parent compound, is most likely to be the effector of apoptosis both *in vitro* and *in vivo*.

SULINDAC METABOLITES: SULINDAC SULPHIDE VERSUS SULINDAC SULPHONE AS ANTINEOPLASTIC AGENTS

The work of Piazza and colleagues[49] has shown unequivocally that both metabolites of sulindac, the COX-active sulphide and the COX-inactive sulphone, have antineoplastic activity in laboratory animals and in cultured neoplastic cells. Moreover, both appear to be chemopreventive agents in humans. Sulindac sulphide and sulindac sulphone both inhibit azoxymethane-induced tumorigenesis in rodents[43,49]. From a clinical standpoint this finding is important since the sulphide, a COX-1/COX-2 inhibitor, is ulcerogenic, whereas sulindac sulphone is non-ulcerogenic. However, Reddy and colleagues[43] have demonstrated that sulindac sulphone is only effective when given during the initiation stage of azoxymethane-induced tumorigenesis. In contrast, sulindac sulphide inhibits tumours when given at all stages of azoxymethane-induced tumorigenesis, including late stages of adenoma progression. Additionally, sulindac, via its sulphide metabolite, causes intestinal tumour regression in APC mutant mice, whereas the sulphone is ineffective in reducing polyps in this model[47,48]. Hence, the antineoplastic mechanisms of sulindac sulphide and sulindac sulphone appear to be separable and distinct.

In tissue culture, the sulphide, not the sulphone, is invariably the more potent sulindac metabolite at inducing apoptosis or inhibiting cell growth. The difference in potency between the two compounds can be tenfold or more. In fact, in some cells, such as transformed murine fibroblasts, the sulphone actually stimulates cell growth rather than inhibiting it (unpublished data). Differences in dose needed to inhibit cell/tumour growth, combined with the ability of the sulphide to induce apoptosis in cells where the sulphone is ineffective is consistent with the concept that the antineoplastic activities of the two sulindac metabolites are not identical.

Because the ulcerogenic sulindac sulphide metabolite has not been tested extensively in humans, little data exist to support the conclusion that the sulphide is solely responsible for the chemopreventive/tumour regressive properties of sulindac. That the sulphide metabolite is important to the anti-tumour effect of sulindac is supported by animal studies. In these experiments either sulindac, which the animal metabolizes to the sulphide and sulphone, or sulindac sulphide is significantly more potent than sulindac sulphone in inhibiting growth of tumours[42,43,47-49]. Recently, a randomized, double-blind, placebo-controlled clinical study showed that chronic administration of sulindac sulphone (200 mg b.i.d. for 6 months) failed to show a reduction in colorectal polyps in patients with FAP[50,51]. Higher doses (300 and 400 mg b.i.d.) caused a stabilization in polyp number and produced partial regression in some small polyps, although significant liver toxicity was observed at the 400 mg dose. The anti-tumour effect observed is significantly less than that seen in studies of Giardello[37] and others using smaller doses of sulindac. More recently, sulindac at 150 mg q.i.d. for 18 months produced a 53% reduction in polyp number[52]. As described above, this effect is assumed not to be due to conversion of the sulphone to the sulphide through two metabolic reduction events because of the difficulty of reducing sulphones. One study in rats failed to find sulindac sulphide in the caecal contents of rats fed high levels (1000–2000 p.p.m.) sulindac sulphone[49]. However, these same animals exhibited 82% inhibition of azoxymethane-induced tumorigenesis by sulindac sulphone treatment.

The finding that a COX-inactive metabolite exhibits some of the anti-neoplastic properties of sulindac has raised significant questions regarding the mechanism of sulindac-induced apoptosis and the role that inhibition of COX-1 or COX-2 plays in that process.

PROPOSED BIOCHEMICAL MECHANISMS FOR SULINDAC-INDUCED TUMOUR REGRESSION AND APOPTOSIS

Multiple biochemical mechanisms for sulindac-induced apoptosis have been described and are illustrated in Figure 2. Each is summarized below in the order in which they were first proposed.

Inhibition of prostaglandin synthesis

Waddell[53,54] first proposed a mechanism to explain his initial observation of the antineoplastic activity of sulindac. He noted high prostaglandin E_2 (PGE_2) content in colon polyps and malignant tumours and suggested that chronic high concentrations of PGE_2 could result in desensitization and downregulation of specific PG receptors. This, in turn, could result in inactivation of PG receptor-coupled adenylate cyclase, with a concomitant decline in cAMP[54]. Low cAMP was proposed to result in inhibition of protein kinase A, which would mediate alteration of the MAP kinase cascade through regulation of raf-1 kinase and protein tyrosine phosphatases[54]. Sulindac treatment would result in inhibition of PGE_2 synthesis and a restoration of cAMP to normal levels.

Binding to and inhibition of activated *ras* proto-oncogene products

The c-K-*ras* proto-oncogene is mutationally activated at amino acids 12 or 13 in approximately 50% of human colorectal cancers. These activating mutations are seen less frequently in adenomatous polyps. Transfection of an activated human c-K-*ras* gene into a spontaneously immortalized rat intestinal cell line produced cells that demonstrated significant resistance to sulindac sulphide inhibition of cell growth and the induction of apoptosis[55]. However, the mechanism of this resistance to sulindac sulphide was not defined.

In other studies, activated human H-*ras* was transfected into rat embryo fibroblasts and sulindac sulphide was shown to inhibit focus formation of transfected cells[56]. Moreover, sulindac sulphide was demonstrated to inhibit c-*raf* kinase, the downstream binding partner of the c-H-*ras* protein, p21*ras*.

Figure 2 Potential biochemical mechanisms for induction of apoptosis by sulindac and its metabolites. Currently a unified mechanism for NSAID-induced apoptosis does not exist. Eight separate mechanisms by which sulindac, sulindac sulphide and sulindac sulphone cause apoptosis or inhibit cell growth have been proposed and are illustrated. Each is explained in detail in the text. This figure is expanded and modified from ref. 67.

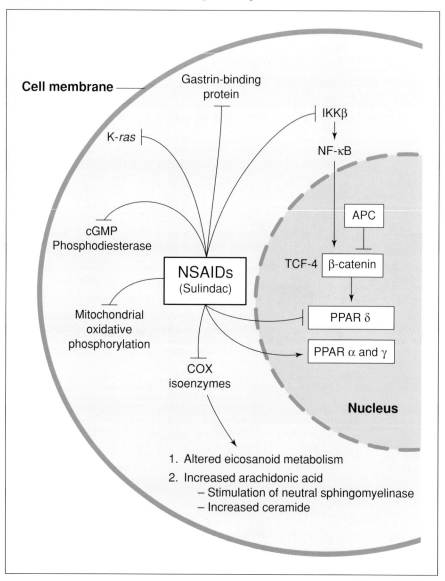

Inhibition of c-*raf* kinase was proposed to occur by direct, reversible interaction of sulindac sulphide with the p21*ras* protein, resulting in its inability to activate c-*raf* kinase. Binding of sulindac sulphide to p21*ras* was reported to result in impairment of this protein's nucleotide exchange as well an acceleration of the protein's GTPase activity by p120GAP. However, concentrations of sulindac needed to affect these changes in p21*ras* activity were high (> 100 μM). Sulindac exhibited only approximately 10–20% of the activity of sulindac sulphide in eliciting these effects. These studies do not explain why sulindac is effective at inhibiting colon polyps in FAP, where activating K-*ras* mutations are uncommon.

Shunting of arachidonic acid to activate ceramide-regulated signal transduction pathways

For many years the effect of inhibiting cyclooxygenases on cellular arachidonic acid pools has been investigated. In theory, inhibition of arachidonic acid metabolizing enzymes such as cyclooxygenases could increase arachidonic acid levels that could activate other arachidonate utilizing enzymes (e.g. lipoxygenases). However, arachidonic acid pools in the cell are poorly understood, and it is unclear how much they are changed by inhibition of COX-1 or COX-2.

Chan et al.[57] proposed that inhibition of COX enzymes by sulindac sulphide in colorectal cell lines HCT116 and SW480 resulted in shunting of arachidonate to activate neutral sphingomyelinase, which metabolizes sphingomyelin to ceramide. Ceramide is a known inducer of apoptosis in some cells[58]. Extracellular addition of high, superphysiological levels (200 μM) of arachidonate to HCT116 and SW480 cells caused increased ceramide levels and apoptosis. Small (two to sixfold) increases in cellular arachidonic acid were also observed following treatment with 125 μM sulindac sulphide and 300 μM indomethacin, which also produced apoptosis.

Binding to and inhibition of IκB kinase β

The transcription factor NF-κB regulates numerous genes in response to a variety of cellular stimuli, including stress and inflammation. It is known to be involved in apoptosis, and mutational disruption of the p65 member of the NF-κB heterodimer results in high levels of hepatic apoptosis. Hence, NF-κB may act as an anti-apoptosis protein in some cells.

In its inactive form, the NF-κB heterodimer is kept sequestered in the cytosol by inhibitor proteins called IκB (α, β and ε). For nuclear translocation of active NF-κB, phosphorylation of specific serines on the N-terminus of IκBβ (IKKβ) occurs, resulting in degradation of the IκB complex and release of active NF-κB. Aspirin and salicylate have been proposed as inhibitors of NF-κB signal transduction, and by this mechanism potentially exert their pharmacological effects[59]. Phosphorylation of IκBβ is carried out by Iκα and Iκβ kinases and this step has been reported to be inhibited by high concentrations of aspirin and salicylate[59]. However, concentrations of aspirin and salicylate needed to be effective in inhibiting NF-κB and IκB kinases were in the 1–10 mM range. In contrast, serum levels in healthy adults given doses of 2 g of aspirin per day were maximally only 600–800 μM[60,61]. Toxic plasma levels of aspirin/salicylate in patients experiencing aspirin/salicylate poisoning are 1.5–2.7 mM[60]. Hence, it is unlikely that this pathway functions at normal, pharmacologically relevant doses of aspirin.

Studies by Yamamoto and colleagues[62] demonstrated that high concentrations of sulindac (1 mM), sulindac sulphone (1 mM) and sulindac sulphide (200 μM) could inhibit NF-κB signal transduction by 75–95%. Moreover, these same concentrations of sulindac and its metabolites inhibited NF-κB translocation and IκB kinase activity in cell extracts and, additionally, inhibited the activity of purified recombinant IκB kinase α. A similar effect was seen with aspirin or salicylate at 5 mM but no effect was seen for indomethacin or ibuprofen at 25 μM. The direct inhibition of IκB kinase α by sulindac led to the conclusion that binding to and inhibition of this enzyme by sulindac and/or its metabolites may be the mechanism by which it exerts its apoptotic effects.

Binding to and inhibition of peroxisome proliferator-activated receptor δ

Peroxisome proliferator-activated receptor (PPAR) receptors are part of the steroid-hormone-receptor family. They are ligand-activated receptors that heterodimerize with retinoid X receptors (RXR) to exert their transcriptional effects by binding to specific direct repeat elements in the 5' controlling regions of genes. Endogenous ligands for PPAR receptors are poorly defined. Eicosanoids (LTB$_4$ and 15-deoxy-$\Delta^{12,14}$-PGJ$_2$, and others) have been proposed as ligands, but at micromolar concentrations that are superphysiological[63,64]. Likewise, NSAIDs such as indomethacin, ibuprofen and fenoprofen bind and activate PPAR receptors α, and γ at concentrations of 100 μM[65,66]. Hence, a wide variety of ligands bind to and activate PPAR receptors at micromolar concentrations, with their commonality being that they are typically amphipathic molecules with a hydrophobic and acetic end.

He and colleagues[67] identified PPARδ as a target of the APC gene. Wild-type APC promotes degradation of β-catenin and thus inhibits the ability of the β-catenin/TCF-4 heterodimer to regulate transcription. The PPARδ gene is a target of the β-catenin/TCF-4 transcription factor and APC mutation in colorectal tumour cells results in upregulation of PPARδ. This, in turn, can result in increased transcription of PPARδ-regulated genes.

By use of a PPARδ reporter construct, He and colleagues demonstrated that sulindac sulphide (100–200 μM) and indomethacin (100–400 μM) inhibited PPARδ activity in HCT116 and SW480 cells. Moreover, over-expression of PPARδ produces nearly a fivefold decrease in apoptosis in HCT116 cells, evoked by treatment with 100 or 125 μM sulindac sulphide.

Unlike PPARα and γ, where NSAIDs appear to bind and activate these receptors, sulindac sulphide (100–300 μM) was found to block binding to its direct repeat of recombinant PPARδ/RXRα heterodimers activated by prostacyclin (10–20 μM). Indomethacin (200–600 μM) and sulindac sulphone (200–600 μM) had a similar but significantly weaker effect. Therefore, induction of apoptosis by sulindac and other NSAIDs was proposed to occur by direct binding to and inhibition of PPARδ[67]. This also would be accompanied by altered eicosanoid metabolism due to inhibition of COX-1 and COX-2.

Uncoupling of oxidative phosphorylation

It has been known for some time that high concentrations (> 50 μM) of indomethacin can result in uncoupling of electron transport in oxidative phosphorylation and release of cytochrome c[68–72]. The same appears to occur with other NSAIDs, including sulindac[68,69]. Such blockage results in production of mitochondrial-initiated apoptosis. However, the precise mechanism by which these drugs uncouple oxidative phosphorylation is unknown. Studies comparing the uncoupler p-nitrophenol with NSAIDs demonstrated that the ability of NSAIDs to cause apoptosis required both uncoupling and COX inhibition[71]. From a structural standpoint, diphenylamine-containing NSAIDs, such as diclofenac and fenamates, have been found to be most potent at uncoupling oxidative phosphorylation[72].

Binding to and inhibition of cGMP phosphodiesterase

Sulindac sulphone (also called exisulind) is in clinical trials under the trade name Aptosyn™[73]. Cell Pathways, the makers of Aptosyn™ state that it is the first of a class of drugs termed 'selective apoptotic antineoplastic drugs' (SAANDs)[73]. Cell Pathways propose that the mechanism of action of Aptosyn is inhibition of cyclic GMP-phosphodiesterase (cGMP-PDE), which is elevated in colon tumour cells[73]. Inhibition of cGMP-PDE results in an increase in cellular cGMP, activation of protein kinase G, decreased β-catenin, and activation of caspases to cause apoptosis. This pathway is independent of Bcl-2, whereas apoptosis induced by other NSAIDs has been shown to be blocked by Bcl-2[74]. This difference is further evidence that the sulindac sulphone-induced pathway of apoptosis is different from the pathway(s) activated by COX-inhibitory NSAIDs.

Binding to and inhibition of 78 kDa gastrin-binding protein

The polypeptide hormone gastrin has a trophic effect in stimulating cells of the GI mucosa[75]. A membrane-bound 78 kDa protein, gastrin-binding protein (GBP) has been reported to bind gastrin and potentially to mediate its effects. GBP binding of endogenous pro-gastrin-derived peptides has been proposed to establish an autocrine growth loop in colorectal carcinomas[76]. Sulindac sulphide and sulindac have been reported to bind GBP with IC_{50} values of 40 μM and 580 μM, respectively. Indomethacin also bound GBP with an IC_{50} value of 150 μM. At 1 mM concentration, sulindac, sulindac sulphide and indomethacin blocked gastrin binding to GBP by 28%, 72% and 55%, respectively. Hence, these drugs would be considered weak antagonists of gastrin binding to GBP.

Sulindac-induced apoptosis: *Bcl-2*, p53, *c-Myc*, caspases, etc.

Because of the differences in NSAIDs, doses and cell types investigated, conflicting data exist over the requirement for major signalling molecules associated with apoptosis. *Bcl-2* was found to block apoptosis in chicken embryo fibroblasts (CEF) upon overexpression, but was unchanged in level during NSAID-induced apoptosis[74,77]. *Bcl-2* was found to be diminished in polyps in *Min* mice after 2–4 days of treatment with sulindac, leading to the conclusion that in intestinal cells it may confer resistance to apoptosis[78]. The pro-apoptotic BAK member of the *Bcl-2* family has been found to be induced following treatment of K-*ras* transformed intestinal cells with sulindac sulphide[55].

p53 expression is unchanged in CEF undergoing NSAID-induced apoptosis, and mutated p53 is not associated with resistance or susceptibility to sulindac-induced apoptosis in human colorectal polyps[32,77]. In contrast, p53 expression has been reported to be upregulated by indomethacin in the MKN28 colorectal cell line, and mutant p53 has been reported to be downregulated by sulindac in another cell line[79,80].

Overexpression of c-*Myc* was found to be essential to NSAID-induced apoptosis in CEF and has also been implicated in NSAID-induced apoptosis in gastric epithelial cells[81,82]. Indomethacin induction of apoptosis has also been shown to result in activation of caspase-3[83].

Treatment of cell lines with sulindac or its metabolites has been reported to result in arrest in the G_1 phase of the cell cycle[41,55]. Cyclin D1 increased in HT-29 colon cells after sulindac sulphide treatment[84], whereas rat intestinal epithelial cells exhibited decreased cyclin D1 expression by COX-2 overexpression[39]. Treatment of the human mammary epithelial cell line MCF-10F with sulindac sulphide resulted in an induction of the CDK inhibitor p21WAF1[41]. Induction of p21WAF1 was also observed upon sulindac sulphide or indomethacin treatment of colorectal cell lines[80].

β-catenin has been found to be downregulated by aspirin and sulindac sulphide during polyp regression in *Min* mice and is downregulated in some colorectal cells during NSAID-induced apoptosis, but not in others[78,85].

The biochemistry of sulindac-induced apoptosis

Studies to date implicate a large number of diverse and perhaps conflicting signal transduction pathways in sulindac-induced apoptosis. The diversity of the pathways identified raises important questions, such as:

1. If p21ras, IκB kinases, PPARδ, cGMP phosphodiesterase and GBP are all binding partners for sulindac sulphide, is this binding specific, or is it due to the well-known ability of sulindac and its metabolites (particularly

sulindac sulphide) to adhere to protein? The concentrations of sulindac sulphide needed to bind directly to the target proteins were greater than 40 μM, and concentrations needed to disrupt function were frequently even higher.

2. Alternatively, does sulindac sulphide mimic in shape and chemistry an endogenous ligand that binds to multiple protein targets in the cell, of which the above may be only a subset? If this is the case, sulindac sulphide would be acting in the above studies as a low affinity, but specific ligand.

3. Does sulindac-induced apoptosis *in vivo* require inhibition of COX enzymes? Clearly the dose levels of sulindac or its metabolites used in virtually all studies of apoptosis to date are superphysiological with regard to blood plasma levels. This assumes administration of sulindac at standard doses of 150–400 mg day^{-1}. In the case of sulindac sulphide dose levels required for apoptosis are 20–60 times higher than the concentrations needed to achieve 50% inhibition of COX-1 and COX-2 (Figure 1), but are similar to the concentrations needed to inhibit 80–100% of the enzyme activity[24]. Recently it has been shown that H-*ras*-transformed-fibroblasts from COX-deficient mice experience sulindac-induced apoptosis at the same concentrations as cells from wild-type mice[86]. This case, and others[87] where sulindac induces apoptosis in cells reported to lack COX enzymes, do not disprove an essential requirement of removal of COX activity by the NSAID to induce apoptosis, since the cells in these studies already lack COX-1 and COX-2. However, they do prove the necessity of inhibiting one or more additional low-affinity sites in order to cause NSAID-induced apoptosis in these *in vitro* models.

In addition to the above mentioned low affinity sites, it is also important to note that a COX with low affinity for NSAIDs has been described in mouse macrophage/monocyte J774.2 cells[88]. This activity, which paralleled induction of COX-2 protein, was induced by treating the cells with high levels (500 μM) of diclofenac, which caused the cells to die by apoptosis. Rapid removal of the drug from these cells revealed a novel COX activity that exhibited markedly reduced sensitivity toward competitively acting NSAIDs such as diclofenac and indomethacin, and insensitivity toward aspirin. It is important to note that in many studies performed on NSAID-induced apoptosis COX-2 protein is induced during apoptosis. Induction of this protein, which correlates with induction of COX-2 activity in J774.2 cells, may be essential to apoptosis. This induction is presumably due to activation of PPARα and γ[65,66]. The phenomenon of COX-2 induction by NSAIDs, first described in CEF transformed with Rous sarcoma virus, can occur maximally at doses as low as 25 μM[77].

4. Because of the high concentrations of sulindac and its metabolites needed to induce apoptosis *in vitro*, is there any relevance to the physiologically observed event of chemoprevention and tumour regression observed *in vivo*? Current data leaves this question open to debate. The unusual conversion of sulindac to its COX-active sulphide metabolite on the lumenal side of the colon may result in regionally high concentrations of this metabolite that could affect colonocytes and colon tumour cells topically. If this is the case, current data are consistent with the notion that sulindac-induced apoptosis results from inhibition of both COX enzymes and interaction with one or more secondary, low-affinity targets, as described above. With the exception of desmoid tumours, which show limited response to sulindac treatment, no evidence to date suggests that NSAIDs cause regression of tumours outside of the GI tract, suggesting that topical contact may be essential for tumour regression. However, chemoprevention by NSAIDs does occur at distant sites[89].

NON-SULINDAC NSAIDS AND APOPTOSIS

Epidemiological evidence dating to the late 1980s suggests that aspirin prevents colorectal cancer[90]. Additionally, numerous animal studies dating back to the 1970s demonstrated that NSAIDs other than sulindac can prevent various types of tumours induced in two-stage models of carcinogenesis and can inhibit metastasis of xenographs implanted in receptive hosts[89]. Hence, it would be expected that other NSAIDs besides sulindac sulphide would cause apoptosis. In 1995, several laboratories showed that many structurally diverse competitively acting NSAIDs cause apoptosis in neoplastic cells[45,77,91]. Lu et al.[77] tested 26 NSAIDs in CEF transformed with a temperature-sensitive mutant of Rous sarcoma virus. The majority of these drugs (18/26) caused inhibition of focus formation and caused apoptosis at doses ranging from 10–100 μM. To date, this is one of the most sensitive cell systems for evaluation of NSAID-induced apoptosis. NSAIDs that were ineffective at inducing apoptosis in this model included prodrugs, such as sulindac, and very weak inhibitors of COX enzymes, such as paracetamol. As in other *in vitro* models of NSAID-induced apoptosis described subsequent to this study, apoptosis was not inhibited by co-administration of PGs, suggesting that inhibition of commonly studied PGs was not sufficient to induce apoptosis.

In CEF and human colorectal cell lines aspirin presented a paradox since it did not induce apoptosis, even at concentrations above 1 mM[77,92]. Yet, at these concentrations COX-1 and COX-2 were fully inhibited. The inability of aspirin to cause apoptosis further underscores the conclusion that simple inhibition of PG synthesis is insufficient to cause apoptosis. Additionally, these data indicate that any secondary site, in addition to COX inhibition, is not fully acted upon by aspirin treatment. Interestingly, aspirin use has been associated epidemiologically with approximately a 50% decrease in the incidence of colon cancer in humans[90]. Because chemopreventive effects do not necessarily require the induction of apoptosis to occur, aspirin may possess chemopreventive properties but lack the ability to induce tumour regression. Such chemopreventive activity may be mediated by the ability of NSAIDs in general to inhibit angiogenesis (see below).

It is now known that a variety of non-sulindac NSAIDs inhibit tumorigenesis in human colon/rectum and in the intestine of APC mutant mice. Small studies have shown piroxicam and indomethacin to be chemopreventive and to cause regression of polyps in patients with FAP. In general, however, these drugs tend to be less effective and to exhibit greater gastric side effects than sulindac. In recent clinical trials, celecoxib, a COX-2 selective inhibitor, administered to FAP patients at 400 mg b.i.d. resulted in a 28% reduction in polyps after 6 months[93]. This study demonstrated that non-acetic, COX-2 selective drugs can inhibit colorectal polyp growth in humans.

COX-2 selective drugs such as MF tricyclic (0.4 mg day^{-1}) also inhibit tumorigenesis in APC mutant mice, such as *Min* mice, by as much as 68%[46]. In contrast, the competitively acting NSAID, piroxicam (0.9 mg day^{-1}), reduces intestinal polyps in these animals by as much as 95%[94,95]. However, this high level of tumour reduction comes at the price of severe ulceration of the GI tract in 100% of the animals treated[95]. Treatment of APC mutant mice with R-flurbiprofen, an enantiomer that shows markedly reduced ability to inhibit COX activity, also showed an ability to inhibit up to 90% of intestinal polyps at the high dose of 20 mg kg^{-1} day^{-1}[96,97]. However, significant ulcerogenicity was also seen in these mice due to epimerization of the R enantiomer to the S form and inhibition of COX-1/COX-2 activity. Hence, significant inhibition of intestinal polyps in APC-deficient mice is frequently associated with ulcerogenesis[96,97]. Ulcerogenic levels of aspirin, a non-competitive COX inhibitor, reduces tumorigenesis by up to 49% in *Min* mice[98,99]. The reduced ability of aspirin to inhibit polyp formation in comparison with competitively acting NSAIDs may reflect a lower ability to induce apoptosis, as demonstrated by *in vitro* studies. An exception to the association of polyp reduction and GI ulceration occurs with COX-2 selective inhibitors which reduce intestinal polyps without ulcerogenesis[48].

DEFINING THE CELLULAR TARGET FOR NSAID-INDUCED APOPTOSIS IN TUMOURS

Several laboratories initially showed that COX-2 was elevated in human colorectal adenomas and carcinomas[100-102]. Since then, COX-2 has been found to be overexpressed in a variety of epithelially derived tumours (see Ristimäki, Chapter 19). It has been logical to assume, therefore, that the antineoplastic effect of NSAIDs may occur at the level of inhibition of COX-2 in the neoplastic epithelial cell. However, inhibition of COX activity could result in apoptosis of the neoplastic cell in several ways (Figure 3):

1. Significant and prolonged inhibition of COX-2 could result in the inability of the cell to live because of depletion of a COX-2 generated survival factor. Such a factor could act on the neoplastic cell in an autocrine fashion. That such a survival aspect of COX-2 exists is suggested by the studies of DuBois and colleagues[91] who demonstrated that COX over-expression could protect rat intestinal epithelial cells from butyrate-induced apoptosis.

2. Tumour cells could undergo apoptosis due to anoxia induced by destruction of the tumour vasculature, as described for cyclophosphamide[15]. Additional studies by DuBois and colleagues demonstrated that elevated levels of PGE_2 synthesized in tumour cells overexpressing COX-2 are angiogenic[103]. In CaCo2 colon carcinoma cells the increased PGE_2 synthesized by elevated levels of COX-2 was found to result in secretion of VEGF, TGF-β, and bFGF, which in turn induced vascular tube formation. In this *in vitro* model, sulindac sulphide and COX-2 selective inhibitors completely inhibit angiogenesis. Further studies by Masferrer and colleagues[104], using *in vivo* models for angiogenesis and the COX-2 selective inhibitor, celecoxib, have confirmed and strengthened the concept that COX-2 in tumours plays a pro-angiogenic role. It is important to note that overexpression of COX-2 in any cell type in the tumour could elicit this pro-angiogenic response. Early studies reported elevated COX-2 to be located primarily in neoplastic epithelial cells of human colorectal tumours[100-102], whereas more recent studies found elevated COX-2 to be located in interstitial macrophages in the same tumour type[105]. Either location would be predicted to be pro-angiogenic since this effect appears to occur through a paracrine action of PGE_2. Additionally, increased COX-2 in tumour endothelial cells resulted in angiogenesis[106]. Thus, COX-2 expression in neoplastic cells invading lymphocytes or stroma, or in the vasculature is proangiogenic.

3. Inhibition of COX-2 could stimulate anti-tumour immunosurveillance. PGE_2 has several inhibitory effects on lymphocytes, including suppressing lymphokine-activated killer cells and cell–cell-mediated tumour cell killing. NSAIDs are potent inhibitors of lung metastasis in rodent xenograph models[107]. Inhibition of PGE_2 synthesis by NSAIDs resulted in increased cell–cell-mediated killing. Since the majority of PGE_2 secreted by tumours appears to be the product of COX-2, COX-2 selective inhibitors may be expected to increase recognition of tumour cells by lymphocytes.

Figure 3 Potential cell targets for NSAIDs in tumours for the induction of apoptosis. NSAIDs may directly inhibit COX enzymes in neoplastic cells to prevent synthesis of PGE_2 or survival factors. Inhibition of PGE_2 results in decreased synthesis of angiogenic factors by the tumour cells and increased immunosurveillance. The former results in tumour cell apoptosis through anoxia or other pathways, and the latter causes tumour cell death through cell–cell-mediated killing. Alternatively, NSAIDs may reduce angiogenesis through inhibition of thromboxane A_2 synthesis in endothelial cells.

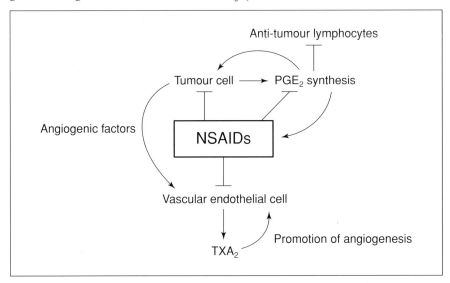

NSAID-INDUCED APOPTOSIS IN CANCER: CONCLUSIONS

Induction of apoptosis by sulindac and other NSAIDs is essential to the ability of these drugs to induce tumour regression, and may also be important to the chemopreventive properties of these drugs. The precise biochemical mechanism(s) by which NSAIDs initiate apoptosis is unclear. Current data are consistent with a requirement for both COX-1 and COX-2 inhibition, as well as inhibition of one or more low-affinity sites. Induction of COX-2 is also a concomitant event of NSAID-induced apoptosis. It is presently unclear what concentrations of NSAIDs are required for apoptosis in colorectal polyps, since tumours are exposed to NSAIDs via the bloodstream and topically.

Of the mechanisms for the antineoplastic effect of NSAIDs that have been proposed, inhibition of angiogenesis resulting in inhibition of tumour growth by anoxia would require the lowest concentrations of NSAID. Inhibition of COX-2 and PGE_2 synthesis in tumours and/or thromboxane A_2 in endothelial cells would require dose levels similar to those required for the anti-inflammatory activity of NSAIDs. For this reason, anti-angiogenesis must be considered as a leading mechanism for tumour chemoprevention by NSAIDs. This is particularly true for tumours exposed solely via the blood.

However, the relatively weak ability of celecoxib at high dose levels to cause tumour regression in the colon/rectum suggests that inhibition of angiogenesis is not the sole mechanism for NSAID-induced tumour regression.

THE CORNEA AND NSAID-INDUCED CELL DEATH

The eye represents another organ, in addition to the GI tract, that is exposed to high NSAID concentrations during medical treatment. Surgery of the cornea, including cataract surgery and corneal refractive surgery to correct myopia (e.g. radial keratotomy, and laser *in situ* keratomileusis (LASIK)) produce local inflammation that is treated with topical NSAIDs and glucocorticoids. In rabbit models, excimer laser ablation or mechanical wounding of the cornea results in a robust increase in PGE_2 synthesis, beginning at 1 h posttreatment, which remains elevated for up to 24 h[108,109]. Leukotriene B_4 synthesis, in contrast, is unaffected by the laser treatment. Fluorometholone (a corticosteroid) and diclofenac inhibit induction of PGE_2 by 50% and 85%, respectively. In one study this induction of PGE_2 has been associated with COX-2 synthesis[109].

Diclofenac and ketorolac have both been formulated for topical treatment of inflammation of the cornea. Both drugs are reported to relieve inflammation and pain after surgery. These NSAIDs, in the form of eye drops, are typically administered during preoperative, perioperative and postoperative periods. The concentration of diclofenac in commercial preparations (e.g. Voltaren Ophthalmic®) is 0.1% or 3.1 mM and the concentration of ketorolac (e.g. Acular®) is 0.5% or 19.6 mM. A reported regimen for administration of these drugs for cataract surgery is to administer them up to 4 times daily for 2–3 days before surgery, administer multiple drops immediately before surgery, and administer 4 times daily for up to 6 weeks after surgery[110]. The majority of ophthalmologists use some regimen of topical NSAID treatment following surgery[110,111].

Topical administration of drugs to the eye results in a modest immediate dilution of the medication by tear fluid. In rabbits an average 25 μl dose is diluted by 7.5 μl of tear fluid[112,113]. Elimination of drug by tear production, tissue absorption and metabolism decrease exposure to the drug. Tear fluid *in vivo* is exchanged at a rate of 9% min⁻¹ (ref. 112). Much of the ability of NSAID solutions to penetrate ocular tissue and, specifically, to reach the anterior compartment of the eye where relief of swelling and inflammation is most important, depends on the compound's lipophilicity (the greater the lipophilicity the greater the penetration) and the vehicle used for formulation.

The high concentration of NSAID in commercially available ocular medications, even upon a tenfold dilution, would be in the range that causes apoptosis in most cell models. The fact that it does not do so in most cases is probably a result of the short period of time the corneal cells are in contact with the drug.

As described above, studies of murine macrophage/monocytes treated with diclofenac produced induction of COX-2 as well as an enormous increase in COX activity that was revealed upon removing the drug and adding arachidonic acid substrate (Figure 4)[88]. NSAID induction of COX-2 is now known to occur also in rabbit corneal cells treated with 30 µM indomethacin or 30 µM flurbiprofen[114]. Induction of COX-2 by NSAID treatment could lead ultimately to hyperinflammation of the cornea and lymphocyte infiltration, as recently proposed by Price[115]. Such a scenario may be evidenced in clinical experience involving Alcon's diclofenac sodium ophthalmic solution (DSOS). This medication was used for relief of ocular inflammation before being removed from the market for side effects. DSOS, and perhaps other topical

Figure 4 Induction of COX activity during NSAID-induced apoptosis. J774.2 cells were treated with diclofenac at the concentrations indicated for 48 h. After treatment, cells were washed twice to remove drug and then exposed to 30 µM arachidonic acid for 15 min. ●, PGE_2 released was estimated by radioimmunoassay and is expressed as ng of PGE_2 ml^{-1} of media times a factor of 10. ▲, values have been recalculated as pg of PGE_2 µg^{-1} of protein to normalize for the large decrease in cell number and mass occurring at higher NSAID concentrations (200 µM or greater). The induced enzyme activity shows reduced sensitivity to competitively acting NSAIDs, is sensitive to paracetamol, and is insensitive to aspirin. (Reproduced from ref. 88.)

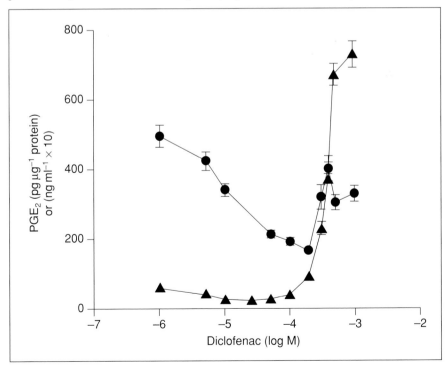

NSAIDs, have been increasingly associated with reports of corneal 'melts', with additional reports of lymphocyte infiltration known as infiltrating keratitis (e.g. regions of intense cellular inflammation). Diclofenac-induced corneal melts, resulting in some cases in perforation of the cornea, are the result of cell death and concomitant thinning of the extracellular components of the cornea. Theoretically, this could be the result of diclofenac-induced apoptosis of corneal cells accompanied by extracellular breakdown. In contrast, corneal infiltrates could be the result of induction of COX-2 in epithelial or other cells with increased COX-2-mediated pro-inflammatory signalling after washout of the drug by tear fluid. In rabbit models, administration of Voltaren Ophthalmic® for 10 h resulted in a demonstrable increase in polymorphonuclear leucocytes in comparison to controls[108].

The onset of these effects, associated primarily with DSOS, may be due to the vehicle used in this preparation, which has been speculated to result in greater time of exposure of the cornea to the drug[110]. Such a condition would favour the twin effects of exposure to high concentrations of NSAIDs: induction of apoptosis and induction of COX-2.

ACKNOWLEDGEMENTS

The authors thank Rachel A. Simmons for assistance in preparing this manuscript and Mark Morris for the preparation of figures. The authors also thank Francis W. Price MD for sharing his ideas regarding diclofenac-induced eye injury and his manuscript on this subject prior to publication. This work was supported by grants AR45296 and AR46688 from the National Institutes of Health.

Address all correspondence to: Daniel L. Simmons, Department of Chemistry and Biochemistry, E280 BNSN, Brigham Young University, Provo, Utah 84604, USA.

REFERENCES

1. Jacobson MD, Weil M, Raff MC. Programmed cell death in animal development. *Cell.* 1997;88:347–54.
2. Vaux DL, Korsmeyer SJ. Cell death in development. *Cell.* 1999;96:245–54.
3. Kuida K, Zheng TS, Na S, Kuan C, Yang D, Karasuyama H et al. Decreased apoptosis in the brain and premature lethality in CPP32-deficient mice. *Nature.* 1996;384:368–72.
4. Kerr JF, Winterford CM. Apoptosis: Its significance in cancer and cancer therapy. *Cancer.* 1994;73:2013–26.
5. Hall PA, Coates PJ, Ansari B, Hopwood D. Regulation of cell number in the mammalian gastrointestinal tract: the importance of apoptosis. *J Cell Sci.* 1994;107:3569–77.

6. Bedi A, Pasricha PJ, Akhtar AJ, Barber JP, Bedi GC, Giardiello FM et al. Inhibition of apoptosis during development of colorectal cancer. *Cancer Res.* 1995;55:1811–6.

7. O'Connor L, Huang D, O'Reilly LA, Strasser A. Apoptosis and cell division. *Curr Opin Cell Biol.* 2000;12:257–63.

8. Agarwal ML, Taylor WR, Chernov MV, Chernova OB, Stark GR. The p53 network. *J Biol Chem.* 1998;273:1–4.

9. Evan G, Littlewood T. A matter of life and cell death. *Science.* 1998;281:1317–22.

10. Guo M, Hay, BA. Cell proliferation and apoptosis. *Cell.* 1999;11:745–52.

11. Song Z, Stellar H. Death by design: mechanism and control of apoptosis. *Trends Biochem Sci.* 1999;24:M49–M52.

12. Basu S, Bayoumy S, Zhang Y, Lozano J, Kolesnick R. BAD enables ceramide to signal apoptosis via Ras and Raf-1. *J Biol Chem.* 1998;273:30419–26.

13. Li P, Nijhawan D, Budihardjo I, Srinivasula SM, Ahmad M, Alnemri ES et al. Cytochrome c and dATP-dependent formation of Apaf-1/caspase-9 complex initiates an apoptotic protease cascade. *Cell.* 1997;91:479–89.

14. Hour TC, Chen L, Lin JK. Suppression of transcription factor NF-κB activity by Bcl-2 protein in NIH3T3 cells: implication of a novel NF-κB p50-Bcl-2 complex for the anti-apoptotic function of Bcl-2. *Eur J Cell Biol.* 2000;79:121–9.

15. Browder T, Butterfield CE, Kräling BM, Shi B, Marshall B, O'Reilly, MS et al. Antiangiogenic scheduling of chemotherapy improves efficacy against experimental drug-resistant cancer. *Cancer Res.* 2000;60:1878–86.

16. Robinson DR. Prostaglandins and the mechanism of action of anti-inflammatory drugs. *Am J Med.* 1983;75:26–31.

17. Davies NM, Watson MS. Clinical pharmacokinetics of sulindac. A dynamic old drug. *Clin Pharmacokinet.* 1997;32:437–59.

18. Russeva VN, Zhivkova ZD. Protein binding of some non-steroidal anti-inflammatory drugs studied by high-performance liquid affinity chromatography. *Int J Pharm.* 1999;180:69–74.

19. Shams-Eldeen MA, Vallner JJ, NeedhamTE. Interaction of sulindac and metabolite with human serum albumin. *J Pharm Sci.* 1978;67:1077–80.

20. Bayley N, Warne RW, Moulds RF, Bury RW. A kinetic study of sulindac in the elderly. *Aust NZ J Med.* 1987;17:39–42.

21. Strong HA, Renwick AG, George CF, Liu YF, Hill MJ. The reduction of sulphinpyrazone and sulindac by intestinal bacteria. *Xenobiotica.*1987;17:685–96.

22. Miller MJ, Bednar MM, McGiff JC. Renal metabolism of sulindac: functional implications. *J Pharmacol Exp Ther.* 1984;231:449–56.

23. Strong HA, Warner NJ, Renwick AG, George CF. Sulindac metabolism: the importance of an intact colon. *Clin Pharmacol Ther.* 1985;38:387–93.

24. Warner TD, Giuliano F, Vojnovic I, Bukasa A, Mitchell JA, Vane JR. Nonsteroid drug selectivities for cyclo-oxygenase-1 rather than cyclo-oxygenase-2 are associated with human gastrointestinal toxicity: a full *in vitro* analysis. *Proc Natl Acad Sci USA.* 1999;96:7563–8.

25. Martel RR, Klicius J. Comparison in rats of the anti-inflammatory and gastric irritant effects of etodolac with several clinically effective anti-inflammatory drugs. *Agents Actions.* 1982;12:295–7.

26. Hamman MA, Hachner-Daniels BD, Wrighton SA, Rettie AE, Hall SD. Stereoselective sulfoxidation of sulindac sulfide by flavin-containing monooxygenases. Comparison of human liver and kidney microsomes and mammalian enzymes. *Biochem Pharmacol.* 2000;60:7–17.

27. Block E. Reactions of organosulfur compounds. In: *Organic Chemistry*, vol. 37. New York: Academic Press; 1978:16–17.

28. Truce WE, Klingler TC, Brand WW. Sulfones and sulfoximines. In: Shigeru O, editor. *Organic Chemistry of Sulfur*. New York: Plenum Press; 1977:572–3.

29. Waddell WR, Loughry RW. Sulindac for polyposis of the colon. *J Surg Oncol.* 1983;24:83–7.

30. Richard CS, Berk T, Bapat BV, Haber G, Cohen Z, Gallinger S. Sulindac for peri-ampullary polyps in FAP patients. *Int J Colorectal Dis.* 1997;12:14–18.

31. Hixson LJ, Earnest DL, Fennerty MB, Sampliner RE. NSAID effect on sporadic colon polyps. *Am J Gastroenterol.* 1993;88:1652–6.

32. Matsuhashi N, Nakajima A, Fukushima Y, Yazaki Y, Oka T. Effects of sulindac on sporadic colorectal adenomatous polyps. *Gut.* 1997;40:344–9.

33. Giardello FM, Hamilton SR, Krush AJ, Piantadosi S, Hylind LM, Celano P et al. Treatment of colonic and rectal adenomas with sulindac in familial adenomatous polyposis. *N Engl J Med.* 1993;328:1313–16.

34. Nugent KP, Farmer KC, Spigelman AD, Williams CB, Phillips RK. Randomized controlled trial of the effect of sulindac on duodenal and rectal polyposis and cell proliferation in patients with familial adenomatous polyposis. *Br J Surg.* 1993;80:1618–19.

35. Windle G, Schmid KW, Brandt B, Muller O, Osswald H. Clinical and genomic influence of sulindac on rectal mucosa in familial adenomatous polyposis. *Dis Colon Rectum.* 1997;40:1156–68.

36. Spagnesi MT, Tonelli F, Dolara P, Caderni G, Valanzano R, Anastasi A et al. Rectal proliferation and polyp occurrence in patients with familial adenomatous polyposis after sulindac treatment. *Gastroenterology.* 1994;106:362–6.

37. Pasricha PJ, Bedi A, O'Connor K, Rashid A, Akhtar AJ, Zahurak ML et al. The effects of sulindac on colorectal proliferation and apoptosis in familial adenomatous polyposis. *Gastroenterology.* 1995;109:994–8.

38. Trifan OC, Smith RM, Thompson BD, Hla T. Overexpression of cyclooxygenase-2 induces cell cycle arrest. *J Biol Chem.* 1999;274:34141–7.

39. DuBois RN, Shao J, Tsujii M, Sheng H, Beauchamp RD. G_1 delay in cells over-expressing prostaglandin endoperoxide synthase-2. *Cancer Res.* 1996;56:733–7.

40. Lim JT, Piazza GA, Han EK, Delohery TM, Li H, Finn TS et al. Sulindac deriv-atives inhibit growth and induce apoptosis in human prostate cancer cell lines. *Biochem Pharmacol.* 1999;58:1097–107.

41. Han EK, Arber N, Yamamoto H, Lim JT, Delohery T, Pamukcu R et al. Effects of sulindac and its metabolites on growth and apoptosis in human mammary epithelial and breast carcinoma cell lines. *Breast Cancer Res Treat.* 1998;48:195–203.

42. Goluboff ET, Shabsigh A, Saidi JA, Weinstein IB, Mitra N, Heitjan D et al. Exisulind (sulindac sulfone) suppresses growth of human prostate cancer in a nude mouse xenograft model by increasing apoptosis. *Urology.* 1999;53:440–5.

43. Reddy BS, Kawamori T, Lubet RA, Steele VE, Kelloff GJ, Rao CV. Chemopreventive efficacy of sulindac sulfone against colon cancer depends on time of administration during carcinogenic process. *Cancer Res.* 1999;59:3387–9.

44. Shiff SJ, Qiao L, Tsai LL, Rigas B. Sulindac sulfide an aspirin-like compound, inhibits proliferation, causes cell cycle quiescence, and induces apoptosis in HT-29 colon adenocarcinoma cells. *J Clin Invest.* 1995;96:491–503.

45. Piazza GA, Rahm AL, Krutzch M, Sperl G, Paranka NS, Gross PH et al.

Antineoplastic drugs sulindac sulfide and sulfone inhibit cell growth by inducing apoptosis. *Cancer Res.* 1995;55:3110–16.

46. Oshima M, Dinchuk JE, Kargman SL, Oshima H, Hancock B, Kwong E et al. Suppression of intestinal polyposis in Apc delta716 knockout mice by inhibition of cyclooxygenase-2 (COX-2). *Cell.* 1996;87:803–9.

47. Chiu CH, McEntee MF, Whelan J. Sulindac causes rapid regression of preexisting tumors in Min/+ mice independent of prostaglandin biosynthesis. *Cancer Res.* 1997;57:4267–73.

48. Mahmoud NN, Boolbol SK, Dannenberg AJ, Mestre JR, Bilinski RT, Martucci C. The sulfide metabolite of sulindac prevents tumors and restores enterocyte apoptosis in a murine model of familial polyposis. *Carcinogenesis.* 1998;19:87–91.

49. Piazza GA, Alberts DS, Hixson LJ, Paranka NS, Li H, Finn T et al. Sulindac sulfone inhibits azoxymethane-induced colon carcinogenesis in rats without reducing prostaglandin levels. *Cancer Res.* 1997;57:2909–15.

50. Stoner GD, Budd GT, Ganapathi R, De Young B, Kresty LA, Nitert M et al. Sulindac sulfone induced regression of rectal polyps in patients with familial adenomatous polyposis. *Adv Exp Med Biol.* 1999;470:45–53.

51. van Stolk R, Stoner G, Hayton WL, Chan K, De Young B, Kresty L et al. Phase I trial of exisulind (sulindac sulfone, FGN-1) as a chemopreventitive agent in patients with familial adenomatous polyposis. *Clin Cancer Res.* 2000;6:78–89.

52. Burke C, van Stolk R, Arber N, Hultcrantz R, Bjork J, Syngal S et al. Exisulind prevents adenoma formation in familial adenomatous polyposis (FAP). *Digestive Diseases Week Meeting,* 2000 May, San Diego.

53. Waddell WR. The effect of sulindac on colon polyps: circumvention of a transformed phenotype – a hypothesis. *J Surg Oncol.* 1994;55:52–5.

54. Waddell WR, Miesfeld RL. Adenomatous polyposis coli, protein kinases, protein tyrosine phosphatase: the effect of sulindac. *J Surg Oncol.* 1995;58:252–6.

55. Arber N, Han EK, Sgambato A, Piazza GA, Delohery TM, Begeman M et al. A K-ras oncogene increases resistance to sulindac-induced apoptosis in rat enterocytes. *Gastroenterology.* 1997;113:1892–900.

56. Herrmann C, Block C, Geisen C, Haas K, Weber C, Winde G et al. Sulindac sulfide inhibits Ras signaling. *Oncogene.* 1998;17:1769–76.

57. Chan TA, Morin PJ, Vogelstein B, Kinzler KW. Mechanisms underlying nonsteroidal antiinflammatory drug-mediated apoptosis. *Proc Natl Acad Sci USA.* 1998;95:681–6.

58. Hannun YA, Luberto C. Ceramide in the eukaryotic stress response. *Trends Cell Biol.* 2000;10:73–80.

59. Kopp E, Ghosh S. Inhibition of NF-Kappa B by sodium salicylate and aspirin. *Science.* 1994;265:956–9.

60. Insel PA. Analgesic-antipyretics and antiinflammatory agents: drugs employed in the treatment of rheumatoid arthritis and gout. In: Gilman AG, Rall TW, Nies AS, Taylor P, editors. *The Pharmacological Basis of Therapeutics,* 8th edition. New York: Pergamon Press; 1990:638–61.

61. McEvoy GK, editor. *AHFS 98 drug information.* Published by the authority of the board of directors of the American Society of Health-System Pharmacists. 1998:1584–664.

62. Yamamoto Y, Yin MJ, Lin KM, Gaynor RB. Sulindac inhibits activation of the NF-kappaB pathway. *J Biol Chem.* 1999;274:27307–14.

63. Yu K, Bayona W, Kallen CB, Harding HP, Ravera CF, McMahon G et al.

Differential activation of peroxisome proliferator-activated receptors by eicosanoids. *J Biol Chem.* 1995;270:23975–83.

64. Rocchi S, Auwerx J. Peroxisome proliferator-activated receptor-gamma: a versatile metabolic regulator. *Ann Med.* 1999;31:342–51.

65. Lehmann JM, Lenhard JM, Oliver BB, Ringold GM, Kliewer SA. Peroxisome proliferator-activated receptors alpha and gamma are activated by indomethacin and other non-steroidal anti-inflammatory drugs. *J Biol Chem.* 1997;272:3406–10.

66. Ledwith BJ, Panley CJ, Wagner LK, Rokos CL, Alberts DW, Manam S. Induction of cyclooxygenase-2 expression by peroxisome proliferators and non-tetradecanoylphorbol 12,13-myristate-type tumor promoters in immortalized mouse liver cells. *J Biol Chem.* 1997;272:3707–14.

67. He TC, Chan TA, Vogestein B, Kinzler KW. PPAR delta is an APC-regulated target of nonsteroidal anti-inflammatory drugs. *Cell.* 1999;99:335–45.

68. Masubuchi Y, Yamada S, Horie T. Possible mechanism of hepatocyte injury induced by diphenylamine and its structurally related nonsteroidal anti-inflammatory drugs. *J Pharmacol Exp Ther.* 2000;292:982–7.

69. Shen TY, Winter CA. Chemical and biological studies on indomethacin, sulindac, and their analogs. *Adv Drug Res.* 1977;12:90–245.

70. Moreno-Sanchez R, Bravo C, Vasquez C, Ayela G, Silveira LH, Martinez-Lavin M. Inhibition and uncoupling of oxidative phosphorylation by nonsteroidal anti-inflammatory drugs: study in mitochondria, submitochondrial particles, cells, and whole heart. *Biochem Pharmacol.* 1999;57:743–52.

71. Somasundaram S, Sigthorsson G, Simpson RJ, Watts J, Jacob M, Tavares IA et al. Uncoupling of intestinal mitochondrial oxidative phosphorylation and inhibition of cyclooxygenase are required for the development of NSAID-enteropathy in the rat. *Aliment Pharmacol Ther.* 2000;14:639–50.

72. Masubuchi Y, Saito H, Horie T. Structural requirements for the hepatotoxicity of nonsteroidal anti-inflammatory drugs in isolated rat hepatocytes. *J Pharmacol Exp Ther.* 1998;287:208–13.

73. Aptosyn™ page. 16 June 2000. Cell Pathways, Inc. <http://www.igi.net/~cell-path/6_APTOSYN/aptosyn.html>

74. Lu X, Fairbairn DW, Bradshaw WS, O'Neill KL, Ewert DL, Simmons DL. NSAID-induced apoptosis in Rous sarcoma virus-transformed chicken embryo fibroblasts is dependent on v-*src* and c-*myc* and is inhibited by *bcl-2*. *Prostaglandins.* 1997;54:549–68.

75. Mu FT, Baldwin G, Weinstock J, Stockman D, Toh BH. Monoclonal antibody to the gastrin receptor on parietal cells recognizes a 78-kDa protein. *Proc Natl Acad Sci USA.* 1987;84:2698–702.

76. Baldwin GS, Rorison KA. Structural requirements for the binding of non-steroidal anti- inflammatory drugs to the 78 kDa gastrin binding protein. *Biochim Biophys Acta.* 1999;1428:68–76.

77. Lu X, Xie W, Reed D, Bradshaw WS, Simmons DL. Nonsteroidal antiinflammatory drugs cause apoptosis and induce cyclooxygenases in chicken embryo fibroblasts. *Proc Natl Acad Sci USA.* 1995;92:7961–5.

78. McEntee MF, Chiu CH, Whelan J. Relationship of beta-catenin and Bcl-2 expression to sulindac-induced regression of intestnal tumors in Min mice. *Carcinogenesis.* 1999;20:635–40.

79. Zhu GH, Wong, BC, Ching CK, Lai KC, Lam SK. Differential apoptosis by indomethacin in gastric epithelial cells through the constitutive expression of

wild-type p53 and/or up- regulation of c-*myc*. *Biochem Pharmacol*. 1999;58:193–200.

80. Goldberg Y, Nassif II, Pittas A, Tsai LL, Dynlacht BD, Rigas B et al. The anti-proliferative effect of sulindac and sulindac sulfide on HT-29 colon cancer cells: alterations in tumor suppressor and cell cycle-regulatory proteins. *Oncogene*. 1996;12:893–901.

81. Zhu GH, Wong BC, Eggo MC, Ching CK, Yuen ST, Chan EY et al. Non-steroidal anti-inflammatory drug-induced apoptosis in gastric cancer cells is blocked by protein kinase C activation through inhibition of c-*myc*. *Br J Cancer*. 1999;79:393–400.

82. Zhu GH, Wong BC, Slosberg ED, Eggo MC, Ching CK, Yuen ST et al. Overexpression of protein kinase C-beta 1 isoenzyme suppresses indomethacin-induced apoptosis in gastric epithelial cells. *Gastroenterology*. 2000;118:507–14.

83. Fujii Y, Matsura T, Kai M, Matsui H, Kawasaki H, Yamada K. Mitochondrial cytochrome c release and caspase-3-like protease activation during indomethacin-induced apoptosis in rat gastric mucosal cells. *Proc Soc Exp Biol Med*. 2000;224:102–8.

84. Qiao L, Shiff SJ, Rigas B. Sulindac sulfide alters the expression of cyclin proteins in HT-29 colon adenocarcinoma cells. *Int J Cancer*. 1998;30:99–104.

85. Smith ML, Hawcroft G, Hull MA. The effect of non-steroidal anti-inflammatory drugs on human colorectal cancer cells: evidence of different mechanisms of action. *Eur J Cancer*. 2000;36:664–74.

86. Zhang X, Morham SG, Langenbach R, Young DA. Malignant transformation and antineoplastic actions of nonsteroidal antiinflammatory drugs (NSAIDs) on cyclooxygenase-null embryo fibroblasts. *J Exp Med*. 1999;190:451–9.

87. Hanif R, Pittas A, Feng Y, Koutsos MI, Qiao L, Staiano-Coico L et al. Effects of nonsteroidal anti-inflammatory drugs on proliferation and on induction of apoptosis in colon cancer cells by a prostaglandin-independent pathway. *Biochem Pharmacol*. 1996;52:237–45.

88. Simmons DL, Botting RM, Robertson PM, Madsen ML, Vane JR. Induction of an acetaminophen-sensitive cyclooxygenase with reduced sensitivity to nonsteroid anti-inflammatory drugs. *Proc Natl Acad Sci USA*. 1999;96:3275–80.

89. Verma AK, Rice HM, Boutwell RK. Prostaglandins and skin tumor promotion: inhibition of tumor promoter-induced ornithine decarboxylase activity in epidermis by inhibitors of prostaglandin synthesis. *Biochem Biophys Res Commun*. 1977;79:1160–6.

90. Potter JD. Colorectal cancer: molecules and populations. *J Natl Cancer Inst*. 1999;91:916–32.

91. Tsujii M, DuBois RN. Alterations in cellular adhesion and apoptosis in epithelial cells overexpressing prostaglandin endoperoxide synthase 2. *Cell*. 1995;83:493–501.

92. Qiao L, Hanif R, Sphicas E, Shiff SJ, Rigas B. Effect of aspirin on induction of apoptosis in HT-29 human colon adenocarcinoma cells. *Biochem Pharmacol*. 1998;55:53–64.

93. Smigel K. Arthritis drug-approved for polyp prevention blazes trail for other prevention trials. *J Natl Cancer Inst*. 2000;92:297–9.

94. Jacoby RF, Cole CE, Tutsch K, Newton MA, Kelloff G, Hawk ET et al. Chemopreventitive efficacy of combined piroxicam and difluoromethylornithine treatment of Apc mutant Min mouse adenomas, and selective toxicity against Apc mutant embryos. *Cancer Res*. 2000;60:1864–70.

95. Ritland SR, Leighton VA, Hirsch RE, Morrow JD, Weaver AL, Gendler SJ. Evaluation of 5-aminosalicylic acid (5-ASA) for cancer chemoprevention: lack of efficacy against nascent ademomatous polyps in the Apc (Min) mouse. *Clin Cancer Res.* 1999;5:853–63.

96. Wechter WJ, Kantoci D, Murray ED, Quiggle DD, Leipold DD, Gibson KM et al. R- flurbiprofen chemoprevention and treatment of intestinal adenomas in the APC (min)/+ mouse model: implications for prophylaxis and treatment of colon cancer. *Cancer Res.* 1997;57:4316–24.

97. Wechter WJ, Murray ED, Kantoci D, Quiggle DD, Leipold DD, Gibson KM et al. Treatment and survival study in the C57BL/6J-APC(Min)/+(Min) mouse with R-flurbiprofen. *Life Sci.* 2000;66:745–53.

98. Barnes CJ, Lee M. Chemoprevention of spontaneous intestinal adenomas in the ademomatous polyposis coli Min mouse model with aspirin. *Gastroenterology.* 1998;114:873–7.

99. Mahmoud NN, Dannenberg AJ, Mestre J, Bilinski RT, Churchhill MR, Martucci C et al. Aspirin prevents tumors in a murine model of familial ademomatous polyposis. *Surgery.* 1998;124:225–31.

100. Eberhart CE, Coffey RJ, Radhika A, Giardiello FM, Ferrenbach S, DuBois RN. Up-regulation of cyclooxygenase 2 gene expression in human colorectal adenomas and adenocarcinomas. *Gastroenterology.* 1994;107:1183–8.

101. Sano H, Kawahito Y, Wilder RL, Hashiramoto A, Mukai S, Asai K et al. Expression of cyclooxygenase-1 and -2 in human colorectal cancer. *Cancer Res.* 1995;55:3785–9.

102. Kargman SL, O'Neill GP, Vickers PJ, Evans JF, Mancini JA, Jothy S. Expression of prostaglandin G/H synthase-1 and -2 protein in human colon cancer. *Cancer Res.* 1995;55:2556–9.

103. Tsujii M, Kawano S, Tsuji S, Sawaoka H, Hori M, Dubois RN. Cyclooxygenase regulates angiogenesis induced by colon cancer cells. *Cell.* 1998;93:705–16.

104. Masferrer JL, Leahy KM, Koki AT, Zweifel BS, Settle SL, Woerner BM et al. Anitiangiogenic and antitumor activities of cyclooxygenase-2 inhibitors. *Cancer Res.* 2000;60:1306–11.

105. Chapple KS, Cartwright EJ, Hawcroft G, Tisbury A, Bonifer C, Scott N et al. Localization of cyclooxygenase-2 in human sporadic colorectal ademomas. *Am J Pathol.* 2000;56:545–53.

106. Daniel TO, Liu H, Morrow JD, Crews BC, Marnett LJ. Thromboxane A_2 is a mediator of cyclooxygenase-2-dependent endothelial migration and angiogenesis. *Cancer Res.* 1999;59:4574–7.

107. Lala PK, Parhar RS, Singh P. Indomethacin therapy abrogates the prostaglandin-mediated suppression of natural killer activity in tumor-bearing mice and prevents tumor metastasis. *Cell Immunol.* 1986;99:108–18.

108. Phillips AF, Szerenyi K, Campos M, Krueger RR, McDonnell PJ. Arachidonic acid metabolites after excimer laser corneal surgery. *Arch Ophthalmol.* 1993;111:1273–8.

109. Jumblatt MM, Willer SS. Corneal endothelial repair. Regulation of prostaglandin E_2 synthesis. *Invest Ophthalmol Vis Sci.* 1996;37:1294–301.

110. Roberts CW. Topical NSAIDs in ophthalmology: current issues. *Ophthamology Times.* 2000;25(1 Suppl):S2–S13.

111. Arshinoff SA, Mills MD, Haber S. Pharmacotherapy of photorefractive keratectomy. *J Cataract Refract Surg.* 1996;22:1037–44.

112. Stevens LE, Missel PJ, Lang JC. Drug release profiles of ophthalmic formulations. 1. Instrumentation. *Anal Chem.* 1992;64:715–23.

113. Keister JC, Cooper ER, Missel PJ, Lang JC, Hager DF. Limits on optimizing ocular drug delivery. *J Pharm Sci.* 1991;80:50–3.

114. Bonazzi A, Mastyugin V, Mieyal PA, Dunn MW, Laniado-Schwartzman M. Regulation of cyclooxygenase-2 by hypoxia and peroxisome proliferators in the corneal epithelium. *J Biol Chem.* 2000;275:2837–44.

115. Price FW. New pieces for the puzzle: nonsteroidal anti-inflammatory drugs and corneal ulcers. *J Cataract Refract Surg.* 2000;26:1263–5.

11 | Cyclooxygenase enzymes and human labour

Victoria Allport and Phillip Bennett

Imperial College School of Medicine, Institute of Reproductive and Developmental Biology, Hammersmith Hospital, Du Cane Road, London W12, UK.

The association between prostaglandins (PG) and successful labour has been recognized for several decades. PGs have been used in clinical practice to induce both second trimester pregnancy termination and labour at term since the 1970s. More recently PGs have become widely used for cervical ripening prior to instrumentation of the non-pregnant uterus and in the first trimester of pregnancy. Inhibition of PG synthesis delays labour at term and, of more clinical relevance, can delay preterm delivery. PGs facilitate the major processes of labour onset and are therefore essential for successful labour and delivery in the human. Specifically, they mediate cervical ripening by increasing the expression of the chemoattractant cytokine interleukin-8 (IL-8)[1] leading to an influx of neutrophils, increased protease activity and tissue remodelling. They also stimulate uterine contractions[2] and synchronize fundally dominant myometrial contractions by the upregulation of both oxytocin receptors and gap junction proteins[3-5].

The onset of human labour requires increased PG synthesis, which in turn drives and forms part of an integrated series of biochemical changes leading to cervical ripening and myometrial contraction. Understanding how PG synthesis is controlled within the uterus would provide clues to the general mechanisms which regulate the length of human pregnancy and allow strategies to be developed for the prediction and prevention of preterm labour.

THE PROCESSES OF LABOUR

The 'progesterone block'

For the first twenty weeks of gestation the uterus grows and expands both by hyperplasia and hypertrophy. For the rest of gestation, however, uterine expansion is due to distension and stretch and the walls of the myometrium become increasingly thinned. Blood vessels within the myometrium also stop growing in the second half of pregnancy and the tight coils that have developed up to this point begin to unwind. There is however no concomitant increase in uterine activity. Painless irregular contractions occur throughout gestation at random sites of pacemaker activity spreading over only a small area of the myometrium but the cervix remains rigid and closed. This phase of pregnancy maintenance is supported by 'pro-pregnancy' factors such as progesterone.

In the human, progesterone is first produced by the corpus luteum which is maintained by the presence of human chorionic gonadatrophin. Luteal regression occurs during the first trimester and progesterone synthesis is continued by the placenta. In humans, unlike other species, there is no decrease in maternal progesterone serum levels prior to the onset of labour. However, there is upregulation of a range of pro-labour genes which are normally repressed by the presence of progesterone[6]. The role of progesterone as an inhibitor of uterine contractions has long been recognized. Csapo introduced the term 'progesterone block' in 1965. The 'progesterone block' opposes the excitatory effect of oestrogen and prevents myometrial responsiveness to uterotonic agents.

In many species there is obvious progesterone withdrawal. In rodents, rabbits, goats and pigs the corpus luteum is the main source of progesterone until term when its regression ('luteolysis') directly causes progesterone withdrawal and labour onset ensues[7]. In sheep, an increase in fetal cortisol induces the activity of the enzyme 17α-hydroxylase which converts progesterone into oestrogen[8]. In guinea-pigs, non-human primates and humans progesterone production is from the placenta and so is not affected in this way by luteolysis. No such shift in steroidogenesis occurs since the 17α-hydroxylase enzyme is not expressed in primate placenta. However, progesterone is essential for pregnancy maintenance and progesterone inhibitors can induce labour onset in humans and other primates.

The mechanisms by which progesterone acts to maintain uterine quiescence have been assessed by studying the biochemical changes which occur in association with labour. In sheep, the timing of gap junction formation corresponds with the changing oestrogen:progesterone ratio[9]. Gap junctions are protein channels between cells formed by the alignment of connexin (Cx) proteins in neighbouring cells. Hendrix et al.[9] followed immunoreactive Cx 43 in rats and found a diffuse staining throughout the cytoplasm several days before the onset of labour which shifted to the Golgi apparatus and was then present in plaques within myometrial cells hours prior to labour onset. Rats in whom progesterone was supplemented and therefore did not undergo a progesterone withdrawal still underwent trafficking of Cx 43 from the endoplasmic reticulum to the Golgi but no further. Junction formation in the myometrial plasma membranes was never achieved. These data demonstrate that one action of progesterone is as a repressor of gap junction formation[10].

Progesterone also represses contractility by desensitizing the uterus to the action of the most powerful uterotonic, oxytocin, through an effect on the oxytocin receptor. Grazzini et al.[11] found that progesterone caused reduced binding of ligand to the oxytocin receptor in rat uteri with no effect on receptor binding affinity. They then used Chinese hamster ovary (CHO) cells expressing the rat oxytocin receptor to demonstrate that this inhibition was achieved through a direct interaction of the oxytocin receptor with progesterone.

Available intracellular calcium levels are also depleted by progesterone[12]. This calcium is not only involved in myosin–actin interactions but may also explain the inhibitory effect of progesterone on the release of arachidonic acid as calcium is required for phospholipase activity[13]. In early pregnancy progesterone also inhibits expression of the inflammatory mediators interleukin-8 (IL-8) and cyclooxygenase-2 (COX-2)[14]. In cattle, antiprogestins induce labour and the animals require less intervention than when administered uterotonics alone. This circumstantial evidence suggests that progesterone does have an inhibitory effect on cervical ripening, which may be mediated by the inhibition of IL-8 and IL-1β. Progesterone therefore functions to repress the translocation of gap junction proteins, the function of the oxytocin receptor, expression of proinflammatory cytokines and the availability of intracellular calcium, each of which is required for the onset of human labour.

Structural changes in cervix, fetal membranes and myometrium

Although progesterone withdrawal has not been shown in primates there is upregulation of cytokines such as IL-8 that are repressed by the presence of progesterone leading to structural changes within the uterus. Interleukin-8 acts as a chemoattractant for neutrophils that invade the cervical tissue, fetal membranes and myometrium. These neutrophils release matrix metalloproteinases (collagenases) which disrupt the collagen structure of the cervix. The proteoglycan concentration increases and the associated increase in hydrophilic glycosaminoglycans increases the water content. The cervix then becomes soft and compliant ready for labour to induce dilation.

The fetal membranes also undergo structural changes particularly at one specific site which will eventually be involved in membrane rupture. This site has been shown to overlay the cervix and the changes involved in this process are so similar to that described for cervical ripening that McLaren and Bell have proposed this as the 'site of fetal membrane ripening'[15-17]. Matrix metalloproteinases disrupt the collagen fibres, there is dissociation of the layers that make up the fetal membranes and a thickening of the spongy layer that separates the amnion from the chorion. Together these structural changes lead to a significantly thinner and weaker region in the fetal membranes. These structural changes appear to begin some 3–4 weeks prior to the onset of labour, at a time when PG synthesis is known to be increasing.

The active phase of labour is recognized by fetal membrane rupture, regular synchronized contractions of the myometrium driven by a single pace-maker, and dilation of the ripened cervix leading to expulsion of the fetus. The contractility of myocytes requires increased intracellular calcium (Ca^{2+}). Calcium forms a complex with calmodulin (CaM); this Ca^{2+}–CaM complex activates the myosin light chain kinase to phosphorylate myosin that enables it to interact with actin. The interaction of myosin and actin shortens the muscle fibrils and therefore shortens the cells. Relaxation is driven by cyclic AMP, which causes the dephosphorylation of the myosin light chain and sub-sequent dissociation from actin. To achieve effective labour these isolated contractile events within each cell must be synchronized across the whole structure of the uterus. Conductivity, or the cell to cell propagation of the action potential is therefore also fundamental to labour onset. Gap junctions are the specialized areas of intimate contact between cells that allows this com-munication to occur. Gap junction formation within the myometrium is repressed by progesterone but increased by oestrogen. A gradual increase in the number of gap junctions in myometrium prior to the onset of labour has been shown in rats and humans as a key step to myometrial conductance and therefore successful labour[18,19].

PROSTAGLANDINS AND LABOUR

Prostaglandin-related mouse knockout experiments

Transgenic mice with knockouts for COX-1 or COX-2 have been reported[20–22]. Surprisingly, COX-1 knockout mice lack the gastrointestinal lesions that would be expected, given the importance of COX-1 mediated PG synthesis in the stomach. This may be because pharmacological inhibition of COX leaves intact the peroxidase activity. The only serious deficiency found in homozygous COX-1 knockout mice was their failure to produce viable off-spring when homozygous mice were cross-bred. Heterozygotes of either sex, when mated with homozygotes, produced litters of normal size and survival, indicating that COX-1 expression in only 50% of pups or their placentas is sufficient for the health of the entire litter. Breeding studies with COX-1 knockout mice ruled out the need for COX-1 during ovulation or spermato-genesis, but suggested an essential requirement for COX-1 during mouse par-turition. Gross et al.[23] reported delayed luteolysis in COX-1 knockouts with no increase in $PGF_{2\alpha}$ production on day 19 that would normally precede luteo-lysis and progesterone withdrawal. There was no effect on PGE_2 production and parturition would continue normally if luteolysis was compensated for.

The first report of a COX-2 knockout mouse by Morham et al.[21] showed that homozygous COX-2 knockout mice begin to die at around 8 weeks of age, with few surviving for as long as 16 weeks. All tissues examined in these mice were normal except the kidney. Nephropathy was seen by 6 weeks in these animals, which increased in severity until death. Examination of COX-2-deleted mice embryos showed that kidney maturation had ceased prematurely after only a small percentage of nephrons had developed, with the vast majority of glomeruli and tubules remaining small and immature. During postnatal life the small number of overworked functional nephrons begin to atrophy, with the development of glomerulosclerosis, interstitial inflammation and fibrosis ultimately leading to kidney failure. In those mice that survived to adulthood, kidney lesions ranged from mild to severe with more severe lesions being more common in female than male homozygotes. This clearly shows an important role for COX-2 in the embryological development of the kidney in mice.

Fertility in COX-2 knockout mice was also dramatically reduced. Lim et al.[22] found that the number of ovulations is reduced in COX-2 knockout mice. Follicular development is normal in these mice but administration of exogenous gonadotrophin did not restore ovulation number. This finding is consistent with previous studies showing that gonadotrophins upregulate COX-2 during follicular development. Transfer of normal mouse blastocysts into COX-2 knockout recipients resulted in implantation failure, as did specific pharmacological inhibition of COX-2 in normal or heterozygous knockout animals, indicating a central role for COX-2 in mouse ovulation, implantation and decidualization.

To define the origin and site of action of PGs involved in stimulation of uterine contractions and cervical ripening and in maintenance of the patency of the ductus arteriosus Reese et al.[24] analysed COX-1-knockout mice and the effect of pharmacological inhibition of COX-2. They found that the mouse uterine epithelium is the major source of PGs during labour and that COX-1-knockout females experience parturition failure that is reversible by exogenous PGs. Using embryo transfer experiments, they showed that successful delivery occurs in COX-1-knockout recipient mothers carrying wild-type pups, showing that fetal PGs are sufficient for parturition. Although patency of the ductus arteriosus is PG dependent, they found neither COX-1 nor COX-2 expression in the fetal or postnatal ductus, although offspring with a double COX-1-knockout died shortly after birth with open ductus arteriosus. These results suggest that mouse ductus arteriosus patency depends on circulating PGs acting on specific receptors within the ductus.

These data suggest that, in mice COX-1 mediates PG synthesis with spontaneous labour onset. Reese et al.[24] suggested that their findings raise concern regarding the use of selective COX inhibitors for the management of preterm labour. Interestingly however, Gross et al.[25] found that specific inhibition of COX-2 inhibited lipopolysaccharide (LPS)-induced preterm labour in the mouse, suggesting that either COX-1 or COX-2 can mediate labour-associated PG synthesis in mice. As will be discussed below, there are major differences between mice and the human, which make conclusions about treatment of human pregnancy from the result of rodent experiments unsafe.

Whilst the respective roles of COX-1 and COX-2 in the menstrual cycle, ovulation and implantation may be similar in mice and humans, there appear to be fundamental differences both in the general mechanism of the onset of parturition and in the roles of COX-1 and COX-2 in parturition between the primate and the rodent. The corpus luteum regresses in the first trimester of human pregnancy and progesterone synthesis is taken over by the placenta. There is no large scale withdrawal of progesterone in the human prior to parturition, although it has been suggested that there may be local withdrawal within the fetal membranes or changes in the expression or activity of the progesterone receptor which leads to 'functional' progesterone withdrawal. Although in the mouse COX-1 mediated PGs appear to be important for progesterone withdrawal at term and the subsequent onset of normal parturition, in the human luteolysis is not the driving force for parturition and it is expression of COX-2 rather than COX-1 which increases within the uterus at term. As discussed below it is doubtful whether COX-1 plays any significant role in the onset of human labour.

PROSTAGLANDIN RECEPTORS

Eight PG receptors (P receptors), have been identified. EP_1–EP_4 show greatest affinity for PGE_2, FP is the $PGF_{2\alpha}$ receptor, TP the thromboxane receptor, IP the prostacyclin receptor, and DP the PGD_2 receptor. These receptors can also be characterized into two groups according to their effect on myometrial contractions. EP_1, EP_3, FP and TP activation result in myometrial contraction, whilst EP_2, EP_4, IP and DP activation results in myometrial relaxation.

Hizaki et al.[26] demonstrated that EP_2 is required for cumulus expansion and successful fertilization using EP_2 knockout mice. Treatment with either PGE_2 or follicle stimulating hormone (FSH) restored expansion, demonstrating that PGs are not solely responsible for this process, although the fertility of these mice was also reduced. After ovulation the cumulus–oocyte complex is no longer under the influence of FSH but is still found to produce PGE_2 via COX-2 expression and continue expansion and fertilization. If this PGE_2 is unable to complete expansion due to the lack of EP_2 receptors or COX-2 the immature oocyte is unable to undergo fertilization. It is clear that FSH can begin cumulus expansion but that in the absence of PGs this is not sustainable and fertilization fails.

FP knockout mice do not undergo luteolysis or the associated withdrawal of progesterone. Oestrogen levels are unaffected, which results in a markedly abnormal oestrogen:progesterone ratio in favour of progesterone. Ovariectomy performed on these mice causes luteolysis, progesterone withdrawal and subsequent labour onset. This suggests that it is $PGF_{2\alpha}$ that is the critical PG involved in luteolysis in mice and that this is produced from the ovary[27]. As discussed above, luteolysis occurs much earlier in human pregnancy than it does in the mouse; however, this is also directed by $PGF_{2\alpha}$ through the FP receptor. The decline in human chronic gonadotrophin (HCG) and rise in progesterone as the corpus luteum ages stimulates increased FP receptor expression and leads to luteolysis[28].

In rats, $PGF_{2\alpha}$ binding to its FP receptor causes activation of phospholipase C, production of IP_3, calcium mobilization and myometrial contraction. However, mRNA for both the FP and the EP_2 receptors were shown to increase towards term, although with labour FP continues to increase whilst the relaxatory EP_2 receptor decreases[29,30]. Progesterone treatment prevents this increase in FP expression, decrease in EP_2 and the onset of labour. Again as in the mouse, ovariectomy will reverse this effect and labour proceeds. The progesterone antagonist RU486 reduced EP_2 and increased FP mRNA expression, whilst an oestrogen inhibitor was able to reduce FP mRNA but had no effect on EP_2 mRNA[30].

In sheep, where labour is preceded by a change in steroidogenesis, there is conflicting data. Ma et al.[31] measured mRNA levels of all the PG receptors by Northern blot analysis and found a labour-associated increase in EP_3, EP_4 and FP receptors. No change in the expression of EP_2 and EP_1 was detected[31]. However, using reverse transcriptase-polymerase chain reaction (RT-PCR), Gyomorey et al.[32] have reported no change in any of the receptors.

Human prostaglandin receptors

In human myometrium the relaxatory EP_2 receptor has been found to decrease through gestation to a minimum at term prior to labour. The contractile receptor FP was also found in higher concentrations preterm and was reported by Brodt-Eppley et al.[33] to decrease with increasing gestational age to term but then to increase significantly in association with the onset of labour. Matsumoto et al.[34] reported that the expression of both contractile receptors FP and EP_3 fell in early pregnancy compared with non-pregnant controls by 55% and 60%, respectively, but that this level was then maintained through gestation. However, they did not study the changes associated with labour onset.

It seems likely that PG receptor expression differs between fundus and lower segment, underlying the different functions of these two areas of uterus. The uterine fundus is the major area of contraction generation whereas the lower segment behaves more like the cervix by stretching and dilating to allow the passage of the fetus. In the baboon, the lower uterine segment was found to contain a higher proportion of the relaxatory EP_2 and lower proportion of the contractile EP_3 receptors compared with the fundus and corpus[35]. In the human both the EP_2 and EP_3 receptors have been identified in the lower segment but, through difficulties in acquiring human tissue, studies have not yet confirmed the distribution pattern of these receptors throughout the entire uterus. Several alternate splice variants of the EP_3 receptor have been described. The EP_{3-1b} splice variant was decreased by misoprostol treatment and it has been suggested that this is the specific subtype involved in human labour onset. In the fetal membranes and decidua the EP_3 receptor is present but does not change with labour but the EP_1 receptor is increased with labour onset[36].

WISH cells, a cell line derived from the amnion, express both EP_1 and EP_3 receptors. IL-1β treatment induces PGE_2 expression and increases the expression of both receptors. Oestrogen causes only a small rise in PGE_2 release and increases only the EP_1 receptor. Aspirin and indomethacin decrease PGE_2 but increase receptor expression by twofold. Corticotrophin releasing hormone (CRH) also increases EP_1 receptor expression in WISH cells, which is not effected by indomethacin, whilst the PGE_2 response is reduced.

The currently available data suggest that it is the relaxatory receptor EP_2 that is required for cervical effacement and the EP_3 receptor and possibly the EP_{3-1b} subtype that is most important for human labour-associated contractions in the myometrium.

PROSTAGLANDIN SYNTHESIS AND METABOLISM

PGs are formed from the precursor arachidonic acid, which is esterified and stored as part of neutral lipids and phospholipids. Liberation of the free/unbound arachidonic acid requires the action of a phospholipase, usually phospholipase A_2 (PLA_2). Five forms of cellular PLA_2 have been identified. Secretory ($sPLA_2$) types I–IV, are low molecular weight enzymes containing several disulphide bridges and require millimolar concentrations of calcium for activity. The fifth form is of larger molecular weight and is a cytosolic enzyme ($cPLA_2$), contains no disulphide bridges and requires only micromolar concentrations of calcium for activity. The phospholipase activity within the uterus has been shown to be due to $sPLA_2$ types II and IV and $cPLA_2$. Secretory PLA_2 type II is the main phospholipase in the placenta and $cPLA_2$ the main constituent of the amnion[37]. Total phospholipase activity has been demonstrated to be two- or threefold higher in the amnion than in choriodecidua or placenta but this does not change with the onset of labour[38]. D. Slater and colleagues (personal communication) have shown that in fetal membranes $cPLA_2$ is the predominant form, whilst in placenta $sPLA_2$ predominates. They found that there is no change in $sPLA_2$ expression within the uterus during pregnancy or with the onset of labour. Skannal et al.[39] found that $cPLA_2$ activity in fetal membranes increases during pregnancy and is highest in anticipation of labour. Together these data suggest that it is $cPLA_2$ and not $sPLA_2$ that mediates the release of bound arachidonic acid in fetal membranes, and specifically the amnion, with the onset of human labour. However, Munns et al.[38] performed activity studies, showing there is no change in phospholipase activity with labour and suggested that previous authors who have demonstrated changes have not used a sensitive enough extraction procedure. There remains doubt therefore about the relative importance of PLA_2 expression of activity in regulation of the PG synthesis associated with labour.

Free arachidonic acid is a substrate for at least three enzyme groups: the COX enzyme pathway, which produces PGs; the lipoxygenase (LOX) enzyme pathway, which produces a series of hydroxyeicosatetraenoic acids (HETEs); and the epoxygenase pathways, producing epoxyeicosatetraenoic acids. Prior to labour endogenous arachidonic acid metabolism in the amnion is principally via the LOX enzyme pathways. With the onset of human labour, there is an increase in arachidonic acid metabolism, a change in the ratio of LOX to COX activity and therefore dramatically increased synthesis of PGE_2 [ref. 40].

COX has a short half-life and undergoes destruction after a limited number of reactions[41]. The evidence that the amnion produces predominately LOX metabolites of arachidonic acid before labour, and the change in the ratio of LOX:COX metabolism with labour, suggests that the activities of the two enzymes COX and PLA_2 must be independently regulated[40,42].

Two COX isoforms are known: the constitutively expressed COX-1 and the inducible COX-2[43,44]. *In situ* hybridization localized the COX-1 isoform to the chorionic mesoderm[45] and COX-2 to the amniotic epithelium and mesoderm. In term human amnion, COX-2 mRNA expression is approximately 100 times higher than COX-1[46]. Slater et al.[46] showed that the mRNA levels of COX-1 do not change significantly through gestation and with labour onset, whereas COX-2 mRNA increases steadily throughout gestation with a significant increase at term. COX-2 protein concentrations in amnion also increased from the first trimester to term with a further increase with the onset of labour (Figures 1, 2 and 3). Interestingly, although COX-1 mRNA concentrations remained very low and did not change with labour, COX-1 protein concentrations were similar to those of COX-2, although there were no gestation or labour associated changes[47]. Both Sawdy et al.[48] and Sadovsky et al.[49] used highly COX-1 and COX-2 selective inhibitors to show that although COX-1 protein is present within the amnion and choriodecidua at term it plays no role in the synthesis of PGs involved in the onset of human labour (Figure 3). Similarly in the mouse, Gross et al.[25] found that specific inhibition of COX-2 inhibited LPS-induced preterm labour.

The increase in COX-2 mRNA, protein and activity begins in the third trimester of pregnancy several weeks before the onset of labour. This demonstrates that the fetal membranes, and in particular the amnion, have the capacity to synthesize PGs several weeks prior to the onset of labour at term (Figure 2). It is likely that this is counterbalanced by the activity of PG dehydrogenase (PGDH) which metabolizes PGs. Within the human uterus oxidation of the

Figure 1 Production of PGE_2 by fetal membranes from endogenous sources. PG production increases from first to third trimester but is decreased in tissues obtained after vaginal delivery. This suggests that the time of maximum PG synthesis in fetal membranes is at term before the clinical onset of labour ($n = 5$ per group, mean $\pm$ SEM, * indicates significantly different to all other groups ($P < 0.05$). (Adapted from ref. 47.)

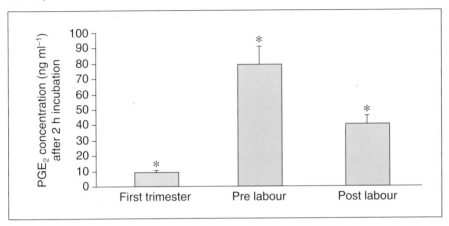

15-hydroxyl group of PGs is catalysed almost entirely by NAD^+-dependent PGDH. Chorionic trophoblast cells are strongly immunoreactive for PGDH[50] and probably inactivate all PGs synthesized by the amnion or chorion and some of those synthesized by decidua during pregnancy. There is now good evidence that fetal membrane PGDH activity is upregulated by progesterone and downregulated by cortisol and by anti-progestagens. Sangha et al.[51] have shown a decrease in expression of PGDH with the onset of labour. This same group have also demonstrated that a subgroup of patients presenting in 'idiopathic' preterm labour have reduced expression of chorionic PGDH both at the mRNA and protein levels. Similarly van Meir et al.[52,53] have shown a labour-associated reduction in PGDH activity in chorion near to the cervix and that chorioamnionitis, leading to preterm delivery, is associated with reduced chorionic PGDH expression. John Challis et al.[51-53] have suggested that PGDH activity in the fetal membranes may be controlled by the opposing effects of progesterone and cortisol acting in both an autocrine and more local paracrine manner.

The regulation of cyclooxygenase-2 within the uterus: the role of NF-κB

The promoter of the human COX-2 gene contains several putative transcription factor binding sites, including a cyclic AMP response element (CRE), a nuclear factor interleukin-6 (NF-IL-6) site and two nuclear factor-kappa (NF-κB) sites (Figure 4). Each of these has been demonstrated in various cells to regulate COX-2 transcription. COX-2 has been shown to

Figure 2 Expression of COX-2 in amnion, choriodecidua and myometrium, throughout pregnancy and before and after labour. Tissues were obtained at term, elective caesarian, emergency caesarian (myometrium) or postdelivery (membranes). Expression measured by qRT-PCR. There is increased COX-2 expression with advancing gestational age and again with the clinical onset of labour. The earlier rise in COX-2 expression may represent the development of a store of enzyme whilst the increase at term and again during labour may represent the need to replace COX-2 at a time of maximum PG synthesis. (Adapted from ref. 47.)

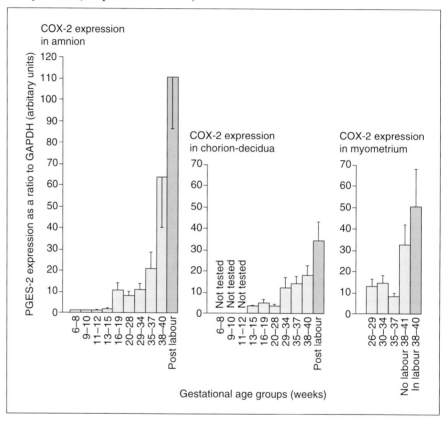

require both the NF-IL-6 and CRE transcription factor binding site for expression after treatment with LPS and phorbol myristate acetate (PMA) in bronchial airway epithelial cells[54] and both the AP-1 and CRE binding proteins are required in human chondrocytes[55]. The transcription factor NF-κB has also been shown to be involved in the regulation of COX-2 transcription in many different cell types including: bronchial epithelial cells[56]; immortalized human myometrial cells[57]; HUVEC and HMEC-1[58]; HERE human brain[59]; and WISH cells, rheumatoid synoviocytes and U937 cells[54].

NF-κB is a transcription factor whose effect on transcription is known to be regulated by cytokines such as IL-1β[60]. NF-κB functions as homo- or heterodimers of the Rel family of proteins, which in vertebrates includes p50,

Figure 3 Production of PGE_2 by intact fetal membranes in tissue culture. Membranes were selected on the basis of high PG production which could not be further stimulated by IL-1β. Membranes cultured with either SC-236 or SC-560 were not simultaneously exposed to IL-1β. IC_{50} indicates the concentration at which 50% enzyme inhibition occurs ($n = 6$ per group, mean ± SEM, * indicates significantly different to control ($P < 0.05$ Student's t test). These data show that COX-1 plays little or no role in the synthesis of PGs in human fetal membranes at term. Similar data, not shown, show that COX-2 is also solely responsible for PG synthesis in fetal membranes collected following preterm labour. (Adapted from ref. 48.)

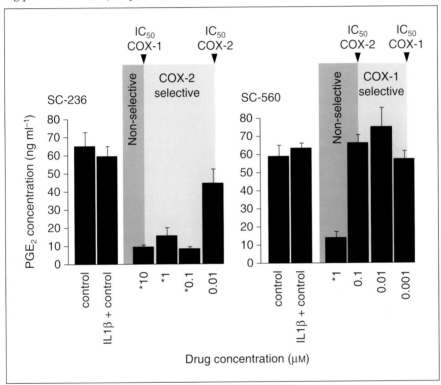

p65, c-Rel, p52 and RelB[61]. The most common combination of subunits is a heterodimer of the p50 and p65 proteins. NF-κB normally exists in the cytoplasm of cells bound by a member of the inhibitor kappa B (IκB) protein family. NF-κB activation by inducers, such as IL-1β leads to phosphorylation and degradation of the IκB protein, allowing NF-κB translocation to the nucleus where it can then bind to specific sites within the promoter sequence of target genes.

Studies in the amnion epithelium derived WISH cell line

To show the induction of PG production in the amnion epithelium-derived WISH cell line by IL-1β, we treated cells with increasing concentrations of IL-1β, which caused a dose-dependent increase in PGE_2 production from

Figure 4 The COX-2 promoter. A schematic diagram representing the COX-2 promoter, which has the features of a rapid response gene including two NF-κB sites and one AP-1 site, and constructs used in transient transfection studies. Putative transcription factor binding sites are represented in the promoter and position in the constructs is represented by a solid line. (Adapted from ref. 76.)

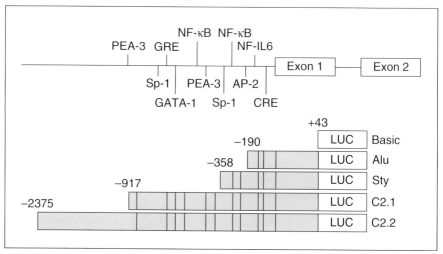

WISH cells. This increase was associated with an increase in COX-2 expression. COX-2 mRNA concentration increased after 15 min, peaking at approximately 1.5 h and maintaining this level up to 24 h of IL-1β treatment (Figure 5). Using a deletion series of the COX-2 promoter in a luciferase (LUC) reporter vector transiently transfected into WISH cells we found that 2.2 kb of upstream DNA is required for reliable upregulation by IL-1β treatment. Western blotting analysis of total protein extracted from WISH cells, which had been either non-stimulated or treated with IL-1β, demonstrated clearly the presence of both the p50 and p65 subunits of NF-κB. Analysis of WISH cells treated with IL-1β over a time course of 90 min showed the degradation and subsequent reappearance of the inhibitor (IκBα) protein, suggesting that with IL-1β treatment NF-κB is activated in WISH cells by the classical mechanism.

To determine whether the putative activation of NF-κB was transcriptionally active in these cells a LUC reporter construct containing six tandem repeats of the consensus NF-κB binding site was transiently transfected into WISH cells. Two control constructs were also used, containing either no transcription factor binding sites or six copies of a mutated consensus NF-κB site. Neither control construct showed any effect of IL-1β treatment but expression from the NF-κB dependent construct demonstrated a threefold increase in reporter expression with IL-1β treatment. Site-directed mutagenesis of the two NF-κB (–222 bp and (470 bp) DNA binding sites in the COX-2 promoter construct was performed. There was a significant reduction in reporter expression caused by mutation of each of the NF-κB sites.

Figure 5 IL-1β treatment of amnion-derived WISH cells increases PG synthesis. WISH cells were either non-stimulated (NS) or treated with a range of concentrations of IL-1β from 0.001 to 100 ng ml⁻¹ for 24 h. PGE_2 production was measured by radio-immunoassay. Data ($n = 6$) each performed in triplicate are expressed as ng PGE_2 μg⁻¹ of total protein and plotted as mean ± SEM.

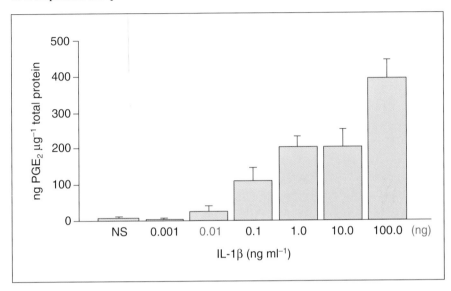

We have concluded that expression of COX-2 in the amnion epithelium-derived WISH cell line is regulated by NF-κB although there are also other factors that bind more upstream to the promoter that also play a role. Either transcription factor(s) bind within the upstream region of the promoter, between −1000 and −2200 bp, to cause transcriptional regulation, or the whole length of the promoter is required for regulation through the cooperative binding of several factors along the entire length of the promoter.

Studies in primary amnion epithelium cells

To assess differences in transcriptional activity due to the transcription factor NF-κB in association with labour in amnion cells we have used an NF-κB dependent LUC reporter construct transiently transfected into amnion cells. In amnion cells taken prior to the onset of labour at term LUC reporter activity is significantly increased with IL-1β treatment compared with non-stimulated cells. In amnion cells taken after spontaneous vaginal delivery at term, non-stimulated NF-κB driven reporter activity is significantly higher than in pre-labour cells but is not further increased by IL-1β treatment. This suggests that there is increased translocation of NF-κB to the nucleus in cells prior to labour which are stimulated with IL-1β and that this NF-κB is able to drive transcription of a synthetic 'promoter.' It also demonstrates that with the onset of labour there is significantly greater availability of NF-κB even in the non-stimulated cells and that this activity is at a maximum as it is not further increased by stimulus.

Electrophoretic mobility shift assays (EMSA) studies using nuclear proteins extracted from amnion cells demonstrate the ability of proteins present in the nucleus to bind to an oligonucleotide of the consensus NF-kB DNA binding site. In pre-labour nuclei there is very little protein binding but this is increased after stimulation with IL-1β. However, in post-labour amnion, protein binding in non-stimulated cells is significantly greater than in pre-labour cells (both with and without stimulation) and is further increased by IL-1β treatment.

There is an apparent discrepancy in post-labour cells between the increased protein binding seen by EMSA analysis after IL-1β treatment and the lack of increase in reporter expression in transfection studies under the same conditions. This may be because the maximum response from the reporter has been reached. Alternatively, the increase in binding seen in the EMSA may be due to the binding of NF-κB that is unable to drive expression of the reporter.

The specific effect of NF-κB on the transcription from the COX-2 promoter has been studied by mutating both of the two NF-κB sites individually within 2200 bp of the human COX-2 promoter. Mutation of the downstream NF-κB DNA binding site showed significantly less reporter expression than the wild-type COX-2 promoter only in post-labour amnion cells. However, mutation of the upstream NF-κB DNA binding site significantly reduced reporter expression in both pre- and post-labour amnion cells. NF-κB therefore appears to be essential for the transcriptional regulation of COX-2 in primary amnion cells both pre- and post-labour.

The increase in NF-κB activity seen within the fetal membranes at term may explain the upregulation of some genes, such as IL-8 whose expression is repressed by progesterone, despite there being no progesterone withdrawal in the human. There is a mutual negative interaction between NF-κB and the progesterone receptor in some cell types[62]. Using co-transfection of a progesterone receptor expression vector with an NF-κB reporter or an NF-κB expression vector with a progesterone receptor reporter we have shown that this mutual repression functions in both amnion and myometrial cells. It is possible that the increased activity of NF-κB seen in amnion cells both increases the expression of COX-2 and other NF-κB dependent genes and contributes to 'functional' progesterone withdrawal through an interaction with the progesterone receptor.

THE CLINICAL USE OF COX-2 SELECTIVE NSAIDS TO PREVENT PRETERM DELIVERY

Preterm labour remains a significant problem in modern obstetric practice. It occurs in up to 10% of all births but accounts for over 85% of perinatal deaths and an unknown proportion of mental and physical handicaps[63]. Although there has been little improvement in therapeutic options to prevent preterm delivery in the last decade, advances in neonatal intensive care have brought improvements in survival rates for preterm infants. However there is an increase in cerebral palsy in low birth-weight infants as a result of improved survival of impaired infants[64]. Perinatal mortality falls after 28 weeks and intact survival rates increase exponentially with increasing gestational age. Reducing the incidence of delivery at gestational ages below 30 weeks would make the largest impact on perinatal mortality and morbidity. There is a degree of overlap between early preterm delivery (i.e. 24–30 weeks) and late second trimester pregnancy loss (i.e. 20–24 weeks). It is likely that the same mechanism acts to cause many cases of both early preterm delivery and late second trimester pregnancy loss.

As discussed above, during pregnancy the uterus expands to accommodate the growing fetus while the cervix remains rigid and closed. Prior to labour the cervix remodels to allow effacement and dilation and the uterus begins to contract. These biochemical events resemble an inflammatory reaction. There is increased synthesis of PGs and of inflammatory cytokines. PGs play a central role in labour – they act to ripen the cervix, relax the lower segment of the uterus and stimulate fundally dominant contractions.

The central role of inflammatory biochemistry in cervical ripening, and myometrial contractility, suggests that NSAIDs may play a role in prevention of late second trimester loss or early preterm delivery. Although their use is limited by fetal side effects, PG synthesis inhibitors are powerful tocolytics[65]. Indomethacin, a COX inhibitor, is highly effective in preventing the contractions that occur during preterm labour. It is more effective in short term prolongation of pregnancy than the sympathomimetics and, unlike sympathomemetics, it can significantly reduce the risk of delivery preterm[64]. The use of indomethacin is limited by fetal side effects. Reduced fetal urine output occurs through reduced renal blood flow and by reduced PGE-mediated inhibition of arginine vasopressin in the collecting duct[66,67]. Constriction of the ductus arteriosus[68,69] is presumably mediated through suppressed synthesis of vasodilator PGs produced either by the ductus or suppressed synthesis of circulating PGs produced elsewhere.

Since all of the PG synthesis within the fetal membranes in the human is via COX-2 whether at term or preterm, it seems probable that COX-2 selective NSAIDs would have the same tocolytic efficacy as indomethacin but might have fewer fetal and maternal side effects through sparing COX-1-mediated PG synthesis.

Nimesulide is an NSAID that shows ten- to 100-fold selectivity for COX-2[70]. We have recently shown that nimesulide is also a calcium channel blocker[71]. We reported the use of nimesulide in prevention of preterm labour in a single case, in the *Lancet* in 1997 in which long term exposure was not associated with significant fetal side effects and the pregnancy outcome was good[72]. Since that time we, and others, have recognized that nimesulide causes oligo-hydramnios in 50% of exposed fetuses, although this takes several weeks to develop. Peruzzi et al.[73] reported prolonged renal failure and immature glomerulogenesis in a premature neonate after prolonged *in utero* exposure to nimesulide and we have also seen a similar case. Fetal or neonatal renal failure may be due to inhibition of fetal renal COX-2 or COX-1. COX-2 appears late in pregnancy in the human fetal kidney and is thought to regulate renal blood flow, whereas COX-1 plays a more important role in glomerulogenesis[74]. Nimesulide has a relatively long plasma half-life and is known to accumulate in tissues. Oligohydramnios may take up to 4 weeks before it appears. This may be due to fetal renal accumulation of nimesulide or to a gradual increase in fetal concentrations secondary to the long half-life. It is possible that tissue or plasma accumulation leads to nimesulide concentrations sufficient to inhibit COX-1.

In patch-clamp experiments we have found that both indomethacin and nimesulide are calcium channel blockers[71]. Whilst this effect is not seen with pharmacologically relevant concentrations of indomethacin, nimesulide treatment probably leads to concentrations sufficient to block calcium channels. It is probably through blockade of calcium channels that both indomethacin and nimesulide inhibit myometrial contractility *in vitro*. In our experience, other NSAIDs have little effect upon spontaneous myometrial contractility *in vitro* at concentrations that should block myometrial PG synthesis. Nimesulide may therefore also reduce fetal renal blood flow through calcium channel blockade-mediated hypotension. It is not certain therefore that the fetal side effects of nimesulide are due solely to inhibition of COX-2.

Despite these fetal side effects nimesulide compares favourably with indomethacin as a long term therapy option. Indomethacin is associated with a 15% incidence of neonatal pulmonary hypertension[75], whereas the fetal renal effects of nimesulide are reversible provided that there is adequate surveil-lance. Nimesulide should be reserved, however, for cases at very high risk of early preterm delivery and should only be used where regular surveillance of amniotic fluid volume can be ensured. Clinical trials are now underway in our unit to determine whether the coxibs, rather than other selective inhibitors of COX-2, may have an improved fetal safety profile. In the longer term it is possible that drugs that specifically target the NF-κB transcription factor system may be used to prevent preterm delivery.

REFERENCES

1. Denison FC, Calder AA, Kelly RW. The action of prostaglandin E$_2$ on the human cervix: stimulation of interleukin 8 and inhibition of secretory leukocyte protease inhibitor. *Am J Obstet Gynecol.* 1999;180:614–20.

2. Crankshaw DJ, Dyal R. Effects of some naturally occurring prostanoids and some cyclooxygenase inhibitors on the contractility of the human lower uterine segment *in vitro*. *Can J Physiol Pharmacol.* 1994;72:870–4.

3. Liggins G. Initiation of labour. *Biology of the neonate.* 1989;55:366–75.

4. Garfield RE, Blennerhassett MG, Miller SM. Control of myometrial contractility: role and regulation of gap junctions. *Oxf Rev Reprod Biol.* 1988;10:436–90.

5. Garfield RE, Hertzberg EL. Cell-to-cell coupling in the myometrium: Emil Bozler's prediction. *Prog Clin Biol Res.* 1990;327:673–81.

6. Lye S. The initiation and inhibition of labour – toward a molecular understanding. *Semin Reprod Endocrinol.* 1994;12:284–94.

7. Turnbull AC. *The Fetus and Birth.* London: Elsevier; 1977.

8. Brooks AN, Challis JR. Regulation of the hypothalamic–pituitary–adrenal axis in birth. *Can J Physiol Pharmacol.* 1988;66:1106–12.

9. Hendrix E, Mao S, Everson W, Larsen W. Myometrial connexin 43 trafficking and gap junction assembly at term and in preterm labor. *Mol Reprod Dev.* 1992;33:27–38.

10. Hendrix E, Myatt L, Sellers S, Russell P, Larsen W. Steroid hormone regulation of rat myometrial gap junction formation: effects on cx43 levels and trafficking. *Biol Reprod.* 1995;52:547–60.

11. Grazzini E, Guillon G, Mouillac B, Zingg H. Inhibition of oxytocin receptor function by direct binding of progesterone. *Nature.* 1998;392:509–12.

12. Carsten ME. Calcium accumulation by human uterine microsomal preparations: effects of progesterone and oxytocin. *Am J Obstet Gynecol.* 1979;133:598–601.

13. Wilson T, Liggins GC, Aimer GP, Watkins EJ. The effect of progesterone on the release of arachidonic acid from human endometrial cells stimulated by histamine. *Prostaglandins.* 1986;31:343–60.

14. Elliott CL, Kelly RW, Critchley HO, Riley SC, Calder AA. Regulation of interleukin 8 production in the term human placenta during labor and by antigestagens. *Am J Obstet Gynecol.* 1998;179:215–20.

15. McLaren J, Malak TM, Bell SC. Structural characteristics of term human fetal membranes prior to labour: identification of an area of altered morphology overlying the cervix. *Hum Reprod.* 1999;14:237–41.

16. McLaren J, Taylor DJ, Bell SC. Increased incidence of apoptosis in non-labour-affected cytotrophoblast cells in term fetal membranes overlying the cervix. *Hum Reprod.* 1999;14:2895–900.

17. McLaren J, Taylor DJ, Bell SC. Increased concentration of pro-matrix metalloproteinase 9 in term fetal membranes overlying the cervix before labor: implications for membrane remodeling and rupture. *Am J Obstet Gynecol.* 2000;182:409–16.

18. Fuchs AR, Fuchs F. Endocrinology of human parturition: a review. *Br J Obstet Gynaecol.* 1984;91:948–67.

19. Garfield RE, Thilander G, Blennerhassett MG, Sakai N. Are gap junctions necessary for cell-to-cell coupling of smooth muscle? An update. *Can J Physiol Pharmacol.* 1992;70:481–90.

20. Langenbach R, Morham SG, Tiano HF, Loftin CD, Ghanayem BI, Chulada PC et al. PG synthase 1 gene disruption in mice reduces arachidonic acid-induced inflammation and indomethacin-induced gastric ulceration. *Cell.* 1995;83:483–92.

21. Morham SG, Langenbach R, Loftin CD, Tiano HF, Vouloumanos N, Jennette JC et al. PG synthase 2 gene disruption causes severe renal pathology in the mouse. *Cell.* 1995;83:473–82.

22. Lim H, Paria BC, Das SK, Dinchuk JE, Langenbach R, Trzaskos JM et al. Multiple female reproductive failures in cyclooxygenase 2-deficient mice. *Cell.* 1997;91:197–208.

23. Gross GA, Imamura T, Luedke C, Vogt SK, Olson LM, Nelson DM et al. Opposing actions of PGs and oxytocin determine the onset of murine labor. *Proc Natl Acad Sci USA.* 1998;95:11875–9.

24. Reese J, Paria BC, Brown N, Zhao X, Morrow JD, Dey SK. Coordinated regulation of fetal and maternal PGs directs successful birth and postnatal adaptation in the mouse. *Proc Natl Acad Sci USA.* 2000;97:9759–64.

25. Gross G, Imamura T, Vogt SK, Wozniak DF, Nelson DM, Sadovsky Y et al. Inhibition of cyclooxygenase-2 prevents inflammation-mediated preterm labor in the mouse. *Am J Physiol.* 2000;278:R1415–23.

26. Hizaki H, Segi E, Sugimoto Y, Hirose M, Saji T, Ushikubi F et al. Abortive expansion of the cumulus and impaired fertility in mice lacking the prostaglandin E receptor subtype EP(2). *Proc Natl Acad Sci USA.* 1999;96:10501–6.

27. Sugimoto Y, Yamasaki A, Segi E, Tsuboi K, Aze Y, Nishimura T et al. Failure of parturition in mice lacking the prostaglandin F receptor. *Science,* 1997;277:681–3.

28. Ottander U, Leung CH, Olofsson JI. Functional evidence for divergent receptor activation mechanisms of luteotrophic and luteolytic events in the human corpus luteum. *Mol Hum Reprod.* 1999;5:391–5.

29. Ou CW, Chen ZQ, Qi S, Lye SJ. Expression and regulation of the messenger ribonucleic acid encoding the prostaglandin F(2alpha) receptor in the rat myometrium during pregnancy and labor. *Am J Obstet Gynecol.* 2000;182:919–25.

30. Dong YL, Yallampalli C. Pregnancy and exogenous steroid treatments modulate the expression of relaxant EP(2) and contractile FP receptors in the rat uterus. *Biol Reprod.* 2000;62:533–9.

31. Ma X, Wu WX, Nathanielsz PW. Differential regulation of prostaglandin EP and FP receptors in pregnant sheep myometrium and endometrium during spontaneous term labor. *Biol Reprod.* 1999;61:1281–6.

32. Gyomorey S, Lye SJ, Gibb W, Challis JR. Fetal-to-maternal progression of prostaglandin H(2) synthase-2 expression in ovine intrauterine tissues during the course of labor. *Biol Reprod.* 2000;62:797–805.

33. Brodt-Eppley J, Myatt L. Prostaglandin receptors in lower segment myometrium during gestation and labor. *Obstet Gynecol.* 1999;93:89–93.

34. Matsumoto T, Sagawa N, Yoshida M, Mori T, Tanaka I, Mukoyama M et al. The prostaglandin E2 and F2 alpha receptor genes are expressed in human myometrium and are down-regulated during pregnancy. *Biochem Biophys Res Commun.* 1997;238:838–41.

35. Smith GC, Baguma-Nibasheka M, Wu WX, Nathanielsz PW. Regional variations in contractile responses to PGs and prostanoid receptor messenger ribonucleic acid in pregnant baboon uterus. *Am J Obstet Gynecol.* 1998;179:1545–52.

36. Spaziani EP, O'Brien WF, Gould SF. The differential expression of CRH induced EP-1 receptors in myometrium. *J Soc Gynecol Invest.* 2000;7:124A.

37. Freed KA, Moses EK, Brennecke SP, Rice GE. Differential expression of type II, IV and cytosolic PLA$_2$ messenger RNA in human intrauterine tissues at term. *Mol Hum Reprod.* 1997;3:493–9.

38. Munns MJ, Farrugia W, King RG, Rice GE. Secretory type II PLA$_2$ immunoreactivity and PLA2 enzymatic activity in human gestational tissues before, during and after spontaneous-onset labour at term. *Placenta.* 1999;20:21–6.

39. Skannal DG, Brockman DE, Eis AL, Xue S, Siddiqi TA, Myatt L. Changes in activity of cytosolic phospholipase A$_2$ in human amnion at parturition. *Am J Obstet Gynecol*. 1997;177:179–84.

40. Bennett PR, Slater D, Sullivan M, Elder MG, Moore GE. Changes in amniotic arachidonic acid metabolism associated with increased cyclo-oxygenase gene expression. *Br J Obstet Gynaecol*. 1993;100:1037–42.

41. Marshall P, Kulmacz R, Lands W. Constraints on PG synthesis in tissues. *J Biol Chem*. 1979;262:3510–17.

42. Bennett PR, Rose MP, Myatt L, Elder MG. Preterm labor: stimulation of arachidonic acid metabolism in human amnion cells by bacterial products. *Am J Obstet Gynecol*. 1987;156:649–55.

43. Hla T, Farrell M, Kumar A, Bailey JM. Isolation of the cDNA for human prostaglandin H synthase. *Prostaglandins*. 1986;32:829–45.

44. O'Banion MK, Sadowski HB, Winn V, Young DA. A serum- and glucocorticoid-regulated 4-kilobase mRNA encodes a cyclooxygenase-related protein. *J Biol Chem*. 1991;266:23261–7.

45. Slater DM, Berger LC, Newton R, Moore GE, Bennett PR. Expression of cyclo-oxygenase types 1 and 2 in human fetal membranes at term. *Am J Obstet Gynecol*. 1995;172:77–82.

46. Slater D, Berger L, Newton R, Moore G, Bennett P. The relative abundance of type 1 to type 2 cyclo-oxygenase mRNA in human amnion at term. *Biochem Biophys Res Commun*. 1994;198:304–8.

47. Slater D, Dennes W, Sawdy R, Allport V, Bennett P. Expression of cyclo-oxygenase types-1 and -2 in human fetal membranes throughout pregnancy. *J Mol Endocrinol*. 1999;22:125–30.

48. Sawdy RJ, Slater DM, Dennes WJ, Sullivan MH, Bennett PR. The roles of the cyclo-oxygenases types one and two in PG synthesis in human fetal membranes at term. *Placenta*. 2000;21:54–7.

49. Sadovsky Y, Nelson DM, Muglia LJ, Gross GA, Harris KC, Koki A et al. Effective diminution of amniotic prostaglandin production by selective inhibitors of cyclo-oxygenase type 2. *Am J Obstet Gynecol*. 2000;182:370–6.

50. Cheung PY, Walton JC, Tai HH, Riley SC, Challis JR. Immunocytochemical distribution and localization of 15-hydroxy prostaglandin dehydrogenase in human fetal membranes, decidua, and placenta. *Am J Obstet Gynecol*. 1990;163:1445–9.

51. Sangha RK, Walton JC, Ensor CM, Tai HH, Challis JR. Immunohistochemical localization, messenger ribonucleic acid abundance, and activity of 15-hydroxy prostaglandin dehydrogenase in placenta and fetal membranes during term and preterm labor. *J Clin Endocrinol Metab*. 1994;78:982–9.

52. Van Meir CA, Ramirez MM, Matthews SG, Calder AA, Keirse MJ, Challis JR. Chorionic prostaglandin catabolism is decreased in the lower uterine segment with term labour. *Placenta*. 1997;18:109–14.

53. Van Meir CA, Sangha RK, Walton JC, Matthews SG, Keirse MJ, Challis JR. Immunoreactive 15-hydroxy prostaglandin dehydrogenase (PGDH) is reduced in fetal membranes from patients at preterm delivery in the presence of infection. *Placenta*. 1996;17:291–7.

54. Inoue H, Tanabe T. Transcriptional role of the nuclear factor kappa B site in the induction by lipopolysaccharide and suppression by dexamethasone of cyclooxygenase-2 in U937 cells. *Biochem Biophys Res Commun*. 1998;244:143–8.

55. Miller C, Zhang M, He Y, Zhao J, Pelletier JP, Martel-Pelletier J, Di Battista JA.

Transcriptional induction of cyclooxygenase-2 gene by okadaic acid inhibition of phosphatase activity in human chondrocytes: co-stimulation of AP-1 and CRE nuclear binding proteins. *J Cell Biochem*. 1998;69:392–413.

56. Newton R, Kuitert LM, Bergmann M, Adcock IM, Barnes PJ. Evidence for involvement of NF-kappaB in the transcriptional control of COX-2 gene expression by IL-1beta. *Biochem Biophys Res Commun*. 1997;237:28–32.

57. Belt AR, Baldassare JJ, Molnar M, Romero R, Hertelendy F. The nuclear transcription factor NF-kappaB mediates interleukin-1beta-induced expression of cyclooxygenase-2 in human myometrial cells. *Am J Obstet Gynecol*. 1999;181:359–66.

58. Schmedtje Jr JF, Ji YS, Liu WL, DuBois RN, Runge MS. Hypoxia induces cyclooxygenase-2 via the NF-kappaB p65 transcription factor in human vascular endothelial cells. *J Biol Chem*. 1997;272:601–8.

59. Lukiw WJ, Bazan G. Strong nuclear factor kappaB-DNA binding parallels cyclooxygenase-2 gene transcription in aging and in sporadic Alzheimer's disease superior temporal lobe neocortex. *J Neurosci Res*. 1998;53:583–92.

60. Croston GE, Cao Z, Goeddel DV. NF-kappa B activation by interleukin-1 (IL-1) requires an IL-1 receptor-associated protein kinase activity. *J Biol Chem*. 1995;270:16514–7.

61. Baldwin Jr AS. The NF-kappa B and I kappa B proteins: new discoveries and insights. *Annu Rev Immunol*. 1996;14:649–83.

62. Kalkhoven E, Wissink S, van der Saag PT, van der Burg B. Negative interaction between the RelA(p65) subunit of NF-kappaB and the progesterone receptor. *J Biol Chem*. 1996;271:6217–24.

63. Martius J, Eschenbach DA. The role of bacterial vaginosis as a cause of amniotic fluid infection, chorioamnionitis and prematurity – a review. *Arch Gynecol Obstet*. 1990;247:1–13.

64. Pharoah PO, Platt MJ, Cooke T. The changing epidemiology of cerebral palsy. *Arch Dis Child Fetal Neonatal Ed*. 1996;75:F169–73.

65. Keirse M. Indomethacin tocolysis in preterm labour. In: *Pregnancy and Childbirth*, Cochrane Database of Systematic Reviews. Oxford: Cochrane Collaboration; 1995:04383.

66. Kirshon B, Moise Jr KJ, Mari G, Willis R. Long-term indomethacin therapy decreases fetal urine output and results in oligohydramnios. *Am J Perinatol*. 1991;8:86–8.

67. Stevenson KM, Lumbers ER. Effects of indomethacin on fetal renal function, renal and umbilicoplacental blood flow and lung liquid production. *J Dev Physiol*. 1992;17:257–64.

68. Moise Jr KJ, Huhta JC, Sharif DS, Ou CN, Kirshon B, Wasserstrum N et al. Indomethacin in the treatment of premature labor. Effects on the fetal ductus arteriosus. *N Engl J Med*. 1988;319:327–31.

69. Moise Jr KJ. Effect of advancing gestational age on the frequency of fetal ductal constriction in association with maternal indomethacin use. *Am J Obstet Gynecol*. 1993;168:1350–3.

70. Vane JR, Bakhle YS, Botting RM. Cyclooxygenases 1 and 2. *Annu Rev Pharmacol Toxicol*. 1998;38:97–120.

71. Sawdy R, Knock GA, Bennett PR, Poston L, Aaronson PI. Effect of nimesulide and indomethacin on contractility and the Ca^{2+} channel current in myometrial smooth muscle from pregnant women. *Br J Pharmacol*. 1998;125:1212–7.

72. Sawdy R, Slater D, Fisk N, Edmonds DK, Bennett P. Use of a cyclo-oxygenase type-2-selective non-steroidal anti-inflammatory agent to prevent preterm delivery [letter]. *Lancet.* 1997;350:265–6.

73. Peruzzi L, Gianoglio B, Porcellini MG, Coppo R. Neonatal end-stage renal failure associated with maternal ingestion of cyclo-oxygenase-type-1 selective inhibitor nimesulide as tocolytic [letter]. *Lancet.* 1999;354:1615.

74. Kömhoff M, Grone HJ, Klein T, Seyberth HW, Nusing RM. Localization of cyclooxygenase-1 and -2 in adult and fetal human kidney: implication for renal function. *Am J Physiol.* 1997;272:460–8.

75. Besinger RE, Niebyl JR, Keyes WG, Johnson TR. Randomized comparative trial of indomethacin and ritodrine for the long-term treatment of preterm labor. *Am J Obstet Gynecol.* 1991;164:981–6.

12 | Cyclooxygenase-2 and the cardiovascular system

Jane A. Mitchell and Salome J. Stanford

Unit of Critical Care Medicine, Royal Brompton Hospital, NHLI Division, Imperial College School of Medicine, Sydney Street, London SW3 6NP, UK.

PROSTAGLANDINS AND CARDIOVASCULAR HOMEOSTASIS

Cell specific prostaglandin production

Following the liberation of the substrate, arachidonic acid, by phospholipase A_2, cyclooxygenases (COX) catalyse the conversion to prostaglandin G_2 (PGG_2) and prostaglandin H_2 (PGH_2). PGH_2 is then converted by downstream synthase enzymes to the full range of COX products[1]. In general, prostacyclin (PGI_2), thromboxane A_2 (TXA_2) and PGE_2 (Figure 1) are the most important COX products in the maintenance of vascular homeostasis. The synthesis of PGI_2 and TXA_2 is regulated by PGI_2 synthase and TXA_2 synthase, respectively. In contrast, PGE_2 can be formed by the action of PGE isomerase/synthase or from PGH_2, independently of a synthase pathway (Figure 2). Thus, in situations where COX is elevated, PGI_2 or TXA_2 synthase may become rate limiting and PGE_2 is produced in higher amounts. For this reason, PGE_2 and not PGI_2 or TXA_2, is often measured as a more direct index of COX activity. Endothelial cells from all sites in the cardiovascular tree express COX-1. In addition, they co-express PGI_2 synthase[2]. Thus, when stimulated, endothelial cells produce high levels of PGI_2 (Figure 2). Platelets, on the other hand, express COX-1 but contain high levels of TXA_2 synthase, with no PGI_2 synthase. Thus, when stimulated, platelets release TXA_2 (Figure 2).

Prostacyclin

PGI_2 activates prostacyclin receptors (IP) that are expressed on numerous cell types, including vascular smooth muscle and platelets. The human IP receptor was cloned and expressed in 1994 by two groups working independently[3,4].

Figure 1 Molecular structures of PGE$_2$, PGI$_2$ and TXA$_2$.

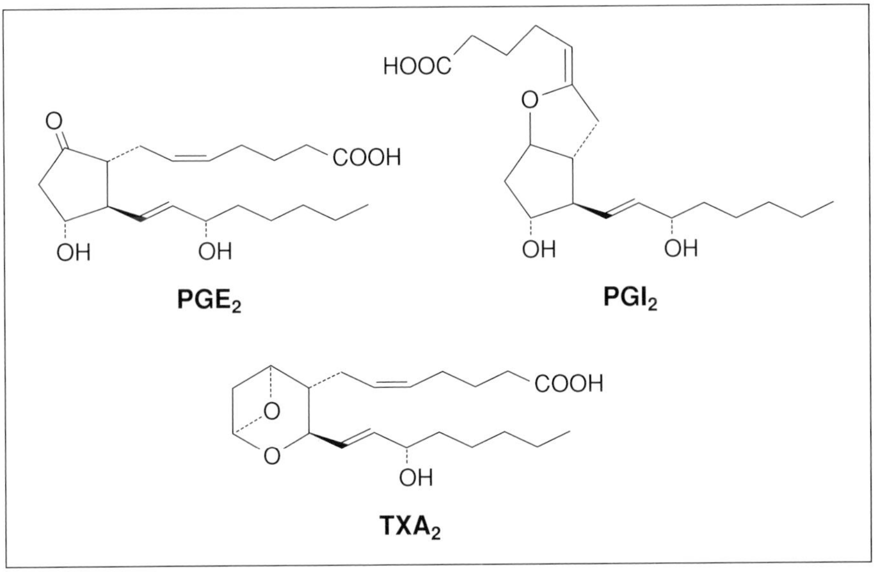

The receptor was found to consist of 386 amino acid residues with a predicted molecular mass of 40961, with seven putative transmembrane domains characteristic of G protein (G$_p$)-coupled receptors. There have been reports showing that, in transformed cells expressing IP receptors, ligand binding leads to activation of the inositol phosphate pathway, via a G$_p$ coupling, with subsequent increases in intracellular calcium. However, it was discovered that this pathway was of minor importance when cells transfected with IP receptors were studied[5]. In addition, IP receptors may couple directly to ion channels such as the ATP-sensitive K$^+$ channel[6], activation of which may account for some of the vasodilator properties of PGI$_2$[7]. Despite the suggested involvement of the inositol phosphate pathway or K$^+$ channels, it is generally accepted that the major intracellular signalling pathway used by PGI$_2$ is activation of adenylate cyclase leading to increases in intracellular cAMP[8,9]. This effect of PGI$_2$ is mediated by IP coupling to G$_s$[10]. Once elevated, cAMP then activates cAMP-dependent protein kinase A. Activation of protein kinase then leads to immediate as well as delayed responses. The immediate cellular changes induced by protein kinase A activation are generally mediated by the activation of calcium sequestration. The delayed responses may be regulated, at least in part, by activation of the putative 'cAMP response unit' that comprises cAMP response elements[11] in the promoter regions of genes.

Role of prostacyclin in vascular homeostasis

PGI$_2$ has a number of cardioprotective actions. It is a vasodilator in many vascular beds and reduces systemic blood pressure. PGI$_2$ also inhibits the

Figure 2 Pathways involved in the synthesis of prostaglandins (PGs), prostacyclin (PGI$_2$) and thromboxanes (TXs) from arachidonic acid. Endothelial cells and platelets express high levels of PGI$_2$ synthase and TXA$_2$ synthase, respectively, and, when stimulated, produce high levels of PGI$_2$ and TXA$_2$.

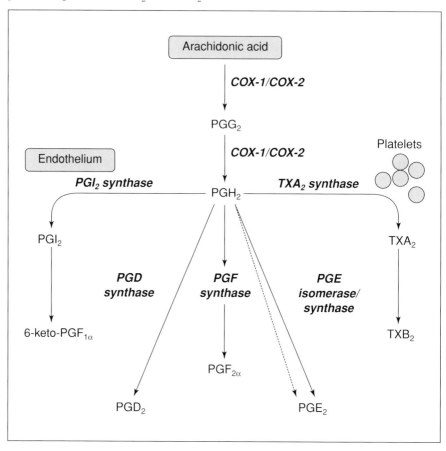

aggregation of platelets and adhesion of leukocytes[12,13]. Moreover, PGI$_2$ is an important inhibitor of atherosclerotic processes. First, it acts at various levels to reduce the ability of smooth muscle cells to take up and accumulate cholesterol. Indeed, in isolated cells in culture, PGI$_2$ inhibits the expression of the low-density lipoprotein (LDL) receptor and the uptake of LDL as well as lowering the intracellular levels of cholesterol ester by stimulating the activity of acid cholesteryl ester hydrolase and neutral cholesteryl ester hydrolase[14-16]. Second, PGI$_2$ inhibits the proliferation of smooth muscle cells isolated from various parts of the vascular tree[17]. This property reduces the propensity for neo-intimal thickening. In line with *in vitro* studies, several groups have shown that administration of prostacyclin *in vivo* preserves vascular function[18,19].

Therapeutic uses of prostacyclin and its analogues

In addition to PGI_2, there are a number of related analogues that activate IP receptors. These include iloprost, cicaprost, octimibate, EPS185 and BMY45778[5]. There have been a number of clinical settings where the administration of PGI_2 or one of its analogues has produced therapeutic benefits. Originally PGI_2 was used clinically in extracorporeal circulation procedures such as cardiopulmonary bypass, charcoal haemoperfusion and haemodialysis[19,20]. Subsequently PGI_2, as well as other IP agonists, were found to be potent therapies in the treatment of peripheral vascular disease[21]. Infusions of PGI_2[21] or, more recently, inhaled iloprost[22], have been used successfully to treat pulmonary hypertension. The use of PGI_2 in clinical settings is limited by its property as a vasodilator and its potential to induce hypotension when given systemically. However, research into the potential therapeutic uses of IP agonists continues.

Cardiovascular implications of IP receptor disruption in mice

Using genetically engineered mice in which the IP receptor was deleted, baseline blood pressure and heart rate were no different from those of control animals[23], indicating that PGI_2 does not function constitutively to regulate vascular reactivity. The IP deficient mice also developed normally, with no apparent cardiovascular problems. However, these mice displayed increased propensity for thrombosis after endothelial cell disruption.

Thromboxane A_2

TXA_2 activates thromboxane receptors (TP) that are expressed on many cell types, including platelets and vascular smooth muscle cells. TP receptors, like IP receptors, are members of the G_p-coupled receptor family. There are two isoforms of TP receptor in man, $TP\alpha$ and $TP\beta$[24,25]. Both forms appear to originate from the same gene and are derived from two spliced variants[25]. $TP\alpha$ and $TP\beta$ are identical for their first 328 amino acids and differ only in the carboxyl-terminal cytoplasmic tail regions[25]. There is evidence that the two TP receptors are co-expressed in some tissues and cells. However, in platelets, it seems that $TP\alpha$ predominates[26]. The major signalling pathway used by TP receptors is activation of G proteins including G_q, $G_{12/13}$ and G_{11}[27-29]. This leads directly to activation of phospholipase $C\beta$, which results in elevation of intracellular levels of calcium followed by stimulation of the cell (i.e. platelets). Most recently it was suggested that activation of G_h could mediate agonist stimulation of $TP\alpha$ but not $TP\beta$[30]. It is not yet clear what physiological roles the two TP receptors share or how they may function independently.

Role of thromboxane A_2 in vascular homeostasis

TXA_2 is one of the most potent endogenous platelet activators. It induces shape change, aggregation and degranulation of platelets. Thus, when TXA_2

is formed appropriately, it is an important mediator in the repair of damaged vessels. However, when platelet activation occurs inappropriately it can induce thrombus formation. In addition to its effects on platelets, TXA_2 induces constriction of blood vessels and airways[31]. Finally, it induces proliferation of vascular smooth muscle cells in culture[31,32]. Thus, the effects of TXA_2 can cause excessive activation of vascular cells leading to thrombus formation, vasospasm and/or remodelling, all of which contribute to the symptoms of various vascular diseases.

Cardiovascular implications of TP receptor disruption in mice

In TP-deficient mice there was an increase in bleeding time and resistance to cardiovascular shock induced by intravenous infusions of the TP agonist U46619. A similar increase in bleeding time is characteristic of a genetic disorder in man where a mutation of the Arg–Leu in the first cytoplasmic loop of the TP receptor occurs, rendering it inactive[33].

Prostaglandin E_2

PGE_2 acts on a range of biologically relevant receptors, designated EP_1, EP_2, EP_3 and EP_4. EP receptors are linked to a diverse range of signalling pathways. Thus, the overall biological effects of increased PGE_2 production will depend not only on the relative release of other products but also on the relative distribution of EP receptor subtypes. In terms of cardiovascular homeostasis, unlike PGI_2 or other IP agonists, there is no clear precedent for either the therapeutic elevation of PGE_2 or the administration of EP agonists. Whether this situation will change with the development of selective ligands for EP receptor subtypes remains to be seen. In fact, for PGE_2, the primary therapeutic direction is for inhibition. Reducing the levels of PGE_2 at the site of inflammation either by COX inhibitors[1] or selective anti-PGE_2 antibodies[34] has well established anti-inflammatory and analgesic benefits.

ISOFORMS OF CYCLOOXYGENASE

Cyclooxygenase-1: the constitutive isoform

COX-1 is expressed in mammalian cells under physiological conditions. However, endothelial cells, platelets and kidney tubule cells express much greater amounts of COX-1 than other cell types[1]. COX-1 was identified and purified in the 1970s from bovine[35] and sheep[36] vesicular glands. This isoform was found to be a membrane bound homo-dimer of 70 kDa. The protein contained both the COX and peroxidase activities required to form PGG_2 and PGH_2, respectively. Either free or protein-bound haem was required for activity. The primary structure of COX-1 was later sequenced and found to comprise a 2.7 kilobase cDNA[37].

Cyclooxygenase-2: the inducible isoform

We now know that COX-2 is responsible for the formation of products under inflammatory conditions. COX-2 was initially identified using Northern blotting techniques in cultured epithelial cells. Two distinct mRNA species were identified in cultured epithelial cells that were recognized by cDNA probes designed for the known COX (COX-1). Using low stringency conditions it was found that the probes hybridized to the predicted 2.8 kilobase mRNA as well as a novel 4.0 kilobase product[38]. Parallel increases in the 4.0 kilobase product with enzymatic activity were measured and the authors concluded that this mRNA would encode for active protein[38]. In a later study the same group confirmed that these epithelial cells did indeed express two distinct forms of COX[39]. In separate studies, Xie and co-workers[40] showed that mitogen-stimulated chicken fibroblasts expressed a 4.1 kilobase mRNA which encoded a protein with 59% homology with the COX identified in sheep seminal vesicles (COX-1). In parallel experiments it was shown that phorbol esters induced mouse fibroblasts to express an inducible COX (TIS10[41]) with striking similarities to that identified in chicken cells[40]. Furthermore the inducible COX gene was demonstrated to encode a protein that had COX activity[42,43].

ROLE OF COX-1 AND COX-2 IN CARDIOVASCULAR HEALTH AND DISEASE

Cyclooxygenase-1 in endothelial cells and platelets

COX-1 is the only isoform of COX that has been identified in the platelet, where its activity regulates TXA_2 release. COX-1 is also expressed in endothelial cells throughout the vasculature, where its activity regulates PGI_2 release. Platelets have no nucleus and so are unable to synthesize new COX-1. By contrast endothelial cells, having a complete nucleus, are able to synthesize COX-1 when required. Thus, when COX-1 is irreversibly blocked it is possible selectively to reduce its activity in platelets and not in endothelial cells. This is the basis of the mechanism of action of low dose aspirin in the prophylactic treatment of cardiovascular disease (Figure 3).

Cyclooxygenase-1 inhibition and low dose aspirin anti-platelet therapy

COX-1 is inhibited by all of the traditional non-steroid anti-inflammatory drugs (NSAIDs[1]). The archetype of the NSAID is aspirin, which is traditionally taken as an analgesic or anti-inflammatory drug. There are several mechanisms by which NSAIDs inhibit COX activity, although only aspirin is able to cause irreversible blockade of the enzyme. It is this property of aspirin that makes it so suitable as anti-platelet therapy. Aspirin irreversibly acetylates the

Figure 3 Diagrammatic representation of the rationale behind 'low dose' aspirin in the prophylactic treatment of cardiovascular disease. At low doses aspirin essentially spares endothelial PGI_2 release whilst irreversibly inhibiting platelet TXA_2 synthesis.

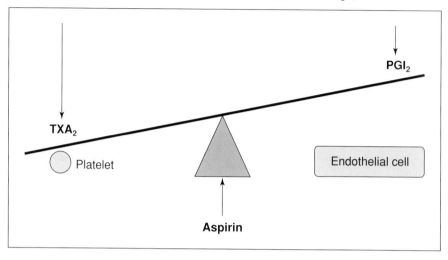

amino acid serine in the active site of COX-1. This prevents the access of the substrate to the catalytic site of the enzyme at tyrosine 385[44] and results in an irreversible inhibition of platelet-dependent TXA_2 formation. Thus, after exposure to aspirin, COX-1 is blocked in platelets for their entire lifetime of approximately 1 week. COX-1 activity in endothelial cells, however, can recover following the synthesis of new protein. It is therefore possible by using carefully balanced doses to inhibit platelet COX-1, and thereby TXA_2 production, with only a partial inhibition of endothelial enzyme and thereby PGI_2 release[44]. The optimal dose of aspirin as an anti-thrombotic drug can differ in different organ circulations. While 100 mg day[-1] is sufficient to prevent thrombus formation in the coronary circulation, higher doses may be required for the prevention of cardiovascular events in the cerebral and peripheral circulations. However, any effective anti-platelet dose of aspirin is associated with an increased risk of bleeding. Therefore, the individual benefit versus risk determines the dose of aspirin administered[44]. Thus, research continues to improve low dose aspirin anti-platelet therapy.

COX-2 IN VASCULAR CELLS

Cyclooxygenase-2 expression *in vitro*
Blood vessels
As in other cell types, COX-2 protein and activity is not normally expressed in rat[45,46] or human[47] vascular tissues, although mRNA may be present. However, after exposure to inducing agents, endothelial cells, as well as the

underlying smooth muscle, express COX-2 and release elevated levels of PGs (Figure 4). In addition to isolated vascular cells in culture, COX-2 is also induced by inflammatory agents in human whole vessels *in vitro*. A wide variety of stimuli have now been shown to induce COX-2 expression in vascular cells and these observations have implicated this enzyme in a number of vascular pathologies. As discussed above, endothelial cells and smooth muscle express PGI_2 synthase, with only very low levels of TXA_2 synthase. Thus, when stimulated to express COX-2, vascular smooth muscle produces levels of PGI_2 that compete with those in endothelial cells[48]. The best studied inducers of COX-2 in vascular cells, as well as in other cell types[1] are the cytokines. In human vascular endothelial cells[49] and smooth muscle cells[47,50] interleukin-1β, together with serum, induces COX-2. Other cytokines and inflammatory agents, including TNFα[50], oncostatin[51], bacterial lipopolysaccharide, growth factors and phorbol esters, induce COX-2 in vascular cells *in vitro*[45,46].

Figure 4 COX-1, present constitutively in endothelial cells (EC) and platelets, releases PGI_2 and TXA_2, respectively. These two prostanoids have opposing actions, PGI_2 causing vasodilation and inhibiting platelet function, and TXA_2 causing vasoconstriction and stimulating platelet aggregation. Both are vital for the normal functioning of the cardiovascular system. Under inflammatory conditions the balance that exists between PGI_2 and TXA_2 is altered. In atherosclerosis the release of protective PGI_2 is compromised due to EC loss. Under these circumstances, in large blood vessels, the induction of COX-2 by smooth muscle cells (SMC) may represent a compensatory mechanism resulting in reduced mitogenesis, cholesterol uptake, cytokine release and adhesion molecule expression.

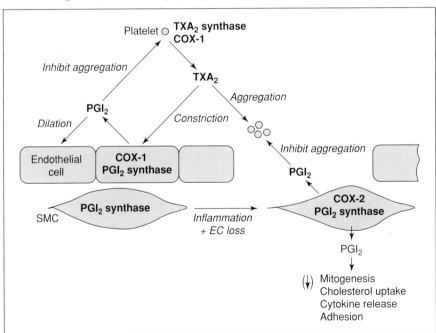

There are now a number of studies identifying specific lipid related agonists as inducers of COX-2 in the vasculature. 25-Hydroxycholesterol, an oxidized derivative of cholesterol that is implicated in the early development of atherosclerosis, increases eicosanoid production and COX-2 expression in rabbit endothelial and vascular smooth muscle cells[52]. Similarly, high-density lipoproteins, which have been known for some time to increase PGI_2 production, do so in part by the induction of COX-2[53,54]. However, cholesterol-loaded vascular smooth muscle cells have a reduced capacity to release PGI_2, a property that was explained by a failing of the cells to express COX-1 and COX-2[55]. Finally, oxidized LDL from macrophage-conditioned medium induces the class A scavenger receptor (SR-A) along with COX-2. These cells are then able to take up unregulated amounts of LDL and ultimately become lipid loaded, a process that was reduced with COX-2 selective inhibitors[56].

Human cytomegalovirus infection of smooth muscle cells generates reactive oxygen species and thereby activates nuclear factor kappa B, which causes expression of viral and cellular genes involved in immune and inflammatory responses. These processes are thought to contribute to the early onset of, and susceptibility to, atherosclerosis. Human cytomegalovirus induces COX-2 expression in vascular smooth muscle cells[57]. Inhibition of COX-2 activity in vascular cells stimulated with cytomegalovirus resulted in a reduction in oxidative stress and thereby inflammatory processes occurring within the cell.

Monocytes/macrophages

COX-2 is expressed in a range of leukocytes, including monocytes[58]. The formation of lipid-laden foam cells, derived from monocyte-derived macrophages, is key to the atherosclerotic process[59]. Thus, the ability of monocytes, macrophages and foam cells, as well as vascular smooth muscle, to express COX-2 may have relevance to the development of atherosclerosis.

Myocytes

COX-2 can be induced *in vitro* in rat neonatal ventricular myocytes, adult rat atrial myocytes or adult ventricular myocytes by phorbol esters, oxidant stress or endotoxin[60,61].

COX-2 EXPRESSION *IN VIVO*

Evidence from laboratory animal models

One of the earliest studies of COX-2 in the vasculature was by Rimarachin and co-workers[46]. In this study it was shown that COX-2 was induced transiently in rat vascular smooth muscle cells *in vitro* after stimulation with serum, platelet-derived growth factor, epidermal growth factor or thrombin. In the same study, COX-2 was induced in blood vessels after physical trauma *in vivo*, and the induction found to be more long lasting[46]. Also in rats, bacterial endotoxin induces COX-2 expression in endothelial cells and vascular smooth muscle cells in the lung[62] and COX-2 activity in atrial and ventricular tissue of the heart[60]. Anoxic stress caused by asphyxia or ischaemia results in COX-2 induction in cerebral arteries and arterioles of pigs[63].

There have been a number of studies suggesting a role for COX-2 in hypertension. Indeed, where hypertension has been induced *in vivo* in rats by the chronic administration of N^G-nitro-L-arginine methyl ester, COX-2 is induced and increases flow in the mesenteric vessels[64]. In contrast, where hypertension is a result of kidney failure or renovascular hypertension, the COX-2 that is induced has been found to contribute to the pathology of the disease[65,66].

In addition to pathophysiological stimuli, there are also physiological insults that appear to induce COX-2 in the vasculature. Indeed, COX-2 appears important in the regulation of closure of fetal ductus arteriosus in lambs[67] and mice[68]. However, in man, the COX-2 inhibitor nimesulide did not constrict the ductus[69]. Whether these apparent differences are due to species or drug dosage variations remains to be established.

Evidence from human studies

In blood vessels of healthy human donors (internal mammary artery or saphenous vein) COX-1 and not COX-2 is mainly expressed. Similarly in blood vessels from healthy laboratory animals it is COX-1 that is principally expressed. However, there is now increasing evidence that COX-2 is present in vessels within atheromatous lesions. In atherosclerotic plaques found in human aortic tissue or plaques obtained after re-vascularization treatment, COX-2 is expressed in macrophages of the shoulder region and lipid core periphery, endothelial cells and smooth muscle of the vasa vasorum in the adventitia as well as in the smooth muscle cells of the intima including the plaque itself[70-72]. COX-2 was also found in similar regions of plaques within human coronary arteries from native and transplanted hearts[73]. Atherosclerosis in carotid vessels similarly contained COX-2, which was expressed in macrophages, smooth muscle cells and endothelial cells[74,75]. Interestingly, in carotid arteries, the endothelium of vasa vasorum in the adventitia of healthy regions of vessel expressed COX-2[74]. Song and co-workers suggest that COX-2 staining in atherosclerotic plaques is associated with areas infected with *Chlamydia pneumoniae*[76].

The expression of matrix metalloproteinases is both an early and ongoing feature of atherosclerosis. Hong and co-workers have recently identified a pattern of co-expression of matrix metalloproteinases and COX-2 in human atherosclerotic plaques, although the role of COX-2 in matrix expression is not clear[72].

In another occlusive disease, moyamoya, where there is a progressive cerebrovascular occlusion that primarily affects children, COX-2 seems to be a feature. The cause is unknown. However, vascular smooth muscle cells cultured from moyamoya patients appear to express more COX-2 and release greater levels of PGs than similarly treated cells from control subjects[77].

In line with animal models of sepsis showing induction of COX-2, McAdam and co-workers have recently demonstrated a similar phenomenon to occur in man[78]. This study implies a role for COX-2 in some of the manifestations of sepsis in man.

COX-2 AND ATHEROSCLEROSIS

As discussed above, there is now sufficient *in vitro* and *in vivo* evidence to show that COX-2 will be an ongoing feature of human atherosclerosis. However, it is not clear what role COX-2 will have under these conditions. There are three possibilities that are currently under debate, which are: (i) COX-2 will do nothing and merely represents a marker of inflammation that has no role in atherosclerosis; (ii) COX-2 activity is deleterious and contributes to the progression of disease; or (iii) COX-2 is expressed as a defence mechanism and its products act to limit the extent of the lesion. It is unlikely that events regulated by COX-2, or any other inflammatory gene, in a biological setting as complex as the atherosclerotic lesion, will fit neatly into a unilateral category. However, there is evidence to suggest that COX-2 activity may be either deleterious or beneficial and current opinion is divided.

Evidence implicating an inflammatory or anti-inflammatory role for cyclooxygenase-2 in atherosclerosis

The processes of atherosclerosis involves a number of key pathological events including: (i) the adhesion and extravasation of blood borne leukocytes; (ii) their differentiation into macrophages; (iii) proliferation of vascular smooth muscle; (iv) the uptake and storage of cholesterol; (v) the expression of specific matrix proteins; and (vi) the production of cytokines and growth factors that propagate the whole process. There are several lines of evidence that have implicated beneficial or causal effects of COX-2 in some of these aspects of atherosclerosis. Undoubtedly the profile of products and the relative level of receptor expression, as would be the case for COX-1, will govern the overall role of COX-2 at a given site. With regard to vascular smooth muscle, we have put forward the hypothesis that COX-2 induction is a protective mechanism to compensate for a failing endothelium[48] (Figure 5). We have come to this conclusion because human vascular smooth muscle cells cultured from several macro vessels produce PGI_2 and PGE_2 but not TXA_2 when COX-2 is induced. Furthermore, in these cells, ligands for IP or EP receptors appear to cause inhibition. Recent evidence in man shows that a similar profile of products is released by COX-2 *in vivo*[71]. Thus, the levels of

Figure 5 COX-2 is induced in a wide range of cell types by inflammatory cytokines such as interleukin-1β (IL-1β). When induced at the site of inflammation COX-2 is associated with deleterious responses such as oedema formation and pain. In large vessels there is evidence that induction of COX-2 may have anti-inflammatory effects. COX-2 products released by smooth muscle cells following endothelial cell dysfunction inhibit proliferation, adhesion molecule expression and cytokine release.

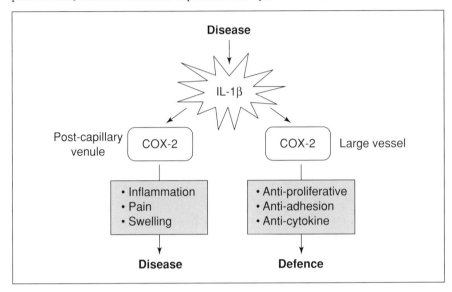

markers of PGI_2 were reduced in healthy volunteers[79-80] or patients with atherosclerosis[71] taking COX-2 selective inhibitors. In contrast, TXA_2 generation in man *in vivo* appears to be regulated exclusively by COX-1[71].

Evidence from our laboratory, as well as from others, has shown an anti-inflammatory or protective role for COX-2 induced in human vascular smooth muscle cells[1,48]. COX-2, induced by interleukin-1β, inhibits the expression of the adhesion molecules ICAM-1 and VCAM-1[81]. This observation suggests that COX-2 activity inhibits the ability of leukocytes to attach to the damaged vessel. In addition, we[47,50] and others[82] have shown that COX-2 induced in human vascular smooth muscle cells inhibits their proliferation. In contrast, Young and co-workers have recently suggested that COX-2 induction is required for tumour necrosis factor alpha (TNF-α) and angiotensin II-mediated proliferation of these cells[83]. The reason for this discrepancy will probably be due to the difference in cell types used. A pro- or anti-proliferative effect of COX-2 will be governed by the products made (i.e. PGI_2 versus TXA_2) and the level of receptors expressed. In Young's study using rat aorta, which is relatively insensitive to PGI_2, the pro-proliferative effects observed may well be due to activation of TP receptors.

We have also shown that COX-2 induced in human vascular smooth muscle cells inhibits the release of granulocyte–macrophage-colony stimulating factor (GM-CSF). GM-CSF is an important cytokine in atherosclerosis where it inhibits the apoptosis of monocytes within the plaque.

Very little evidence exists for the potential role of COX-2 in human vascular smooth muscle in cholesterol uptake and metabolism. Since PGI_2 and other IP agonists inhibit cholesterol uptake and metabolism, one may predict a protective role in this response too. However, Mietus-Snyder and co-workers[56], have recently shown that COX-2 induced in human vascular smooth muscle cells participates in the induction of the scavenger receptor (SR-A) for LDL. In their study, when cells were stimulated with oxidized LDL the SR-A was co-induced with COX-2, resulting in the exaggerated uptake of LDL, a response that was reduced with COX-2 inhibitors.

ROLE OF COX-2 IN ISCHAEMIC DISEASE

Heart disease

Hypoxia, which is associated with heart failure, leads to induction of COX-2 in human umbilical vein endothelial cells. The transactivation factors Sp1 and Sp3 were implicated in this induction[84,85]. Furthermore, Wong and co-workers[86] have shown that COX-2 is expressed in the myocardium of patients with congestive heart failure. They reported increased COX-2 immuno-staining in endothelial cells and myocytes of the infarcted area secondary to heart disease. COX-2 was also evident in myocytes of myocardial fibrosis due to dilating cardiomyopathy. In myocardial sepsis, COX-2 was positively stained in myocytes and inflammatory cells[86]. The potential beneficial or deleterious effects of COX-2 in this setting in man are not clear. However, we have shown that in rat isolated atria, the intrinsic rate of beating is pro-foundly limited by COX-2 activity[60]. In this study we found no role for COX activity in the inotropic responses of atria. This observation establishes a role for COX-2 in the control of myocyte function. In addition, COX-2 expressed in cardiac myocytes inhibits apoptosis of these cells[61]. The control of heart rate as well as myocyte death are vital events in the regulation of homeostasis. The effects of COX-2 in these processes will be dependent upon the nature of the physiological/pathophysiological stimulus to the heart.

Although there is no direct evidence, COX-2 may well be induced in the vasculature during peripheral vascular disease. PGI_2 infusions have proved useful therapies of this disease. Thus, if COX-2 expression in peripheral vascular disease is associated with increased PGI_2 production, its activity will serve a protective role.

Pulmonary hypertension

Pulmonary hypertension is characterized by constriction of the pulmonary circulation and vascular re-modelling. Cytokines and growth factors are elevated in the lungs of hypertensive patients. Thus, it is likely that COX-2 may be expressed in this setting. We have shown that when COX-2 is induced in human pulmonary vascular smooth muscle cells, PGI_2 and PGE_2 are produced. Moreover, the induction of COX-2 in these cells profoundly inhibited mitogenesis[50]. Infusion of PGI_2 is one of the most successful treatments for pulmonary hypertension. Thus, we suggest that if COX-2 is expressed in the pulmonary vasculature of patients with pulmonary hypertension, its activity is likely to be protective.

CONCLUDING REMARKS

There is now no doubt that COX-2 will feature in cardiovascular inflammation. Nevertheless, how it mediates events has yet to be elucidated. We have hypothesized that its presence in some diseases will be protective and that COX-2 selective inhibitors may exacerbate symptoms. However, the pathophysiological role of COX-2 in any biological setting will depend on four main points, which are: (i) the amount of products formed, which is dependent upon the levels of phospholipase activity at the site; (ii) the profile of COX products produced, for example, the level of PGI_2 versus thromboxane or atypical products such as 15-HETE or isoprostanes; (iii) the level and distribution of prostanoid receptors expressed on target cells; and (iv) the level and nature of other inflammatory/vasoactive mediators present. The same four conditions will, of course, influence the end result of COX-1 activity in a given tissue. Thus, with such an array of complicated factors governing the effects of COX-2 (or COX-1), it is difficult to put forward a unifying hypothesis on the beneficial or deleterious effects of COX-2 in cardiovascular disease. However, information from two trials has recently been released with contradictory results on the effects of COX-2 selective inhibitors on cardiovascular events. Data from the CLASS trial reporting the effects of celecoxib in osteoarthritis and rheumatoid arthritis showed no increase in cardiovascular events in patients taking the COX-2 selective NSAID[87]. However, a press release in April 2000 reported increased thromboembolic events in a group of arthritis patients taking rofecoxib compared with a similar group taking the COX-1 selective NSAID naproxen. Thus, in order to understand fully the role of COX-2 in all cardiovascular diseases that afflict man, specific experiments will have to be done and clinical data from trials with selective drugs carefully analysed.

Address all correspondence to: Dr Jane A. Mitchell, Unit of Critical Care Medicine, Royal Brompton Hospital, NHLI Division, Imperial College School of Medicine, Sydney Street, London SW3 6NP, UK.

REFERENCES

1. Mitchell JA, Warner TD. Cyclo-oxygenase-2: pharmacology, physiology, biochemistry and relevance to NSAID therapy. *Br J Pharmacol.* 1999;128:1121–32.
2. Tabanbe T, Ullrich V. Prostacyclin and thromboxane synthases. *J Lipid Mediat Cell Signal.* 1995;12:243–55.
3. Katsuyama M, Sugimoto Y, Namba T, Irie A, Negishi M, Narumiya S et al. Cloning and expression of a cDNA for the human prostacyclin receptor. *FEBS Lett.* 1994;344:74–8.
4. Boie Y, Rushmore TH, Darmon-Goodwin A, Grygorczyk R, Slipetz DM, Metters KM et al. Cloning and expression of a cDNA for the human prostanoid IP receptor. *J Biol Chem.* 1994;269:12173–8.
5. Wise H, Jones RL. Focus on prostacyclin and its novel mimetics. *Trends Pharmacol Sci.* 1996;17:17–21.
6. Siegel G, Carl A, Adler A, Stock G. Effect of the prostacyclin analogue iloprost on K^+ permeability in the smooth muscle cells of the canine carotid artery. *Eicosanoids.* 1989;2:213–22.
7. Merritt JE, Brown AM, Bund S, Cooper DG, Egan JW, Hallam TJ et al. Primate vascular responses to octimibate, a non-prostanoid agonist at the prostacyclin receptor. *Br J Pharmacol.* 1991;102:260–6.
8. Gorman RR, Bunting S, Miller OV. Modulation of human platelet adenylate cyclase by prostacyclin (PGX). *Prostaglandins.* 1977;13:377–88.
9. Hashimoto H, Negishi M, Ichikawa A. Identification of a prostacyclin receptor coupled to the adenylate cyclase system via a stimulatory GTP-binding protein in mouse mastocytoma P-815 cells. *Prostaglandins.* 1990;40:491–505.
10. Namba T, Oida H, Sugimoto Y, Kakizuka A, Negishi M, Ichikawa A et al. cDNA cloning of a mouse prostacyclin receptor. Multiple signaling pathways and expression in thymic medulla. *J Biol Chem.* 1994;269:9986–92.
11. Roesler WJ. What is a cAMP response unit? *Mol Cell Endocrinol.* 2000;162:1–7.
12. Moncada S, Vane JR. Prostacyclin and its clinical applications. *Ann Clin Res.* 1984;16:241–52.
13. Vane JR, Botting RM. Pharmacodynamic profile of prostacyclin. *Am J Cardiol.* 1995;75:3A–10A.
14. Hajjar DP, Pomerantz KB. Eicosanoids and their role in atherosclerosis. *Arch Mal Coeur Vaiss.* 1989;82:21–6.
15. Krone W, Klass A, Nagele H, Behnke B, Greten H. Effects of prostaglandins on LDL receptor activity and cholesterol synthesis in freshly isolated mononuclear leukocytes. *J Lipid Res.* 1988;29:1663–9.
16. Sinzinger H, Rogatti W. Prostaglandins and arterial wall lipid metabolism *in vitro, ex vivo* and *in vivo* radioisotopic studies. *J Physiol Pharmacol.* 1994;45:27–40.
17. Schrör K, Weber AA. Roles of vasodilatory prostaglandins in mitogenesis of vascular smooth muscle cells. *Agents Actions.* 1997;48:63–91.
18. Braun M, Hohlfeld T, Kienbaum P, Weber AA, Sarbia M, Schrör K. Antiatherosclerotic effects of oral cicaprost in experimental hypercholesterolemia in rabbits. *Atherosclerosis.* 1993;103:93–105.
19. Hohlfeld T, Weber A, Schrör K. Oral cicaprost reduces platelet and neutrophil activation in experimental hypercholesterolemia. *Agents Actions.* 1992;37:289–96.
20. Moncada S, Vane JR. Prostacyclin: its biosynthesis, actions and clinical potential *Phil Trans R Soc Lond B* 1981;294:305–29.

21. Sinzinger H, Virolini I, O'Grady J. Clinical trials of PGE_1, PGI_2 and mimetics in patients with peripheral vascular disease. *Prog Clin Biol Res.* 1989;301;85–96.

22. Hoeper MM, Schwarze M, Ehlerding S, Adler-Schuermeyer A, Spiekerkoetter E, Niedermeyer J et al. Long-term treatment of primary pulmonary hypertension with aerosolized iloprost, a prostacyclin analogue. *N Engl J Med.* 2000;342:1866–70.

23. Yukihiko S, Narumiya S, Ichikawa A. Distribution and function of prostanoid receptors: studies from knockout mice. *Prog Lipid Res.* 2000;39:289–314.

24. Hirata M, Hayashi Y, Ushikubi F, Yokota Y, Kageyama R, Nakanishi S et al. Cloning and expression of cDNA for a human thromboxane A_2 receptor. *Nature.* 1991;349:617–20.

25. Raychowdhury MK, Yukawa M, Collins LJ, McGrail SH, Kent KC, Ware JA Alternative splicing produces a divergent cytoplasmic tail in the human endothelial thromboxane A_2 receptor. *J Biol Chem.* 1994;269:19256–61.

26. Habib A, FitzGerald GA, Maclouf J. Phosphorylation of the thromboxane receptor alpha, the predominant isoform expressed in human platelets. *J Biol Chem.* 1999;274:2645–51.

27. Kinsella BT, O'Mahony DJ, Fitzgerald GA. The human thromboxane A_2 receptor alpha isoform (TP alpha) functionally couples to the G proteins Gq and G11 *in vivo* and is activated by the isoprostane 8-epi prostaglandin F_2 alpha. *J Pharmacol Exp Ther.* 1997;281:957–64.

28. Allan CJ, Higashiura K, Martin M, Morinelli TA, Kurtz DT, Geoffroy O et al. Characterization of the cloned HEL cell thromboxane A_2 receptor: evidence that the affinity state can be altered by G alpha 13 and G alpha q. *J Pharmacol Exp Ther.* 1996;277:1132–9.

29. Offermanns S, Laugwitz KL, Spicher K, Schultz G. G proteins of the G12 family are activated via thromboxane A_2 and thrombin receptors in human platelets. *Proc Natl Acad Sci USA.* 1994;91:504–8.

30. Vezza R, Habib A, FitzGerald GA. Differential signaling by the thromboxane receptor isoforms via the novel GTP-binding protein, G_h. *J Biol Chem.* 1999;274:12774–9.

31. Schrör K. The effect of prostaglandins and thromboxane A_2 on coronary vessel tone: mechanisms of action and therapeutic implications. *Eur Heart J.* 1993;14:34–41.

32. Baldenkov GN, Akopov SE, Ryong LH, Orekhov AN. Prostacyclin, thromboxane A_2 and calcium antagonists: effects on atherosclerotic characteristics of vascular cells. *Biomed Biochim Acta.* 1988;47:S324–7.

33. Sugimoto Y, Narumiya S, Ichikawa A. Distribution and function of prostanoid receptors: studies from knockout mice. *Prog Lipid Res.* 2000;39:289–314.

34. Portanova JP, Zhang Y, Anderson GD, Hauser SD, Masferrer JL, Seibert K et al. Selective neutralization of prostaglandin E_2 blocks inflammation, hyperalgesia, and interleukin 6 production *in vivo*. *J Exp Med.* 1996;84:883–91.

35. Miyamoto T, Ogino N, Yamamoto S, Hayaishi O. Purification of prostaglandin endoperoxide synthetase from bovine vesicular gland microsomes. *J. Biol. Chem.* 1976;251:2629–36.

36. Hemler M, Lands WE. Purification of the cyclooxygenase that forms prostaglandins. Demonstration of two forms of iron in the holoenzyme. *J Biol Chem.* 1976;251:5575–9.

37. DeWitt DL, Smith WL. Primary structure of prostaglandin G/H synthase from sheep vesicular gland determined from the complementary DNA sequence. *Proc Natl Acad Sci USA.* 1988;85:1412–6.

38. Rosen GD, Birkenmeier TM, Raz A, Holtzman MJ. Identification of a cyclooxy-genase-related gene and its potential role in prostaglandin formation. *Biochem Biophys Res Commun.* 1989;164:1358–65.

39. Holtzman MJ, Turk J, Shornick LP. Identification of a pharmacologically distinct prostaglandin H synthase in cultured epithelial cells. *J Biol Chem.* 1992:267:21438–45.

40. Xie WL, Chipman JG, Robertson DL, Erikson RL, Simmons DL. Expression of a mitogen-responsive gene encoding prostaglandin synthase is regulated by mRNA splicing. *Proc Natl Acad Sci USA.* 1991;88:2692–6.

41. Kujubu DA, Fletcher BS, Varnum BC, Lim RW, Herschman HR. TIS10, a phorbol ester tumor promoter-inducible mRNA from Swiss 3T3 cells, encodes a novel prostaglandin synthase/cyclo-oxygenase homolog. *J Biol Chem.* 1991;266; 12866–72.

42. Fletcher BS, Kujubu DA, Perrin DM, Herschman HR. Structure of the mitogen-inducible TIS10 gene and demonstration that the TIS10-encoded protein is a func-tional prostaglandin G/H synthase. *J Biol Chem.* 1992;267:4338–44.

43. O'Banion MK, Winn VD, Young DA. cDNA cloning and functional activity of a glucocorticoid-regulated inflammatory cyclooxygenase. *Proc Natl Acad Sci USA.* 1992;89:4888–92.

44. Schrör K. Aspirin and platelets: the antiplatelet action of aspirin and its role in thrombosis treatment and prophylaxis. *Semin Thromb Hemostasis.* 1997;23:349–56.

45. Bishop-Bailey D, Larkin SL, Williams TJ, Pepper J, Mitchell JA. Characterisation of the induction of nitric oxide synthase and cyclo-oxygenase in rat aorta in organ culture. *Br J Pharmacol.* 1997;121:125–33.

46. Rimarachin JA, Jacobson JA, Szabo P, Maclouf J, Creminon C, Weksler BB. Regulation of cyclooxygenase-2 expression in aortic smooth muscle cells. *Arterioscler Thromb Vasc Biol.* 1994;14:1021–31.

47. Bishop-Bailey D, Pepper JR, Haddad EB, Newton R, Larkin SW, Mitchell JA. Induction of cyclo-oxygenase-2 in human saphenous vein and internal mammary artery. *Arterioscler Thromb Vasc Biol.* 1997;17:1644–8.

48. Mitchell JA, Evans TW. Cyclooxygenase-2 as a therapeutic target. *Inflamm Res.* 1998;47(Suppl 2):S88–92.

49. Hla T, Neilson K. Human cyclooxygenase-2 cDNA. *Proc Natl Acad Sci USA.* 1992;89:7384–8.

50. Jourdan KB, Evans TW, Lamb NJ, Goldstraw P, Mitchell JA. Autocrine function of inducible nitric oxide synthase and cyclooxygenase-2 in proliferation of human and rat pulmonary artery smooth-muscle cells. Species variation. *Am J Respir Cell Mol Biol.* 1999;21:105–10.

51. Pourtau J, Mirshahi F, Li H, Muraine M, Vincent L, Tedgui A et al. Cyclooxygenase-2 activity is necessary for the angiogenic properties of oncostatin M. *FEBS Lett.* 1999;459:453–7.

52. Wohlfeil ER, Campbell WB. 25-Hydroxycholesterol increases eicosanoids and alters morphology in cultured pulmonary artery smooth muscle and endothelial cells. *Arterioscler Thromb Vasc Biol.* 1999;19:2901–8.

53. Vinals M, Martinez-Gonzalez J, Badimon JJ, Badimon L. HDL-induced prosta-cyclin release in smooth muscle cells is dependent on cyclooxygenase-2 (COX-2). *Arterioscler Thromb Vasc Biol.* 1997;17:3481–8.

54. Vinals M, Martinez-Gonzales J, Badimon L. Regulatory effects of HDL on smooth muscle cell prostacyclin release. *Arterioscler Thromb Vasc Biol.* 1999;19:204–11.

55. Pomerantz KB, Summers B, Hajjar DP. Eicosanoid metabolism in cholesterol-enriched arterial smooth muscle cells. Evidence for reduced post-transcriptional processing of cyclooxygenase I and reduced cyclooxygenase II gene expression. *Biochemistry.* 1993;32:13624–35.

56. Mietus-Snyder M, Gowri MS, Pitas RE. Class A scavenger receptor up-regulation in smooth muscle cells by oxidized low density lipoprotein: enhancement by calcium flux and concurrent cyclooxygenase-2 up-regulation. *J Biol Chem.* 2000;275:17661–70.

57. Speir E, Yu ZX, Ferrans VJ, Huang ES, Epstein SE. Aspirin attenuates cytomegalovirus infectivity and gene expression mediated by cyclooxygenase-2 in coronary artery smooth muscle cells. *Circ Res.* 1998;83:210–6.

58. Niiro H, Otsuka T, Tanabe T, Hara S, Kuga S, Nemoto Y et al. Inhibition by inter-leukin-10 of inducible cyclooxygenase expression in lipopolysaccharide-stimulated monocytes: its underlying mechanism in comparison with interleukin-4. *Blood.* 1995;85:3736–45.

59. Yamashita S, Maruyama T, Hirano K, Sakai N, Nakajima N, Matsuzawa Y. Molecular mechanisms, lipoprotein abnormalities and atherogenicity of hyperal-phalipoproteinemia. *Atherosclerosis.* 2000;152:271–85.

60. Price S, Evans TW, Warner TD, Mitchell JA. Role of COX activity in the chronotropic responses to ET-1 in the rat isolated atria. *Br J Pharmacol.* 2001; in press.

61. Adderly S, Fitzgerald DJ. Oxidative damage of cardiomyocytes is limited by ERK1/2-mediated induction of cyclooxygenase-2. *J Biol Chem.* 1999;274:5038–46.

62. Ermert L, Ermert M, Merkle M, Goppelt-Struebe M, Duncker HR, Grimminger F et al. Rat pulmonary cyclooxygenase-2 expression response to endotoxin challenge: differential regulation in the various types of cells in the lung. *Am J Pathol.* 2000:156;1275–87.

63. Busija DW, Thore C, Beasley T, Bari F. Induction of cyclooxygenase-2 following anoxic stress in piglet cerebral arteries. *Microcirculation.* 1996;3:379–86.

64. Henrion D, Dechaux E, Dowell FJ, Maclouf J, Samuel JL, Levy BI et al. Alteration of flow-induced dilation in mesenteric resistance arteries of L-NAME treated rats and its partial association with induction of cyclo-oxygenase-2. *Br J Pharmacol.* 1997;121:83–90.

65. Sanchez PL, Salgado LM, Ferreri NR, Escalante B. Effect of cyclooxygenase-2 inhi-bition on renal function after renal ablation. *Hypertension.* 1999;34:848–53.

66. Wang JL, Cheng HF, Shappell S, Harris RC. A selective cyclooxygenase-2 inhibitor decreases proteinuria and retards progressive renal injury in rats. *Kidney Int.* 2000;57:2334–42.

67. Takahashi Y, Roman C, Chemtob S, Tse MM, Lin E, Heymann MA et al. Cyclooxygenase-2 inhibitors constrict the fetal lamb ductus arteriosus both *in vitro* and *in vivo*. *Am J Physiol Regul Integr Comp Physiol.* 2000;278:R496–R505.

68. Reese J, Paria BC, Brown N, Zhao X, Morrow JD, Dey SK. Coordinated regula-tion of fetal and maternal prostaglandins directs successful birth and postnatal adap-tation in the mouse. *Proc Natl Acad Sci USA.* 2000;97:9759–64.

69. Sawdy R, Slater DM, Fisk NM, Edmonds DK, Bennett PR. Use of a cyclooxy-genase type-2 selective NSAI to prevent preterm delivery. *Lancet.* 1997;350:265–6.

70. Schonbeck U, Sukhova GK, Graber P, Coulter S, Libby P. Augmented expression of cyclooxygenase-2 in human atherosclerotic lesions. *Am J Pathol.* 1999;155:1281–91.

71. Belton O, Byrne D, Kearney D, Leahy A, Fitzgerald DJ. Cyclooxygenase-1 and -2 dependent prostacyclin formation in patients with atherosclerosis. *Circulation.* 2000;102:840–5.

72. Hong BK, Kwon HM, Lee BK, Kim D, Kim IJ, Kang SM et al. Coexpression of cyclooxygenase-2 and matrix metalloproteinases in human aortic atherosclerotic lesions. *Yonsei Med J.* 2000;41:82–8.

73. Baker CS, Hall RJ, Evans TJ, Pomerance A, Maclouf J, Creminon C et al. Cyclooxygenase-2 is widely expressed in atherosclerotic lesions affecting native and transplanted human coronary arteries and colocalizes with inducible nitric oxide synthase and nitrotyrosine particularly in macrophages. *Arterioscler Thromb Vasc Biol.* 1999;19:646–55.

74. Stemme V, Swedenborg J, Claesson H, Hansson GK. Expression of cyclo-oxygenase-2 in human atherosclerotic carotid arteries. *Eur J Vasc Endovasc Surg.* 2000;20:146–52.

75. Schonbeck U, Sukhova GK, Graber P, Coulter S, Libby P. Augmented expression of cyclooxygenase-2 in human atherosclerotic lesions. *Am J Pathol.* 1999;155:1281–91.

76. Song YG, Kwon HM, Kim JM, Hong BK, Kim DS, Huh AJ et al. Serologic and histopathologic study of *Chlamydia pneumoniae* infection in atherosclerosis: possible pathogenetic mechanism of atherosclerosis induced by *Chlamydia pneumoniae.* *Yonsei Med J.* 2000;41:319–27.

77. Yamamoto M, Aoyagi M, Fukai N, Matsushima Y, Yamamoto K. Increase in prostaglandin E_2 production by interleukin-1β in arterial smooth muscle cells derived from patients with moyamoya disease. *Circ Res.* 1999;85:912–18.

78. McAdam BF, Catella-Lawson F, Mardini IA. Systemic biosynthesis of prostacyclin by cyclooxygenase (COX)-2: the human pharmacology of a selective inhibitor of COX-2. *Proc Natl Acad Sci USA.* 1999;96:272–7.

79. Cullen L, Kelly L, O'Connor S. Selective cyclooxygenase-2 inhibition by nimesulide in man. *J Pharmacol Exp Ther.* 1998;287:578–82.

80. Catella-Lawson F, McAdam BH, Morrison BW. Effects of specific inhibition of cyclooxygenase-2 on sodium balance, hemodynamics and vasoactive eicosanoids. *J Pharmacol Exp Ther.* 1999;289:735–41.

81. Bishop-Bailey D, Burk-Gaffty A, Hellewell P, Mitchell JA. Role of cyclo-oxygenase-2 in the regulation of adhesion receptors on human vascular smooth muscle. *Biochem Biophys Res Commun.* 1998;249:44–7.

82. Bornfeldt KE, Campbell JS, Koyama H, Argast GM, Leslie CC, Raines EW et al. The mitogen-activated protein kinase pathway can mediate growth inhibition and proliferation in smooth muscle cells. Dependence on the availability of downstream targets. *J Clin Invest.* 1997;100:875–85.

83. Young W, Mahboubi K, Haider A, Li I, Ferreri NR. Cyclooxygenase-2 is required for tumor necrosis factor-alpha- and angiotensin II-mediated proliferation of vascular smooth muscle cells. *Circ Res.* 2000;86:906–14.

84. Schmedtje JF, Ji YS, Liu WL, DuBois RN, Runge MS. Hypoxia induces cyclooxygenase-2 via the NF-kappaB p65 transcription factor in human vascular endothelial cells. *J Biol Chem.* 1997;272:601–8.

85. Xu Q, Ji Y-S, Schedtje JF. Sp1 increases expression of cyclooxygenase-2 in hypoxic vascular endothelium: implications for the mechanisms of aortic aneurysm and heart failure. *J Biol Chem.* 2000;275;24583–9.

86. Wong SC, Fukuchi M, Melnyk P, Rodger I, Giaid A. Induction of cyclooxygenase-

2 and activation of nuclear factor-kB in the myocardium of patients with congestive heart failure. *Circulation.* 1998;98:100–3.

87. Silverstein FE, Faich G, Goldstein JL, Simon LS, Pincus T, Whelton A et al. Gastrointestinal toxicity with celecoxib vs nonsteroidal anti-inflammatory drugs for osteoarthritis and rheumatoid arthritis: the CLASS study: a randomized controlled trial. Celecoxib Long-term Arthritis Safety Study. *J Am Med Assoc.* 2000;284:1247–55.

13 | Expression and regulation of cyclooxygenase-2 in synovial tissues

LESLIE J. CROFFORD

Department of Internal Medicine, Division of Rheumatology, University of Michigan, Ann Arbor, MI 48109, USA.

Use of cyclooxygenase (COX) inhibitors in the treatment of arthritis is almost universal and illustrates the important role played by prostaglandins (PGs) in the symptoms of these diseases. It has been known that PGs were increased in the synovial fluids and tissues of patients with rheumatoid arthritis (RA) since the mid-1970s. PGs are key mediators of inflammation and also have the potential to stimulate production of matrix metalloproteinases and erosion of bone[1,2]. As early as 1977, the observation was made that PG production could be stimulated in rheumatoid synovial cells by a factor derived from mononuclear cells[3]. However, at that time, upregulated PG production was thought to be due to increased availability of the arachidonic acid substrate for COX. Inhibition of PG production by glucocorticoids was thought to be due to inhibition of phospholipase activity by annexin-1 (lipocortin-1)[4].

A major change in thinking about PG production came with the demonstration that COX activity could be increased by proinflammatory stimuli *in vitro* and *in vivo*[5,6]. These observations were followed shortly by the molecular cloning of COX-2 as a gene that was upregulated after stimulation by serum[7], cellular transformation by a viral oncogene[8], or stimulation with a tumour promoter[9]. The general observation that COX-2 was upregulated by inflammation was quickly followed by studies demonstrating increased COX-2 in animal models of arthritis and patients with inflammatory arthritis[10,11].

ANIMAL MODELS OF ARTHRITIS

The first studies demonstrating upregulated immunostaining of COX in the joints of rats with adjuvant-induced or streptococcal cell wall-induced arthritis were performed with antibodies that did not discriminate between COX-1 and COX-2[10]. Staining for COX was increased prior to the onset of clinical arthritis, marking one of the earliest observable changes in joint tissues. Treatment with glucocorticoids completely eliminated upregulated expression[10]. COX-1 mRNA was unchanged in these joint tissues suggesting that the increase of COX immunostaining was due to COX-2.

With the availability of COX-2 sequence information and specific antibodies, it was demonstrated conclusively that the upregulated protein species was in fact COX-2[12]. In addition, COX-2 mRNA was also increased in joint tissues of animals with adjuvant arthritis[12,13]. Increased expression of COX-2 mRNA and protein in these studies occurred just prior to or concomitant with the development of arthritis and concurrent with increased PGE_2 levels (Table 1)[12].

In addition to upregulation of COX-2 in joint tissues, COX-2 expression is increased in the spinal cord of animals with arthritis. In a model of acute arthritis induced by intra-articular injection of kaolin and carrageenan, COX-2, but not COX-1, protein was increased as early as 3 h after induction of arthritis with maximum elevation after 12 hours[14]. Expression of PGE_2 was evaluated by antibody microprobes and was slightly elevated compared with basal production after about 3 h and markedly elevated after about 8 hours. Evaluation of the spinal cords of rats with adjuvant arthritis demonstrated an early twofold upregulation of COX-2 mRNA associated with injection of adjuvant that returned to baseline by day three after injection (when clinical arthritis is absent)[15]. During the chronic phase of arthritis, COX-2 mRNA and protein were also elevated.

To determine if upregulated COX-2 was responsible for the clinical expression of adjuvant arthritis, animals were treated with selective COX-2 inhibitors[12]. Treatment of arthritic animals suppressed paw swelling by 80–85%, similar to the effect of the non-specific COX inhibitor indomethacin. Dexamethasone, which blocks upregulation of COX-2 in addition to its other anti-inflammatory activities, inhibited paw oedema by 95–100%. Inhibition

Table 1 Expression and regulation of COX-2 in animal models of arthritis

Models	Adjuvant-induced arthritis[10,12,13,16]
	Streptococcal cell wall arthritis[10]
COX-2 mRNA	Increased in joint tissues[12,13,16]
	Increased in spinal cord[15]
COX-2 protein	Increased in joint tissues[10,12,13,16]
	Increased in spinal cord[15]
PGE_2 tissue levels	Increased in joint tissues[12]
Effects of treatment	COX-2 protein and/or arthritis inhibited by glucocorticoids[10,12]
	Arthritis reduced by selective COX-2 inhibitors[12]
	Arthritis blocked by COX-2 selective oligodeoxy nucleotides[16]

of PGE_2 by the selective COX-2 inhibitor resulted in a reduction of the inflammatory cell infiltrate, reduced COX-2 expression, and reduced interleukin 6 (IL-6) expression[12]. Inhibition of COX-2 in the adjuvant model was further explored using antisense (AS) oligodeoxynucleotides (ODN) to specifically block increased expression of COX-2[16]. In these experiments, AS ODN suppressed COX-2 mRNA and protein expression and induction of arthritis in a dose-dependent manner whereas sense or scrambled ODN had no effect. COX-2 inhibition also inhibits formation of IgG antibodies but not the delayed hypersensitivity reaction to *Mycobacteria butyricum* in adjuvant arthritis[17]. Finally, mice engineered to be deficient in COX-2 were resistant to the development of experimental arthritis (see L. Ballou et al., Chapter 6). Taken together, these data implicate COX-2 in the inflammation associated with animal models of arthritis.

EXPRESSION OF COX-2 IN SYNOVIAL TISSUES OF PATIENTS WITH ARTHRITIS

The first reports of COX immunostaining in rheumatoid arthritis (RA) and osteoarthritis (OA) used antibodies detecting both COX-1 and COX-2 and revealed increased staining in RA tissues compared with OA tissues[10]. Availability of specific antibodies allowed more precise localization of the COX isoforms. In RA, most COX-2 was found in vascular endothelium, infiltrating mononuclear inflammatory cells, and sub-lining synovial fibroblast-like cells (Figure 1)[13,18,19]. COX-2 was increased in the more inflammatory forms of arthritis, RA and ankylosing spondylitis, compared with the less inflammatory OA[19]. There was little expression of COX-2 in normal human synovial tissue[13].

COX-1 is expressed in synovial lining, but not increased in inflammatory versus non-inflammatory forms of arthritis[19]. The fact that COX-2 mRNA was less abundant than COX-1 mRNA in patients with RA may reflect rapid degradation of COX-2 transcripts[18,20].

REGULATION OF COX-2 IN SYNOVIAL CELLS AND TISSUES *IN VITRO*

Synovial tissues explanted from patients with RA release large amounts of PGE_2 and prostacyclin, particularly after stimulation with interleukin-1β (IL-1β). Synovial explants contain type A (macrophage-like) and type B (fibroblast-like) synoviocytes as well as other cell types found *in vivo*. Treatment of synovial explant tissues with agents that selectively inhibit COX-2 effectively blocks PG release[21]. Metabolic labelling of newly synthesized proteins demonstrates that COX-2 synthesis is minimal under *ex vivo* conditions unless synovial explant tissues are stimulated with IL-1β or phorbol ester, emphasizing

Figure 1 Immunostaining of rheumatoid synovium with anti-COX-2 antisera. (a) Representative synovial tissue section of synovium from a patient with rheumatoid arthritis stained with anti-COX-2 antisera (630×). Positive staining is indicated by brownish-black deposits. (b) Adjacent section stained with non-immune rabbit serum (630×). BV = blood vessels; MNC = mononuclear inflammatory cells. Also stained are sub-synovial fibroblast-like cells. (Reprinted from ref. 10 with permission.)

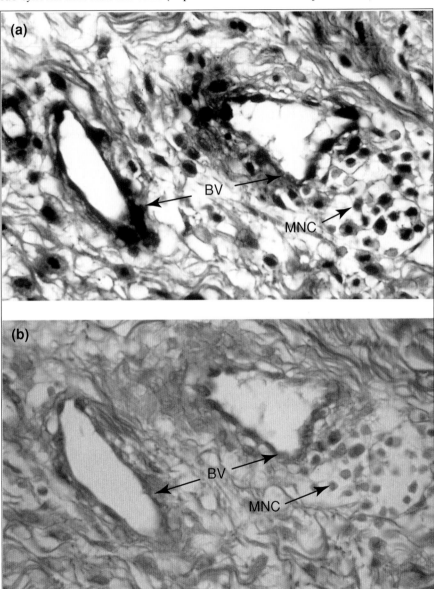

the need for ongoing stimulation to maintain expression[18]. In contrast, synthesis of COX-1 is present under basal conditions and unaffected by treatment with proinflammatory or mitogenic agents. Upregulated expression of COX-2, but not COX-1, is blocked by dexamethasone in a dose-dependent fashion[18].

Cultured synoviocytes (type B fibroblast-like cells) can be grown from human synovial tissues and passaged *in vitro* while maintaining some characteristic phenotypes of the cells found *in vivo* in RA[22]. Synoviocytes from patients with RA and OA behave similarly *in vitro* with respect to COX-2 regulation. These primary cells have been used further to define the regulation of COX-2 (Table 2). Similar to other cell types IL-1β increases expression of COX-2 mRNA (Figure 2) and protein[11,18,23-26]. Glucocorticoids inhibit basal and cytokine-stimulated COX-2 expression[11]. Interleukins IL-4, IL-13, and IL-10 have been reported to inhibit tumour necrosis factor (TNF-α)-stimulated COX-2 expression in cultured synoviocytes[26].

In addition to proinflammatory cytokines, a number of other stimuli that affect similar intracellular signalling pathways also stimulate COX-2 expression. When synoviocytes are stimulated with interferon (IFN-γ), class II MHC expression is increased[27,28]. Engagement of class II MHC on IFN-γ-treated synoviocytes by staphylococcal superantigen leads to increased expression of COX-2 and increased PGE_2 production[28]. IL-4, TGF-β and dexamethasone block the superantigen-induced expression of COX-2[29]. Synoviocyte and T-lymphocyte co-culture leads to increased PGE_2 production that is inhibited by antibodies to class II MHC and CD11a/CD18 (D. A. Fox, personal communication). Although not shown yet in synovial tissues, CD40–CD40 ligand interactions stimulate COX-2[31,32]. Stimulation of synoviocyte cell surface integrins also stimulates COX-2 expression[33]. These observations suggest that in addition to cytokines, cell–cell and cell–matrix interactions may regulate COX-2 expression in these cells.

Table 2 Regulation of COX-2 in synoviocytes or chondrocytes

Increased COX-2	Proinflammatory cytokines: IL-1, TNF-α[11,18,23-26]; IL-6 (chondrocytes)[41]
	Tumour promoters: phorbol ester (synovial explants)[11]
	Superantigens: staphylococcal superantigen, in IFN-γ-treated synoviocytes[28]
	Binding to cell-surface integrins: adenovirus (synoviocytes)[33]; defined matrices (synoviocytes) (L. J. Crofford, unpublished data)
	Growth factors: platelet-derived growth factor[37]
Decreased COX-2	Glucocorticoids[11,18,41]
	Inhibitory cytokines: IL-4, IL-13, IL-10 (synoviocytes)[26]
	Nitric oxide: inhibits activity (OA cartilage, macrophages)[39,40]

Figure2 Reverse transcriptase-polymerase chain reaction (RT-PCR) for COX-2 in cultured synoviocytes treated with IL-1β. Synoviocytes show rapid upregulation of COX-2 mRNA after stimulation by IL-1β beginning by 30 min after treatment. The control housekeeping gene *G3PDH* is unchanged.

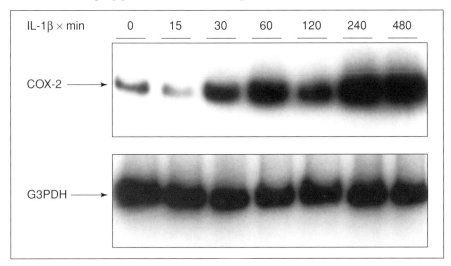

In many cell systems, growth factors stimulate COX-2 expression. Though there are no published reports specific to synoviocytes, the principal synovio-cyte growth factor platelet-derived growth factor (PDGF), increases COX-2 expression and expression of other enzymes critical for PG production in many cell populations[34-36]. PDGF alone is a poor stimulus for PGE$_2$ production in synovial cells. However, PDGF can act synergistically with IL-1β to increase PGE$_2$ production when these factors are provided together[37]. PGE$_2$ itself inhibits synoviocyte proliferation and IL-1-induced PGE$_2$ blunts the proliferative signal of PDGF[37]. Normal growth of mesenchymal cells may incorporate transient upregulation of PG production leading to increased cAMP and subsequent growth inhibition. Dysregulated synovial cell growth in RA may involve aberrant operation of these overlapping growth regulatory pathways.

EXPRESSION AND REGULATION OF COX-2 IN OSTEOARTHRITIC CARTILAGE AND CHONDROCYTES

Different pathogenic mechanisms are involved in RA and OA. While RA is a disease process of synovial pannus tissue, the initial and predominant site of pathology in OA is the cartilage. To be sure, synovial inflammation is present in OA. However, the synovial tissue does not invade articular cartilage or juxta-articular bone. OA-affected cartilage in *ex vivo* conditions spontaneously releases detectable amounts of PGE$_2$ due to upregulation of COX-2[38,39]. Additionally, OA-affected cartilage releases IL-1β in sufficient quantity to stimulate endogenous PGE$_2$[38].

There is evidence that PGE_2 production in OA cartilage is influenced by nitric oxide (NO), also produced spontaneously by OA-affected cartilage[39]. In OA cartilage, NO attenuated the production of COX-2-derived PGE_2. Further studies suggested a potential mechanism for this effect since NO induces nitration of COX-2 in lipopolysaccharide-stimulated macrophages[40]. This physical change in the COX-2 protein was associated with inhibition of PGE_2 production. NO stimulates PGE_2 production via COX-1.

In cultured primary chondrocytes, COX-2 and PGE_2 were stimulated by the proinflammatory cytokines, IL-1β, TNF-α and IL-6[41]. Dexamethasone completely inhibited IL-1β-induced COX-2 mRNA expression[41].

SIGNAL TRANSDUCTION PATHWAYS

There is enormous complexity in the intracellular signalling pathways that mediate regulation of COX-2 expression (Figure 3). In addition, there are tissue and species-specific differences. For example, whereas nuclear factor-κB (NF-κB) is important for early upregulation of COX-2 in synovial cells as well as other human cells[24,25], NF-κB appears to be unimportant in murine tissues. Since IL-1β is the most potent inducer of COX-2 in cultured human synoviocytes, signal transduction pathways stimulated by IL-1β have been examined. After stimulation with IL-1β, the inhibitory protein IκBα is phosphorylated, dissociates from NF-κB and becomes ubiquitinated and degraded. NF-κB moves into the nucleus and binds to specific elements

Figure 3 Regulatory regions of COX-2. Both the 5′ and 3′ regions contain sequences that promote the rapid increase of COX-2 transcripts. GAS = γ-interferon activated sequence; NF-κB = binding site for nuclear factor-κB; c/EBP = binding site for CAAT element binding protein; CRE = cAMP responsive element; AUUUA = mRNA sequence associated with transcript instability.

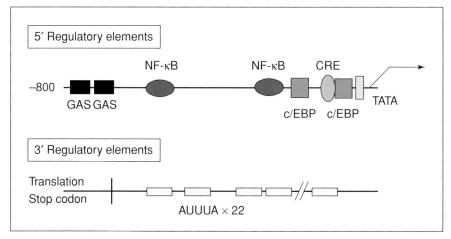

located in the COX-2 promoter[25]. Inhibiting NF-κB binding by AS ODN to the p65 subunit of NF-κB blocks the early upregulation of COX-2 and PGE_2 production[24,25].

IL-1β also stimulates phosphorylation of mitogen activated protein kinases (MAPK). There are three main MAPK pathways activated by IL-1β in these cells: the extracellular receptor-activated kinase (ERK-1/-2); p38 MAPK; and c-Jun kinase (JUNK) or stress-activated protein kinase (SAPK). Inhibitors of ERK phosphorylation or p38 activity block IL-1β-induced upregulation of COX-2 in synoviocytes as in other cell types[42-44]. The p38 pathway is also likely to be involved in the IL-1β-induced stabilization of COX-2 mRNA[20,43,44].

In chondrocytes, similar pathways are involved. Inhibitors of protein tyrosine kinases block IL-1β-induced COX-2 expression while inhibitors of protein kinase C and protein kinase A had no effect[41]. Phosphatase inhibitors induce COX-2 expression[45]. The transcription factors involved are likely to be in the AP-1 family of proteins binding to a cyclic AMP responsive element (CRE) in the COX-2 promoter[45]. The CAAT enhancer binding proteins c/EBPβ and c/EBPδ also play a role in induction of the human COX-2 promoter in rabbit articular chondrocytes[46]. There is also evidence for involvement of c/EBP in regulation of COX-2 in synoviocytes since TNF-stimulated induction of c/EBP is diminished by IL-4 and IL-13, which in turn inhibits stimulated COX-2 expression[26].

Thus, multiple signalling pathways and transcription factors interact to provide full stimulation of COX-2 expression in synoviocytes and chondrocytes. mRNA stability, due to the presence of sequences in the 3′ untranslated region, is also controlled[20]. Together, these molecular mechanisms provide for tightly regulated COX-2 expression in joint tissues.

IMPLICATIONS FOR THE TREATMENT OF ARTHRITIS WITH SELECTIVE COX-2 INHIBITORS

Data from cultured synoviocytes, explanted cultures of synovial tissues or articular cartilage, and animal models implicate COX-2 in the stimulated production of PGs in arthritis (Figure 4). To the extent that PGs are responsible for symptoms of arthritis (pain, swelling, stiffness), inhibition of COX-2 activity would be predicted to provide therapeutic efficacy in the treatment of arthritis[47]. However, it must be remembered that the role of PGs in arthritis is pleiotropic[48]. While there is no doubt that inhibition of PG production reduces the symptoms of arthritis, therapeutic administration of PGE_1 also blocks signs and symptoms of arthritis[49,50]. PGE-induced production of cAMP in cells involved in inflammatory arthritis leads to modulation of many immune mechanisms, including cytokine production and regulation of neutrophil and lymphocyte proliferation[48]. In addition, other PG products may be

Figure 4 Role of COX-2 in arthritis. Increased transcription and translation are stimulated by proinflammatory cytokines and other stimuli. PGs mediate inflammation and may contribute to tissue remodelling by stimulating angiogenesis or production of metalloproteinases. PGs also affect function of immune and inflammatory cells.

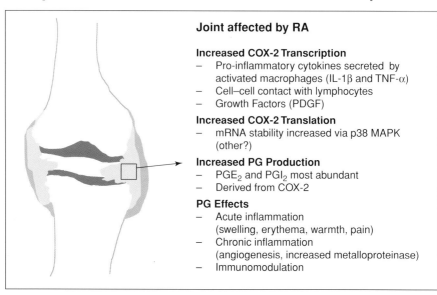

Joint affected by RA

Increased COX-2 Transcription
— Pro-inflammatory cytokines secreted by activated macrophages (IL-1β and TNF-α)
— Cell–cell contact with lymphocytes
— Growth Factors (PDGF)

Increased COX-2 Translation
— mRNA stability increased via p38 MAPK (other?)

Increased PG Production
— PGE_2 and PGI_2 most abundant
— Derived from COX-2

PG Effects
— Acute inflammation (swelling, erythema, warmth, pain)
— Chronic inflammation (angiogenesis, increased metalloproteinase)
— Immunomodulation

involved in the resolution phase of inflammation in certain settings (see D. Willoughby et al., Chapter 5). Nevertheless, clinical trials using selective COX-2 inhibitors in patients with arthritis demonstrate equal efficacy with traditional NSAIDs in all studies so far, confirming the dominant role for COX-2 in excess PG production associated with arthritis[51].

Address all correspondence to: Leslie J. Crofford MD, University of Michigan, Room 5510E, MSRB I, 1150 West Medical Center Drive, Ann Arbor, MI 48109-0680, USA.

REFERENCES

1. Robinson DR, Tashijian AHJ, Levine L. Prostaglandin-stimulated bone resorption by rheumatoid synovia: a possible mechanism for bone destruction in rheumatoid arthritis. *J Clin Invest.* 1975;56:1181–88.
2. Dayer J-M, Krane SM, Russell RGG, Robinson DR. Production of collagenase and prostaglandins by isolated adherent rheumatoid synovial cells. *Proc Natl Acad Sci USA.* 1976;73:945–9.
3. Dayer J-M, Robinson DR, Krane SM. Prostaglandin production by rheumatoid synovial cells: stimulation by a factor from human mononuclear cells. *J Exp Med.* 1977;145:1399–404.
4. Flower RJ. Lipocortin. *Prog Clin Biol Res.* 1990;349:11–25.

5. Raz A, Wyche A, Siegel N, Needleman P. Regulation of fibroblast cyclooxygenase synthesis by interleukin-1. *J Biol Chem.* 1988;263:3022–8.

6. Masferrer JL, Zweifel BS, Seibert K, Needleman P. Selective regulation of cellular cyclooxygenase by dexamethasone and endotoxin in mice. *J Clin Invest.* 1990;86:1375–9.

7. O'Banion MK, Sadowski HB, Winn V, Young DA. A serum- and glucocorticoid-regulated 4-kilobase mRNA encodes a cyclooxygenase-related protein. *J Biol Chem.* 1991;266:23261–7.

8. Xie W, Chipman JG, Robertson DL, Erikson RL, Simmons DL. Expression of a mitogen-responsive gene encoding prostaglandin synthase is regulated by mRNA splicing. *Proc Natl Acad Sci USA.* 1991;88:2692–6.

9. Kujubu DA, Fletcher BS, Varnum BC, Lim RW, Herschman HR. TIS10, a phorbol ester tumor promoter-inducible mRNA from Swiss 3T3 cells, encodes a novel prostaglandin synthase/cyclooxygenase homologue. *J Biol Chem.* 1991;266:12866–72.

10. Sano H, Hla T, Maier JAM, Crofford LJ, Case JP, Maciag T et al. *In vivo* cyclooxygenase expression in synovial tissues of patients with rheumatoid arthritis and osteoarthritis and rats with adjuvant and streptococcal cell wall arthritis. *J Clin Invest.* 1992;89:97–108.

11. Crofford LJ, Wilder RL, Ristimäki AP, Remmers EF, Epps HR, Hla T. Cyclooxygenase-1 and -2 expression in rheumatoid synovial tissues: effects of interleukin-1β, phorbol ester, and corticosteroids. *J Clin Invest.* 1994;93:1095–101.

12. Anderson GD, Hauser SD, Bremer ME, McGarity KL, Isakson PC, Gregory SA. Selective inhibition of cyclooxygenase-2 reverses inflammation and expression of COX-2 and IL-6 in rat adjuvant arthritis. *J Clin Invest.* 1996;97:2672–9.

13. Kang RY, Freire-Moar J, Sigal E, Chu CQ. Expression of cyclooxygenase-2 in human and an animal model of rheumatoid arthritis. *Br J Rheumatol.* 1996;35:711–8.

14. Ebersberger A, Grubb BD, Willingale HL, Gardiner NJ, Nebe J, Schaible HG. The intraspinal release of prostaglandin E_2 in a model of acute arthritis is accompanied by an up-regulation of cyclo-oxygenase-2 in the spinal cord. *Neuroscience.* 1999;93:775–81.

15. Beiche F, Scheuerer S, Brune K, Geisslinger G, Goppelt-Struebe M. Up-regulation of cyclooxygenase-2 mRNA in the rat spinal cord following peripheral inflammation. *FEBS Letts.* 1996;390:165–9.

16. Yamada R, Sano H, Hla T, Hashiramoto A, Kawahito Y, Mukai S et al. Selective inhibition of cyclooxygenase-2 with antisense oligodeoxynucleotide restricts induction of rat adjuvant-induced arthritis. *Biochem Biophys Res Commun.* 2000;269:415–21.

17. Turull A, Queralt J. Selective cycloxygenase-2 (COX-2) inhibitors reduce anti-*Mycobacterium* antibodies in adjuvant arthritic rats. *Immunopharmacology.* 2000;46:71–7.

18. Crofford LJ. Expression and regulation of COX-2 in synovial tissues of arthritis patients. In: Vane J, Botting J, Botting R, editors. *Improved Non-Steroid Anti-Inflammatory Drugs. COX-2 Enzyme Inhibitors.* London: Kluwer Academic Publishers and William Harvey Press; 1996:133–43.

19. Siegle I, Klein T, Backman JT, Saal JG, Nüsing RM, Fritz P. Expression of cyclooxygenase 1 and cyclooxygenase 2 in human synovial tissue. Differential elevation of cyclooxygenase 2 in inflammatory joint diseases. *Arthritis Rheum.* 1998;41:122–29.

20. Ristimäki A, Garfinkel S, Wessendorf J, Maciag T, Hla T. Induction of cyclo-oxygenase-2 by interleukin-1 alpha. Evidence for post-transcriptional regulation. *J Biol Chem.* 1994;269:11769–75.

21. Tan B, Brock TG, Peters-Golden M, Crofford LJ. Prostaglandin (PG) production in rheumatoid synovial explants and cultured synovial fibroblast-like cells (synoviocytes) is dependent on cyclooxygenase (COX)-2 [abstract]. *Arthritis Rheum.* 1998;41(Suppl):S161.

22. Lafyatis R, Remmers EF, Roberts AB, Yocum DE, Sporn MB, Wilder RL. Anchorage-independent growth of synoviocytes from arthritic and normal joints: stimulation by exogenous platelet derived growth factor and inhibition by transforming growth factor-beta and retinoids. *J Clin Invest.* 1989;83:1267–76.

23. Hulkower KI, Wertheimer SJ, Levin W, Coffey JW, Anderson CM, Chen T et al. Interleukin-1β induces cytosolic phospholipase A$_2$ and prostaglandin H synthase in rheumatoid synovial fibroblasts. Evidence for their roles in the production of prostaglandin E$_2$. *Arthritis Rheum.* 1994;37:653–61.

24. Roshak AK, Jackson JR, McGough K, Chabot-Fletcher M, Mochan E, Marshall LA. Manipulation of distinct NFκB proteins alters interleukin-1β-induced human rheumatoid synovial fibroblast prostaglandin E$_2$ formation. *J Biol Chem.* 1996;271:31496–501.

25. Crofford LJ, Tan B, McCarthy CJ, Hla T. NF-κB is involved in the regulation of cyclooxygenase-2 expression by interleukin-1β in rheumatoid synoviocytes. *Arthritis Rheum.* 1997;40:226–36.

26. Alaaeddine N, Di Battista JA, Pelletier JP, Kiansa K, Cloutier JM, Martel-Pelletier J. Inhibition of tumor necrosis factor alpha-induced prostaglandin E$_2$ production by the antiinflammatory cytokines interleukin-4, interleukin-10, and interleukin-13 in osteoarthritic synovial fibroblasts: distinct targeting in the signaling pathways. *Arthritis Rheum.* 1999;42:710–18.

27. Tsai C, Diaz LA, Singer NG, Li LL, Kirsch AH, Mitra R et al. Responsiveness of human T lymphocytes to bacterial superantigens presented by cultured rheumatoid arthritis synoviocytes. *Arthritis Rheum.* 1996;39:125–36.

28. Mehindate K, Al-Daccak R, Dayer J-M, Kennedy BP, Kris C, Borgeat P et al. Superantigen-induced collagenase gene expression in human IFN-γ-treated fibroblast-like synoviocytes involves prostaglandin E$_2$. *J Immunol.* 1995;155:3570–7.

29. Mehindate K, al-Daccak R, Aoudjit F, Damdoumi F, Fortier M, Borgeat P et al. Interleukin-4, transforming growth factor beta 1, and dexamethasone inhibit superantigen-induced prostaglandin E$_2$-dependent collagenase gene expression through their action on cyclooxygenase-2 and cytosolic phospholipase A$_2$. *Lab Invest.* 1996;75:529–38.

30. Yamamura Y, Diaz Jr. LA, He SX, Fox DA. Activation of fibroblastic synoviocytes by subsets of resting T cells [abstract]. *Arthritis Rheum.* 1999;42(Suppl):S89.

31. Zhang Y, Cao HJ, Graf B, Meekings H, Smith TJ, Phipps RP. CD40 engagement up-regulates cyclooxygenase-2 expression and prostaglandin E$_2$ production in human lung fibroblasts. *J Immunol.* 1998;160:1053–7.

32. Cao HJ, Wang HS, Zhang Y, Lin HY, Phipps RP, Smith TJ. Activation of human orbital fibroblasts through CD40 engagement results in a dramatic induction of hyaluronan synthesis and prostaglandin endoperoxide H synthase-2 expression. Insights into potential pathogenic mechanisms of thyroid-associated ophthalmopathy. *J Biol Chem.* 1998;273:29615–25.

33. Crofford LJ, Bian H, Petruzelli LM, McDonagh KT, Roessler BJ. Adenovirus bind-

ing to cultured synoviocytes triggers signalling through the MAPK pathway and induces expression of cyclooxygenase-2 and interleukin-8 [abstract]. *Arthritis Rheum.* 1999;42(Suppl):S164.

34. Xie W, Herschman HR. Transcriptional regulation of prostaglandin synthase 2 gene expression by platelet-derived growth factor and serum. *J Biol Chem.* 1996;271:31742–8.

35. Chen QR, Miyaura C, Higashi S, Murakami M, Kudo I, Saito S et al. Activation of cytosolic phospholipase A_2 by platelet-derived growth factor is essential for cyclooxygenase-2-dependent prostaglandin E_2 synthesis in mouse osteoblasts cultured with interleukin-1. *J Biol Chem.* 1997;272:5952–8.

36. Goppelt-Struebe M, Stroebel M, Hoppe J. Regulation of platelet-derived growth factor isoform-mediated expression of prostaglandin G/H synthase in mesangial cells. *Kidney Intl.* 1996;50:71–8.

37. Kumkumian GK, Lafyatis R, Remmers EF, Case JP, Kim S-J, Wilder RL. Platelet-derived growth factor and IL-1 interactions in rheumatoid arthritis. Regulation of synoviocyte proliferation, prostaglandin production, and collagenase transcription. *J Immunol.* 1989;143:833–7.

38. Attur MG, Patel IR, Patel RN, Abramson SB, Amin AR. Autocrine production of IL-1 beta by human osteoarthritis-affected cartilage and differential regulation of endogenous nitric oxide, IL-6, PGE_2, and IL-8. *Proc Assoc Am Physicians.* 1998;110:65–72.

39. Amin AR, Attur M, Patel RN, Thakker GD, Marshall PJ, Rediske J et al. Superinduction of cyclooxygenase-2 activity in human osteoarthritis-affected carti-lage. *J Clin Invest.* 1997;99:1231–7.

40. Clancy R, Varenika B, Huang W, Ballou L, Attur M, Amin AR et al. Nitric oxide synthase/COX cross-talk: nitric oxide activates COX-1 but inhibits COX-2-derived prostaglandin production. *J Immunol.* 2000;165:1582–7.

41. Geng Y, Blance FJ, Cornelisson M, Lotz M. Regulation of cyclooxygenase-2 expres-sion in normal human articular chondrocytes. *J Immunol.* 1995;155:796–801.

42. Guan Z, Buckman SY, Miller BW, Springer LD, Morrison AR. Interleukin-1beta-induced cyclooxygenase-2 expression requires activation of both c-Jun NH_2-termi-nal kinase and p38 MAPK signal pathways in rat renal mesangial cells. *J Biol Chem.* 1998;273:28670–6.

43. Lasa M, Mahtani KR, Finch A, Brewer G, Saklatvala J, Clark AR. Regulation of cyclooxygenase 2 mRNA stability by the mitogen-activated protein kinase p38 signaling cascade. *Mol Cell Biol.* 2000;20:4265–74.

44. Wadleigh DJ, Reddy ST, Kopp E, Ghosh S, Herschman HR. Transcriptional acti-vation of the cyclooxygenase-2 gene in endotoxin-treated RAW 264.7 macrophages. *J Biol Chem.* 2000;275:6259–66.

45. Miller C, Zhang M, He Y, Zhao J, Pelletier JP, Martel-Pelletier J et al. Transcriptional induction of cyclooxygenase-2 gene by okadaic acid inhibition of phosphatase activity in human chondrocytes: co-stimulation of AP-1 and CRE nuclear binding proteins. *J Cell Biol.* 1998;69:392–413.

46. Thomas B, Berenbaum F, Humbert L, Bian H, Bereziat G, Crofford L et al. Critical role of C/EBPδ and C/EBPβ factors in the stimulation of the cyclooxygenase-2 gene transcription by interleukin-1β in articular chondrocytes. *Eur J Biochem.* 2000;267:6798–809.

47. Crofford LJ. COX-1 and COX-2 tissue expression: implications and predictions. *J Rheumatol.* 1997;24(Suppl 49):15–19.

48. Weissmann G. Prostaglandins as modulators rather than mediators of inflammation. *J Lipid Mediators.* 1993;6:275–86.

49. Zurier RB, Quagliata F. Effect of prostaglandin E_1 on adjuvant arthritis. *Nature.* 1971;234:304–5.

50. Moriuchi-Murakami E, Yamada H, Ishii O, Kikukawa T, Igarashi R. Treatment of established collagen induced arthritis with prostaglandin E_1 incorporated in lipid microspheres. *J Rheumatol.* 2000;27:2389–96.

51. Crofford LJ, Lipsky PE, Brooks P, Abramson SB, Simon LS, van de Putte LBA. Basic biology and clinical application of specific COX-2 inhibitors. *Arthritis Rheum.* 2000;43:4–13.

14 | Cyclooxygenase-2 and bone turnover

CAROL C. PILBEAM AND YOSUKE OKADA

University of Connecticut Health Center, Farmington, CT 06030, USA.

ROLE OF COX-2 IN BONE TURNOVER

Coupling of resorption and formation

There are two major lineages of cells involved in bone turnover (Figure 1). Osteoclasts are the bone-resorbing cells. They differentiate from haematopoietic stem cells in the bone marrow, fuse into multinuclear cells which can resorb mineralized bone matrix, and eventually undergo apoptosis. Osteoblasts, the bone-forming cells, differentiate from a stromal stem cell in the bone marrow. Osteoblastic cells at various stages of differentiation generate local factors which regulate the differentiation and activity of the osteoclastic lineage. Although osteoclasts appear to initiate the turnover cycle by resorbing mineralized bone, the differentiation of mature osteoclasts from haematopoietic stem cells is dependent on contact of osteoclastic precursors with cells of the osteoblastic lineage (Figure 1). Mature osteoblasts produce the bone matrix, consisting largely of type I collagen, which will subsequently become mineralized. Some mature osteoblasts will then undergo apoptosis, some may become cells lining the newly formed matrix, and some will become incorporated into the newly formed matrix as an interconnecting network of terminally differentiated cells called osteocytes. Osteocytes are said to be the cells that sense strains in the mineralized matrix and send out signals that result in adaptive bone remodelling in response to mechanical loading.

The turnover cycle results in net bone loss when resorption is greater than formation. Both resorption and formation are dependent on the numbers of mature cells that differentiate from bone marrow progenitors and on the activity of these cells. Differentiation and activity of both osteoclasts and osteoblasts are governed by systemic hormones, such as parathyroid hormone (PTH), and by local factors, such as prostaglandins (PG). It is therapeutically

307

Figure 1 Schematic diagram of the turnover cycle on trabecular and endosteal surfaces of bone which interface with bone marrow. The bone-resorbing osteoclast differentiates from a haematopoietic stem cell in the marrow. The bone-forming osteoblast differentiates from a stromal stem cell in the marrow. Contact between the two lineages is necessary to form mature osteoclasts. Newly formed unmineralized matrix is shown in dark grey. Mineralized matrix containing the terminally differentiated osteocytes is in light grey.

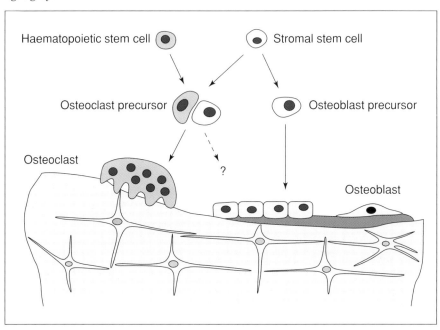

important to inhibit osteoclastic activity if net turnover is negative, since the turnover cycle is initiated by osteoclastic resorption. In addition, if osteoclasts completely erode through a trabecular bridge, then there is no template on which the osteoblasts can produce replacement matrix, and bone may be irretrievably lost. Hence, our current therapies, which act largely to inhibit bone resorption, are useful in slowing or preventing bone loss. However, once bone is lost, our current therapies have very limited ability to restore lost bone. We are clearly in need of new therapies to increase bone formation, particularly in the elderly who have lost significant bone mass.

Expression and regulation of cyclooxygenase-2 in osteoblasts

PGs can act on cells in both osteoclastic and osteoblastic lineages and are among the factors that couple resorption and formation. PGs are produced by cells of the osteoblastic lineage. COX-2 expression is generally undetectable in osteoblasts under unstimulated conditions but can be rapidly and transiently induced by many agents. COX-1 is constitutively expressed in osteoblastic cells and little affected by regulators of COX-2 expression.

COX-2 is the enzyme largely responsible for stimulated PG responses in bone cells[1]. Agonists which induce COX-2 expression in osteoblasts include cytokines, interleukin-1 (IL-1)[2–6], tumour necrosis factor-α (TNF-α)[4], and IL-6[7]; growth factors, transforming growth factor-β (TGF-β)[5,8], TGF-α[2,5], and basic fibroblast growth factor (FGF-2)[9]; and hormones PTH[3,10] and 1,25(OH)$_2$ vitamin D$_3$[11]. PGs themselves induce COX-2 and can therefore amplify PG responses to other agonists[3,12]. Serum is also a potent stimulator of COX-2 expression and PG production in cultured osteoblasts[8]. Hence, the agonists for COX-2 include not only inflammatory agents, such as cytokines, but also the major physiological regulators of bone turnover.

Fewer inhibitors of COX-2 expression have been identified. Gluco-corticoids are potent inhibitors of stimulated PG production by multiple agonists in osteoblastic cells, and their major inhibitory effect is on COX-2 expression[3,8]. IL-4 and IL-13 also inhibit COX-2 expression and PG production in bone organ and cell cultures[13]. We have found that retinoic acid is a transcriptional inhibitor of COX-2 gene expression and PG production in osteoblasts[14]. As noted above, PGs themselves can induce COX-2 expression and, hence, non-steroid anti-inflammatory drugs (NSAIDs) which inhibit COX activity can also decrease COX-2 expression in cases where PGs are being produced abundantly[3,12].

For most agonists, COX-2 behaves like a primary gene response in osteoblasts, with the induction of mRNA expression being rapid, transient and independent of new protein production[5,6,8,9]. The transcriptional regulation of COX-2 induction has been studied using murine COX-2 promoter–luciferase reporter assays. In murine osteoblastic cells transfected with these promoter–reporter constructs, we have found that a short portion of the 5′-flanking COX-2 gene, the 371 bp proximal to the transcription start site, is adequate to mediate induction by many of the agonists discussed above[5,7,9,10,15–17]. In this short region of the murine COX-2 promoter, there are many putative *cis*-acting sequences, identified by computer DNA sequence analysis, including a shear stress response element (SSRE), a cyclic AMP response element (CRE) and an activator protein-1 (AP-1 or Fos/Jun) binding site (Figure 2).

For several agents studied, including IL-1, serum, phorbol ester, forskolin and FGF-2, sequential deletion analysis indicated that major *cis*-acting sites mediating murine COX-2 promoter activity lie between −40 and −150 bp[5,17,18]. For FGF-2, phorbol ester and serum, specific induction of luciferase activity in murine osteoblastic cells is mediated by the AP-1 binding site and the neigh-bouring CRE[17,19] (Figure 2). The function of this AP-1 site has only been studied in osteoblasts. However, a recent study in human chondrocytes showed that okadaic acid induced COX-2 expression and stimulated binding to an AP-1 consensus sequence[20]. The AP-1 binding site 5′-aGAGTCA-3′ at −69/−63 bp in the murine COX-2 5′-flanking region is similar to the

Figure 2 Putative *cis*-acting regions in the $-371/+70$ bp 5'-flanking DNA of the murine COX-2 gene. The DNA sequences are written from 5' to 3' bp. Small letters denote differences from the accepted consensus sequences.

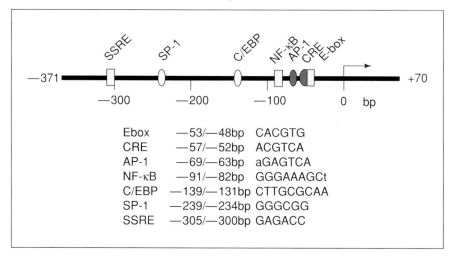

Ebox	$-53/-48$bp	CACGTG
CRE	$-57/-52$bp	ACGTCA
AP-1	$-69/-63$bp	aGAGTCA
NF-κB	$-91/-82$bp	GGGAAAGCt
C/EBP	$-139/-131$bp	CTTGCGCAA
SP-1	$-239/-234$bp	GGGCGG
SSRE	$-305/-300$bp	GAGACC

sequence 5'-acAGTCA-3' found at $-68/-62$ bp in the rat and human COX-2 genes[21,22], suggesting that this motif may be important for regulating these genes as well. The AP-1 complex is involved in cellular proliferation, tumorigenesis and inflammation in multiple tissues and might be implicated in the increased COX-2 expression found in tumorigenesis and inflammation. In mice with collagen-induced arthritis, bone resorption and synovial overgrowth at joints can be inhibited by administering short, double stranded AP-1 DNA oligonucleotides to compete for the binding of AP-1 *in vivo*[23]. Moreover, the anti-inflammatory actions of glucocorticoids may be mediated in part by interactions of glucocorticoid receptors with AP-1 proteins[24].

TGF-β appears to induce COX-2 expression in osteoblasts independently of the AP-1 and CRE sites. A 90% drop in luciferase activity occurred with deletion of the region from -371 to -213 bp of the COX-2 promoter[5]. Perhaps because it involves a site distant from that of the other agonists, the stimulation of luciferase activity and COX-2 expression by TGF-β is additive to the stimulation of several other agonists, including IL-1, forskolin and phorbol ester[5].

To study the transcriptional regulation of COX-2 *in vivo*, we generated mice transgenic for $-371/+70$ bp of the COX-2 promoter DNA fused to a luciferase reporter[16]. When these mice are injected with lipopolysaccharide (LPS), a potent inflammatory mediator, COX-2 mRNA and luciferase activity are induced in multiple tissues. The LPS induction of both luciferase activity and of endogenous COX-2 mRNA in calvarial bone, chosen because it contains little bone marrow, was among the highest of all the tissues sampled, including brain, colon, heart, lung and uterus. Hence, bone cells may be an important, and overlooked, source of PGs *in vivo*, and PGs produced by bone cells may influence neighbouring cells in the bone marrow and in the vascular network.

Role of cyclooxygenase-2 in osteoclast formation and bone resorption

As noted above, osteoclast differentiation is highly dependent on osteoblasts. Osteoblasts are not only the source of many local factors known to regulate the resorption process, but they also have the receptors for most of the local and systemic factors that regulate resorption. It has recently become clear that formation of mature bone-resorbing osteoclasts requires a contact-dependent interaction between osteoclastic precursor cells and cells of the osteoblastic lineage[25–27] (Figure 3). The molecule mediating this interaction was originally cloned as receptor activator of NF-κB (RANK) ligand (RANKL)[28] and found to be identical to TNF-related activation induced cytokine (TRANCE)[29]. RANKL is also a ligand for osteoprotegerin (OPG), a soluble receptor for RANKL which acts as a 'decoy' receptor, preventing binding of RANKL to its active receptor RANK[30]. Osteoblastic cells produce both RANKL and

Figure 3 Schematic representation of interactions between the osteoclastic and osteoblastic lineages, which regulate osteoclastogenesis. Cells of the osteoblastic lineage produce M-CSF and RANK ligand (RANKL), both of which are necessary for osteoclastogenesis. They also produce OPG, a decoy receptor for RANKL. Resorption agonists, including IL-1, PTH, PGE_2 and $1,25(OH)_2$ vitamin D_3, act on osteoblastic cells to increase RANKL and inhibit OPG expression. Osteoclastic cells produce the receptor for RANKL, RANK. Mature osteoclasts are identified as multinucleated, tartrate-resistant acid phosphatase positive (TRAP+) cells, which express calcitonin receptors (CTR+) and resorb mineralized bone. Please see text for definition of terms.

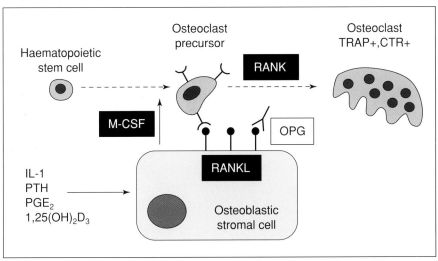

OPG, as well as macrophage colony stimulating factor (M-CSF), which is also required for osteoclastogenesis, while osteoclastic cells express RANK (Figure 3). The only resorption agonist that has been reported to be able to induce osteoclastogenesis in the absence of RANKL is TNF[31]. Mice with the gene for the RANK receptor disrupted have absent bone resorption and develop osteopetrosis[32], and mice with the gene for OPG disrupted resorb too much bone and develop osteoporosis[33]. In general, the ability of an agonist to stimulate resorption can be thought of as proportional to its ability to stimulate RANKL expression and inhibit OPG expression.

PGs of the E series are potent stimulators of bone resorption in organ culture and PGE_1 and PGE_2, but not $PGF_{2\alpha}$, stimulate osteoclast formation in marrow cultures[34]. Many factors that stimulate PG production also stimulate resorption in organ culture, and the resorption stimulated by such factors can be mediated in part by PG production[35–39]. However, the dependence of resorption in organ culture on stimulated PG production is quite variable[1]. In contrast, studies in marrow culture generally demonstrate a dependence of osteoclast formation on stimulated PG production. Agonists that have been reported to stimulate PG-dependent osteoclast formation include IL-1[37,40,41], $TNF\alpha$[41], PTH[42,43], $1,25(OH)_2$ vitamin D3[44], IL-11[45,46], IL-6[7], IL-17[47], phorbol ester[48], and FGF-2[49]. Hence, the most important role for PGs in bone resorption may be in the regulation of osteoclast formation and differentiation.

We examined the effect of disruption of both alleles for COX-2 or for COX-1 on osteoclast formation in murine marrow cultures[11]. As noted above, marrow cultures contain precursors for both osteoblasts and osteoclasts. *In vitro*, few osteoclasts are formed in the absence of resorption agonists. We used $1,25(OH)_2D_3$ and PTH as stimulators of osteoclast formation since they are the major systemic physiological regulators of bone resorption. Osteoclast formation, whether stimulated by $1,25(OH)_2D_3$ or by PTH, was reduced 60–70% in COX-2$^{-/-}$ cultures compared with COX-2$^{+/+}$ cultures. PGE_2 production was significantly reduced in marrow cultures from mice lacking the COX-2 gene compared with cultures from wild-type mice. Decreased osteoclastogenesis in COX-2$^{-/-}$ cultures was reversed by exogenous PGE_2. Treatment of normal cultures with COX inhibitors (indomethacin and NS-398, a selective inhibitor of COX-2) mimicked the results observed in cultures from COX-2 mice. The reduced response to $1,25(OH)_2D_3$ and PTH hormone in COX-2$^{-/-}$ cultures was associated with reduced expression of RANKL by osteoblastic cells secondary to decreased PG production in the absence of COX-2. These data are consistent with other studies showing that PGE_2 increases the expression of RANKL in osteoblastic cells while decreasing the expression in those same cells of the inhibitory OPG[30,50] (Figure 4). We found no effect of COX-1 disruption on stimulated PG production or osteoclastogenesis.

Figure 4 Schematic representation of the role of COX-2 in osteoclastogenesis. Agonists, including PGE_2, act on osteoblastic cells to induce COX-2 expression and PGE_2 production. PGE_2 acts via the prostaglandin receptors EP_2 and EP_4, to increase RANKL expression and, perhaps, to decrease OPG expression in osteoblastic cells. PGE_2 also acts, probably via the EP_2 receptor, to decrease expression of GM-CSF, an inhibitor of osteoclastogenesis, in haematopoietic cells. In contrast to these stimulatory effects, PGE_2 can have a transient inhibitory effect on mature osteoclast activity. Please see text for definition of terms.

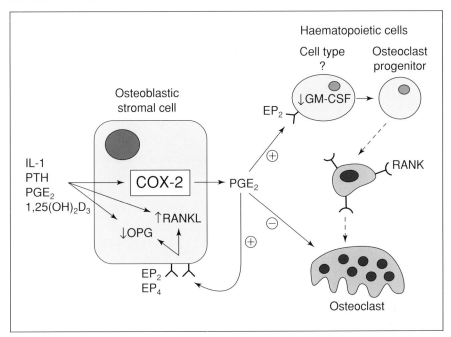

In addition to acting on osteoblastic cells, PGs may also act on osteoclastic progenitors among the haematopoietic cells to influence the formation and activity of osteoclasts. PGs can transiently inhibit the resorbing activity of isolated osteoclasts[51], but the physiological relevance of this observation is unknown. Osteoclasts can be formed in spleen cultures, which contain osteoclast precursors but no osteoblasts, if the cultures are treated with M-CSF and soluble RANKL to replace the need for supporting osteoblastic cells. PGE_2 has been shown to synergize with RANKL and M-CSF in stimulating osteoclast formation in spleen culture systems[52]. In such a system, we found that osteoclast formation was reduced 50% when spleen cells came from COX-2$^{-/-}$ mice compared with cells from COX-2$^{+/+}$ mice[11]. This reduction was due to increased expression of granulocyte macrophage colony stimulating factor (GM-CSF), an inhibitor of osteoclast formation in these cultures[11]. GM-CSF may act by diverting progenitor cells into the macrophage pathway that might otherwise differentiate into osteoclasts. Hence, PGs can enhance osteoclastogenesis by acting on osteoclast supporting cells to increase RANKL and on haematopoietic cells to decrease GM-CSF (Figure 4).

There are at least four classes of receptors for PGE_2, two of which, EP_2 and EP_4, act via stimulating cAMP[53]. Both of these receptors have been shown to be involved in the PGE_2 stimulation of osteoclast formation supported by osteoblasts[54–56]. The EP_2 receptor appears to be the receptor that mediates the effect of PGE_2 on the haematopoietic cells[56].

Although it is clear that PGs produced by COX-2 are necessary for maximal stimulation of osteoclastogenesis *in vitro*, little is known about the role of COX-2 in bone resorption *in vivo*. Clearly COX-2 is not required for bone resorption since COX-2$^{-/-}$ mice do not develop osteopetrosis[11]. We speculate that a role for COX-2 in bone resorption may be most evident when resorption is rapid, such as in inflammation, and the ability to form new osteoclasts becomes the factor limiting the rate of resorption. To study this possibility, we injected PTH at high dose above the calvaria of COX-2$^{-/-}$ mice and their wild-type littermates[11]. This protocol has been shown to result in localized resorption at the site of injection, which is reflected by systemic hypercalcaemia[57]. After 3 days of injection, PTH caused hyper-calcaemia in the wild-type mice but not in the COX-2$^{-/-}$ mice, indicating that resorption in response to PTH was inhibited in the COX-2$^{-/-}$ mice. Hence, the absence of COX-2 limits the maximal resorption response to PTH *in vivo* and the maximal osteoclastogenesis response to PTH *in vitro*. We have found similar results for IL-1 both *in vitro* and *in vivo* (unpublished data).

Role of cyclooxygenase-2 in osteoblast formation and bone formation

The effects of exogenous prostaglandins on bone formation *in vitro* are complex[1]. PGs can stimulate DNA synthesis and cell replication in bone cell and organ cultures[58]. In organ culture the mitogenic effect of PGE_2 appears to be selective for preosteoblasts[59]. Exposure time and dose may be important. In periosteal cells from embryonic chick calvariae, the mitogenic effect of PGE_2 is greatest after brief exposure and decreases with prolonged exposure[60]. A dose-related biphasic effect has been reported in cultured human bone cells with stimulation of mitogenesis at 10^{-9} M and inhibition at 10^{-6} M PGE_2[61]. PGs can both stimulate and inhibit collagen synthesis. The inhibitory effect appears to be a transcriptional effect on the collagen promoter[62]. In organ culture, the anabolic effect is best seen in the presence of glucocorticoids[63,64]. In marrow stromal cell and primary calvarial cell cultures designed to study differentiation of osteoblasts from progenitors, PGE_2 stimulates the forma-tion of colony-forming units and mineralized nodules[65–67]. We have recently shown that marrow stromal cells or primary osteoblasts cultured from mice with the COX-2 gene disrupted have significantly delayed osteoblastic differentiation compared with cultures from wild-type mice[68]. Hence, it seems likely that, similar to their effects on the osteoclast lineage, PGs enhance the differentiation of osteoblastic progenitors but can inhibit the function of mature osteoblasts.

In vivo, many animal experiments have shown that prolonged administration of PGE_2 stimulates both endosteal and periosteal new bone formation[69,70]. This effect does not require prior bone resorption[71]. In addition, PGE_2 given *in vivo* enhances osteoblastic differentiation in explanted marrow stromal cells[72]. Little is known about the role of endogenous PGs *in vivo*.

COX-2 AND MECHANICAL LOADING OF BONE

Responses of bone to mechanical loading
One of the major physiological roles for prostaglandins in bone may be to mediate effects of mechanical loading on bone. Bone is a dynamic tissue that responds to mechanical stress with changes in mass and structure, to achieve a better balance between stress and load-bearing capacity. The predictable increase in bone remodelling to applied forces underlies therapeutic modalities in contemporary orthodontics and orthopaedics. PGs have been demonstrated to mediate effects of mechanical loading on bone in multiple studies. Some of these effects appear to be related to the ability of PGs to stimulate resorption, while others reflect the anabolic effect of PGs. Orthodontic movement of teeth stimulates PG production, and endogenous or exogenous PGs enhance the rate of tooth movement[73-78]. This enhancement is presumably the result, at least in part, of PG-stimulated bone resorption.

Mechanical loading can also stimulate new bone formation and/or prevent bone loss. Because of this observation, protocols for skeletal loading are part of osteoporosis prevention and therapy programmes. Moderate exercise programmes have been shown to increase bone density by 5–7%[79-83]. Excess loading may even lead to bone hypertrophy, as in the arms of professional tennis players or in the spinal osteophytic processes in the elderly. Unloading, as with immobilization or during space flight, can increase bone loss and the risk for osteoporotic fracture[84-88].

Role of prostaglandins in the anabolic effects of mechanical loading
PGs are thought to mediate some of the anabolic effects of mechanical loading. Mechanical loading of bone explants increased PG production and resulted in new bone formation[89-91]. Loading of an isolated avian ulna preparation stimulated transformation of a quiescent periosteum into one actively forming new bone; the new bone formation was blocked by a non-selective NSAID[92]. In a model in which tail vertebrae of rats were externally loaded *in*

vivo, loading increased bone formation and a non-selective NSAID blocked the increase[93]. In humans, *in situ* microdialysis showed a 2.5–3.5-fold increase in the release of PGE_2 in the tibial metaphysis after loading[94].

Although PGs may mediate anabolic effects of loading, they may also mediate catabolic effects of unloading. A study using tenotomy to immobilize mice found that bone loss of tenotomy was prevented by treatment with a non-selective NSAID[95]. Similarly, a non-selective NSAID prevented disuse-induced bone loss in the tail suspension model of immobilization in rats[96].

It is hypothesized that COX-2 plays a major role in the production of PGs involved in mediating the effects of increased mechanical loading. For example, a single short period of bending applied to rat tibiae can increase endosteal bone formation[97], and this increase is prevented by a selective COX-2 inhibitor (NS-398)[98]. Although it is not known how mechanical loading is coupled to cellular responses in bone, fluid flow is likely to play an important role. Normal activities, such as walking and chewing, cause small cyclic displacements in the mineralized matrix of bone which generate inter-stitial fluid flow in the lacunar–canalicular network. Shear stress (force per unit area) is exerted in the direction of the flow on membranes of cells lining the surfaces, and this fluid shear stress induces PG production[99,100]. The PGE_2 release which occurs within minutes of applied fluid shear is probably due to an early release of arachidonic acid that is converted to PGs by the con-stitutively expressed COX-1, while the sustained production of PGs is due to fluid shear stress induced COX-2 mRNA expression[100].

Because of the importance of mechanical loading in therapeutic protocols and in normal skeletal adaptation, it is important to consider the possibility that selective COX-2 inhibitors might affect the skeletal response to mechanical loading.

EFFECTS OF NSAIDS ON BONE TURNOVER

Role of prostaglandins in inflammatory bone loss

A number of studies have reported that PG production is increased in inflam-matory processes, such as rheumatoid arthritis[101]. In the rat carrageenan footpad model of acute inflammation, COX-2 expression is elevated, and selective inhibition of COX-2 activity inhibited oedema and hyperalgesia[102]. Because of this association of PG production with inflammation, and because PGs are potent stimulators of bone resorption, it is often assumed that PGs contribute to the bone loss and cartilage destruction associated with inflam-matory diseases. There are a few studies showing that NSAIDs decrease alveolar bone loss in peridontitis to support this conclusion[103-105]. Patients with rheumatoid arthritis can have systemic bone changes[106], but these changes may reflect the direct effects of other factors, such as cytokines, levels of which are elevated in the disease process. Proinflammatory agents, such as cytokines and LPS, are themselves potent inducers of bone resorption; their effects are enhanced by PGs but are not dependent on PGs. In addition, cytokines can inhibit bone matrix proteins independently of cytokine-induced PG production[107]. Hence, it is not clear that PGs are simply mediators of catabolic effects on the skeleton in inflammatory diseases; their potential role to stimulate osteoblastic differentiation might have a protective effect.

Effects of NSAIDs on bone mineral density

Measurements of bone mineral density (BMD) are now accepted as the basis for assessing the risk for osteoporotic fracture. Only a few studies have examined the effects of NSAIDs on BMD in animals or humans. NSAIDs were found to slow bone loss in ovariectomized rats, but the effect was transient[108]. In a study of postmenopausal women, 65 years of age or older, there was no significant difference found in N-telopeptide cross-link excretion (NTX), a marker of bone resorption, between self-reported users of NSAIDs or aspirin, compared with non-users[109]. In a similar cohort, the use of aspirin or NSAIDs was found to be associated with a small but significant increase in hip and spine BMD, but there was no clinically significant protective effect on risk of fracture[110]. In a more recent study of older women from Rancho Bernardo, CA, the regular use of propionic acid NSAIDs (ibuprofen, naproxen, ketoprofen), but not acetic acid NSAIDs (indomethacin, diclofenac, sulindac, tolmetin), was associated with higher BMD at multiple skeletal sites[111]. When women with self-reported osteoarthritis were excluded, significantly higher BMD was observed in the hip in propionic acid NSAID users. Those who concurrently used oestrogen and propionic acid NSAIDs had the highest BMD at all sites. There are no published studies examining the effects of selective COX-2 inhibitors on BMD.

Other effects of NSAIDs on bone

Heterotropic ossification is a complication of hip arthroplasty that can adversely affect the outcome. Several studies have shown that perioperative treatment with aspirin or non-selective NSAIDs can prevent this complication[112–114], suggesting that the problem is caused by PG-mediated bone formation.

Because PGs may enhance the bone remodeling needed for fracture healing, there is concern that NSAIDs might adversely affect fracture healing. Studies suggest that some NSAIDs can inhibit repair of fractured femurs[115–116] and spinal fusions[117] in rats and the fixation of implants in femora of rabbits[118], while exogenously applied PGs can stimulate callus formation in rabbits[119]. Ultrasound stimulation can enhance bone healing, and studies have suggested both that ultrasound acts by decreasing PG production[120] and by stimulating COX-2 induction and associated PG production[121].

INTERACTIONS OF NITRIC OXIDE SYNTHASE WITH COX-2

There are at least three isoforms of nitric oxide (NO) synthase (NOS): neuronal NOS (NOS1), inducible NOS (NOS2), and endothelial NOS (NOS3). NOS1 and NOS3 are expressed constitutively and are dependent on Ca^{2+}. NOS2 is induced in macrophages, neutrophils and chondrocytes by cytokines. NOS2 and NOS3 are expressed in both osteoblastic and in osteoclastic cells[122–126]. Many studies have noted coordinate regulation of NOS2 and COX-2 by inflammatory agents. In models of inflammation, studies suggest that constitutive NOS can activate COX-1 enzyme and that inducible NOS can activate COX-2[127,128]. In addition, selective inhibitors of inducible NOS can exert anti-inflammatory actions by inhibiting both NO and PG production[129]. Some studies find that NO also increases COX-2 expression[130], while other studies find that NO inhibits COX-2 expression[131].

As is true for COX-2, there are conflicting data on the role of NO in bone turnover. A number of studies indicate that NO promotes bone formation. Intermittent use of nitrates has been shown to increase BMD in elderly women[132]. There are several studies in cultured osteoblastic cells showing that NO enhances osteoblastic differentiation[133,134]. An inhibitor of inducible NOS decreased bone formation in rats[135]. NO was produced by bone during fracture healing and suppression of NOS impaired fracture healing[136]. Many studies have demonstrated that NO inhibits osteoclast formation and bone resorption[123,137–142]. On the other hand, in an animal model of inflammation-induced osteoporosis, NOS inhibitors reversed the decrease in osteoblast numbers, the increase in osteoclast numbers, and the reduction in bone mass caused by inflammation[143].

The relationship of the effects of NO on bone cells to the possible NO-enhanced PG production by these cells is unclear. In the majority of studies on osteoclastogenesis, NO inhibits and PGs stimulate. However, it has been suggested that NO has biphasic effects on bone, stimulating both formation and resorption at low concentrations and inhibiting both at high concentrations[144]. To disentangle these two pathways, it might be helpful to determine if selective COX-2 inhibitors block the effects of NO, to study the effects of NO in COX-2 knockout mice, and to study the effects of COX-2 agonists in NOS2 and NOS3 knockout mice.

SUMMARY

The role of PGs in skeletal metabolism is complex. COX-2 is the major regulatory enzyme for acute PG responses in bone. Previous studies using non-selective NSAIDs may not have been able to attain continuous inhibition of COX-2 activity because of toxic side effects. *In vitro* studies indicate that

NSAIDs can have biphasic effects – low concentrations can increase, rather than decrease, PG production[145,146]. Studies with the new selective inhibitors of COX-2 may help to clarify the role of COX-2 in bone metabolism. Whether the results of inhibiting COX-2 are catabolic or anabolic in bone may depend on the amplitude and duration of COX-2 expression and activity, as well as on the current state of remodelling. We speculate that inhibition of COX-2 in inflammation or other states of high resorption activity will protect bone, but that chronic inhibition of COX-2 might reduce the formation response to resorption and result in bone loss.

Address all correspondence to: Carol C. Pilbeam, University of Connecticut Health Center, Farmington, CT 06030, USA.

REFERENCES

1. Pilbeam CC, Harrison JR, Raisz LG. Prostaglandins and bone metabolism. In: Bilezikian JP, Raisz LG, Rodan GA, editors. *Principles of Bone Biology*. New York: Academic Press; 1996; 715–28.
2. Harrison JR, Lorenzo JA, Kawaguchi H, Raisz LG, Pilbeam CC. Stimulation of prostaglandin E_2 production by interleukin-1 and transforming growth factor-α in osteoblastic MC3T3-E1 cells. *J Bone Miner Res*. 1994;9:817–23.
3. Kawaguchi H, Raisz LG, Voznesensky OS, Alander CB, Hakeda Y, Pilbeam CC. Regulation of the two prostaglandin G/H synthases by parathyroid hormone, inter-leukin-1, cortisol and prostaglandin E_2 in cultured neonatal mouse calvariae. *Endocrinology*. 1994;135:1157–64.
4. Kawaguchi H, Nemoto K, Raisz LG, Harrison JR, Voznesensky OS, Alander CB et al. Interleukin-4 inhibits prostaglandin G/H synthase-2 and cytosolic phospholi-pase A_2 induction in neonatal mouse parietal bone cultures. *J Bone Miner Res*. 1996;11:358–66.
5. Pilbeam C, Rao Y, Voznesensky O, Kawaguchi H, Alander C, Raisz LG et al. Transforming growth factor-β1 regulation of prostaglandin G/H synthase-2 expres-sion in osteoblastic MC3T3-E1 cells. *Endocrinology*. 1997;138:4672–82.
6. Min YK, Rao Y, Okada Y, Raisz LG, Pilbeam CC. Regulation of prostaglandin G/H synthase-2 expression by interleukin-1 in human osteoblast-like cells. *J Bone Miner Res*. 1998;13:1066–75.
7. Tai H, Miyaura C, Pilbeam CC, Tamura T, Ohsugi Y, Koishihara Y et al. Transcriptional induction of cyclooxygenase-2 in osteoblasts is involved in inter-leukin-6-induced osteoclast formation. *Endocrinology*. 1997;138:2372–9.
8. Pilbeam CC, Kawaguchi H, Hakeda Y, Voznesensky O, Alander CB, Raisz LG. Differential regulation of inducible and constitutive prostaglandin endoperoxide synthase in osteoblastic MC3T3-E1 cells. *J Biol Chem*. 1993;268:25643–9.
9. Kawaguchi H, Pilbeam CC, Gronowicz G, Abreu C, Fletcher BS, Herschman HR et al. Regulation of inducible prostaglandin G/H synthase mRNA levels and promoter activity by basic fibroblast growth factor in osteoblastic cells. *J Clin Invest*. 1995;96:923–30.
10. Tetradis S, Pilbeam CC, Liu Y, Herschman HR, Kream BE. Parathyroid hormone

increases prostaglandin G/H synthase-2 transcription by a cyclic adenosine 3′,5′-monophosphate-mediated pathway in murine osteoblastic MC3T3-E1 cells. *Endocrinology.* 1997;138:3594–600.

11. Okada Y, Lorenzo JA, Freeman AM, Tomita M, Morham SG, Raisz LG et al. Prostaglandin G/H synthase-2 is required for maximal formation of osteoclast-like cells in culture. *J Clin Invest.* 2000;105:823–32.

12. Pilbeam CC, Raisz LG, Voznesensky O, Alander CB, Delman BN, Kawaguchi K. Autoregulation of inducible prostaglandin G/H synthase in osteoblastic cells by prostaglandins. *J Bone Miner Res.* 1994;10:406–14.

13. Onoe Y, Miyaura C, Kaminakayashiki T, Nagai Y, Noguchi K, Chen QR et al. IL-13 and IL-4 inhibit bone resorption by suppressing cyclooxygenase-2-dependent prostaglandin synthesis in osteoblasts. *J Immunol.* 1996;156:758–64.

14. Pilbeam C, Bernecker P, Harrison J, Alander C, Voznesensky O, Herschman H et al. Retinoic acid inhibits induction of prostaglandin G/H synthase-2 mRNA and promoter activity in MC3T3-E1 osteoblastic cells. *J Bone Miner Res.* 1995;10(S1):S496.

15. Pilbeam CC, Kawaguchi H, Voznesensky OS, Alander CB, Raisz LG. Regulation of inducible prostaglandin G/H synthase by interleukin-1, transforming growth factors-alpha and -beta, and prostaglandins in bone cells. *Adv Exp Med Biol.* 1997;400B:617–23.

16. Freeman A, Mallico E, Voznesensky O, Bhatt A, Clark S, Pilbeam C. Transcriptional regulation of prostaglandin G/H synthase-2 in transgenic mice. *J Bone Miner Res.* 1999;14S:S472.

17. Okada Y, Voznesensky O, Herschman H, Harrison J, Pilbeam C. Identification of multiple *cis*-acting elements mediating the induction of prostaglandin G/H synthase-2 by phorbol ester in murine osteoblastic cells. *J Cell Biochem.* 2000;78:197–209.

18. Harrison JR, Kelly PL, Pilbeam CC. Involvement of C/EBP transcription factors in prostaglandin G/H synthase-2 gene induction by interleukin-1 in osteoblastic MC3T3-E1 cells. *J Bone Miner Res.* 2000;15:1138–46.

19. Okada Y, Tetradis S, Voznesensky O, Kream BE, Herschman HR, Hurley MM et al. AP-1 and CRE sites jointly mediate the induction of prostaglandin G/H synthase-2 promoter activity by basic fibroblast growth factor in osteoblastic MC3T3-E1 cells. *Bone.* 1998;23(S5): S245.

20. Miller C, Zhang M, He Y, Zhao J, Pelletier JP, Martel-Pelletier J et al. Transcriptional induction of cyclooxygenase-2 gene by okadaic acid inhibition of phosphatase activity in human chondrocytes: co-stimulation of AP-1 and CRE nuclear binding proteins. *J Cell Biochem.* 1998;69:392–413.

21. Kosaka T, Miyata A, Ihara H, Hara S, Sugimoto T, Takeda O et al. Characterization of the human gene (PTGS2) encoding prostaglandin-endoperoxide synthase 2. *Eur J Biochem.* 1994;221:889–97.

22. Sirois J, Richards JS. Transcriptional regulation of the rat prostaglandin endoperoxide synthase 2 gene in granulosa cells. Evidence for the role of a *cis*-acting C/EBP beta promoter element. *J Biol Chem.* 1993;268:21931–8.

23. Shiozawa S, Shimizu K, Tanaka K, Hino K. Studies on the contribution of c-fos/AP-1 to arthritic joint destruction. *J Clin Invest.* 1997;99:1210–16.

24. Krane SM. Some molecular mechanisms of glucocorticoid action. *Br J Rheumatol.* 1993;32(Suppl 2):3–5.

25. Martin T, Udagawa N. Hormonal regulation of osteoclast function. *Trends Endocrinol Metab.* 1998;9:6–12.

26. Reddy SV, Roodman GD. Control of osteoclast differentiation. *Crit Rev Eukaryot Gene Expr.* 1998;8:1–17.

27. Suda T, Takahashi N, Udagawa N, Jimi E, Gillespie MT, Martin TJ. Modulation of osteoclast differentiation and function by the new members of the tumor necrosis factor receptor and ligand families. *Endocr Rev.* 1999;20:345–57.

28. Anderson DM, Maraskovsky E, Billingsley WL, Dougall WC, Tometsko ME, Roux ER et al. A homologue of the TNF receptor and its ligand enhance T-cell growth and dendritic-cell function. *Nature.* 1997;390:175–9.

29. Wong BR, Rho J, Arron J, Robinson E, Orlinick J, Chao M et al. TRANCE is a novel ligand of the tumor necrosis factor receptor family that activates c-Jun N-terminal kinase in T cells. *J Biol Chem.* 1997;272:25190–4.

30. Yasuda H, Shima N, Nakagawa N, Yamaguchi K, Kinosaki M, Mochizuki S et al. Osteoclast differentiation factor is a ligand for osteoprotegerin/osteoclastogenesis-inhibitory factor and is identical to TRANCE/RANKL. *Proc Natl Acad Sci USA.* 1998;95:3597–602.

31. Kobayashi K, Takahashi N, Jimi E, Udagawa N, Takami M, Kotake S et al. Tumor necrosis factor alpha stimulates osteoclast differentiation by a mechanism independent of the ODF/RANKL-RANK interaction. *J Exp Med.* 2000;191:275–86.

32. Li J, Sarosi I, Yan XQ, Morony S, Capparelli C, Tan HL et al. RANK is the intrinsic hematopoietic cell surface receptor that controls osteoclastogenesis and regulation of bone mass and calcium metabolism. *Proc Natl Acad Sci USA.* 2000;97:1566–71.

33. Bucay N, Sarosi I, Dunstan CR, Morony S, Tarpley J, Capparelli C et al. Osteoprotegerin-deficient mice develop early onset osteoporosis and arterial calcification. *Genes Dev.* 1998;12:1260–8.

34. Klein DC, Raisz LG. Prostaglandins: stimulation of bone resorption in tissue culture. *Endocrinology.* 1970;86:1436–40.

35. Tashjian AHJ, Hohmann EL, Antoniades HN, Levine L. Platelet-derived growth factor stimulates bone resorption via a prostaglandin-mediated mechanism. *Endocrinology.* 1982;111:118–24.

36. Sato K, Fujii Y, Kasono K, Saji M, Tsushima T, Shizume K. Stimulation of prostaglandin E_2 and bone resorption by recombinant human interleukin 1 alpha in fetal long bone. *Biochem Biophys Res Commun.* 1986;138:618–24.

37. Akatsu T, Takahashi N, Udagawa N, Imamura K, Yamaguchi A, Sato K et al. Role of prostaglandins in interleukin-1-induced bone resorption in mice *in vitro. J Bone Miner Res.* 1991;6:183–9.

38. Stern PH, Krieger NS, Nissenson RA, Williams RD, Winkler ME, Derynck R et al. Human transforming growth factor-alpha stimulates bone resorption *in vitro. J Clin Invest.* 1985;76:2016–19.

39. Tashjian AH, Voelkel EF, Lazzaro M, Goad D, Bosma T, Levine L. Tumor necrosis factor-α (cachectin) stimulates bone resorption in mouse calvaria via a prostaglandin-mediated mechanism. *Endocrinology.* 1987;120:2029–36.

40. Sato T, Morita I, Sakaguchi K, Nakahama KI, Smith WL, DeWitt DL et al. Involvement of prostaglandin endoperoxide H synthase-2 in osteoclast-like cell formation induced by interleukin-1 beta. *J Bone Miner Res.* 1996;11:392–400.

41. Lader CS, Flanagan AM. Prostaglandin E_2, interleukin 1α, and tumor necrosis factor-α increase human osteoclast formation and bone resorption *in vitro. Endocrinology.* 1998;139:3157–64.

42. Inoue H, Tanaka N, Uchiyama C. Parathyroid hormone increases the number of

tartrate-resistant acid phosphatase-positive cells through prostaglandin E$_2$ synthesis in adherent cell culture of neonatal rat bones. *Endocrinology.* 1995;136:3648–56.

43. Sato T, Morita I, Murota S. Prostaglandin E$_2$ mediates parathyroid hormone induced osteoclast formation by cyclic AMP independent mechanism. *Adv Exp Med Biol.* 1997;407:383–6.

44. Collins DA, Chambers TJ. Prostaglandin E$_2$ promotes osteoclast formation in murine hematopoietic cultures through an action on hematopoietic cells. *J Bone Miner Res.* 1992;7:555–61.

45. Girasole G, Passeri G, Jilka RL, Manolagas SC. Interleukin-11: a new cytokine critical for osteoclast development. *J Clin Invest.* 1994;93:1516–24.

46. Morinaga Y, Fujita N, Ohishi K, Zhang Y, Tsuruo T. Suppression of interleukin-11-mediated bone resorption by cyclooxygenases inhibitors. *J Cell Physiol.* 1998;175:247–54.

47. Kotake S, Udagawa N, Takahashi N, Matsuzaki K, Itoh K, Ishiyama S et al. IL-17 in synovial fluids from patients with rheumatoid arthritis is a potent stimulator of osteoclastogenesis. *J Clin Invest.* 1999;103:1345–52.

48. Amano S, Hanazawa S, Kawata Y, Nakada Y, Miyata Y, Kitano S. Phorbol myristate acetate stimulates osteoclast formation in 1 alpha,25-dihydroxyvitamin D$_3$-primed mouse embryonic calvarial cells by a prostaglandin-dependent mechanism. *J Bone Miner Res.* 1994;9:465–72.

49. Hurley MM, Lee SK, Raisz LG, Bernecker P, Lorenzo J. Basic fibroblast growth factor induces osteoclast formation in murine bone marrow cultures. *Bone.* 1998;22:309–16.

50. Tsukii K, Shima N, Mochizuki S, Yamaguchi K, Kinosaki M, Yano K et al. Osteoclast differentiation factor mediates an essential signal for bone resorption induced by 1 alpha,25-dihydroxyvitamin D$_3$, prostaglandin E$_2$, or parathyroid hormone in the microenvironment of bone. *Biochem Biophys Res Commun.* 1998;246:337–41.

51. Chambers TJ, McSheehy PM, Thomson BM, Fuller K. The effect of calcium-regulating hormones and prostaglandins on bone resorption by osteoclasts disaggregated from neonatal rabbit bones. *Endocrinology.* 1985;116:234–9.

52. Wani MR, Fuller K, Kim NS, Choi Y, Chambers T. Prostaglandin E$_2$ cooperates with TRANCE in osteoclast induction from hemopoietic precursors: synergistic activation of differentiation, cell spreading, and fusion. *Endocrinology.* 1999;140:1927–35.

53. Coleman RA, Smith WL, Narumiya S. International Union of Pharmacology classification of prostanoid receptors: properties, distribution, and structure of the receptors and their subtypes. *Pharm Rev.* 1994;46:205–20.

54. Ono K, Akatsu T, Murakami T, Nishikawa M, Yamamoto M, Kugai N et al. Important role of EP$_4$, a subtype of prostaglandin (PG) E receptor in osteoclast-like cell formation from mouse bone marrow cells induced by PGE$_2$. J Endocrinol. 1995;158:R1–R5.

55. Sakuma Y, Tanaka K, Suda M, Yasoda A, Tanaka L, Ushikubi F et al. Defective osteoclast formation by prostaglandin E$_2$, IL-1α, TNFα, basic FGF, TGFβ in mice deficient in EP$_4$ subtype of PGE receptor. *Bone.* 1998;23:S215.

56. Li X, Okada Y, Pilbeam CC, Lorenzo JA, Kennedy CR, Breyer RM et al. Knockout of the murine prostaglandin EP$_2$ receptor impairs osteoclastogenesis *in vitro*. *Endocrinology.* 2000;141:2054–61.

57. Zhao W, Byrne MH, Boyce BF, Krane SM. Bone resorption induced by parathyroid

hormone is strikingly diminished in collagenase-resistant mutant mice. *J Clin Invest.* 1999;103:517–24.

58. Woodiel FN, Fall PM, Raisz LG. Anabolic effects of prostaglandins in cultured fetal rat calvariae: structure–activity relations and signal transduction pathway. *J Bone Miner Res.* 1996;11:1249–55.

59. Gronowicz GA, Fall PM, Raisz LG. Prostaglandin E_2 stimulates preosteoblast replication: an autoradiographic study in cultured fetal rat calvariae. *Exp Cell Res.* 1994; 212:314–20.

60. Scutt A, Duvos C, Lauber J, Mayer H. Time-dependent effects of parathyroid hormone and prostaglandin E_2 on DNA synthesis by periosteal cells from embryonic chick calvaria. *Calcif Tissue Int.* 1994;55:208–15.

61. Baylink TM, Mohan S, Fitzsimmons RJ, Baylink DJ. Evaluation of signal transduction mechanisms for the mitogenic effects of prostaglandin E_2 in normal human bone cells *in vitro*. *J Bone Miner Res.* 1996;11:1413–18.

62. Fall PM, Breault DT, Raisz LG. Inhibition of collagen synthesis by prostaglandins in the immortalized rat osteoblastic cell line, Py1a: structure activity relations and signal transduction mechanisms. *J Bone Miner Res.* 1994;9:1935–43.

63. Chyun YS, Raisz LG. Stimulation of bone formation by prostaglandin E_2. *Prostaglandins.* 1984;27:97–103.

64. Raisz LG, Fall PM. Biphasic effects of prostaglandin E_2 on bone formation in cultured fetal rat calvariae: interaction with cortisol. *Endocrinology.* 1990;128:1654–9.

65. Flanagan AM, Chambers TJ. Stimulation of bone nodule formation *in vitro* by prostaglandins E_1 and E_2. *Endocrinology.* 1992;130:443–8.

66. Scutt A, Bertram P. Bone marrow cells are targets for the anabolic actions of prostaglandin E_2 on bone: induction of a transition from nonadherent to adherent osteoblast precursors. *J Bone Miner Res.* 1995;10:474–87.

67. Nagata T, Kaho K, Nishikawa S, Shinohara H, Wakano Y, Ishida H. Effect of prostaglandin E_2 on mineralization of bone nodules formed by fetal rat calvarial cells. *Calcif Tissue Int.* 1994;55:451–7.

68. Okada Y, Tomita M, Tsurukami H, Nakamura T, Alander C, Sohn J et al. Effects of prostaglandin G/H synthase-2 knockout on bone. *J Bone Miner Res.* 1999;14(S1):S173.

69. Jee WS, Ma YF. The *in vivo* anabolic actions of prostaglandins in bone. *Bone.* 1997;21:297–304.

70. Suponitzky I, Weinreb M. Differential effects of systemic prostaglandin E_2 on bone mass in rat long bones and calvariae. *J Endocrinol.* 1998;156:51–7.

71. Lin BY, Jee WSS, Ma YF, Ke HZ, Kimmel DB, Li XJ. Effects of prostaglandin E_2 and risedronate administration on cancellous bone in older female rats. *Bone.* 1994;15:489–96.

72. Weinreb M, Suponitzky I, Keila S. Systemic administration of an anabolic dose of PGE_2 in young rats increases the osteogenic capacity of bone marrow. *Bone.* 1997;20:521–6.

73. Saito M, Saito S, Ngan PW, Shanfeld J, Davidovitch Z. Interleukin 1 beta and prostaglandin E are involved in the response of periodontal cells to mechanical stress *in vivo* and *in vitro*. *Am J Orthod Dentofacial Orthop.* 1991;99:226–40.

74. Sandy JR, Farndale RW, Meikle MC. Recent advances in understanding mechanically induced bone remodeling and their relevance to orthodontic theory and practice. *Am J Orthod Dentofacial Orthop.* 1993;103:212–22.

75. Grieve WG III, Johnson GK, Moore RN, Reinhardt RA, DuBois LM. Prostaglandin E (PGE) and interleukin-1 beta (IL-1 beta) levels in gingival crevicular fluid during human orthodontic tooth movement. *Am J Orthod Dentofacial Orthop.* 1994;105:369–74.

76. Giunta D, Keller J, Nielsen FF, Melsen B. Influence of indomethacin on bone turnover related to orthodontic tooth movement in miniature pigs. *Am J Orthod Dentofacial Orthop.* 1995;108:361–6.

77. Leiker BJ, Nanda RS, Currier GF, Howes RI, Sinha PK. The effects of exogenous prostaglandins on orthodontic tooth movement in rats. *Am J Orthod Dentofacial Orthop.* 1995;108:380–8.

78. Kehoe MJ, Cohen SM, Zarrinnia K, Cowan A. The effect of acetaminophen, ibuprofen, and misoprostol on prostaglandin E_2 synthesis and the degree and rate of orthodontic tooth movement. *Am J Orthod.* 1996;66:339–49.

79. Dalsky GP, Stocke KS, Ehsani AA, Slatopolsky E, Lee WC, Birge SJ. Weight-bearing exercise training and lumbar bone mineral content in postmenopausal women. *Ann Int Med.* 1988;108:824–8.

80. Raab DM, Crenshaw TD, Kimmel DB, Smith EL. A histomorphometric study of cortical bone activity during increased weight-bearing exercise. *J Bone Miner Res.* 1991;6:741–9.

81. Rubin CT, Gross TS, McLeod KJ, Bain SD. Morphologic stages in lamellar bone formation stimulated by a potent mechanical stimulus. *J Bone Miner Res.* 1995;10:488–95.

82. Harter LV, Hruska KA, Duncan RL. Human osteoblast-like cells respond to mechanical strain with increased bone matrix protein production independent of hormonal regulation. *Endocrinology.* 1995;136:528–35.

83. Sun Y-Q, McLeod KJ, Rubin CT. Mechanically induced periosteal bone formation is paralleled by the upregulation of collagen type I mRNA in osteocytes as measured by in situ reverse transcript-polymerase chain reaction. *Calcif Tissue Int.* 1995;57:456–62.

84. Globus RK, Bikle DD, Morey-Holton E. The temporal response of bone to unloading. *Endocrinology.* 1986;118:733–42.

85. Weinreb M, Rodan GA, Thompson DD. Osteopenia in the immobilized rat hind limb is associated with increased bone resorption and decreased bone formation. *Bone.* 1989;10:187–94.

86. Leblanc AD, Schneider VS, Evans HJ, Engelbretson DA, Krebs JM. Bone mineral loss and recovery after 17 weeks of bed rest. *J Bone Miner Res.* 1990;5:843–50.

87. Wakley GK, Portwood JS, Turner RT. Disuse osteopenia is accompanied by down-regulation of gene expression for bone proteins in growing rats. *Am J Physiol.* 1992;263:E1029–34.

88. Gross TS, Rubin CT. Uniformity of resorptive bone loss induced by disuse. *J Orthop Res.* 1995;13:708–14.

89. Rawlinson SCF, El-Haj AJ, Minter SL, Tavares IA, Bennett A, Lanyon LE. Loading-related increases in prostaglandin production in cores of adult canine cancellous bone *in vitro*: A role for prostacyclin in adaptive bone remodeling? *J Bone Miner Res.* 1991;6:1345–52.

90. Lanyon LE. Control of bone architecture by functional load bearing. *J Bone Miner Res.* 1992;7:S369–75.

91. Cheng MZ, Zaman G, Rawlinson SC, Pitsillides AA, Suswillo RF, Lanyon LE. Enhancement by sex hormones of the osteoregulatory effects of mechanical

loading and prostaglandins in explants of rat ulnae. *J Bone Miner Res.* 1997;12:1424–30.

92. Pead MJ, Lanyon LE. Indomethacin modulation of load-related stimulation of new bone formation *in vivo*. *Calcif Tissue Int.* 1989;45:34–40.

93. Chow JW, Chambers TJ. Indomethacin has distinct early and late actions on bone formation induced by mechanical stimulation. *Am J Physiol.* 1994;267:E287–92.

94. Thorsen K, Kristoffersson AO, Lerner UH, Lorentzon RP. *In situ* microdialysis in bone tissue: stimulation of prostaglandin E_2 release by weight-bearing mechanical loading. *J Clin Invest.* 1997;98:2446–9.

95. Thompson DD, Rodan GA. Indomethacin inhibition of tenotomy-induced bone resorption in rats. *J Bone Miner Res.* 1988;3:409–14.

96. Fiorentino S, Melillo G, Fedele G, Clavenna G, D'Agostino C, Mainetti E. Ketoprofen lysine salt inhibits disuse-induced osteopenia in a new non- traumatic immobilization model in the rat. *Pharmacol Res.* 1996;33:277–81.

97. Forwood MR, Owan I, Takano Y, Turner CH. Increased bone formation in rat tibiae after a single short period of dynamic loading *in vivo*. *Am J Physiol.* 1996;270:E419–23.

98. Forwood MR. Inducible cyclooxygenase (COX-2) mediates the induction of bone formation by mechanical loading *in vivo*. *J Bone Miner Res.* 1996;11:1688–93.

99. Reich KM, Frangos JA. Protein kinase C mediates flow-induced prostaglandin E_2 production in osteoblasts. *Calcif Tissue Int.* 1993;52:62–66.

100. Klein-Nulend J, Burger EH, Semeins CM, Raisz LG, Pilbeam CC. Pulsating fluid flow stimulates prostaglandin release and inducible prostaglandin G/H synthase mRNA expression in primary mouse bone cells. *J Bone Miner Res.* 1997;12:45–51.

101. Crofford LJ, Wilder RL, Ristimaki AP, Sano H, Remmers EF, Epps HR et al. Cyclooxygenase-1 and -2 expression in rheumatoid synovial tissues. *J Clin Invest.* 1994;93:1095–101.

102. Seibert K, Zhang Y, Leahy K, Hauser S, Masferrer J, Perkins W et al. Pharmacological and biochemical demonstration of the role of cyclooxygenase 2 in inflammation and pain. *Proc Natl Acad Sci USA.* 1994;91:12013–7.

103. Howell TH, Jeffcoat MK, Goldhaber P, Reddy MS, Kaplan ML, Johnson HG et al. Inhibition of alveolar bone loss in beagles with the NSAID naproxen. *J Periodontal Res.* 1991;26:498–501.

104. Jeffcoat MK, Reddy MS, Moreland LW, Koopman WJ. Effects of nonsteroidal antiinflammatory drugs on bone loss in chronic inflammatory disease. *Ann NY Acad Sci.* 1993;696:292–302.

105. Cavanaugh PFJ, Meredith MP, Buchanan W, Doyle MJ, Reddy MS, Jeffcoat MK. Coordinate production of PGE_2 and IL-1 beta in the gingival crevicular fluid of adults with periodontitis: its relationship to alveolar bone loss and disruption by twice daily treatment with ketorolac tromethamine oral rinse. *J Periodontal Res.* 1998;33:75–82.

106. Pitt P, Compston J, Trivedi P, Salisbury J, Berry H, Moniz C et al. Systemic bone changes accompanying early rheumatoid arthritis in patients treated with nonsteroidal antiinflammatory drugs alone. *Clin Orthop.* 1994;250–8.

107. Rosenquist JB, Ohlin A, Lerner UH. Cytokine-induced inhibition of bone matrix proteins is not mediated by prostaglandins. *Inflamm Res.* 1996;45:457–63.

108. Kimmel DB, Coble T, Lane N. Long-term effect of naproxen on cancellous bone in ovariectomized rats. *Bone.* 1992;13:167–72.

109. Lane NE, Bauer DC, Nevitt MC, Pressman AR, Cummings SR. Aspirin and non-steroidal antiinflammatory drug use in elderly women: effects on a marker of bone resorption. Study of Osteoporotic Fractures Research Group. *J Rheumatol.* 1997;24:1132–6.

110. Bauer DC, Orwoll ES, Fox KM, Vogt TM, Lane NE, Hochberg MC et al. Aspirin and NSAID use in older women: effect on bone mineral density and fracture risk. Study of Osteoporotic Fractures Research Group. *J Bone Miner Res.* 1996;11:29–35.

111. Morton DJ, Barrett-Connor EL, Schneider DL. Nonsteroidal anti-inflammatory drugs and bone mineral density in older women: the Rancho Bernardo study. *J Bone Miner Res.* 1998;13:1924–31.

112. Kienapfel H, Koller M, Wust A, Sprey C, Merte H, Engenhart-Cabillic R et al. Prevention of heterotopic bone formation after total hip arthroplasty: a prospective randomised study comparing postoperative radiation therapy with indomethacin medication. *Arch Orthop Trauma Surg.* 1999;119:296–302.

113. Nilsson OS, Persson PE. Heterotropic bone formation after joint replacement. *Curr Opin Rheumatol.* 1999;11:127–31.

114. Neal BC, Rodgers A, Clark T, Gray H, Reid IR, Dunn L et al. A systematic survey of 13 randomized trials of non-steroidal anti-inflammatory drugs for the prevention of heterotopic bone formation after major hip surgery. *Acta Orthop Scand.* 2000;71:122–8.

115. Altman RD, Latta LL, Keer R, Renfree K, Hornicek FJ, Banovac K. Effect of nonsteroidal antiinflammatory drugs on fracture healing: a laboratory study in rats. *J Orthop Trauma.* 1995;9:392–400.

116. Reikeraas O, Engebretsen L. Effects of ketorolac tromethamine and indomethacin on primary and secondary bone healing. An experimental study in rats. *Arch Orthop Trauma Surg.* 1998;118:50–2.

117. Dimar JR, Ante WA, Zhang YP, Glassman SD. The effects of nonsteroidal anti-inflammatory drugs on posterior spinal fusions in the rat. *Spine.* 1996;21:1870–976.

118. Jacobsson SA, Djerf K, Ivarsson I, Wahlstrom O. Effect of diclofenac on fixation of hydroxyapatite-coated implants. An experimental study. *J Bone Jt Surg Br Vol.* 1994;76:831–3.

119. Keller J, Klamer A, Bak B, Suder P. Effect of local prostaglandin E_2 on fracture callus in rabbits. *Acta Orthop Scand.* 1993;64:59–63.

120. Sun JS, Tsuang YH, Lin FH, Liu HC, Tsai CZ, Chang WH. Bone defect healing enhanced by ultrasound stimulation: an *in vitro* tissue culture model. *J Biomed Mater Res.* 1999;46:253–61.

121. Kokubu T, Matsui N, Fujioka H, Tsunoda M , Mizuno K. Low intensity pulsed ultrasound exposure increases prostaglandin E_2 production via the induction of cyclooxygenase-2 mRNA in mouse osteoblasts. *Biochem Biophys Res Commun.* 1999;256:284–7.

122. Hukkanen M, Hughes FJ, Buttery LD, Gross SS, Evans TJ, Seddon S et al. Cytokine-stimulated expression of inducible nitric oxide synthase by mouse, rat, and human osteoblast-like cells and its functional role in osteoblast metabolic activity. *Endocrinology.* 1995;136:5445–53.

123. Sunyer T, Rothe L, Kirsch D, Jiang X, Anderson F, Osdoby P et al. Ca^{2+} or phorbol ester but not inflammatory stimuli elevate inducible nitric oxide synthase messenger ribonucleic acid and nitric oxide (NO) release in avian osteoclasts:

autocrine NO mediates Ca²⁺-inhibited bone resorption. *Endocrinology.* 1997;138:2148–62.

124. Armour KE, Ralston SH. Estrogen upregulates endothelial constitutive nitric oxide synthase expression in human osteoblast-like cells. *Endocrinology.* 1998;139:799–802.

125. Fox SW, Chow JW. Nitric oxide synthase expression in bone cells. *Bone.* 1998;23:1–6.

126. Hukkanen MV, Platts LA, Fernandez DMI, O'Shaughnessy M, MacIntyre I, Polak JM. Developmental regulation of nitric oxide synthase expression in rat skeletal bone. *J Bone Miner Res.* 1999;14:868–77.

127. Salvemini D, Misko TP, Masferrer JL, Seibert K, Currie MG, Needleman P. Nitric oxide activates cyclooxygenase enzymes. *Proc Natl Acad Sci USA.* 1993;90:7240–4.

128. Salvemini D, Seibert K, Masferrer JL, Misko TP, Currie MG, Needleman P. Endogenous nitric oxide enhances prostaglandin production in a model of renal inflammation. *J Clin Invest.* 1994;93:1940–7.

129. Salvemini D, Manning PT, Zweifel BS, Seibert K, Connor J, Currie MG et al. Dual inhibition of nitric oxide and prostaglandin production contributes to the antiinflammatory properties of nitric oxide synthase inhibitors. *J Clin Invest.* 1995;96:301–8.

130. Hughes FJ, Buttery LD, Hukkanen MV, O'Donnell A, Maclouf J, Polak JM. Cytokine-induced prostaglandin E₂ synthesis and cyclooxygenase-2 activity are regulated both by a nitric oxide-dependent and -independent mechanism in rat osteoblasts *in vitro*. *J Biol Chem.* 1999;274:1776–82.

131. Habib A, Bernard C, Lebret M, Creminon C , Esposito B, Tedgui A et al. Regulation of the expression of cyclooxygenase-2 by nitric oxide in rat peritoneal macrophages. *J Immunol.* 1997;158:3845–51.

132. Jamal SA, Browner WS, Bauer DC, Cummings SR. Intermittent use of nitrates increases bone mineral density: the study of osteoporotic fractures. *J Bone Miner Res.* 1998;13:1755–9.

133. Otsuka E, Hirano K, Matsushita S, Inoue A, Hirose S, Yamaguchi A et al. Effects of nitric oxide from exogenous nitric oxide donors on osteoblastic metabolism. *Eur J Pharmacol.* 1998;349:345–50.

134. Koyama A, Otsuka E, Inoue A, Hirose S, Hagiwara H. Nitric oxide accelerates the ascorbic acid-induced osteoblastic differentiation of mouse stromal ST2 cells by stimulating the production of prostaglandin E(2). *Eur J Pharmacol.* 2000;391:225–31.

135. Turner CH, Owan I, Jacob DS, McClintock R, Peacock M. Effects of nitric oxide synthase inhibitors on bone formation in rats. *Bone.* 1997;21:487–90.

136. Diwan AD, Wang MX, Jang D, Zhu W, Murrell GA. Nitric oxide modulates fracture healing. *J Bone Miner Res.* 2000;15:342–51.

137. MacIntyre I, Zaidi M, Alam AS, Datta HK, Moonga BS, Lidbury PS et al. Osteoclastic inhibition: an action of nitric oxide not mediated by cyclic GMP. *Proc Natl Acad Sci USA.* 1991;88:2936–40.

138. Lowik CW, Nibbering PH, van de Ruit RM, Papapoulos SE. Inducible production of nitric oxide in osteoblast-like cells and in fetal mouse bone explants is associated with suppression of osteoclastic bone resorption. *J Clin Invest.* 1994;93:1465–72.

139. Kasten TP, Collin-Osdoby P, Patel N, Osdoby P, Krukowski M, Misko TP et al.

Potentiation of osteoclast bone-resorption activity by inhibition of nitric oxide synthase. *Proc Natl Acad Sci USA.* 1994;91:3569–73.

140. Brandi ML, Hukkanen M, Umeda T, Moradi-Bidhendi N, Bianchi S, Gross SS et al. Bidirectional regulation of osteoclast function by nitric oxide synthase isoforms. *Proc Natl Acad Sci USA.* 1995;92:2954–8.

141. Holliday LS, Dean AD, Lin RH, Greenwald JE, Gluck SL. Low NO concentrations inhibit osteoclast formation in mouse marrow cultures by cGMP-dependent mechanism. *Am J Physiol.* 1997;272:F283–91.

142. Collin-Osdoby P, Rothe L, Bekker S, Anderson F, Osdoby P. Decreased nitric oxide levels stimulate osteoclastogenesis and bone resorption both *in vitro* and *in vivo* on the chick chorioallantoic membrane in association with neoangiogenesis. *J Bone Miner Res.* 2000;15:474–88.

143. Armour KE, Van'T Hof RJ, Grabowski PS, Reid DM, Ralston SH. Evidence for a pathogenic role of nitric oxide in inflammation-induced osteoporosis. *J Bone Miner Res.* 1999;14:2137–42.

144. Evans DM, Ralston SH. Nitric oxide and bone. *J Bone Miner Res.* 1996;11:300–5.

145. Raisz LG, Simmons HA, Fall PM. Biphasic effects of nonsteroidal anti-inflammatory drugs on prostaglandin production by cultured rat calvariae. *Prostaglandins.* 1989;37:559–65.

146. Lindsley HB, Smith DD. Enhanced prostaglandin E_2 secretion by cytokine-stimulated human synoviocytes in the presence of subtherapeutic concentrations of nonsteroidal antiinflammatory drugs. *Arthritis Rheum.* 1990;33:1162–9.

15 | Basis of gastrointestinal toxicity of non-steroid anti-inflammatory drugs

BRENDAN J. R. WHITTLE

William Harvey Research Institute, St Bartholomew's & The Royal London School of Medicine & Dentistry, Charterhouse Square, London EC1M 6BQ, UK.

The pharmacological quest to minimize the gastric mucosal injury provoked by non-steroid anti-inflammatory drugs (NSAIDs) has been of major clinical and pharmaceutical interest over the past 40 years. Apart from buffering or reducing the acidity of the stomach contents, one major strategy to achieve this aim has involved the concurrent use of additional pharmacological agents to protect the gastrointestinal (GI) mucosa from the injurious actions of the NSAIDs. The latter approach has had limited success, at least from the clinical perspective, despite ample demonstration of efficacy of a number of drug combinations in a wide range of experimental studies.

Another key strategy has focused on reducing the inherent ability of the agents to provoke injury, utilizing the evolving knowledge of the pathological mechanisms underlying such toxicity of these agents. Chemical manipulation of existing agents, and the identification of novel chemical classes exhibiting anti-inflammatory properties, suggested from early studies that a more favourable safety profile than the classical NSAIDs could be achieved. Such an approach has culminated in the very recent advent of the cyclooxygenase (COX)-2-selective inhibitors, celecoxib and rofecoxib, designed to eliminate the GI toxicity by reducing one key element of the pathological process of mucosal damage. This latter approach is already having a significant impact on current clinical prescribing practice following the launch of these two products.

CLINICAL BACKGROUND

The introduction of salicylates into therapeutic practice at the start of the 20th century, was soon followed by reports, mostly anecdotal, of their side effects on the stomach. Over the past 20 years, however, considerable evidence from clinical studies, both direct patient trials and retrospective surveys, have confirmed that chronic use of aspirin and NSAIDs gives rise to serious toxic actions in the GI tract including haemorrhage and ulcers in a large proportion of the patient population. Major epidemiological studies have well-documented the so-called stealth epidemic of the gastropathy that has developed over the period since the non-aspirin NSAIDs were introduced[1, 2].

The massive growth of the market for such products, which has involved different patient populations and the prescription of high doses, has led to the current substantial problem of some 103 000 hospitalizations and 16500 deaths per year in the US alone. The impact of such events on health-care budgets is therefore substantial, and the risk of serious side effects from these NSAIDs is an important consideration in long-term anti-inflammatory therapy, especially in the elderly.

Early gastroscopic studies on the effect of aspirin on the human stomach reported the injurious properties of this compound on the gastric mucosa[3]. Extensive studies have since demonstrated the damaging actions of many of the clinically well-used anti-inflammatory agents, including aspirin, naproxen and indomethacin, using endoscopic observations of the gastric mucosa[4,5]. All of these compounds cause visible gastric mucosal damage and erosion formation to various degrees, depending on the dosage regimen employed. Such direct determination of the potential to provoke injurious actions has become an important feature of the development of novel anti-inflammatory agents.

These relatively recent advances in clinical knowledge and recognition of the magnitude of the problems associated with such compounds have been accompanied by a significant change in our understanding of the basic mechanisms underlying these damaging actions. Acquisition of such mechanistic information has allowed and promoted the development of new pharmacological strategies for reducing or eliminating this widespread iatrogenic disease.

GASTRIC MUCOSAL IRRITATION

A major concept concerning the effects of topically applied salicylates on the gastric mucosa was developed in the mid-1960s by Davenport and colleagues[6]. The ability of topically administered aspirin and related salicylates to promote acid back-diffusion into the canine gastric mucosa was clearly demonstrated in early experiments[6] and has subsequently been amply confirmed by many workers using different species and models, both *in vivo* and *in vitro*. The measurable increase in acid loss is accompanied by an increase in luminal sodium ion concentration and the efflux of potassium ions into the gastric human lumen, while the transmucosal flux of non-ionic moieties is also enhanced by topical irritants (Figure 1).

Figure 1 The back-diffusion of acid and the flux of sodium and potassium ions across the gastric mucosa under physiological conditions is limited by epithelial integrity, as well as by the presence of a mucus–alkaline layer. Under pathological conditions following topical irritation such as that provoked by many NSAIDs, acid diffuses readily into the mucosal tissue.

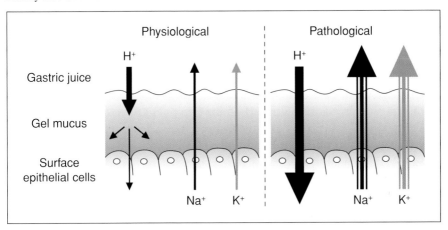

The electrical potential difference (PD) across the gastric mucosa has been extensively used as an index of the integrity of the gastric mucosa in experimental studies in animals[7]. A reduction in gastric PD can also be observed after the topical application of irritants such as aspirin in man and these occur concurrently with the other characteristics of gastric 'barrier' damage such as the acid back-diffusion from the gastric lumen into the mucosa[8]. These changes correlate with histologically demonstrable damage to the human mucosa after aspirin ingestion[8].

The changes in PD are considered to reflect injury to the epithelial cells, allowing the unregulated flux of ionic moieties. Following mucosal injury, the restoration of PD reflects the process of rapid restitution, which re-establishes the continuity of the damaged epithelial layer that follows superficial local damage[7]. The transmucosal flux of non-ionic species is also enhanced, as determined by the passage of albumin, or the permeability markers, inulin and dextran. These latter changes reflect not only disruption to the epithelium, but also increases in microvascular permeability to large molecules such as plasma protein.

These vascular responses could reflect the intramucosal release of pro-inflammatory mediators such as histamine, 5-hydroxytryptamine or platelet activating factor, either from invading or resident inflammatory cells or from local tissue. These mediators, once released into the interstitial areas, would be expected to perpetuate the tissue injury[9]. Furthermore, such cellular perturbation and the change in intramucosal pH would lead to the release and subsequent activation of tissue-destructive lysosomal enzymes and proteases, as well as pepsinogen. These enzymes would provoke autodigestion of the tissue and hence augment the cellular damage and necrosis[9].

Mechanisms of mucosal irritation

The barrier changes following application of aspirin or salicylate to the mucosa are also observed with many other NSAIDs. However, intravenous administration of aspirin to animals or humans failed to elicit barrier damage[10], as determined by luminal acid-loss or potential difference measurements. These findings suggested that the observed superficial barrier injury is the result of local contact with the mucosa tissue and not a reflection of a generalized biochemical and pharmacological response such as COX inhibition.

Early studies indicated that the barrier-breaking activities of aspirin and salicylate occurred under acid conditions in the stomach. Thus it was proposed that absorption of the unionized form of these carboxylic acids was involved with the damage, although the presence of hydrogen ions in the gastric lumen appears very important. Other early studies utilizing radio-labelled material suggested that the salicylate anion could be trapped in the mucosal cells during absorption, but its contribution to the process of mucosal injury was not established[9].

Further work indicated that the barrier-breaking activity of these drugs resulted from epithelial disruption, with actions on the cellular tight-junctions. Such effects may be the consequence of local metabolic actions, including the uncoupling of oxidative phosphorylation in the epithelium that can be achieved at high concentrations of salicylates and other NSAIDs[11,12]. A number of early studies in a number of different paradigms demonstrated actions of aspirin and salicylate on mucosal ATP and phosphocreatine levels or on the oxidative phosphorylation process[11]. More recently, this concept has been revived and additional supportive evidence for actions of a wide range of the newer NSAIDs on the energy pathways have been provided, with effects on ATP synthesis and mitochondrial respiration being demonstrated[13,14].

As a consequence of acid back-diffusion, acidification of the mucosal interstitial tissue following challenge with NSAIDs could thus occur. Such changes in interstitial pH, if sustained by, for example, a concurrent reduction in mucosal blood flow, would lead to the observed intramucosal cellular damage and necrosis.

Luminal surface layers

The mucus layer offers little buffering capacity and appears readily permeable to acid[15]. However, it can act as a lubricant and barrier to physical damage such as that induced by local tissue contact with fragments of anti-inflammatory tablets. This layer can also impede the back-diffusion of hydrogen ions creating an unstirred layer of water and electrolytes, notably bicarbonate, at the apical membrane[15]. It has been suggested that NSAIDs may affect mucus biosynthesis[16], as well as alkaline secretion, and could therefore contribute to the process of ulceration by attenuating the elaboration of this local more alkaline environment, making the underlying tissue more susceptible to damage.

Early investigations showed that aspirin could affect mucus biosynthesis in epithelial and mucus neck cells, while inhibition of the biosynthesis of sulphated gastric mucus glycoproteins by NSAIDs has been shown. It has also been demonstrated in early work that aspirin could alter the physicochemical properties of mucus with a reduction in its viscosity[9]. A number of studies have demonstrated that NSAIDs could affect the secretion of bicarbonate in different experimental systems. Such actions not only could reduce the alkaline buffering layer, but could also affect the protective mucoid cap that forms after superficial injury to the mucosa[15]. The pH gradient across this cap is dissipated following administration of NSAIDs and thus impedes the rapid repair process of restitution to the epithelium[7].

It has also been proposed that the mucosa is protected from attack by luminal acid by the water-repellent properties of the luminal surface. The hydrophobicity of the mucosal surface, previously attributed to a layer of surface-active phospholipids, has now been shown to be largely dependent on surface mucus gel[17]. The hydrophobicity can be substantially reduced by topical application of aspirin, which may reflect to some extent the inhibition of mucus and bicarbonate secretion[18]. Such changes could thus augment acid back-diffusion and contribute to the local irritant actions of aspirin and other NSAIDs.

PROTECTION AGAINST INJURY

Acid inhibition

Since the back-diffusion of acid is a key factor promoting the tissue injury, early strategies for therapeutic intervention focused on the reduction in concentration of luminal acid. Thus, treatment with antacid buffers, histamine H_2-receptor antagonists, proton pump inhibitors and prostaglandins in antisecretory doses have all been shown to attenuate the mucosal injury following challenge with various NSAIDs in both experimental and clinical studies[19–22].

In a number of large-scale long-term studies, the proton pump inhibitor omeprazole has been shown to be effective as prophylaxis against the development of gastroduodenal ulcers from NSAIDs, being more effective than the H_2-receptor antagonist ranitidine[19,20]. In a 6-month comparative study in 935 patients, the efficacy of omeprazole has been compared with the prostaglandin E_1 analogue misoprostol in antisecretory doses[21]. The overall rate of successful prevention of the ulcers and erosions caused by NSAIDs was similar, whereas maintenance with misoprostol had a higher rate of relapse and was less well tolerated than omeprazole. The combination of misoprostol with the NSAID diclofenac is currently available as a formulated product.

Pharmaceutical and chemical modification

More direct approaches to reducing the direct topical gastric damage of the NSAIDs have involved pharmaceutical formulation to prevent direct contact with the gastric mucosa. Such so-called enteric coated preparations found some favour for many years, although the evidence for their superior safety profile was not extensive and such preparations have been largely superseded.

Early chemical modifications to minimize the irritant actions of the acidic class of NSAIDs involved manipulation of the free acidic carboxyl substituents, which have been implicated as a factor in these toxic actions. Esterification of this moiety, as in methyl aspirin, has provided compounds with less ulcerogenic actions following intragastric administration, while anti-inflammatory activity is retained, presumably following liberation of the free acid by the action of plasma esterases[12]. While such modifications may reduce direct local irritancy, these chemically modified compounds, once activated in the systemic circulation, by de-esterification for example, could retain their biochemical actions, including actions on gastric COX, that may lead to more chronic development of gastrointestinal disturbances.

This chemical masking of the free carboxylic acid grouping may also contribute, in part, to the gastric mucosal-sparing actions of the nitric oxide (NO)-containing NSAIDs, which contain the nitroxybutyl ester[23,24]. The contribution of such a chemical manipulation of these agents to their overall safety profile awaits experimental evaluation. Thus, it may be possible to substitute non-reactive NO chemical groups, or groups that do not contain NO, and retain anti-inflammatory activity with good safety characteristics.

Luminal protection

Other approaches to the prevention of mucosal damage by NSAIDs have utilized locally acting protective agents. One such product is sucralfate[25], which has been demonstrated to exert protective actions in a number of models of gastric injury. The protective action of sucralfate may involve the local stimulation of the biosynthesis of the endogenous protective mediators prostanoids and NO. In clinical studies, although sucralfate did not attenuate the acute gastric injury provoked by aspirin challenge over 3 days, it did reduce the accompanying bleeding[26]. In another clinical study over a 4–8 week period in patients who had developed gastric ulcer following NSAIDs, sucralfate did bring about ulcer healing, but was less effective than omeprazole[27].

It has also been demonstrated in experimental studies that the chemical complex of certain NSAIDs with zwitterionic phospholipids can reduce their topical irritant actions[28]. Such actions, as with the buffered formulations and enteric-coated NSAIDs, may be effective under conditions of acute or sub-chronic administration, but may not yield safer agents for long-term therapy. Indeed, it is known from experimental studies that the degree of local irritant activity on the gastric mucosa may diminish on prolonged therapy with classical NSAIDs[9]. Thus, development of such tolerance may minimize the therapeutic impact of strategies aimed solely at reducing such local mucosal injury.

Protective mediators: prostanoids

Endogenous metabolites of arachidonic acid, formed predominantly by the cyclooxygenase enzyme, COX-1, have been implicated as local mediators or modulators of gastric mucosal function. Prostaglandins of the E and I series – PGE_2 and prostacyclin (PGI_2), respectively – are formed by gastric mucosal tissue[29]. These prostanoids can inhibit gastric acid secretion and stimulate both gastric bicarbonate and mucus secretion, as well as affect sodium and chloride ionic flux across the injured mucosa. In addition, these prostanoids induce vasodilation in the mucosal microcirculation, and can also prevent the vascular stasis that is induced by a range of damaging agents[29].

Early studies had characterized the potent anti-ulcer activity of the prostanoids and their analogues in a number of experimental ulcer models[29,30]. Further studies also indicated that these lipids could protect the gastric mucosa against injury provoked by a wide range of challenging agents. This property, often referred to by the term 'cytoprotection'[30], may be brought about by the effect of these prostanoids on several of these beneficial parameters, acting in concert[22,29,30].

The changes in the mucosal barrier parameters characteristic of topical injury by NSAIDs have been shown to be attenuated by a number of endogenously occurring prostaglandins and their synthetic analogues. These prostanoids also prevent the development of erosive injury induced by a range of NSAIDs in experimental models, an effect that has been confirmed clinically[22].

Protective mediators: nitric oxide

Like the endogenous prostanoid PGI_2, NO is formed in vascular tissue where it exerts a key vasodilator role and can prevent cellular adhesion to the endothelium[31]. In addition, like the prostanoids, NO is also formed in other mucosal cells, including the epithelium, where it can stimulate mucus and electrolyte secretion[31]. Agents that can release NO, the NO donors, exert protective actions against mucosal injury in a range of experimental models[31,32]. However, under experimental conditions, very high doses of NO donors can provoke or exacerbate mucosal damage, an effect associated with the cytotoxic actions of NO at high concentrations, particularly in combination with reactive oxygen species[33].

Clinical support for the concept that NO donors can protect against the damage induced by NSAIDs has come from recent epidemiological studies. Thus a recent survey has shown that the use of nitrovasodilators is associated with a reduced risk of upper GI bleeding with NSAIDs[34].

Nitric oxide-containing NSAIDs

As a result of the NO-bearing subsituent, usually a nitroxybutyl ester, the NO-NSAIDs exhibit a pharmacological profile distinct from the parent compounds from which they have been derived[23,24]. However, unlike the classical nitrovasodilators, the mechanism of the potential involvement of NO in the protective actions of the NO-NSAIDs is not clear. Thus, the NO-NSAIDs may release low levels of NO in the microenvironment where cellular injury is usually initiated by NSAIDs, thus offsetting the cytotoxic process. However, whether these agents have a more unique profile of pharmacological activity remains to be established fully.

CYCLOOXYGENASE INHIBITION AND GASTRIC INJURY

Whereas it is clear that NSAIDs exert local injuries on the gastric mucosa after luminal or oral administration, it is also apparent that these agents can provoke gastric mucosal toxicity by systemic mechanisms. Thus, many of these agents cause extensive mucosal injury following parenteral administration. The mechanisms of such systemic actions are known to involve the inhibition of the COX enzymes[35] reducing the production of protective prostanoids such as PGE_2 and PGI_2[29].

Since prostanoids were known to exert such potent actions on various key aspects of gastric function and integrity, it was proposed, from the time of the original discovery of COX inhibition by NSAIDs, that a reduction in local prostaglandin formation is a likely mechanism underlying gastric damage and disease[35]. Although there was initial reluctance to accept this hypothesis, it has become apparent from extensive experimentation that inhibition of COX is a critical step in the development of gastric injury and ulceration by the classical NSAIDs[9,36]. The cascade of events that follow inhibition of COX, and the reduction of constitutively formed prostanoids, generated predominantly by COX-1 in the gastric mucosa, appear to involve actions on the microcirculation, inflammatory cells and the release of local injurious mediators[9]. Such events arising from cellular injury deep in the mucosa would lead to erosion and eventual ulceration.

Role of mucosal blood flow

Early studies on the effects of NSAIDs on mucosal function after local application indicated that marked changes in the gastric microcirculation were evident, although the direct irritation of the mucosa precluded clear interpretation of the actions as a consequence of COX inhibition. In studies conducted some 30 years ago in the rat, a substantial fall in mucosal blood flow was observed following parenteral injection of indomethacin[37]. Many subsequent studies using a variety of techniques supported the observations that blood flow is reduced by NSAIDs[38,39], findings that have again been confirmed in the year 2000[40].

While the relative ischaemia produced by such a fall in blood flow in the microcirculation could itself provoke mucosal injury, this change may not be sufficient to account for the degree of mucosal injury observed with NSAIDs. Such a compromise in the mucosal perfusion would, however, be of significant importance under conditions where the mucosa is under concurrent challenge, such as that following topical irritation of the surface epithelium with increased acid back-diffusion[41]. Under these conditions, the protective hyperaemia that is known to accompany this enhanced acid load in the mucosal tissue would be also attenuated, thus allowing acid to accumulate in the mucosal tissue without being cleared by the vascular perfusion[41]. Such actions could underlie the observed synergistic interactions between topical irritation of NSAIDs and their actions to inhibit COX[9]. Thus, agents that exhibit both properties on oral administration will have a substantially greater propensity to provoke gastric mucosal injury than agents that have either a reduced ability to cause topical damage or do not inhibit COX in the mucosa.

Role of leukocytes and ischaemia

A significant finding in the understanding of the mechanism underlying the mucosal damage by NSAIDs was the involvement of inflammatory cells, particularly neutrophils, in the initiating process leading to mucosal injury[42,43]. Subsequent studies indicated that modulation of leukocyte adhesion factors that would prevent neutrophil adhesion to the gastric microcirculation would also prevent NSAID-induced gastric injury[43-46].

The proinflammatory cytokine tumour necrosis factor (TNF-α) can potently upregulate the production of adhesion proteins, and agents that can interfere with the actions of this cytokine, such as pentoxyphyline and thalidomide, can also reduce NSAID-induced gastric injury[47]. Thus, such cytokines appear to be involved in the initiation of injurious processes that leads to the production of mucosal lesions.

The mechanism by which adhering neutrophils could initiate mucosal injury through actions on the microcirculation may involve the release of cytotoxic radicals such as superoxide, following activation of the cells during the process of adherence[48]. Such a concept is supported by a wealth of literature, much of which preceded these findings, that has demonstrated the protective actions of broad range scavengers of oxygen reactive species on NSAID-induced gastric injury[9,49]. Thus, such injury with NSAIDs shares several of the key characteristics of the mucosal damage that are known to follow local ischaemia with a re-perfusion of the tissue. Moreover, NSAIDs, can aggravate the gastric injury that follows ischaemia re-perfusion procedures in the rat[50].

Despite the substantial pharmacological support for the involvement of neutrophil adhesion in the mucosal microcirculation as an important feature of tissue injury, there is limited direct evidence derived from detailed histological studies of the gastric mucosa following challenge with NSAIDs. Many of the observations on cell adherence have come from studies on the intestinal circulation, and these have utilized relatively large vessels, rather than those of the gastric mucosal microcirculation. Thus, using *in situ* intestinal vascular models, superfusion of the vessels with aspirin or indomethacin has been shown to enhance leukocyte adherence, an effect attenuated by perfusion with prostanoids[51]. While the evidence produced is convincing, these would be reinforced by more detailed observations in gastric mucosal preparations.

Early studies on the actions of local superfusion of aspirin on the gastric microcirculation did report the occurrence of white bodies, although whether these were platelets or leukocytes was not established[52]. Indeed, it would be of interest to know whether any inflammatory cell aggregates are found in the microcirculation of other vascular beds after systemic administration of NSAIDs, and lead to tissue injury. It is not known whether the more chronic administration of NSAIDs, including the coxibs, have shown evidence of cellular aggregates in the microcirculation in longer-term safety studies, although it could be argued that such events are only initiating mechanisms of injury and would not be seen at a later stage. It is not clear, however, whether the adhering cells would themselves provide sufficient mass in the mucosal microcirculation to occlude the mucosal microcirculation, hence further promoting tissue ischaemia and injury.

Role of local mediator release

In addition to oxygen free radicals and related moieties[48,49], there has been much debate as to whether products of the lipoxygenase pathways could be involved in the damage process. Thus, an early hypothesis was that inhibition of COX led to a diversion of the substrate, arachidonate, to the lipoxygenase enzymes. This was an attractive concept, especially as one key product, leukotriene B_4, is a potent chemoattractant, while leukotriene C_4 is a powerful vasoconstrictor in the gastric microcirculation[9]. However, studies with a range of agents, including selective 5-lipoxygenase inhibitors and leukotriene antagonists, have not produced any clear or consistent evidence to support this suggestion[9].

Additional mechanisms contributing to damage
Epithelial integrity
It is also possible that prostanoid inhibition may additionally affect the integrity of the superficial epithelial layer through actions on the overlying protective mucus–bicarbonate layer[15]. In addition, inhibition of COX may affect the biosynthesis and properties of the surface-active phospholipids that regulate the hydrophobicity of the mucosa[53].

Effects on haemostasis

The ability of aspirin and other NSAIDs to prevent the synthesis of thromboxane A_2 by platelets and reduce their aggregation has long been considered to contribute to the process of GI bleeding. However, production of platelet-like microthombi, following application of acidified aspirin to the gastric mucosal microcirculation[52], may reflect direct local vascular actions, including inhibition of PGI_2 formation, rather than effects on platelet function. In an experimental study on bleeding time in the gastric mucosa of the rat, rabbit and dog, neither topical aspirin nor parenteral indomethacin augmented the rates of bleeding. Indeed, known anti-platelet agents such as PGI_2 and thromboxane synthase inhibitors had no effect, whereas heparin substantially augmented the bleeding time in this model[54].

Studies in humans have produced inconsistent findings; an early study demonstrating that acute or chronic administration of aspirin, in doses sufficient to prolong skin bleeding time, did not prolong bleeding from a mucosal biopsy site[55]. Other studies have shown, however, that administration of low-dose aspirin can augment bleeding from biopsy sites[26]. Thus, although actions on haemostasis may not be involved in the early pathogenesis of mucosal injury, it could affect existing GI ulcer sites, and hence the contribution of this additional tendency for bleeding to the overall safety profile of NSAIDs cannot be excluded.

Changes in motility

Studies in the rat have suggested that local changes in gastric motility may contribute to the process of mucosal injury by indomethacin and other NSAIDs[49]. Indeed it is feasible that changes in smooth muscle contractility of the underlying gastric muscle could lead to alterations in the mucosal microcirculation through physical changes.

Effects on restitution and healing

The restitution of the epithelial continuity that follows topical irritation and lesion formation is an integral feature of the rapid repair of the barrier characteristic of the gastric mucosa[7]. This process, which involves the rapid migration of deeper epithelial cells to align across the denuded surface, is stimulated by a number of growth factors and cytokines. This process may be affected by inhibition of prostanoid biosynthesis, although there is scant evidence for a direct action on epithelial movement. Inhibition of COX may affect the response of the intermediates, while the removal of the neutral environment of the overlying mucoid cap by reducing prostanoid stimulation of bicarbonate or mucus secretion would also retard repair[7].

The involvement of apoptosis in the injurious process provoked by NSAIDs *in vivo* has not yet been established. However, a number of studies have demonstrated that NSAIDs can delay the healing of experimental ulcers, as well as the process of angiogenesis involved with tissue re-modelling[56,57].

SITE-SELECTIVE INHIBITION OF CYCLOOXYGENASE

In experimental studies conducted some 20 years ago on the possible differential inhibition of COX, it was demonstrated that prostanoid production at inflammatory sites could be inhibited without affecting prostanoid generation in the gastric mucosa[58]. Moreover, selective inhibition in the inflammatory areas by the prototypic anti-inflammatory agents was not accompanied by gastric mucosal injury (Figure 2). In addition, the findings suggested that sodium salicylate could act as a selective inhibitor of COX at the inflammatory site[58]. Such findings may be related to the more recent observations that salicylate can act as suppressor of COX-2 gene transcription[59].

It was proposed from these early studies that there may be different iso-forms of COX, at the inflammatory sites and in the gastric mucosa, that would be susceptible to pharmacological exploitation. The contribution of any pharma-

Figure 2 Early studies demonstrating the site-selective inhibition of COX products in inflammatory exudates and the rat gastric mucosa, in relation to gastric mucosal damage. The NSAIDs and the experimental compound BW755C were administered orally three times over 24 h, and PGI_2 formation in gastric mucosal strips *ex vivo* and PGE_2 levels in carrageenan-induced inflammatory exudate in an implanted sponge was determined. Gastric mucosal damage was assessed macroscopically in terms of a damage score. Results are shown as mean $\pm$ SEM of 5–12 experiments where significant difference from control is shown as $^\star P < 0.01$. (Data are adapted from the studies of Whittle et al., 1980[58].)

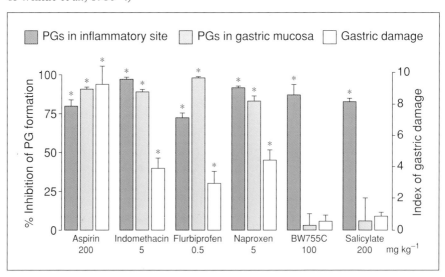

cokinetic disposition to the site-selectivity of the agents studied was not known, or whether it reflected uptake or selectivity of action of the agents by the inflammatory cells. However, the findings did indicate the potential for site-selective COX inhibitors to yield anti-inflammatory agents with less GI toxicity[58].

Cyclooxygenase-2 selective agents

The biochemical rationale for the development of COX-2 selective drugs arose some 10 years later from an understanding of the molecular biology of COX, with the identification of two distinct isoforms[60-62]. These seminal studies have emphasized the importance of molecular techniques in enzyme targeting and drug design. The COX-1 isoform present in the GI mucosa, renal systems and platelets was identified as a constitutive enzyme. The prostanoids synthesized by this COX-1 enzyme control many physiological functions, including microvascular blood flow, platelet aggregation, renal tubular functions, as well as the regulation of gastric acid production and mucosal integrity.

The second isoform, COX-2, was found to be inducible, being expressed within 4–24 h in a number of cell systems following challenge with inflammatory mediators such as interleukin-1, lipopolysaccharide and various mitogens[60-63]. This isoform is considered to be the primary source of the proinflammatory prostanoids making it an appropriate target for drug development[64-68].

However, this working hypothesis will require some modification as it is unlikely that such discrete functions are only served by the products of either isoform, especially as in many situations the products of the respective COX activity are the same. Thus, the COX-2 isoform can apparently also occur constitutively in some tissues in physiological situations, and may also play a defensive role in the gut and kidney[63]. In the gastric mucosa, COX-2 inhibitors can aggravate the damage provoked by ischaemia reperfusion[49] and can attenuate the protective response elicited by mild irritants to more severe subsequent challenge[69]. Moreover, this isoform may have a functional role in the healing of mucosal ulcers[56,57,70]. Similarly, products of the inducible COX may exert anti-inflammatory actions[71], while COX-1 products can play a role in the inflammatory response, at least in experimental models[72].

Despite these challenges to the concept of selective roles of COX-1 and COX-2 products in physiology and pathology, evaluation of the pharmacological profile of COX-2 selective inhibitors has supported their development as effective anti-inflammatory agents. Indeed, preclinical evaluation of the coxibs has clearly demonstrated that, in contrast to the classical NSAIDs, they do not provoke gastric mucosal injury in a number of experimental settings[65,73].

Interactions between cyclooxygenase-1 and cyclooxygenase-2 in gastric injury

Early confirmation that interference with the COX products in the gastric mucosa, other than by the use of NSAIDs, could lead to gastric damage came from work with specific antibodies raised to prostaglandins. Thus, active immunization with a prostanoid conjugate induced endoscopic evidence of gastric and duodenal ulceration in experimental models, as did passive sensitization by challenge with prostanoid antibodies[74]. Such findings established a role for endogenous COX-derived products in the protection against injury sustained under physiological conditions. As with the studies with NSAIDs, such investigations could not define the cellular location of the prostanoids or their COX-isoform source.

In an attempt to evaluate the role of COX-1 in inflammation and gastric pathology, studies have been conducted in animals in which the COX-1 gene had been deleted[75]. It is clear, however, from work in many genetically manipulated animals, that the phenotype may well be altered and other processes may subserve the function played by the original mediator. Thus, these COX-1 knockout mice did not develop spontaneous gastric lesions. Although a compensatory increase in mucosal prostanoid production was not noted, it is likely that any upregulation of gastric COX-2 activity under these conditions would not have been detected. Moreover, other studies have demonstrated that following acute inhibition of COX, the mucosa can be protected from acute injury by the other endogenous mediators, NO or calcitonin gene-related peptide[76]. Support for such a protective process is suggested by the findings that, in comparison with the wild-type animals, the COX-1 knockout animals had a reduced propensity for gastric lesion formation with an intermediate dose of indomethacin.

Recent studies with the selective COX-2 inhibitors suggest that these agents, like the classical NSAIDs, can cause leukocyte adhesion in rat intestinal vascular preparations following local superfusion[40]. However, these agents did not cause gastric mucosal injury in parallel studies in the rat. Thus, whether such events seen in the mesenteric preparation reflect the actions of these agents in the gastric microcirculation is unknown, but could also suggest that leukocyte adhesion alone does not necessarily lead to mucosal injury.

As with the standard NSAIDs, studies with a selective COX-1 inhibitor showed a substantial reduction in mucosal blood flow in the rat. This effect on blood flow was not exhibited by the selective COX-2 inhibitors and, as found with the COX-2 inhibitors, the COX-1 inhibitors alone did not cause acute gastric mucosal injury[40]. These studies thus suggest that inhibition of both isoforms may be necessary to produce acute gastric injury in the rat, although further evaluation will be required using additional highly selective agents for both isoforms and specific COX-gene deleted animals. These findings could therefore reflect a minimum requirement for concurrent actions on both leukocyte adhesion and blood flow in the microcirculation, for tissue damage to be initiated by COX inhibitors.

CYCLOOXYGENASE INHIBITION AND INTESTINAL INJURY

In addition to the actions of non-selective COX-1 inhibitors on the gastric mucosa, such agents promote damage in the small and large intestine in experimental studies[77,78]. Moreover, oral ingestion of aspirin, ibuprofen or indomethacin by healthy volunteers and patients increased the permeability of the small intestine to radiolabelled markers[79,80]. This effect was also observed after rectal administration of these agents, indicating that this was a systemic action and not just a reflection of any local irritation. In addition, in studies on patients receiving NSAIDs for the treatment of rheumatoid arthritis or osteoarthritis, over 60% exhibited blood and protein loss with demonstrable inflammation of the small intestine[81].

As in the gastric mucosa, local irritant actions on the intestinal mucosa involving inhibition of oxidative phosphorylation and COX inhibition have been proposed to explain the injurious actions[80,82]. The early suggestion of a role for the enterohepatic recirculation of a number of these NSAIDs, at least in the rat, has been confirmed[83]. Such a process would allow prolonged exposure of the small bowel to the NSAID and its metabolites.

Role of nitric oxide in intestinal injury

More recent experimental studies have also indicated a role of the inducible isoform of NO synthase (iNOS) that can generate sustained excessive levels of nitric oxide. Such NO can act in concert with superoxide to form the cytotoxic species peroxynitrite[84]. Such a role of NO moieties, formed by iNOS, contrasts with the protective actions of NO, formed by constitutive NO synthase enzymes, under more physiological conditions in the intestine. Indeed, experimental studies using superoxide dismutase indicate that peroxynitrite rather than NO itself is the damaging species in the model.

The slow onset of intestinal lesions following these NSAIDs appears to involve gut bacteria that release an endotoxin following translocation into the intestinal tissue. This endotoxin appears to provoke the stimulation of iNOS expression, probably though a process involving the release of cytokines. Thus, antibacterial agents, as well as polymixin B which binds and inactivates lipopolysaccharide, can reduce both the induction of iNOS and the intestinal inflammation and vascular leakage that follows NSAID administration[84]. The induction of iNOS and the subsequent development of vascular leakage and tissue injury is site-specific, occurring predominantly in the jejunal region[85]. The early events that give rise to the breach in the mucosal defence mechanisms, allowing the ingress of luminal bacteria into the small bowel, appear to involve the inhibition of COX-1 and epithelial dysfunction[84] (Figure 3). However, as with the recent findings on the gastric mucosa, it is possible that inhibition of both COX-1 and COX-2 are required for the initiation of intestinal injury, although agents that do not inhibit COX-1 such as the coxibs will still be free of this intestinal damage.

Evidence so far from experimental and clinical studies on faecal blood loss as an index of haemorrhagic injury in the gut has suggested that COX-2 inhibitors do not provoke intestinal injury, a finding supported by the use of specific permeability markers[86,87].

Thus, whereas gastroduodenal injury from standard NSAIDs can be attenuated by the use of gastric mucosal protective agents and by gastric acid suppressors, particularly proton pump inhibitors, these latter agents are unlikely to be effective against intestinal injury. In contrast, the COX-2 selective agents appear to provide a more comprehensive reduction in the ability to provoke GI damage. Likewise, the NO-NSAIDs appear to have a relatively low risk of causing intestinal injury, at least in short-term experimental studies[23].

CLINICAL FINDINGS WITH SELECTIVE CYCLOOXYGENASE INHIBITORS

A number of clinical studies with NSAIDs proposed to have selectivity on gastroduodenal or inflammatory COX activity have been conducted over the

Figure 3 Sequence of events leading to the production of intestinal lesions in the rat following administration of NSAIDs. The process involves initial inhibition of COX, allowing bacterial translocation into the intestinal tissue, following concurrent epithelial disruption. The release of lipopolysaccharide leads to the expression of iNOS, with the NO so produced combining with superoxide to form the damaging species peroxynitrite. (The diagram is based on the findings from Whittle and colleagues[84,85].)

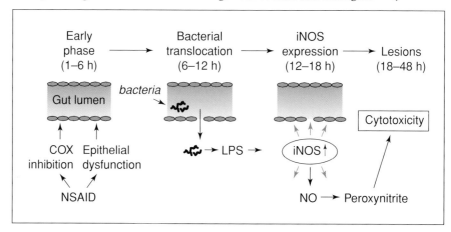

past 10 years. Thus, therapeutic doses of etodolac, which shows some selectivity for the COX-2 isoform in *in vitro* studies, did not suppress gastric or duodenal prostanoid biosynthesis and had a favourable GI side-effect profile in humans[5]. Studies using nimesulide have also reported less suppression of gastric mucosal prostanoid production *ex vivo*, as well as thromboxane production in whole blood, than the standard NSAID, naproxen, but nimesulide was more potent than naproxen on COX-2 dependent PGE_2 production in whole blood[88].

The findings from clinical trials generally support the favourable side-effect profile of these agents exhibiting preferential inhibition of the COX-2 isoform. Thus, a meta-analysis of controlled trials with nimesulide indicated that it had a better risk–benefit ratio than the standard NSAIDs[89]. In a 3-month comparative study in osteoarthritic patients, there was no difference between the incidence and severity of GI side effects with nimesulide and etodolac[90]. In other studies, etodolac has produced a reduced side effect profile on the gut compared with standard NSAIDs[91], but had a similar GI safety profile as nabumetone[92], another agent claimed to exhibit site-selective actions on COX. In the MELISSA and SELECT trials in osteoarthritic patients with meloxicam, an anti-inflammatory agent with preferential *in vitro* selectivity for the COX-2 isoform, a significantly reduced incidence of side effects was noted in the meloxicam group compared with the comparators diclofenac and piroxicam, respectively, but with comparable clinical efficacy[93,94].

The clinical promise of the coxibs was indeed upheld by the recent clinical studies published over the past 2 years. Thus, celecoxib was approved for the treatment of rheumatoid arthritis and osteoarthritis, based on submitted findings from 5285 patients in controlled trials. In one 24-week study in rheumatoid arthritic patients, it produced comparable sustained management of pain and inflammation as the comparator, diclofenac, but with reduced gastroduodenal ulceration and less withdrawal from that treatment because of GI side effects[95]. In a further study in rheumatoid patients, both celecoxib and naproxen improved the signs and symptoms of arthritis, whereas the incidence of endoscopically assessed gastroduodenal ulceration with celecoxib was the same as the placebo group, and was substantially less than that observed in the naproxen group[96].

Rofecoxib has also demonstrated efficacy as an anti-inflammatory agent in a number of clinical studies, with once daily treatment. In a comparison of eight studies involving 5435 patients with osteoarthritis, rofecoxib was associated with an overall significantly lower incidence of upper GI tract bleeding than the comparators NSAIDs, including diclofenac and ibuprofen[97]. In a further study in osteoarthritis, using ibuprofen as the comparator, the incidence of ulcers with rofecoxib was significantly lower than with the higher dose of ibuprofen at 12 and 24 weeks[98]. More recently, in addition to a number of other clinical studies with these agents, two extensive studies with coxibs have recently been presented, the VIGOR study with rofecoxib[99] and the CLASS study with celecoxib[100], supporting the therapeutic efficacy and reduced GI side effect profile of these coxibs.

CONCLUSIONS

It will be apparent, therefore, that the mechanisms underlying the GI injury by NSAIDs are complex, while the processes for gastric and intestinal damage are distinct (Figure 3 and 4). However, the mechanisms of injury at both sites appear to involve the inhibition of COX, although other processes, including local topical irritancy on the gastric mucosa and iNOS expression in the intestine, play interactive roles in the pathogenesis of the tissue damage. Such findings predict, however, that the COX-2 selective inhibitory agents should have beneficial anti-inflammatory actions with reduced propensity for gut toxicity, as has now been established in extensive clinical studies. The pharmacokinetic distribution of these agents in the body, along with their ability to provoke topical mucosal irritation, will also have some influence on the therapeutic ratio of these agents between the anti-inflammatory actions and the incidence of GI erosion and ulceration.

Although recent experimental studies suggest that inhibition of both isoforms is necessary to produce acute gastric injury in the rat[40], whether this

Figure 4 Interactive mechanisms in the pathogenesis of gastric mucosal damage induced by NSAIDs. The diagram shows the topical irritant actions of agents on the surface epithelium, allowing the back-diffusion of acid. Inhibition of COX-1, the predominant isoform in the gastric mucosa, can affect the microvasculature, leading to changes in local blood flow, while white cell adhesion may also result from COX inhibition. Such actions can initiate the production of gastric lesions. In addition, topical damage and COX-inhibition can synergistically interact to provoke extensive mucosal damage.

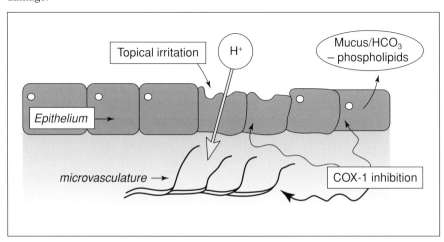

is also the case following chronic administration of these inhibitors awaits further study. It is not known how such findings reflect the protective inter-active roles of COX-1 and COX-2 in the GI tract of humans. Moreover, the possible requirement for both COX isoforms to be inhibited to produce GI injury does not limit or obviate the therapeutic potential of the coxibs as anti-inflammatory drugs free of these side effects, although it may require some reinterpretation of the underlying principle of such agents.

The pharmacological profile of these agents as anti-inflammatory anal-gesics will need to be explored fully in the therapeutic setting, and their safety and efficacy established in long-term clinical studies in patients, especially those most at risk such as the elderly. Thus, it is not known yet whether such prolonged suppression of COX-2 will affect physiological responses, as this enzyme can be expressed constitutively. In the gut, COX-2 appears to be involved in the healing of experimental peptic ulcers and in the associated process of angiogensis, at least in experimental models[57,58]. Although the exist-ing clinical data with these agents do not suggest a major problem over that anticipated with other NSAIDs, direct studies will reveal whether COX-2-selective inhibitors will affect healing in patients with pre-existing gastric or duodenal ulcers.

Whether coxibs, like other NSAIDs, will be contraindicated in patients with inflammatory bowel diseases has not been established in appropriate clinical studies. Exacerbation with a range of COX-2-selective inhibitors in experimental colonic inflammation has been reported[101], and such agents do not appear to offer anti-inflammatory benefit in colitis models[102].

The findings of large scale studies have suggested that the long-term use of coxibs, which unlike classical NSAIDs do not inhibit thromboxane pro-duction and hence lack this beneficial anti-platelet, anti-thrombotic activity, will need further consideration and study in patients at cardiovascular risk. Although the coxibs may reduce the production of vascular PGI_2[103], which would theoretically promote platelet aggregability, whether the lack of action on platelet and haemostatic function contributes to the reduction in peptic ulcer bleeds with these agents requires consideration. Indeed, it will be impor-tant to establish fully whether concurrent administration of low-dose aspirin to restore the anti-thrombotic cover in patients taking coxibs for long-term periods, will tend to offset any therapeutic gain observed from GI bleeds.

Whereas the more established NSAIDs will continue to be used in the clinic for some time, strategies for the limitation of their gastric side effects may be increasingly employed, such as the use of mucosal protective agents or, more likely, concomitant acid anti-secretory therapy. However, it remains to be established whether the pharmaco-economics of such combination therapy will compete with the costs or efficacy of the COX-2 inhibitors for long term therapy. The therapeutic potential of NO-NSAIDs that exhibit reduced gastric mucosal injury under experimental conditions is currently under clinical investigation[25]. Such agents, if proved to be effective in patients and to show diminished GI toxicity, as well as a satisfactory general safety profile, could provide an alternative therapeutic strategy to the use of COX-2 selective agents.

Advances in our understanding of the biochemical and pharmacological processes underlying the development of GI injury by NSAIDs have successfully prompted new pharmaceutical initiatives in this area. These pharmacological strategies have allowed the development of a range of novel agents that are proving to be clinically acceptable alternatives to the classical NSAIDs. Thus, some 250 years after the identification of the therapeutic properties of salicylate, we have now the possibility to provide effective anti-inflammatory and analgesic relief without compromising the GI tract of the recipients.

REFERENCES

1. Fries JF, Miller SR, Spitz PW, Williams CA, Hubert HB, Bloch DA. Toward an epidemiology of gastropathy associated with nonsteroidal anti-inflammatory drug use. *Gastroenterology.* 1989;96:647–55.
2. Langman MJ, Weil J, Wainwright P, Lawson DH, Rawlins MD, Logan RF et al. Risks of bleeding peptic ulcer associated with individual nonsteriodal anti-inflammatory drugs. *Lancet.* 1994;343:1075–8.
3. Douthwaite AH, Lintott GM. Gastroscopic observation of the effects of aspirin and certain other substances on the stomach. *Lancet.* 1935;ii:1222–5.
4. Caruso I, Bianchi Porro G. Gastroscopic evaluation of anti-inflammatory agents. *Br Med J.* 1980;280:75–8.
5. Russell RI. Endoscopic evaluation of etodolac and naproxen, and their relative effects on gastric and duodenal prostaglandins. *Rheumatol Int.* 1990;10:17–21.
6. Davenport HW. Gastric mucosal injury by fatty and acetylsalicylic acids. *Gastroenterology.* 1964;46:245–53.
7. Wallace JL, Whittle BJR. Role of mucus in the repair of gastric epithelial cell damage in the rat. *Gastroenterology.* 1986;91:603–11.
8. Bowen BK, Krause WJ, Ivey KJ. Effect of sodium bicarbonate on aspirin-induced damage and potential difference changes in human gastric mucosa. *Br Med J.* 1977;2:1052–4.
9. Whittle BJR. Unwanted effects of aspirin and related agents in the gastrointestinal tract. In: Vane JR, Botting RM, editors. *Aspirin and Other Salicylates.* London: Chapman & Hall; 1992:465–509.
10. Grossman MI, Matsumota KK, Lichter RJ. Fecal blood loss by oral and intravenous administration of various salicylates. *Gastroenterology.* 1961;40:383–8.
11. Skidmore IF, Whitehouse MW. Concerning the regulation of some diverse biochemical reactions underlying the inflammatory response by salicylic acid, phenylbutazone and other acidic antirheumatic drugs. *J Pharm Pharmacol.* 1966;18:558–60.
12. Rainsford KD, Whitehouse MW. Anti-inflammatory anti-pyretic salicylic acid esters, with low gastric ulcerogenic activity. *Agents Actions.* 1980;10:451–6.
13. Somasundaram S, Hayllar H, Rafi S, Wrigglesworth JM, Macpherson AJ, Bjarnason

I. The biochemical basis of non-steroidal anti-inflammatory drug-induced damage to the gastrointestinal tract: a review and a hypothesis. *Scand J Gastroenterol.* 1995;30:289–99.

14. Moreno-Sanchez R, Bravo C, Vasquez C, Ayala G, Silveira LH, Martinez-Lavin M. Inhibition and uncoupling of oxidative phosphorylation by nonsteroidal anti-inflammatory drugs: study in mitochondria, submitochondrial particle, cells and whole heart. *Biochem Pharmacol.* 1999;57:743–52.

15. Allen A, Garner A. Mucus and bicarbonate secretion in the stomach and their possible role in mucosal protection. *Gut.* 1980;21:249–62.

16. Rainsford KD. The effects of aspirin and other nonsteroidal anti-inflammatory/analgesics drugs on gastrointestinal mucus glycoprotein biosynthesis in vivo: relationship to ulcerogenic actions. *Biochem Pharmacol.* 1978;27:877–85.

17. Goddard PJ, Kao YJ, Lichtenberger LM. Luminal surface hydrophobicity of canine gastric mucosa is dependent on a surface mucous gel. *Gastroenterology.* 1990;98:361–70.

18. Lichtenberger LM, Ulloa C, Romero JJ, Vanous AL, Illich PA, Dial EJ. Nonsteroidal anti-inflammatory drug and phospholipid prodrugs: combination therapy with antisecretory agents in rats. *Gastroenterology.* 1996;111:990–5.

19. Hawkey CJ. Progress in prophylaxis against nonsteroidal anti-inflammatory drug-associated ulcers and erosions. Omeprazole NSAID Steering Committee. *Am J Med.* 1998;104:67S–74S.

20. Bianchi Porro G, Parente F, Imbesi V, Montrone F, Caruso I. Role of *Helicobacter pylori* in ulcer healing and recurrence of gastric and duodenal ulcers in longterm NSAID users. Response to omeprazole dual therapy. *Gut.* 1996;39:22–6.

21. Hawkey CJ, Karrasch JA, Szczepanski L, Walker DG, Barkun A, Swannell AJ et al. Omeprazole compared with misoprostol for ulcers associated with nonsteroidal anti-inflammatory drugs. Omeprazole versus Misoprostol for NSAID-induced Ulcer Management (OMNIUM) study group. *N Engl J Med.* 1998;338:727–34.

22. Hawkey CJ, Whittle BJR. Prostaglandins in the management of gastroduodenal ulceration. In: Vane JR, O'Grady J, editors. *Therapeutic Applications of Prostaglandins.* London: Edward Arnold; 1993:122–40.

23. Wallace JL. Non-steroidal anti-inflammatory drugs and gastroenteropathy: the second hundred years. *Gastroenterology.* 1997;112:1000–16.

24. Wallace JL, Reuter B, Cicala C, McKnight W, Grisham M, Cirino G. A diclofenac derivative without ulcerogenic properties. *Eur J Pharmacol.* 1994;257:249–55.

25. Ardizzone S, Bianchi Porro G. Prevention of NSAID-gastropathy. *Ital J Gastroenterol.* 1996;28(Suppl 4):33–6.

26. Hudson N, Murray FE, Cole AT, Filippowicz B, Hawkey CJ. Effect of sucralfate on aspirin induced mucosal injury and impaired haemostasis in humans. *Gut.* 1997;41:19–23.

27. Bianchi Porro G, Lazzaroni M, Manzionna G, Petrillo M. Omeprazole and sucralfate in the treatment of NSAID-induced gastric and duodenal ulcer. *Aliment Pharmacol Ther.* 1998;12:355–60.

28. Lichtenberger LM, Wang Z-M, Romero JJ, Ulloa C, Perez JC, Giraud M-N et al. Nonsteroidal anti-inflammatory drugs (NSAIDs) associate with zwitterionic phospholipids: insight into the mechanism and reversal of NSAID-induced gastrointestinal injury. *Nature Med.* 1995;1:154–8.

29. Whittle BJR, Vane JR. Prostanoids as regulators of gastrointestinal function. In: Johnson LR, editor. *Physiology of the Gastrointestinal Tract* (2nd edn). New York: Raven Press; 1987:143–80.

30. Robert A, Nezamis JE, Lancaster C, Hanchar AJ. Cytoprotection by prostaglandins in rats – prevention of gastric necrosis produced by alcohol, HCl, NaOH, hypertonic NaCl and thermal injury. *Gastroenterology*. 1979;77:433–43.

31. Whittle BJR. Nitric oxide in gastrointestinal physiology and pathology. In: Johnson LR, editor. *Physiology of the Gastrointestinal Tract* (3rd edn). New York: Raven Press; 1994:267–94.

32. Barrachino MD, Calatayud S, Canet A, Esplugues JV. Transdermal nitroglycerin prevents nonsteriodal anti-inflammatory drug gastropathy. *Eur J Pharmacol*. 1995;281:R3–4.

33. Whittle BJR. Nitric oxide – a mediator of inflammation or mucosal defence. *Eur J Gastro Hepato*. 1997;9:1026–32.

34. Lanas A, Bajador E, Serrano P, Fuentes J, Carreno S, Guardia J et al. Nitrovasodilators, low-dose aspirin, other nonsteroidal antiinflammatory drugs, and the risk of upper gastrointestinal bleeding. *N Engl J Med*. 2000;343:834–9.

35. Vane JR. Inhibition of prostaglandin synthesis as a mechanism of action of aspirin-like drugs. *Nature New Biol*. 1971;231:232–5.

36. Rainsford KD. An analysis of the gastrointestinal side-effects of non-steroidal anti-inflammatory drugs, with particular reference to comparative studies in man and laboratory species. *Rheumatol Int*. 1982;2:1–10.

37. Main IHM, Whittle BJR. Investigation of the vasodilator and antisecretory role of prostaglandins in the rat gastric mucosa by use of non-steroidal anti-inflammatory drugs. *Br J Pharmacol*. 1975;53:217–24.

38. Ashley SW, Sonnenschein LA, Cheung LY. Focal gastric mucosal blood flow at the site of aspirin-induced ulceration. *Am J Surg*. 1985;149:53–9.

39. Gana TJ, Huhlewych R, Koo J. Focal gastric mucosal blood flow in aspirin-induced ulceration. *Ann Surg*. 1987;205:399–403.

40. Wallace JL, McKnight W, Reuter BK, Vergnolle N. NSAID-induced gastric damage in rats: requirement for inhibition of both cyclooxygenase 1 and 2. *Gastroenterology*. 2000;119:705–14.

41. Whittle BJR. Mechanisms underlying gastric mucosal damage induced by indomethacin and bile salt, and the actions of prostaglandins. *Br J Pharmacol*. 1977;60:455–60.

42. Wallace JL, Keenan CM, Granger DN. Gastric ulceration induced by non-steroidal anti-inflammatory drugs is a neutrophil-dependent process. *Am J Physiol*. 1990;259:G462–7.

43. Wallace JL, McKnight W, Miyasaka M, Tamatani T, Paulson J, Anderson DC et al. Role of endothelial adhesion molecules in NSAID-induced gastric mucosal injury. *Am J Physiol*. 1993;265:G993–8.

44. Wallace JL, Arfors K-E, McKnight GW. A monoclonal antibody against the CD18 leukocyte adhesion molecule prevents indomethacin-induced gastric damage in the rabbit. *Gastroenterology*. 1991;100:878–83.

45. Lee M, Aldred K, Lee E, Feldman M. Aspirin-induced acute gastric mucosal injury is a neutrophil-dependent process in rats. *Am J Physiol*. 1992;263:G920–6.

46. Andrews FJ, Malcontenti-Wilson C, O'Brien PE. Effect of nonsteroidal anti-inflammatory drugs on LFA-1 and ICAM-1 expression in gastric mucosa. *Am J Physiol*. 1994;266:G657–64.

47. Santucci L, Fiorucci S, Di Matteo FM. Role of tumour necrosis factor alfa release and leucocyte margination in indomethacin-induced gastric injury in rats. *Gastroenterology*. 1995;108:393–401.

48. Vaananen PM, Meddings JB, Wallace JL. Role of oxygen-derived free radicals in indomethacin-induced gastric injury. *Am J Physiol.* 1991;261:G470–5.

49. Takeuchi K, Ueshima K, Hironaka Y, Fujioka Y, Matsumoto J, Okabe S. Oxygen free radicals and lipid peroxidation in the pathogenesis of gastric mucosal lesions induced by indomethacin in rats. Relation to gastric hypermotility. *Digestion.* 1991;49:175–84.

50. Maricic N, Ehrlich K, Gretzer B, Schuliogi R, Respondek M, Peskar BM. Selective cyclo-oxygenase-2 inhibitors aggravate ischaemia-reperfusion injury in the rat stomach. *Br J Pharmacol.* 1999;128:1659–66.

51. Asako H, Kubes P, Wallace JL, Wolf RE, Granger DN. Modulation of leukocyte adhesion in rat mesenteric venules by aspirin and salicylate. *Gastroenterology.* 1992;103:146–52.

52. Kitahora T, Guth PH. Effect of aspirin plus hydrochloric acid on the gastric mucosal microcirculation. *Gastroenterology.* 1987;93:810–17.

53. Giraud MN, Motta C, Romero JJ, Bommelaer G, Lichtenberger LM. Interaction of indomethacin and naproxen with gastric surface-active phospholipids: a possible mechanism form the gastric toxicity of nonsteroidal anti-inflammatory drugs (NSAIDs). *Biochem Pharmacol.* 1999;57:247–54.

54. Whittle BJR, Kauffman GL, Moncada S. Hemostatic mechanisms, independent of platelet aggregation, arrest gastric mucosal bleeding. *Proc Natl Acad Sci USA.* 1986;83:5683–7.

55. O'Laughlin JC, Hoftiezer JW, Mahoney JP, Ivey KI. Does aspirin prolong the bleeding from gastric biopsies in man? *Gastrointest Endosc.* 1981;27:1–5.

56. Schmassmann A, Peskar BM, Stettler C, Netzer P, Stroff T, Flogerzi B et al. Effects of inhibition of prostaglandin endoperoxide synthase-2 in chronic gastro-intestinal ulcer models in rats. *Br J Pharmacol.* 1998;123:795–804.

57. Jones MK, Wang H, Peskar BM, Levin EM, Itani RM, Sarfeh IJ et al. Inhibition of angiogenesis by nonsteroidal anti-inflammatory drugs: insight into mechanisms and implications for cancer growth and ulcer healing. *Nat Med.* 1999;5:1418–23.

58. Whittle BJR, Higgs GA, Eakins KE, Moncada S, Vane JR. Selective inhibition of prostaglandin production in inflammatory exudates and gastric mucosa. *Nature.* 1980;284:271–3.

59. Xu XM, Sansores-Garcia L, Chen XM, Matijevic-Aleksic N, Du M, Wu KK. Suppression of inducible cyclo-oxygenase 2 gene transcription by aspirin and sodium salicylate. *Proc Natl Acad Sci USA.* 1999;96:5292–7.

60. Fu J-Y, Masferrer JL, Seibert K, Raz A, Needleman P. The induction and suppression of prostaglandin H_2 synthase (cyclooxygenase) in human monocytes. *J Biol Chem.* 1990;265:16737–40.

61. Xie W, Chipman JG, Robertson DL, Erikson RL, Simmons DL. Expression of a mitogen-responsive gene encoding prostaglandin synthase is regulated by mRNA splicing. *Proc Natl Acad Sci USA.* 1991;88:2692–6.

62. O'Banion MK, Sadowski HB, Winn V, Young DA. A serum- and glucocorticoid-regulated 4-kilobase mRNA encodes a cyclooxygenase-related protein. *J Biol Chem.* 1991;266:23261–7.

63. Mitchell JA, Warner TD. Cyclo-oxygenase-2: pharmacology, physiology, biochemistry and relevance to NSAID therapy. *Br J Pharmacol.* 1999;128:1121–32.

64. Vane JR, Mitchell JA, Appleton I, Tomlinson A, Bishop-Bailey D, Croxtall J et al. Inducible isoforms of cyclo-oxygenase and nitric-oxide synthase in inflammation. *Proc Natl Acad Sci USA.* 1994;91:2046–50.

65. Masferrer JL, Zweifel BS, Manning PT, Hauser SD, Leahy KM, Smith WG et al. Selective inhibition of inducible cyclooxygenase 2 in vivo is antiinflammatory and nonulcerogenic. *Proc Natl Acad Sci USA.* 1994;91:3228–32.

66. Smith CJ, Zhang Y, Koboldt CM, Muhammad J, Zweifel BS, Schaffer A et al. Pharmacological analysis of cyclooxygenase-1 in inflammation. *Proc Natl Acad Sci USA.* 1998;95:13313–18.

67. Hawkey CJ. COX-2 inhibitors. *Lancet.* 1999;353:307–14.

68. Warner T, Giuliano F, Vojnovic I, Bukasa A, Mitchell JA, Vane JR. Nonsteroid drug selectivities for cyclo-oxygenase-1 rather than cyclo-oxygenase-2 are associated with human gastrointestinal toxicity: a full *in vitro* analysis. *Proc Natl Acad Sci USA.* 1999;96:7563–8.

69. Gretzer B, Ehrlich K, Maricic N, Lambrecht N, Respondek M, Peskar BM. Selective cyclo-oxygenase-2 inhibitors and their influence on the protective effect of a mild irritant on the stomach. *Br J Pharmacol.* 1998;123:927–35.

70. Kishimoto Y, Wada K, Nakamoto K, Kawasaki H, Hasegawa J. Levels of cyclo-oxygenase-1 and -2 mRNA expression at various stages of acute gastric injury induced by ischemia-reperfusion in rats. *Arch Biochem Biophys.* 1998;352:153–7.

71. Gilroy DW, Colville-Nash PR, Willis D, Chivers J, Paul-Clark MJ, Willoughby DA. Inducible cyclo-oxygenase may have anti-inflammatory properties. *Nature Med.* 1999;5:698–701.

72. Wallace JL, Bak A, McKnight W, Asfaha S, Sharkey A, MacNaughton WK. Cyclo-oxygenase-1 contributes to inflammatory responses in rats and mice: implications for gastrointestinal toxicity. *Gastroenterology.* 1998;115:101–9.

73. Chan CC, Boyce S, Brideau C, Charleson S, Cromlish W, Ethier D et al. Rofecoxib [Vioxx®, MK-0966; 4-(-4'-methylsulfonylphenyl)-3-phenyl-2-(5H)-furanone]: a potent and orally active cyclooxygenase-2 inhibitor. Pharmacological and biochemical profiles. *J Pharmacol Exp Ther.* 1999;290:551–60.

74. Redfern JS, Feldman M. Role of endogenous prostaglandins in preventing gastrointestinal ulceration: induction of ulcers by antibodies to prostaglandins. *Gastroenterology.* 1989;96(Suppl):596–605.

75. Langenbach R, Morham SG, Tiano HF, Loftin CD, Ghanayem BI, Chulada PC et al. Prostaglandin synthase 1 gene disruption in mice reduces arachidonic acid-induced inflammation and indomethacin-induced gastric ulceration. *Cell.* 1995;83:483–92.

76. Whittle BJR. Thirteenth Gaddum Memorial Lecture. Neuronal and endothelium-derived mediators in the modulation of the gastric microcirculation: integrity in the balance. *Br J Pharmacol.* 1993;110:3–17.

77. Robert A. An intestinal disease produced experimentally by a prostaglandin deficiency. *Gastroenterology.* 1975;69:1045–7.

78. Whittle BJR. Temporal relationship between cyclo-oxygenase inhibition, as measured by prostacyclin biosynthesis, and the gastrointestinal damage induced by indomethacin in the rat. *Gastroenterology.* 1981;80:94–8.

79. Bjarnason I, Zanelli G, Smith T, Prouse P, Williams P, Smethurst P et al. Non-steroidal anti-inflammatory drug-induced intestinal inflammation in humans. *Gastroenterology.* 1987;93:480–9.

80. Bjarnason I, MacPherson A, Hollander D. Intestinal permeability: an overview. *Gastroenterology.* 1995;108:1566–81.

81. Sigthorsson G, Tibble J, Hayllar J, Menzies I, Macpherson A, Moots R et al. Intestinal permeability and inflammation in patients on NSAIDs. *Gut.* 1998;43:506–11.

82. Sigthorsson G, Jacob M, Wrigglesworth J, Somasundaram S, Tavares I, Foster R et al. Comparison of indomethacin and nimesulide, a selective cyclo-oxygenase-2 inhibitor, on key pathophysiologic steps in enteropathy. *Scand J Gastroenterol.* 1998;33:728–35.

83. Reuter BK, Davies NM, Wallace JL. Nonsteroidal anti-inflammatory drug enteropathy in rats: role of permeability, bacteria, and enterohepatic circulation. *Gastroenterology.* 1997;112:109–17.

84. Whittle BJR, Laszlo F, Evans SM, Moncada S. Induction of nitric oxide synthase and microvascular injury in the rat jejunum provoked by indomethacin. *Br J Pharmacol.* 1995;116:2286–90.

85. Evans SM, Laszlo F, Whittle BJ. Site-specific lesion formation, inflammation and inducible nitric oxide synthase expression by indomethacin in the rat intestine. *Eur J Pharmacol.* 2000;388:281–5.

86. Bjarnason I. Forthcoming non-steroidal anti-inflammatory drugs: are they really devoid of side effects? *Ital J Gastroenterol Hepatol.* 1999;31:27–36.

87. Sigthorsson G, Crane R, Simon T, Hoover M, Quan H, Bolognese J et al. COX-2 inhibition with rofecoxib does not increase intestinal permeability in healthy subjects: a double blind crossover study comparing rofecoxib with placebo and indomethacin. *Gut.* 2000;47:527–32.

88. Shah AA, Murray FE, Fitzgerald DJ. The *in vivo* assessment of nimesulide cyclo-oxygenase-2 selectivity. *Rheumatology.* 1999;38:19–23.

89. Wober W. Comparative efficacy and safety of nimesulide and diclofenac in patients with acute shoulder, and a meta-analysis of controlled studies with nimesulide. *Rheumatology.* 1999:38:33–8.

90. Lucker PW, Pawlowski C, Friedrich I, Faiella F, Magni E. Double-blind randomised, multi-centre clinical study evaluating the efficacy and tolerability of nimesulide in comparison with etodolac in patients suffering from osteoarthritis of the knee. *Eur J Rheumatol Inflamm.* 1994;14:29–38.

91. Schnitzer TJ, Constantine G. Etodolac (Lodine) in the treatment of osteoarthritis: recent studies. *J Rheumatol Suppl.* 1997;47:23–31.

92. Schnitzer TJ, Ballard IM, Constantine G, McDonald P. Double-blind, placebo-controlled comparison of the safety and efficacy of orally administered etodolac and nabumetone in patients with active osteoarthritis of the knee. *Clin Ther.* 1995;17:602–12.

93. Hawkey C, Kahan A, Steinbruck K, Alegre C, Baumelou E, Begaud B et al. and the Melissa International Study Group. Gastrointestinal tolerability of meloxicam compared to diclofenac in osteoarthritis patients. *Br J Rheumatol.* 1998;37:937–45.

94. Dequeker J, Hawkey C, Kahan A, Steinbruck K, Alegre C, Baumelou E et al. Improvement in gastrointestinal tolerability of the selective cyclo-oxygenase (COX)-2 inhibitor, meloxicam, compared with piroxicam: results of the safety and efficacy large-scale evaluation of COX-inhibiting therapies (SELECT) trial in osteoarthritis. *Br J Rheumatol.* 1998;37:946–51.

95. Emery P, Zeidler, H, Kvien TK, Guslandi M, Naudin R, Stead H et al. Celecoxib versus diclofenac in long-term management of rheumatoid arthritis: randomised double-blind comparison. *Lancet.* 1999;354:2106–11.

96. Simon LS, Weaver AL, Graham DY, Kivitz AJ, Lipsky PE, Hubbard RC et al. Anti-inflammatory and upper gastrointestinal effects of celecoxib in rheumatoid arthritis: a randomized controlled trial. *J Am Med Ass.* 1999;242:1921–8.

97. Langman MJ, Jensen DM, Watson DJ, Harper SE, Zhao PL, Quan H et al. Adverse

upper gastrointestinal effects of rofecoxib compared with NSAIDs. *J Am Med Ass.* 1999;282:1929–33.

98. Laine L, Harper S, Simon T, Bath R, Johanson J, Schwartz H et al. A randomized trial comparing the effect of rofecoxib, a cyclo-oxygenase 2-specific inhibitor, with that of ibuprofen on the gastroduodenal mucosa of patients with osteoarthritis. *Gastroenterology.* 1999;117:776–83.

99. Bombardier C, Laine L, Reicin A, Shapiro D, Burgos-Vargas R, Davis B et al. Comparison of upper gastrointestinal toxicity of rofecoxib and naproxen in patients with rheumatoid arthritis. *N Engl J Med.* 2000;343:1520–8.

100. Silverstein FE, Faich G, Goldstein JL, Simon LS, Pincus T, Whelton A et al. Gastrointestinal toxicity with celecoxib vs nonsteroidal anti-inflammatory drugs for osteoarthritis and rheumatoid arthritis: the CLASS study: a randomized controlled trial. Celecoxib Long-term Arthritis Safety Study. *J Am Med Ass.* 2000;284:1247–55.

101. Reuter BK, Asfaha S, Buret A, Sharkey KA, Wallace JL. Exacerbation of inflammation-associated colonic injury in rat through inhibition of cyclo-oxygenase-2. *J Clin Invest.* 1996;98:2076–85.

102. Lesch CA, Kraus ER, Sanchez B, Gilbertsen R, Guglietta A. Lack of beneficial effect of COX-2 inhibitors in an experimental model of colitis. *Methods Find Exp Clin Pharmacol.* 1999;21:99–104.

103. McAdam BF, Catella-Lawson F, Mardini IA, Kapoor S, Lawson JA, FitzGerald GA. Systemic biosynthesis of prostacyclin by cyclo-oxygenase (COX)-2: the human pharmacology of a selective inhibitor of COX-2. *Proc Natl Acad Sci USA.* 1999;96:5890.

16 | Gastrointestinal toxicity of non-steroid anti-inflammatory drugs

C. J. HAWKEY

Division of Gastroenterology, Queen's Medical Centre,
University Hospital Nottingham, Nottingham NG7 2UH, UK.

For many years salicylic acid, an extract of willow bark, was used as a non-steroid anti-inflammatory drug (NSAID)[1]. Nowadays salicylic acid is seldom used for this purpose. Its main utility in clinical practice is as a topical inorganic acid that dissolves cutaneous warts. This property emphasizes the intrinsic toxicity of salicylic acid. However, within the stomach, salicylic acid may cause mucosal reddening (due to vasodilation) but erosion and ulceration are infrequent. It is likely that this is because salicylic acid provokes reactive synthesis of mucosal prostaglandins (PGs)[2] which protect the mucosa by orchestrating a number of defensive functions[3]. These include increased mucosal blood flow, secretion of mucus and bicarbonate and possibly enhancement of surface hydrophobicity.

When Felix Hoffman was asked by his father to synthesize a more palatable derivative of salicylic acid he achieved this by acetylating it to produce aspirin. It became apparent that aspirin, unlike salicylic acid, frequently caused acute mucosal erosions and chronic gastroduodenal ulcers[4]. The discovery that aspirin inhibited PG synthesis and could thereby abrogate the reactive synthesis of protective PGs in response to salicylate injury provided a rational explanation for these observations. The marked accompanying reduction in dyspepsia implies PG synthesis is involved in its mediation[5], presumably because PGs are involved in pain perception. It also emphasizes the disjunction between symptoms and injury and illustrates one of the major problems in clinical management of NSAID users – that dyspepsia is not a reliable index of mucosal ulceration[6].

GASTROINTESTINAL MANIFESTATIONS OF NSAID USE

Although toxic effects of NSAIDs on the stomach and the duodenum were the first and are by far the best recognized consequences of NSAID ingestion, it is clear that they are toxic to the entire gastrointestinal (GI) tract. Chronic NSAID use is associated with oesophageal disease[6–8], although acute injury is seldom evident microscopically and the importance of PG synthesis in pathogenesis uncertain. At least some NSAIDs damage the small bowel acutely and result in intestinal ulceration[6,7,9–15]. This is associated with active inflammation, chronic blood loss and perforation. Small bowel damage is particularly characteristic of NSAIDs that undergo enterohepatic circulation[13] and is seen more floridly in rat models than in human disease. Whether inhibition of PG synthesis or other mechanisms are most central to NSAID-induced enteric injury is uncertain.

NSAIDs probably also enhance large bowel permeability[16] and growing data associate them with development of inflammation here too[17–21]. Evidence principally comes from epidemiological studies, associating NSAID use with relapse or development of ulcerative colitis[17–19]. It seems likely that this is causal but mechanisms are unclear (particularly the contribution of COX-1 or COX-2 – see below), a consequential relationship has not definitively been excluded, estimates of risk vary substantially and the longest established specific relationship is for paracetamol rather then NSAIDs[17]. NSAIDs also cause colonic ulcers[20], though probably rarely, and contribute significantly to the development of diverticular perforation[21].

OESOPHAGEAL DISEASE: CONTINUING CONUNDRUMS

Several studies suggest an association between NSAID use and oesophageal injury[6–8]. These have included heartburn, stricture and erosive oesophagitis[7,15,22–30]. Oesophagitis has been associated with diseases treated with NSAIDs[30–32]. However, these findings have not received widespread support. There are several reasons for this:

1. Some of the studies are uncontrolled and/or unblinded.
2. There is suspicion that NSAID use might be a marker for disease associated problems[30], for example reduced epidermal growth factor[31], either because of salivary gland disease or reduced mastication in NSAID users[32].
3. A plausible mechanism for NSAID damage has yet to emerge convincingly.

The last is probably the most important reason. In general, PGs reduce both peristalsis in the lower oesophagus and oesophageal sphincter pressure[33,34] whilst NSAIDs enhance tone and sphincter pressure[35], or prevent acid-induced sphincter hypotension[36]. However, effects may be transient[35] and negative studies have been reported[37]. Moreover, PGs have been shown to cause paradoxical prejunctional enhancement of cholinergic transmission[38].

Likewise, there are more animal data suggesting benefit from NSAIDs than harm. Microscopic improvement and/or protection has been seen with acid-induced injury[36] and radiation[39] and indomethacin can prevent radiation mucositis[40,41], as well as abrogating oesophageal tumour development[42,43]. Moreover, numerous short-term studies show very little injury, in contrast to stomach and duodenum.

To these apparently paradoxical findings that NSAIDs may protect against acid reflux and have beneficial effects at mucosal level must be added a third set of observations. Oesophageal mucosa is squamous in origin and, unlike the stomach, a lipoxygenase metabolite[44] (probably 12-hydroxy eicosatetra-noic acid[45]) appears to be the main product of arachidonic acid metabolism, rather than a PG. Several studies have suggested that reflux is not associated with the enhancement in PG synthesis that might be expected with inflam-mation[46–48], whilst leukotriene B_4 does appear to be elevated[49]. Moreover, one animal study showed more protection against acid injury by the combined PG and leukotriene inhibitor BW755C than indomethacin[50]. Indeed, acid may inhibit PG release, though acid pepsin injury causes its enhancement[51]. Under some circumstances PGs can be protective, for example against caustic injury[52], and a local alkaline tide[53] and possible abrogation of the enhanced permeability seen with (even parenteral) aspirin[54] maybe responsible.

Assessment

The multiple internal contradictions in the data have inhibited a consensus about the role of NSAIDs and PGs in oesophagitis. Nevertheless informal observations continue to suggest an association of heartburn and oesophagitis with their use. Recent large trials of prophylaxis in NSAID users have shown a 25% incidence of heartburn which is effectively treated with omeprazole[55]. What seems most needed is an epidemiological study, which would have to be large because of the multiple other influences on oesophagitis, on a case control basis to establish whether degrees of oesophageal reflux falling short of oesophageal structuring are or are not truly associated with NSAID use.

GASTRODUODENAL ULCERATION

This is the most well recognized adverse property of NSAIDs.

Pathogenesis

(i) Prostaglandin synthesis
Central to gastroduodenal ulceration is the ability of NSAIDs to inhibit gastro-duodenal PG synthesis[56–62] and abrogate PG-dependent defence mechanisms. Many studies have reported that aspirin and non-aspirin NSAIDs reduce

gastric mucosal synthesis of PGs by more than 50%. However most studies are not comparable because a wide variety of methods have been used. Processing of biopsy samples inevitably stimulates PG synthesis, making it doubtful that it is possible to measure mucosal levels. There is an enormous variation in the absolute values that have been reported and this partly reflects differences in biopsy processing. However, in some studies, the amount of PG synthesis that has been reported has exceeded whole body basal daily production.

These problems are stimulating the emergence of a consensus on methods to compare individual patients and the *in vitro* and *ex vivo* effects of NSAIDs. These methods use vortexing of suspended biopsy samples to provide a standardized stimulus to PG synthesis by gastric or duodenal mucosa and are based upon a method originally described by Whittle et al.[56].

This method results in synthesis of levels of PGs that are low enough to be a realistic reflection of *in vivo* capacity, and is responsive to inhibition by NSAIDs both *in vivo* and *in vitro*. Recently, we and others have further refined this method, reducing variability to a coefficient of variation of approximately 30%[58,59]. At endoscopy, 12 individual mucosal biopsy samples are collected into polypropylene vials containing 1 ml Tris HCl buffer, minced for 10 s and, after several washes, vortexed for 3 min before centrifuging and transfer of supernatant to a stop tube containing 100 μg of indomethacin. When used to investigate the effect of naproxen 500 μg b.i.d., this method showed a 65% (53–74%) inhibition of *ex vivo* PGE_2 synthesis compared with placebo[61]. This method has also been used to show dose-dependent inhibition of PG synthesis with doses of aspirin as low as 10 mg[62].

(ii) Other mechanisms
NSAIDs have other actions that may contribute to gastroduodenal mucosal injury including:

PERMEABILITY

NSAIDs cause increased permeability in the stomach[63] as they do in the rest of the GI tract. This has been described as 'breaking the mucosal barrier'. Indeed this was one of the earliest identified toxic mechanisms[64], but is not a sufficient factor since salicylic acid also breaks the mucosal barrier without possessing the ulcerogenic properties of aspirin. However, once PG synthesis is inhibited, enhanced permeability possibly contributes to mucosal injury.

TOPICAL TOXICITY

Local actions, not dependent upon inhibition of PG synthesis, may occur because weakly acidic NSAIDs become ionized and trapped in the mucosa at high concentrations. There have actually been few demonstrations that this theoretical phenomenon occurs, although it has been demonstrated for aspirin and sodium salicylate[65]. Non PG-dependent properties that may come into play at relatively high concentrations include a direct effect on enzyme activity, uncoupling of oxidative phosphorylation and inhibition of fatty acid metabolism[66–68]. The contribution of these effects of NSAIDs – together with their relationship to the concept of breaking of the gastric mucosal barrier – are controversial, but the fact that aspirin is clearly much more toxic than salicylic acid implies a pre-eminent role for inhibition of PG synthesis. In addition, many observations show, for doses which have equivalent bio-availability, that the gastroduodenal toxicity of NSAIDs in humans is not significantly abrogated by systemic or remote administration[69].

INFLAMMATORY RESPONSES

Animal data suggest that neutrophils are important in initiating NSAID damage[70,71]. In humans however, there is seldom an excess of neutrophils in the mucosa in the absence of *H. pylori* infection. It may be that there is a species difference or that human studies concern a later consequence of NSAID-associated injury.

PROLIFERATION AND APOPTOSIS

Both proliferation and apoptosis are probably influenced by NSAIDs[67–78]. The results from different investigators vary and it can be difficult to distinguish cause and consequence. In animal studies, both mucosal erosion and mucosal hyperplasia have been reported[75,76]. Clinically, hyperplasia may be relevant to Type C gastritis which is characterized by epithelial, endothelial and myofibrillar hyperplasia[79].

MOTILITY

NSAIDs have been associated with altered gastroduodenal motility[80], although a consistent pattern has not emerged. It is possible that impaired antral emptying and consequent biliary reflux may contribute to the changes seen in type C gastritis, which are also seen in patients not using NSAIDs who have primary or secondary bile acid reflux.

(iii) Effect on healing mechanisms

ACUTE RESTITUTION

As well as promoting mucosal injury, NSAIDs also inhibit the healing of ulcers[81,82] although the mechanisms are much less well understood. Within minutes of GI mucosal injury, a restitutive process dependent principally upon epithelial migration occurs to restore epithelial continuity[78]. Subepithelial myofibroblasts may play a critical role in this process[83] which is influenced by a large number of cytokines and growth factors. PG synthesis probably plays a minor role[83,84].

CHRONIC PROLIFERATION

Chronic administration of PGs[84] has been shown to enhance – and NSAIDs to inhibit – a proliferation of epithelial cells in gastric glands.

ANGIOGENESIS

NSAIDs are associated with reduced vascularity of ulcers and impairment of (possibly COX-2-dependent) angiogenic responses[72–74].

(iv) Effects on thromboxane

Aspirin is well known to produce a prolonged reduction of serum thromboxane, associated with interference with platelet function and increased bleeding time, via its irreversible acetylation of the platelet COX enzyme[48,57,85]. An effect of non-aspirin NSAIDs on thromboxane[86] and bleeding time[87] is also well recognized, although this has received less attention and may play an important role when patients present clinically with bleeding peptic ulcers[87]. With interest in possible differences between COX-2 inhibitors and non-selective NSAIDs in their effects on thrombotic processes, there is a growing awareness that non-aspirin NSAIDs may differ significantly in their ability to inhibit platelet thromboxane across their whole dosing period. In one study, the geometric mean percentage inhibition from baseline over 5 days was: 7.1% with placebo and 94.2% with naproxen (1 g day^{-1}) treatment, respectively[57]. Inhibition of thromboxane synthesis and platelet function may therefore also contribute when patients taking non-aspirin NSAIDs present clinically with bleeding peptic ulcers.

Manifestations of gastroduodenal NSAID injury

(i) Acute mucosal injury

ASPIRIN

Ingestion of 600 mg of aspirin is followed in nearly all subjects by the development of intragastric petechiae and erosions within an hour or so[58]. With ingestion of aspirin 1.8–2.4 g day^{-1} over a few days, subjects would typically have about ten intragastric erosions. The effects of aspirin appear to be dose-dependent, and only 30–40% of subjects taking aspirin 75 mg have erosions acutely[86].

ADAPTATION

With continued ingestion of aspirin or, probably, other NSAIDs over several weeks, the number of erosions may diminish by some process of adaptation[88–92]. The extent of adaptation may depend upon the dosing interval in relation to drug elimination half-life[92].

NON-ASPIRIN NSAIDS

The onset of mucosal injury with non-aspirin NSAIDs tends to be slower. Dose dependence is much less well established. A number of authors have reported that erosions were diminished by a process of adaptation similar to that observed with aspirin, though this is less well established[91,92].

RISK FACTORS

The patient-associated risk factors for acute mucosal injury are not well understood. A number of studies show more mucosal injury in those infected with *H. pylori*[93,94]. However, this appears to be because in positive studies, *H. pylori* causes baseline injury rather than enhancing the effect of NSAIDs. Older patients do not appear more vulnerable to aspirin-induced injury than younger patients[95,96].

(ii) Ulceration

With continued ingestion, excavated ulcers develop and are seen in the stomach and to a lesser extent in the duodenum of patients taking both aspirin and non-aspirin NSAIDs. It is clear that this arises in part because these drugs not only damage the mucosa but also retard ulcer healing[12,13]. There is some evidence that progression from superficial erosions to deep mucosal injury is an acid-peptic process[97].

(iii) Dyspepsia

In addition, NSAIDs not only mask ulcer pain, but commonly cause non-ulcer drug-related dyspepsia[98–100]. Whilst this is well recognized clinically, reports associating NSAID use with dyspepsia at a population level have varied in their assessment of the strength of association. This may be because a high level of initially experienced dyspepsia leads many susceptible patients to stop using NSAIDs.

The seeming paradox of (relatively) silent ulceration and enhanced drug-induced dyspepsia can be reconciled if it is assumed that non-aspirin NSAIDs would, like salicylic acid, cause even more dyspepsia, because of their irritant actions, if they did not inhibit PG synthesis. In addition, NSAID-associated dyspepsia is a poorly understood entity that may be heterogeneous, involving different mechanisms and causing symptoms that are different from typical ulcer pain.

(iv) Histological changes

Chronic NSAID use is commonly associated with antral changes described as type C gastritis[79]. Type C gastritis is characterized by epithelial, endothelial and muscular hyperplasia and is unfortunately named since an inflammatory component is absent. There is no evidence that type C gastritis causes clinically evident symptoms or pathology.

Risks of NSAID ulcer disease

(i) Endoscopic studies of patients

Many cross-sectional studies of patients taking aspirin or non-aspirin NSAIDs have shown a very high prevalence of peptic ulceration, amounting to approximately one in five patients[101–104]. Whilst individual studies have varied, there is usually a predominance of gastric over duodenal ulcers. Clinical trials in which patients are screened for trial suitability have confirmed the high prevalence of ulcers in relatively unselected patients taking NSAIDs, and have also shown that ulcers can develop in a substantial number of patients given NSAIDs for periods of 1–6 months[104–113].

RISK FACTORS

Patients infected with *H. pylori* are more likely than those not infected to develop endoscopic ulcers when taking NSAIDs[114]. Amongst those who have had previous ulcers, this past history becomes a dominant influence: the effects of *H. pylori* are no longer seen[105–107].

Past history is exerted in a highly site specific manner so that those who have previous gastric ulcers are much more likely to have gastric than duodenal ulcers and vice versa[106,107,115,116]. One interesting observation to emerge from recent studies concerning COX-2 inhibitors (where a number of patients are taken off NSAIDs and placed either on a COX-2-selective inhibitor or placebo) is that the increased risk associated with previous ulceration appears to persist even in those who take placebo[116]. This cannot be explained adequately by *H. pylori* infection and may indicate that some NSAID users develop local mucosal injury and have a persisting ulcer risk once the NSAID is stopped. Given the opportunity represented by COX-2 inhibitors (see below) to take patients at high risk off NSAIDs, the possibility that NSAIDs can induce irreversible changes and that the risk may persist deserves further investigation.

During healing or prophylaxis of NSAID-associated ulcers, the influences of *H. pylori* and past history are further complicated by the specific effects of the healing or prophylactic agent and its particular interaction with them (see below)[106,107].

Mucosal erosions have generally been dismissed as of little intrinsic significance and value in clinical management, although there has been limited evidence. However, recent data have shown patients with mucosal erosions to be at increased risk of later ulcers (as well as subsequent erosions) compared with those without[116]. Other influences on endoscopically detected ulcers are less well established. Potential factors that have been reported as associated with NSAID-induced ulceration are smoking, male sex (duodenal lesions, apparently independent of *H. pylori* status), age and NSAID dose (particularly gastric ulcers)[117]. Although endoscopic ulceration is more common in elderly compared with younger patients, the differences are not so great as for ulcer complications[106,107,116,118,119] (see below). Interestingly, acute studies in healthy elderly volunteers have not found increased mucosal injury compared with younger volunteers[95,96] (even though it is possible that such patients have lower mucosal PG levels)[120].

(ii) Epidemiological studies of ulcer complications

A large industry confirming and re-confirming an association between NSAID use and ulcer complications has developed.

ABSOLUTE RISKS

In unselected populations, the excess rate of hospitalization has been estimated to lie between two and 20 per 1000 patient years[121-132]. Several estimates of the number of patients dying per annum as a result of NSAID ulcer complications have been made. In the USA these estimates have ranged between 5000 and 16500 deaths per annum. In the UK, the range lies between 200 and 3500, a recent paper estimating the risk as 2000 deaths per annum in the UK[132]. Higher estimates of risk seem unlikely since there are only approximately 4000 ulcer deaths per annum and relatively few misclassifications[133,134]. The attributable risk of ulcer complications probably lies between 25% and 35% for all NSAID users[127,135,136]. Assuming the attributable rate for complications and death is similar, these figures imply 1200 deaths per annum in the UK from non-aspirin NSAIDs. Comparable pro rata estimates have been made for the USA. Increasingly, use of low-dose aspirin for cardiovascular prophylaxis is an additional factor leading to ulcer bleeding[137,138].

RELATIVE RISKS

Numerous studies have suggested an approximately four-fold enhancement of the risk of ulcer bleeding, perforation and death in elderly patients taking non-aspirin NSAIDs[127,130,134-147]. These studies have also identified non-drug risk factors which synergize to place patients at particularly high risk. Well established risk factors include past history, age over 60 years, NSAID dose and concurrent use of corticosteroids or anticoagulants. It has also emerged that, at commonly used doses, NSAIDs vary fairly consistently in the strength of association between their use and ulcer complications. In particular, ibuprofen at doses of 1200 mg day^{-1} or less is associated with relatively low risks, whilst azapropazone and piroxicam are often associated with relatively high risks[147]. It is not clear how much these differences reflect differences in intrinsic drug toxicity or the effective drug dose.

RISK MODIFIERS: MAGNITUDE AND MECHANISMS

Duration of use. Early studies suggested risk was higher in the first 3 months of NSAID use[134,139] than later, but more recent studies have failed to support this[140].

Age. The risk of developing ulcers and their complications rises in older patients irrespective of NSAID use[148]. The association between old age and NSAID ulcer complications almost certainly arises because a higher background risk is magnified to an extent similar to that seen in younger patients rather than because the magnification itself is greater[148]. This is in line with endoscopic and bleeding studies that do not show old patients as a group are especially vulnerable to NSAIDs[95,96]. It seems more likely that old age acts as a marker for an increased likelihood of an ulcer diathesis.

Whatever the mechanism, age and NSAID use represents a potent mixture for NSAID-associated ulcer complications. In one study, patients over the age of 60 years who were not taking NSAIDs had a 3.7 (2.6–5.4)-fold increase in the risk of ulcer bleeding compared with younger patients[140]. The overall risk associated with NSAIDs was 4.7 (3.8–5.7). When these factors interacted together, old patients taking NSAIDs had a 13.2 (10.0–17.1) odds ratio for ulcer bleeding compared with younger patients not taking NSAIDs.

Past history. As with endoscopic studies, past history is a strong risk factor, whether or not patients take NSAIDs. Past history and NSAID use interact positively. One study has reported an odds ratio of 17.1 (10.0–29.6) for NSAID users with a past history compared with patients without either risk factor[140]. A growing number of observations also suggest that past history is site specific for ulcer complications as it is for endoscopic ulcers, implying that it is mediated via a local mucosal change that is exacerbated by NSAID use[117].

Mucosal erosions. One recent study has reported that the risk of later ulcer complications is apparently much higher in patients with erosions, compared with those with a clean mucosa[117]. More research is needed, but the conventional wisdom that erosions are clinically irrelevant may be misplaced.

NSAID dose. Many studies show that the risk of ulcer complications with NSAIDs is dose dependent[137,139–141,144,147] and that there appears not to be a ceiling for this effect. A dose-dependent effect on ulcer complications seems to apply to all NSAIDs that have been investigated. Relatively low toxicity NSAIDs, such as ibuprofen, are associated with more ulcer complications when used at higher doses.

Anticoagulants. NSAID users who are anticoagulated are at substantially increased risk of ulcer haemorrhage[146]. This presumably occurs because anti-aggregatory and anticoagulant actions have an enhanced anti-haemostatic effect.

Corticosteroids. There is a long running debate as to whether corticosteroids are ulcerogenic or not. A breakthrough in the early 1990s was the observation that most corticosteroid-associated risks could be attributed to an enhancement of risks in patients who were also taking NSAIDs[145]. In one study, the relative risk of ulcer haemorrhage was 4.4 in NSAID users who were not taking corticosteroids and 14.6 in those who were[145]. Corticosteroids on their own did not enhance risk. Unfortunately, this topic remains controversial. One study has failed to show an interaction between corticosteroids and

NSAIDs, whilst another has recently supported the view that corticosteroids themselves may still be associated with enhanced risks of ulcer complication, even in the absence of NSAID use[143,144].

Individual NSAIDs. Ibuprofen at doses of 1200 mg day^{-1} or less has consistently been associated with fewer ulcer complications than other NSAIDs[147] (Figure 1). It also appears that some NSAIDs such as azapropazone or piroxicam are associated with greater than average risks. These differences may in part be associated with differences in effective dose but the factors such as short half-life or differences in pK_a may also contribute[149].

Helicobacter pylori. Whether *Helicobacter pylori* enhances NSAID risk has been hotly debated. It seems plausible that it would do so by a mechanism of 'double trouble', particularly in the light of endoscopic studies showing increased levels of ulceration in those who start to take NSAIDs when they are *H. pylori* positive[114]. However, its effects on PG synthesis are opposite to those of NSAIDs[150], and acid-suppressing drugs are more effective in *H. pylori* positive patients[151]. It is thus theoretically possible that risks could be un-enhanced or even abrogated, under some circumstances.

In fact, of several epidemiological studies to investigate whether *H. pylori* enhances the risk of NSAID-associated ulcer complications, one has shown a slight enhancement of risk[152], three have shown no effect[153–155] and three have reported a slight reduction in risk[137,156,157]. Whilst opinion may vary as to whether there is an effect of *H. pylori* on NSAID-associated risk or not,

Figure 1 Relative risks of ulcer complications with individual NSAIDs. Data are expressed relative to ibuprofen (which itself is increased approximately twofold at a dose of ≤1200 mg daily, compared with placebo). (Data derived from ref. 147 and reproduced by kind permission.)

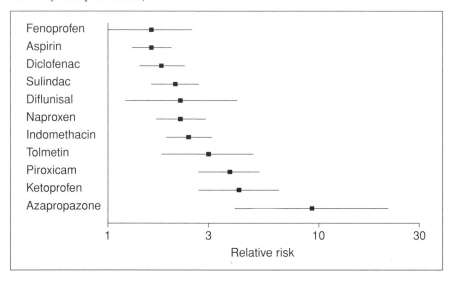

these studies have led most to conclude that any effect of *H. pylori* infection upon NSAID-associated risk in patients not taking anti-ulcer treatment is at most limited.

Occult aspirin use. Where over-the-counter use of aspirin is common, this appears to be a factor that enhances the risk of presentation with ulcer complications. It may also be important in patients with ulcers that are resistant to healing[158].

Paracetamol. Whether the analgesic drug paracetamol might also cause ulcer complications is currently controversial. Previous studies have shown an increased risk of ulcer complications in patients taking paracetamol but this was attributed to selective use of paracetamol[159] in higher risk patients or spontaneous use in response to dyspeptic symptoms[160]. A recent study suggests there may be a dose-dependent increase in ulcer complications with paracetamol implying a causal effect (L. García Rodriguez, personal communication).

Treatment and prevention
(i) Targets for therapy
Understanding the way in which NSAIDs affect the gastric mucosa and their interaction with epidemiological factors suggest a number of obvious targets for treatment.

PROSTAGLANDIN REPLACEMENT
Replacement of depleted endogenous gastric mucosal PGs from an exogenous source is an obvious strategy that has resulted in the development of the PGE_1 derivative misoprostol.

ACID SUPPRESSION
Acid causes NSAID-induced mucosal erosions to deepen and become ulcers suggesting that acid suppression would be an effective strategy. However, animal studies would predict a lesser effect on acute erosions than on ulcers and a need for sustained elevation of intragastric pH to 4 or above.

ENTERIC COATING
The fact that some NSAIDs have a strong topical component to their mucosal injury would suggest enteric coating might be beneficial, at least in those NSAIDs where this is a dominant mechanism compared with systemic inhibition of PG synthesis.

H. PYLORI ERADICATION
Mechanistic and clinical/epidemiological observations suggest that this may be a less effective strategy, at least in those with established ulcers.

(ii) Management of established NSAID ulcers

Several studies suggest that NSAIDs retard active healing of ulcers, at least with H_2 antagonists[81,82]. In general, where possible, stopping the NSAID is regarded as a responsible approach in those who present with NSAID ulcers clinically.

HEALING WITH MISOPROSTOL

There are relatively few data on the ability of misoprostol to heal NSAID-associated ulcers[107,152]. They suggest that misoprostol can heal ulcers, though less well than it heals erosions and less well than can be achieved with proton pump inhibitors[107] (Figure 2).

Figure 2 Studies comparing healing of gastric and duodenal ulcers and gastroduodenal erosions with omeprazole and misoprostol (OMNIUM study) or omeprazole and ranitidine (ASTRONAUT study). (Reproduced from refs 106 and 107, with permission.)

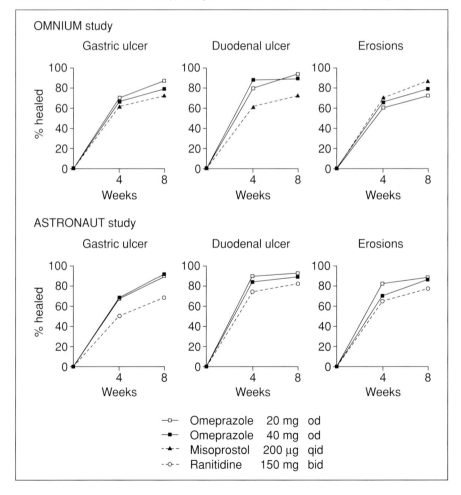

H_2 ANTAGONISTS

Whilst normal doses of H_2 antagonists can cause healing of peptic ulcers whilst NSAIDs are continued, this is retarded both for gastric and duodenal ulcers compared with the healing rate seen if NSAIDs are stopped[107,161]. It is not known whether this retardation can be overcome by use of higher doses of H_2 antagonist, although one small study suggests that this is possible[105], and pro-phylactic efficacy is greater at higher doses[162].

PROTON PUMP INHIBITORS

Several studies show that proton pump inhibitors are effective agents for healing of both gastric and duodenal ulcers[106,107,163–165]. Comparative studies suggest that they are more effective than misoprostol for healing of duodenal ulcers and more effective than standard doses of ranitidine for healing of both gastric and duodenal ulcers (Figure 3). Interestingly, in view of the different effects of PGs and acid suppression in animal studies, they appear to be less effective than misoprostol in healing acute superficial erosive injury occurring in the absence of ulceration.

OTHER AGENTS

Acute volunteer studies have shown some beneficial effects of both sucralfate and bismuth based compounds[166,167], but there are no data as to whether these translate into a favourable effect on NSAID-associated ulcer healing.

H. PYLORI ERADICATION

The effect of *H. pylori* eradication on ulcer healing with proton pump inhibitors has been investigated in three studies[108,154,155]. In all of these studies, *H. pylori* eradication had no demonstrable beneficial effect. In fact, in all three studies ulcer healing was retarded in those receiving eradication therapy, although this was only significant in one study[108]. Similarly, for both ranitidine and omeprazole, healing of gastric ulcers was significantly faster for individuals who were naturally *H. pylori* infected compared with uninfected individuals[106,107]. This difference was seen neither for healing with misoprostol[107], where, if anything, there was an opposite influence, nor for healing of duodenal ulcers (with any agent).

HEALING OF ASPIRIN-INDUCED ULCERS

There have been few studies of the healing of ulcers in patients who continue to take aspirin and none so far specifically investigating ulcer healing in patients taking low (cardiovascular) doses of aspirin. Roth and his colleagues studied 239 patients with active rheumatoid arthritis in whom treatment with aspirin 3.9 g daily was associated with ulceration or lesser degrees of mucosal damage[161]. In patients receiving misoprostol 200 µg q.d.s., 68% of gastro-duodenal ulcers healed by 8 weeks compared with 26% of those given

Figure 3 Studies comparing omeprazole 20 mg with misoprostol 200 μg b.i.d. (OMNIUM study), ranitidine 150 mg b.i.d. (ASTRONAUT study) or placebo (SCUR and OPPULENT studies), as prophylaxis against a combined end-point of development of an ulcer or >10 erosions or moderate or severe dyspepsia. The end-point for SCUR and OPPULENT studies was a simple development of an ulcer. (Reproduced with permission from ref. 238.)

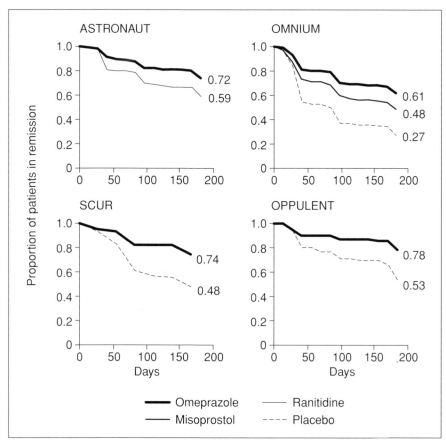

placebo. However, misoprostol was far from perfect in preventing gastric ulcers since new ulcers developed in those receiving both misoprostol and placebo.

PROGNOSTIC FACTORS FOR HEALING OF NSAID-ASSOCIATED ULCERS
In patients who continue to take NSAIDs, healing takes longer with gastric than duodenal ulcers[106]. Large gastric ulcers take longer to heal than small ones, whilst healing by acid suppression is faster in patients who are *H. pylori* positive than negative. In comparative studies, healing of gastric ulcers by omeprazole was faster than by ranitidine[108]. Healing of duodenal ulcers by

omeprazole was faster than by misoprostol. Conversely, healing of erosions without ulcers by misoprostol was faster than by omeprazole[107]. Lansoprazole (15 mg and 30 mg o.d.) was more effective than ranitidine (150 mg b.i.d.) for gastric ulcer healing[165].

(iii) Prophylactic measures

Until the advent of COX-2 inhibitors, management of patients at high risk of NSAID complications involved stopping the NSAID and/or co-prescription of a prophylactic anti-ulcer drug[168]. Conceptually, management might differ for those who have had a proven ulcer (secondary prophylaxis/ maintenance) compared with those who have not (primary prophylaxis). However, relatively little attention has been paid to this issue. A recent meta-analysis identified 34 randomized controlled trials that qualified for a systematic analysis[169].

MISOPROSTOL

Nearly all studies have investigated primary prophylaxis[168–172]. Misoprostol significantly reduced the risk of patients developing endoscopic ulcers and this was dose-dependent for gastric (though not duodenal) ulcers, with miso-prostol 800 μg day^{-1} being superior to 400 μg day^{-1} (L. García Rodriguez, personal communication). In a direct comparative study as well as a meta-analysis, misoprostol was more effective than ranitidine in preventing NSAID-associated gastric ulcers[169]. In a maintenance study comparing misoprostol with omeprazole, misoprostol was less effective than omeprazole against a composite end-point of no ulcer, five erosions and no more than mild dys-pepsia[107] (Figure 3). When the individual mode of relapse was investigated, duodenal ulcers and dyspepsia were more common with misoprostol whilst gastric ulcers were more common with omeprazole, especially in H. pylori negative individuals.

OUTCOME STUDIES

Misoprostol was investigated in a large outcome study, the MUCOSA study[173]. In this study, 8842 patients were randomized to receive misoprostol 600 to 800 μg daily or placebo. Over 6 months, treatment with misoprostol was associated with a 40% reduction in serious GI complications compared with placebo. In this study, those with a past history had a higher level of ulcer complications than those without but the protective effects of misoprostol we had also seen in these patients. Conversely, when misoprostol 400 μg daily was used as maintenance prophylaxis in patients receiving naproxen (0.5–1.0 g daily), there was a high rate of recurrent gastric ulcer bleeding (20%) over 6 months in H. pylori negative patients versus 9% with nabumetone (1.0–1.5 g daily) with no co-prophylaxis[174,175].

ADVERSE EFFECTS

Unfortunately, misoprostol has a high rate of adverse effects, principally abdominal pain and diarrhoea[176,177]. These appear to be dose-related, like the therapeutic benefits of misoprostol.

H_2 ANTAGONISTS

Ten trials have investigated the ability of standard doses of H_2 receptor antagonists to prevent endoscopic ulcers over 1 to 3 months or longer[104,162,169]. These studies show that H_2 antagonists could effectively reduce the likelihood of duodenal ulcer development by two thirds to three quarters but had no significant effect on the risk of developing gastric ulcers. In contrast, when the dose of H_2 antagonist was doubled there was a significant reduction in the risk of both duodenal and gastric ulcers. There have been no outcome studies of the effect of H_2 antagonists on development of ulcer complications in patients taking NSAIDs. Thus, although H_2 antagonists are popular because they are well tolerated and reduce NSAID-associated dyspepsia, they are of unproven efficacy, particularly for prevention of gastric ulcers. Indeed, there is a possibility that, by masking symptoms but not preventing ulcers, there may be an increased risk of ulcer bleeding in patients taking these drugs[177].

PROTON PUMP INHIBITORS

Five large studies have investigated the ability of proton pump inhibitors (omeprazole or lansoprazole) to prevent ulcer development in patients taking NSAIDs or reduce the chances of relapse after healing[106,107,109,110,169,178]. In these studies, proton pump inhibitors significantly reduce the risk of both gastric and duodenal ulcers. This ability was seen in both a primary[109] and secondary[106,107,110,178] prophylaxis setting. Comparative studies suggested that omeprazole was superior to ranitidine as maintenance treatment (Figure 3). Compared with misoprostol, it altered the pattern of relapse and was more effective in preventing duodenal ulcers and dyspepsia than gastric ulcers, and in preventing relapse of *H. pylori* positive than negative patients[107].

OUTCOME STUDIES

Primary prophylaxis with omeprazole against ulcer complications has not been investigated. When used as secondary prophylaxis in *H. pylori* positive patients who have presented with bleeding gastric ulcers, omeprazole appeared to be highly effective in preventing subsequent ulcer bleeding over 6 months. This was seen in 2% of the patients taking omeprazole compared with 20% of patients who underwent *H. pylori* eradication and have no protective co-prescription[179].

OTHER ANTI-ULCER DRUGS
There is no body of evidence supporting use of other anti-ulcer drugs for prophylaxis.

H. PYLORI ERADICATION
One study has reported that eradication of *H. pylori* with a bismuth based regime reduces the risk of gastric ulcer in patients starting naproxen 750 mg b.i.d. from 26% to 3%[113]. This was an interesting study since the patients selected were unlikely to have had previous ulcer disease. In contrast, a study of patients in whom previous ulcer disease and/or moderate or severe dyspepsia had been objectively established prior to trial entry, *H. pylori* eradication alone had no effect on the risk of relapse[108]. There have been no long-term studies of the effect of combining *H. pylori* eradication with anti-ulcer prophylaxis but, amongst those naturally infected, there is some evidence that acid suppression is more rather than less effective[106,107].

PROGNOSTIC FACTORS DURING MAINTENANCE TREATMENT
Site-specific injury is the dominant influence on relapse[106]. Having an ulcer doubles the chances of getting one again – most ulcers replicate the site (body versus antrum versus duodenum) of the initial lesion. An ulcer that took a long time to heal initially is more likely to relapse, and there is some evidence that relapse is higher in smokers than non-smokers. As with healing, there is an interaction between *H. pylori* and the prophylactic agent used. Proton pump inhibitors are more effective at maintaining remission in *H. pylori* positive than negative patients, whilst the converse tends to be true for miso-prostol (at least for gastric ulcers).

(iv) The problem of low dose aspirin
Although aspirin has an immediate and reproducible effect in inducing acute gastroduodenal damage, it was widely expected that the low doses that are used for prophylaxis of cardiovascular disease would have little or no effect on ulcer risks. This has turned out not to be the case[180,181]. One study reported that low-dose aspirin approximately doubled risk at 75 mg, trebled it at 150 mg and quadrupled it at 300 mg[181]. The relative contribution of aspirin as an anti-haemostatic or ulcerogenic agent is not clear. Since the former properties are maximal by 75 mg daily[182], the increased risk of ulcer compli-cations with higher doses of aspirin imply a contribution of its ulcerogenic effects, at least at higher prophylactic doses. These relationships also stress that restriction of dose to 75–82.5 mg daily would reduce the risks of ulcer bleeding with aspirin. This is important because ulcer bleeding from use of aspirin for cardiovascular prophylaxis has become an important public health issue, with some studies associating more ulcer bleeding with low dose aspirin than with all non-aspirin NSAIDs[137].

RISK FACTORS

Risk factors for ulcer bleeding with low dose aspirin are only now starting to be defined. They appear to be similar to risks for non-aspirin NSAIDs, with an increase in patients with a past history[183]. The relationship with *H. pylori* may be less complex than for non-aspirin NSAIDs[184], with both factors together tending to increase risk compared with either alone.

PROPHYLACTIC MEASURES

Prophylactic strategies for prevention of ulcer complications with low dose aspirin are not fully developed. Measures that have proved successful in preventing ulcers associated with non-aspirin NSAIDs, such as proton pump inhibitors or misoprostol, have also been shown to prevent short-term injury with aspirin[185,186]. Both misoprostol and proton pump inhibitors have been quite effective, whilst H_2 antagonists seemed less so. Doses of prophylactic agents for prevention of low dose aspirin injury may be different than for high dose injury. Thus one volunteer study suggests that misoprostol 100 μg daily was able to prevent mucosal injury from aspirin 300 mg daily over 28 days[186]. However longer term patient-based trials are needed, and the possibility that haemostasis rather than ulceration is at least in part a target should be considered.

SMALL BOWEL DAMAGE

Small intestinal injury by NSAIDs, though less investigated than gastroduodenal injury, undoubtedly occurs in many patients[9–15,187–198]. It contributes to clinically significant morbidity and mortality, although the extent of the problem is less well defined than for gastroduodenal ulcer disease.

Pathogenesis

Animal studies suggest that there may be a topical component to NSAID enteropathy, since it is seen with NSAIDs that undergo enterohepatic circulation and can be prevented by interrupting this. Injury is focused on the terminal ileum where compounds that undergo enterohepatic circulation are reabsorbed[199]. As in the stomach, this leads to enhanced permeability[200], possibly because of high mucosal concentrations. Secondary infection contributes substantially to injury, and antibiotics can ameliorate it[199].

Observational studies in humans suggest that similar mechanisms may be at play. NSAIDs that undergo enterohepatic circulation reliably abrogate intestinal barrier function, causing increased permeability to tracer molecules and resulting in increased influx of neutrophils to the intestinal mucosa with subsequent loss into the lumen[189,190].

Clinical presentation

Approximately 10% of patients taking NSAIDs who undergo enteroscopy have small intestinal ulcers[187]. These are generally relatively small and superficial. Similar observations come from postmortem examination of NSAID users dying for other reasons[188]. It should also be stressed that their distribution throughout the jejunum and ileum is quite different from that seen in animal studies where deep ileal ulceration is associated with local perforation, sepsis and death.

A number of patients develop more serious ileal lesions that all closely reflect animal disease. There are a number of case reports, most/all involving NSAIDs that undergo enterohepatic circulation, of deeper ileal ulceration[13], associated with intense neutrophil accumulation[14]. Several epidemiological studies show that NSAID use is associated with an increased risk of perforation of both the small and large bowel, including pre-existing lesions such as diverticula[21,196]. Finally, some patients taking NSAIDs develop valve-like intestinal strictures which can cause obstruction, which may require surgery and have a mortality[194,198].

It seems likely that lower level NSAID enteropathy contributes to ill health. There is evidence that these patients have a protein-losing enteropathy and microbleeding. Misoprostol increases haemoglobin in such patients, implying that significant blood loss contributes to anaemia[201]. Whether hypoalbuminaemia can be reversed by protective effects against NSAID enteropathy is not known.

Treatment

This is a poorly investigated area. The observation that misoprostol can lead to a rise in haemoglobin supports a protective effect. There is also some short-term evidence that sulphasalazine can protect against NSAID enteropathy[202]. However, there is a need for studies that investigate clinically important endpoints on a systematic rigorous basis.

COLONIC DISEASE

NSAIDs have been shown to inhibit eicosanoid synthesis[203], increase colonic permeability[16], cause isolated colonic ulcers[20] and possibly induce relapse of inflammatory bowel disease[17–19,194].

Pathogenesis

In animal studies, colonic disease with NSAIDs is rare and much less florid than ileal disease. NSAIDs reduce colon PG production and limited evidence suggests that they enhance permeability[16,203].

Clinical presentation

COLONIC ULCERATION

There are sporadic reports of colonic ulcers in patients using NSAIDs[20,195]. They are sufficient to establish that this is a relatively rare complication and insufficient to establish whether they are clinically significant.

COLONIC PERFORATION

As with small bowel disease, epidemiological studies report an increased incidence of colonic perforation, for example through diverticula[21].

RELAPSE OF ULCERATIVE COLITIS

Several epidemiological studies associate use of analgesic drugs with relapse of ulcerative colitis[17,19,204,205]. The first such study amalgamated NSAIDs and paracetamol for the purposes of analysis[17]. Amongst individual drugs it was only paracetamol that showed a significant association with relapse. Nevertheless, on the basis of suspicion and informal clinical evaluation, most gastroenterologists have been convinced that a subgroup of patients exists who have an increased tendency to relapse when they take NSAIDs. Several epidemiological studies have suggested this is a true association, though estimates of risk have varied substantially. A very recent epidemiological study, however, again associated use of paracetamol rather than NSAIDs with relapse of ulcerative colitis[204].

This is, therefore, an uncertain area and the issues that need to be resolved are whether analgesic drug use occurs in response to early symptoms of relapse and is just a marker for it and what the relative risks of paracetamol and NSAIDs are. In contrast to ulcerative colitis, there are few data associating relapse of Crohn's disease with NSAID use, although studies are also fewer.

THE PROMISE OF COX-2 INHIBITORS

For many years the principle of no therapeutic gain without adverse event pain, based upon the belief that there was only one cyclooxygenase enzyme, persisted[206]. The discovery of a second inducible cyclooxygenase, COX-2, represented an appealing target for drug development that has progressed from initial discovery to validation in large outcomes studies[207,208] in the remarkably short period of 9 years. Compared with anti-ulcer prophylaxis, substitution of a COX-2 inhibitor for a non-selective NSAID has the potential to reduce injury to the lower GI tract as well as the stomach and duodenum.

Currently there are two available tricyclic compounds[209,210] developed specifically to inhibit COX-2 selectively, as a result of binding within the COX-2 pocket[211]. A number of existing drugs that are structurally different, and/or may act in a different manner, have selectivity for COX-2[212-218].

Biochemical effects

(i) Assessing selectivity

A consensus has not emerged on a single method to compare individual drug selectivity. Selectivity ratios in recombinant enzyme assays tend to be much higher than they are in whole-blood assays[206]. One large comparative study using a modified whole-blood COX-2 assay reported a selectivity ratio of 75 for rofecoxib[218]. Celecoxib, etodolac, meloxicam and nimesulide showed a lower degree of selectivity. These studies are complemented by *ex vivo* assessments that show that even high doses of rofecoxib have no effect on thromboxane synthesis[219]. There is little or no effect of celecoxib on thromboxane synthesis[220]. Relatively high doses of meloxicam and nimesulide caused some inhibition of thromboxane formation[85,221].

(ii) Gastric prostaglandins

In two studies, rofecoxib 25 and 50 mg daily over 7 days has been shown not to inhibit human gastric mucosal PG synthesis[57,59], in contrast to a 70% reduction with naproxen 500 mg b.i.d., based upon *ex vivo* vortex assay. Similar data have not been published for celecoxib.

Meloxicam has been reported not to affect gastric PG synthesis[213] although the authors raised questions about the validity of their method. Etodolac and nimesulide also had little effect on PG synthesis, although a vortex method was not used and there were relatively high PG levels[214-216].

(iii) Acute mucosal injury

When given to volunteers for 7 days, a very high daily dose of rofecoxib (250 mg daily) only caused erosions in 12% of subjects (compared with 8% with placebo, 83% with ibuprofen and over 90% with aspirin[222]). Likewise, celecoxib at doses up to 400 mg day^{-1} did not significantly enhance acute injury, whilst naproxen did[223].

Meloxicam 7.5 mg causes less acute mucosal injury than piroxicam, although 15 mg causes more than 7.5 mg[212]. In acute studies, nimesulide and etodolac caused less injury than diclofenac or naproxen[215,217,224].

(iv) Endoscopy studies in patients

Both rofecoxib[225,226] and celecoxib[227,228] have been subject to an extensive programme of evaluation in endoscopy studies lasting up to 6 months. When compared directly with placebo, these drugs have shown no increase in the incidence of ulcers (Figure 4). With one exception, all studies have shown a substantial 50–80% reduction in ulcers compared with NSAID comparators. Patients with mucosal erosions at baseline and those with a past history of ulcer disease were at increased risk of ulcer development. This is also seen in patients given placebo and was not further magnified by drug use.

Meloxicam, nimesulide and etodolac have not been systematically

Figure 4 Cumulative ulcer incidence with placebo, ibuprofen, rofecoxib (25 mg and 50 mg); combined data from two identical studies that enrolled 1516 patients. The 12-week ulcer rates on rofecoxib 25 mg were statistically equivalent to placebo and those on rofecoxib 50 mg were not significantly different from placebo. The reduction in ulceration compared with ibuprofen, with rofecoxib was highly significant. (Reproduced from ref. 226, with permission.) Similar reductions compared with non-selective NSAIDs have also been reported for celecoxib.

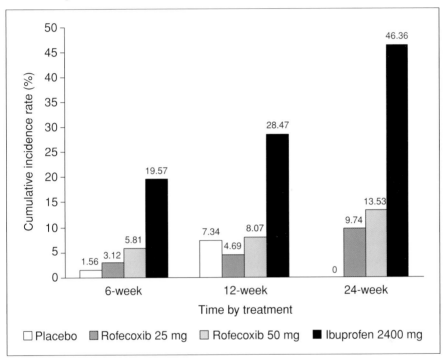

investigated in large perspective endoscopic studies in patients to the same extent as the coxibs.

(v) Effects on ulcer complications

For rofecoxib and celecoxib, endoscopic studies were not sufficient to persuade regulatory authorities to alter traditional NSAID warning labels. Accordingly, the effects of both rofecoxib and celecoxib on ulcer complications have been evaluated. This has been achieved both by a structured analysis of clinically important events – perforations, ulcers, obstructions and bleeds (PUBs) – occurring during phase IIb–III studies[229–231], as well as larger prospective studies specifically designed to investigate the hypothesis that clinically significant ulcers would be reduced by COX-2 inhibitors compared with non-selective NSAIDs[207,208].

Phase IIb–III studies. In studies covering 1428 patient years of exposure, rofecoxib was reported to result in a diminution by 51% in the number of patients presenting with perforations, ulcers and bleeds compared with comparator NSAIDs (ibuprofen 2.4 g daily, diclofenac 150 mg daily, nabumetone 1.5 g daily)[230]. Similarly, in 1020 patient years of celecoxib use (25–400 mg b.i.d.), there were only two perforations, obstructions and bleeds compared with nine with comparator NSAIDs in 535 patient years[231]. Because of differences in end-points, results with rofecoxib and celecoxib cannot be compared directly.

Outcome studies. Recently two large outcome studies have been completed in which the incidence of clinically significant or complicated upper GI ulcers/events in patients taking rofecoxib[207] or celecoxib[208] were compared with naproxen, ibuprofen or diclofenac (Table 1). To achieve sufficient power, these studies each randomized 8000 patients, as shown in Table 1, and followed them for an average of 9 months.

In the VIGOR[207] study, there was a 54% reduction in all confirmed clinical events, 57% in complicated events and 62% in all ulcer bleeds (upper and lower intestinal). In this study, the five commonest symptomatic adverse events were upper gastrointestinal and there was a significant reduction with rofecoxib compared with naproxen.

In the CLASS[208] study of celecoxib versus ibuprofen or diclofenac, patients were, by contrast with the VIGOR study, allowed to take aspirin at cardiovascular protective doses. An unexpectedly large number of such patients (21%) took aspirin in this study. In all patients (including those taking aspirin), there was a reduction in all ulcers (from 3.54% to 2.08% per annum) and in complicated ulcers (the primary end-point), although the latter did not

Table 1 Comparison of the VIGOR and CLASS outcome studies. These comparisons are based on oral presentations and may not be complete

VIGOR	*Rofecoxib 50 mg o.d.*	*CLASS Celecoxib 400 mg b.i.d.*
Patients	8076 RA	~7980 OA (72%) + RA
Aspirin allowed	no	yes
NSAIDs	Naproxen 1 g	Diclofenac 150 mg Ibuprofen 2.4 g
Duration (months)	9.2 (13)	~9 (13)
Primary end-point	Clinically significant UGI events	Complicated ulcers
Secondary end-point	Complicated events	Clinically significant ulcers
Analysis	ITT (life table)	Crude, censored (3 days–6 months)

achieve statistical significance (1.54% to 0.76%, $P = 0.09$). When patients taking low dose aspirin were excluded, differences were larger and all significant. Importantly, amongst those taking low dose aspirin there were no differences between celecoxib and NSAIDs (2.01% versus 2.12% for complicated ulcers, 4.70% versus 6.0% for all ulcers).

CARDIOVASCULAR EVENTS

One of the early concerns was that a lack of the ability of non-selective NSAIDs to inhibit platelet COX-1 might lead to a higher risk of thrombotic cardiovascular disease compared with non-selective NSAIDs. Initial data were reassuring. Thus, in the phase IIb–III studies of rofecoxib, there was an apparent reduction rather than an increase in mortality from myocardial infarction compared with the non-selective NSAIDs ibuprofen, diclofenac and nabumetone[231]. More recently, in the VIGOR study, naproxen 1 g daily was associated with significantly fewer myocardial infarcts than rofecoxib 50 mg[207]. A similar difference between the coxib and non-selective NSAIDs was not seen in the CLASS study[208]. However the crude event rates for rofecoxib, celecoxib and non-selective NSAIDs other than naproxen were fairly similar across these two studies. It is possible that naproxen, because of its powerful prolonged inhibition of thromboxane synthesis[57] and platelet function discussed earlier, may differ from many non-selective NSAIDs in acting as an aspirin-like drug. More research is needed. If there are circumstances where the benefits of a COX-2 inhibitor on NSAID gastropathy are counterbalanced by comparatively adverse effects on thrombotic complications of vascular disease, it is likely that coadministration of aspirin (75 mg) would be a more appropriate choice than a non-selective NSAID[182].

GASTROINTESTINAL OUTCOMES WITH OTHER DRUGS

There have been no formal outcome studies of meloxicam, nimesulide or etodolac. In two large short-term studies of all adverse effects of meloxicam versus diclofenac or piroxicam, there appeared to be some reduction in admission for PUBs with meloxicam[118,119]. However, the studies were not set up to investigate this, or powered to detect it, and differences may have arisen by chance.

Future issues with COX-2 inhibitors. Recently, animal studies have suggested that inhibition of COX-1 and COX-2 appears to be necessary for development of gastroduodenal erosions in rats[232]. However this appears to be at variance with human experience so far. Because COX-2 is induced at the rim of ulcers[234] and in animal studies COX-2 inhibitors may retard ulcer healing[233,235], it is possible that the same will be seen in human studies. However, there are no reasons to believe that this will be any greater than the retardation known to occur with non-selective NSAIDs[81,82]. By the same criteria, it seems likely that there will be no inhibition of ulcer healing by proton pump inhibitors[82]. Likewise, COX-2 inhibitors could share the association seen between NSAIDs and relapse of inflammatory bowel disease[17-19], although this is not necessarily the case. It depends upon whether the effects of non-selective NSAIDs are to inhibit COX-1 during remission and thus induce relapse, or to inhibit COX-2, delay healing and thus cause relapse. A concern with regard to COX-2 inhibitors relates to non-GI effects, in particular their ability to cause salt and water retention[236,237] like non-selective NSAIDs.

SYNOPSIS

NSAIDs have effects throughout the GI tract and represent a major public health problem. By not inhibiting COX-1, COX-2 inhibitors spare GI mucosal PG synthesis and have less adverse toxic effects on the GI tract. However, patients with established vascular disease need aspirin to prevent its thrombotic complications and these patients may lose all or part of the GI safety advantage of COX-2 inhibitors, although this is currently an area of uncertainty.

Address all correspondence to: C. J. Hawkey, Division of Gastroenterology, Queen's Medical Centre, University Hospital Nottingham, Nottingham NG7 2UH, UK.

REFERENCES

1. Vane JR, Flower RJ, Botting RM. History of aspirin and its mechanism of action. *Stroke.* 1990;21;12–23.
2. Vane JR. Inhibition of prostaglandin synthesis as a mechanism of action for aspirin-like drugs. *Nature.* 1971;231:232–5.
3. Wallace JL, Bell CJ. Gastric mucosal defence. *Curr Opin Gastroenterol.* 1996;12:503–11.
4. Douthwaite AH, Lintott SAM. Gastroscopic observation of the effect of aspirin and certain other substances on the stomach. *Lancet.* 1938;2:1222–5.
5. Ferreira SH. Prostaglandins, aspirin-like drugs and analgesia. *Nature New Biol.* 1972;240:200–3.
6. Wolfe MM, Lichtenstein DR, Sing G. Gastrointestinal toxicity of non-steroidal anti-inflammatory drugs. *N Engl J Med.* 1999;340:1888–99.
7. Bjorkman D. Nonsteroidal anti-inflammatory drug-associated toxicity of the liver, lower gastrointestinal tract, and esophagus. *Am J Med.* 1998;105:17S–21S.
8. Mason JC. NSAIDs and the oesophagus. *Eur J Gastroenterol Hepatol.* 1999;11:369–73.
9. Bjarnason I, Hayllar J, MacPherson AJ, Russell AS. Side effects of non-steroidal anti-inflammatory drugs on the small and large intestine in humans. *Gastroenterology.* 1993;104:1832–47.
10. Schneider AR, Benz C, Riemann JF. Adverse effects of non-steroidal anti-inflammatory drugs on the small and large bowel. *Endoscopy.* 1999;31:761–7.

11. Aabakken L. Small-bowel side-effects of non-steroidal anti-inflammatory drugs. *Eur J Gastroenterol Hepatol.* 1999;11:383–8.

12. Morris AJ. Non-steroidal anti-inflammatory drug enteropathy. *Gastrointest Endosc Clin North America.* 1999;9:125–33.

13. Hudson N, Wilkinson MJ, Swannell AJ, Steele RJ, Hawkey CJ. Ileo-caecal ulceration associated with the use of diclofenac retard. *Aliment Pharmacol Ther.* 1993;7:197–200.

14. Sigthorsson G, Tibble J, Hayllar J, Menzies I, Macpherson A, Moots R et al. Intestinal permeability and inflammation in patients on NSAIDs. *Gut.* 1998;43:506–11.

15. Somasundaram S, Rafi S, Hayllar J, Sigthorsson G, Jacob M, Price AB et al. Mitochondrial damage: a possible mechanism of the 'topical' phase of NSAID induced injury to the rat intestine. *Gut.* 1997;41:344–53.

16. Jenkins AP, Trew DR, Crump BJ, Nukajam WS, Foley JA, Menzies IS et al. Do non-steroidal anti-inflammatory drugs increase colonic permeability? *Gut.* 1991;32:66–9.

17. Rampton DS, McNeil NI, Sarner M. Analgesic ingestion and other factors preceding relapse in ulcerative colitis. *Gut.* 1983;24:187–9.

18. Evans JM, McMahon AD, Murray FE, McDevitt DG, MacDonald TM. Non-steroidal anti-inflammatory drugs are associated with emergency admission to hospital for colitis due to inflammatory bowel disease. *Gut.* 1997;40:619–22.

19. Gleeson MH, Lim SH, Spencer D. Non-steroidal anti-inflammatory drugs, salicylates, and colitis [letter]. *Lancet.* 1996;347:904–5.

20. Stamm C, Burkhalter E, Pearce W, Larsen B, Willis M, Kikendall JW et al. Benign colonic ulcers associated with nonsteroidal antiinflammatory drugs ingestion. *Am J Gastroenterol.* 1994;89:2230–3.

21. Campbell K, Steele RJ. Use of anti-inflammatory drugs and complicated diverticular disease: a case-control study. *Br J Surgery.* 1991;78:190–1.

22. Heller SR, Fellows IW, Ogilvie AL, Atkinson M. Non steroidal anti inflammatory drugs and benign oesophageal stricture. *Br Med J.* 1982;285:167–8.

23. Tympner F. Gastroscopic findings after therapy with non-steroidal anti-rheumatic drugs. *Z Rheumatol.* 1981;40:179–81.

24. Semble EL, Wu WC, Castell DO. Non steroidal anti inflammatory drugs and oesophageal injury. *Semin Arthritis Rheum.* 1989;19:99–109.

25. Shallcross TM, Wyatt JI, Rathbone BJ, Heatley RV. Non steroidal anti inflammatory drugs, hiatus hernia and *Helicobacter pylori* in patients with oesophageal ulceration. *Br J Rheumatol.* 1990;29:288–90.

26. Purushotham AD, Gray GR, Hansell DT. Prostaglandins in the treatment of reflux oesophagitis: double-blind placebo controlled clinical trial. *J Roy Coll Surgeons Edinburgh.* 1991;36:216–8.

27. Bellary SV, Isaacs PET, Lee FI. Upper gastrointestinal lesions in elderly patients presenting for endoscopy: relevance of NSAID usage. *Am J Gastroenterol.* 1991;86:961–4.

28. Ecker GA, Karsh J. Naproxen induced ulcerative oesophagitis. *J Rheumatol.* 1992;19:646–7.

29. Matikainen M. Is there a relationship between the use of analgesics and non-steroidal anti-inflammatory drugs and acute upper gastrointestinal bleeding? A Finnish case control study. *Scand J Gastroenterol.* 1996;31:912–6.

30. El Serag HB, Sonnenberg A. Association of esophagitis and esophageal strictures

with diseases treated with non steroidal anti inflammatory drugs. *Am J Gastroenterol.* 1997;92;52–6.

31. Rourk RM, Namiot Z, Edmunds MC, Sarosiek J, Yu Z, McCallum RW. Diminished luminal release of esophageal epidermal growth factor in patients with reflux esophagitis. *Am J Gastroenterol.* 1994;89:1177–84.

32. Sarosiek J, Scheurich CJ, Marcinkiewicz M, McCallum RW. Enhancement of salivary esophagoprotection. Rationale for a physiological approach to gastro-esophageal reflux disease. *Gastroenterology.* 1996;110:675–81.

33. Sinar DR, Fletcher JR, Castell DO. Prostaglandin E_1 effects of resting and cholinergically stimulated lower esophageal sphincter pressure in cats. *Prostaglandins.* 1981;21:581–90.

34. Sinar DR, Cordovan CM, Fletcher JR, Castell DO. Decreased esophageal peristaltic amplitude in response to prostaglandin E_1 and prostacyclin in the baboon. *Dig Dis Sci.* 1982;27:1067–72.

35. Tottrup A, Forman A, Raundahl U, Andersson KE. Effects of prostanoids and indomethacin on isolated smooth muscle from the human lower oesophagus. *Pharmacol Toxiolol.* 1992;71:65–74.

36. Eastwood GL, Beck BD, Castell DO, Brown FC, Fletcher JR. Beneficial effect of indomethacin on acid induced esophagitis in cats. *Dig Dis Sci.* 1981;26:601–8.

37. Scheiman JM, Patel PM, Henson EK, Nostrant TT. Effect of naproxen on gastroesophageal function: A randomized double blind placebo controlled study. *Am J Gastroenterol.* 1995;90:754–7.

38. Kamikawa V, Shimo Y. Modulating effects of opiods, purine compounds, 5-hydroxytryptamine and prostaglandin E_2 on cholinergic neurotransmission in a guinea pig oesophagus preparation. *J Pharm Pharmacol.* 1982;34:794–7.

39. Northway MG, Libshitz HI, Osbourne BM, Feldman MS, Mamel JJ, West JH et al. Radiation esophagitis in the opossum: radioprotection with indomethacin. *Gastroenterology.* 1980;78;883–92.

40. Pillsbury HC III, Webster WP, Rosenman J. Prostaglandin inhibitor and radiotherapy in advanced head and neck cancers. *Arch Otolaryngol – Head & Neck Surg.* 1986;112:552–3.

41. Tochner Z, Barnes M, Mitchell JB, Orr K, Glatstein E, Russo A. Protection by indomethacin against acute radiation oesophagitis. *Digestion.* 1990;47:81–7.

42. Rubio CA. Further studies on the therapeutic effect of indomethacin on oesophageal tumours. *Cancer.* 1986;58;1029–31.

43. Morgan G. Beneficial effects of NSAIDs in the gastrointestinal tract. *Eur J Gastroenterol Hepatol.* 1999;11:393–400.

44. Stein BE, Schwartzman ML, Carroll MA, Rosenthal WA. Rabbit oesophagus metabolizes arachidonic acid predominantly via a lipoxygenase pathway. *Prostaglandin Leukotriene Essent Fatty Acid.* 1988;34:75–80.

45. Moussard C, Alber D, Henry JC. Profiles of eicosanoid production from 14C – arachidonic acid and prostaglandin metabolism by rabbit oesophageal mucosa and muscularis. *Prostaglandins Leukotrienes Med.* 1988;31:31–9.

46. Ottignon Y, Alber D, Moussard C, Deschamps JP, Carayon P, Henry JC. Oesophageal mucosal prostaglandin E_2 levels in health and in gastro-oesophageal reflux disease. *Prostaglandins Leukotrienes Med.* 1987;29:141–51.

47. Sarosiek J, McCallum RW. Esophago protection by prostaglandins: How far are we from reaching a verdict? *Am J Gastroenterol.* 1995;90:847–9.

48. Tihanyi K, Rozsa I, Banai J, Dobo I, Bajtai A. Tissue concentrations and correla-

tions of prostaglandins in healthy and inflamed human oesophageal and jejunal mucosa. *J Gastroenterol.* 1996;31:149–52.

49. Triadafilopoulos G, Kaczynska M, Iwane M. Esophageal mucosal eicosanoids in gastroesophageal reflux disease and Barrett's esophagus. *Am J Gastroenterol.* 1996;91:65–74.

50. Stein BE, Schwartzman ML, Carroll MA, Stahl RE, Rosenthal WS. Role of arachidonic acid metabolites in acid pepsin injury to rabbit esophagus. *Gastroenterology.* 1989;97:278–83.

51. Sarosiek J, Yu Z, Namiot Z, Rourk RM, Hetzel DP, McCallum RW. Impact of acid and pepsin on human esophageal prostaglandins. *Am J Gastroenterol.* 1994;89:588–94.

52. Sinar DR, Fletcher JR, Castell DO, The beneficial effect of methyl PGE$_2$ to diminish caustic esophageal injury. *Clin Res.* 1982;30:498A.

53. McGreevy JM, Moody FG. A mechanism for prostaglandin cytoprotection. *Br J Surg.* 1980;67:873–6.

54. Lanas AI, Sousa FL, Ortego J, Esteva F, Blas JM, Soria J et al. Aspirin renders the oesophageal mucosa more permeable to acid and pepsin. *Eur J Gastroenterol Hepatol.* 1995;11:1065–72.

55. Hawkey CJ, Swannell AJ, Yeomans ND, Langstrom G, Lofberg I, Taure E. Site specific ulcer relapse in non steroidal anti inflammatory drug (NSAID) users: improved prognosis with *H. pylori* and with omeprazole compared to misoprostol. *Gut.* 1996;39:A149.

56. Whittle BJ. Temporal relationship between cyclooxygenase inhibition, as measured by prostacyclin biosynthesis, and the gastrointestinal damage induced by indomethacin in the rat. *Gastroenterology.* 1981;80:94–8.

57. Wight NJ, Garlick N, Calder N, Dallob A, Gottesdiener K, Hawkey CJ. Evidence that the COX-2 specific inhibitor rofecoxib at 50 mg spares gastric mucosal prostaglandin synthesis in humans. *Gut.* 1999;45(Suppl.V);30.03.

58. Hawkey CJ, Hawthorne AB, Hudson N, Cole AT, Mahida YR, Daneshmend TK. Separation of aspirin's impairment of haemostasis from mucosal injury in the human stomach. *Clin Sci.* 1991; 81: 565–73.

59. Cryer B, Gottesdiener K, Gertz B, Wong P, Dallob A, Feldman M. *In vivo* effects of rofecoxib, a new cyclooxygenase (COX)-2 inhibitor, on gastric mucosal prostaglandin (PG) and serum thromboxane B$_2$ (TXB$_2$) synthesis in healthy humans. *Gastroenterology.* 1999;116:A141.

60. Laine L, Cominelli F, Sloane R, Casini-Raggi V, Marin-Sorensen M, Weinstein WM. Interaction of NSAIDs and *Helicobacter pylori* on gastrointestinal injury and prostaglandin production: a controlled double-blind trial. *Aliment Pharmacol Ther.* 1995;9:127–35.

61. Hawkey CJ, O'Morain C, Murray FE, McCarthy C, Tiernay D, Devane J. Two comparative endoscopic evaluations of naprelan. *Am J Orthopedics.* 1996;25(9S):30–6.

62. Cryer B, Feldman M. Effects of very low dose daily, long-term aspirin therapy on gastric, duodenal, and rectal prostaglandin levels and on mucosal injury in healthy humans. *Gastroenterology.* 1999;117:17–25.

63. Sutherland LR, Verhoef M, Wallace JL, Van Rosendaal G, Crutcher R, Meddings JB. A simple, non-invasive marker of gastric damage: sucrose permeability. *Lancet.* 1994;343:998–1000.

64. Davenport HW. Gastric mucosal injury by fatty acid and acetyl-salicylic acids. *Gastroenterology.* 1964;93:245–53.

65. Garner A. Mechanisms of action of aspirin on the gastric mucosa of the guinea pig. *Acta Physiol Scand Suppl.* 1978;103:101–10.
66. Smith MJH, Dawkins PD. Salicylates and enzymes. *J Pharm Pharmacol.* 1971;23:729–44.
67. Jorgensen TG, Weis-Fogh US, Nielsen HH, Olesen HP. Salicylate and aspirin-induced uncoupling of oxidative phosphorylation in mitochondria isolated from the mucosal membrane of the stomach. *Scand J Clin Lab Invest.* 1976;36:649–54.
68. Roediger WEW, Mollard S. Selective inhibition of fatty acid oxidation in colonocytes by ibuprofen: a cause of colitis? *Gut.* 1995;36:55–9.
69. Kelly JP, Kaufman DW, Jurgelon JM, Sheehan J, Koff RS, Shapiro S. Risk of aspirin associated major upper-gastrointestinal bleeding with enteric-coated or buffered product. *Lancet.* 1996;348:1413–6. Comment in: *Lancet.* 1996;348:1394–5.
70. Appleyard CB, McCafferty DM, Tigley AW, Swain MG, Wallace JL. Tumor necrosis factor mediation of NSAID-induced gastric damage: role of leukocyte adherence. *Am J Physiol.* 1996;270:G42–G48.
71. Levi S, Goodlad RA, Lee CY, Stamp G, Walport MG, Wright NA et al. Inhibitory effect of non-steroidal anti-inflammatory drugs on mucosal cell proliferation associated with gastric ulcer bleeding. *Lancet.* 1990;336:841–3.
72. Hudson N, Balsitis M, Everitt S, Hawkey CJ. Angiogenesis in gastric ulcers: impaired in patients taking non-steroidal anti-inflammatory drugs. *Gut.* 1995;37:191–4.
73. Hull MA, Brough JL, Hawkey CJ. Expression of cyclooxygenase-1 and -2 by human gastric endothelial cells. *Gut.* 1999;45:529–36.
74. Jones MK, Wang H, Peskar BM, Levin E, Itani RM, Sarfeh IJ et al. Inhibition of angiogenesis by nonsteroidal anti-inflammatory drugs: insight into mechanisms and implications for cancer growth and ulcer healing. *Nat Med.* 1999;5:1418–23.
75. Uribe A, Johansson C, Rubio C. Cell proliferation of the rat gastrointestinal mucosa after treatment with E_2 prostaglandins and indomethacin. *Digestion.* 1987;36:238–45.
76. Baumgartner A, Koelz HR, Halter F. Indomethacin and turnover of gastric mucosal cells in the rat. *Am J Physiol.* 1986;250:G830–5.
77. Zhu GH, Yang XL, Lai KC, Ching CK, Wong BC, Yuen St et al. Nonsteroidal antiiflammatory drugs could reverse *Helicobacter pylori*-induced apoptosis and proliferation in gastric epithelial cells. *Dig Dis Sci.* 1998;43:1957–63.
78. Lacy ER. Rapid epithelial restitution in the stomach: an updated perspective. *Scand J Gastroenterol.* 1995;210:6–8.
79. Voutilainen M, Sokka T, Juhola M, Farkkila M, Hannonen P. Nonsteroidal anti-inflammatory drug-associated upper gastrointestinal lesions in rheumatoid arthritis patients. Relationships to gastric histology, *Helicobacter pylori* infection, and other risk factors for peptic ulcer. *Scand J Gastroenterol.* 1998;33:811–16.
80. Bassotti G, Bucaneve G, Furno P, Morelli A, Del Favero A. Double-blind, placebo-controlled study on effects of diclofenac sodium and indomethacin on postprandial gastric motility in man. *Dig Dis Sci.* 1998;43:1172–6.
81. Lancaster-Smith MJ, Jaderberg ME, Jackson DA. Ranitidine in the treatment of non-steroidal anti-inflammatory drug-associated gastric and duodenal ulcers. *Gut.* 1991:32:252–5.
82. Walan A, Bader JP, Classen M, Lamers CB, Piper DW, Rutgersson K et al. Effect of omeprazole and ranitidine on ulcer healing and relapse rates in patients with benign gastric ulcer. *N Engl J Med.* 1989;320:69–75.

83. Beltinger J, McKaig BC, Makh S, Stack WA, Hawkey CJ, Mahida YR. Human colonic subepithelial myofibroblasts modulate transepithelial resistance and secretory response. *Am J Physiol.* 1999;277: C271–C279.

84. Hawkey CJ. Nonsteroidal anti-inflammatory drug gastropathy. *Gastroenterology.* 2000;119:521–35.

85. Patrignani P, Panara MR, Sciulli MG, Santini G, Renda G, Patrono C. Differential inhibition of human prostaglandin endoperoxide synthase-1 and -2 by nonsteroidal anti-inflammatory drugs. *J Physiol Pharmacol.* 1997;48:623–31.

86. Cole AT, Hudson N, Liew LCW, Murray FE, Hawkey CJ, Heptinstall S. Protection of human gastric mucosa against aspirin – enteric coating or dose reduction? *Aliment Pharmacol Ther.* 1999;13:187–93.

87. Day JP, Lanas A, Rustagi P, Hirschowitz GI. Reversible prolonged skin bleeding time in acute gastrointestinal bleeding presumed due to NSAIDs. *J Clin Gastroenterol.* 1996;22:96–103.

88. Graham DY, Smith JL, Dobbs SM. Gastric adaptation occurs with aspirin administration in man. *Dig Dis Sci.* 1983;28:1–6.

89. Graham DY, Smith JL, Spjut HJ, Torres E. Gastric adaptation. Studies in humans during continuous aspirin administration. *Gastroenterology.* 1998;95:327–33.

90. Olivero JJ, Graham DY. Gastric adaption to nonsteroidal anti-inflammatory drugs in man. *Scand J Gastroenterol.* 1992;27:53–8.

91. Lipscomb GR, Wallis N, Armstrong G, Goodman MJ, Rees WD. Gastric mucosal adaptation to etodolac and naproxen. *Aliment Pharmacol Ther.* 1995;9:379–85.

92. Skeljo MV, Cook GA, Elliott SL, Giraud AS, Yeomans ND. Gastric mucosal adaptation to diclofenac injury. *Dig Dis Sci.* 1996;41:32–9.

93. Heresbach D, Raoul JL, Bretagne JF, Minet J, Donnio PY, Ramee MP et al. *Helicobacter pylori*: a risk and severity factor of non-steroidal anti-inflammatory drug induced gastropathy. *Gut.* 1992;33:1608–11.

94. Taha AS, Dahill S, Morran C, Hudson N, Hawkey CJ, Lee FD et al. Neutrophils, *Helicobacter pylori*, and nonsteroidal anti-inflammatory drug ulcers. *Gastroenterology.* 1999;116:254–8.

95. Johnson PC. Gastrointestinal consequences of treatment with drugs in elderly patients. *J Am Geriatr Soc.* 1982;30:S52–S57.

96. Moore JG, Bjorkman DJ, Mitchell MD, Avots-Avotins A. Age does not influence acute aspirin-induced gastric mucosal damage. *Gastroenterology.* 1991;100:1626–9.

97. Elliot SL, Ferris RJ, Giraud AS, Cook GA, Skeljo MV, Yeomans ND. Indomethacin damage to rat gastric mucosa is markedly dependent on luminal pH. *Clin Exp Pharmacol Physiol.* 1996;23:432–4.

98. Goggin PM, Collins DA, Jazrawi RP, Jackson PA, Corbishley CM, Bourke BE et al. Prevalence of *Helicobacter pylori* infection and its effect on symptoms and non-steroidal anti-inflammatory drug induced gastrointestinal damage in patients with rheumatoid arthritis. *Gut.* 1993;34:1677–80.

99. Jones ST, Clague RB, Eldridge J, Jones DM. Serological evidence of infection with *Helicobacter pylori* may predict gastrointestinal intolerance to non-steroidal anti-inflammatory drug (NSAID) treatment in rheumatoid arthritis. *Br J Rheumatol.* 1991;30:16–20.

100. Hawkey CJ, Hudson N. Mucosal injury caused by drugs, chemicals and stress. In: Haubrich WS, Schaffner F, Berk JE, editors. *Bockus Gastroenterology*, vol.2, 5th edition. Philadelphia: W. B. Saunders; 1994:656–99.

101. Sun DCH, Roth SH, Mitchell CS, Englund DW. Upper gastrointestinal disease in rheumatoid arthritis. *Dig Dis.* 1974;19:405–10.

102. Biewer W, Buschmeier B, Bolten W. Risk factors of gastrointestinal injury: prospective multicentre study on 497 rheumatic patients. *Gut.* 1990;31:A1176.

103. Geis GS, Stead H, Wallenmark C-B, Nicholson PA. Prevalence of mucosal lesions in the stomach and duodenum due to chronic use of NSAID in patients with rheumatoid arthritis or osteoarthritis, and interim report on prevention by misoprostol of diclofenac associated lesions. *J Rheumatol Suppl.* 1991;28:11–4.

104. Taha AS, Hudson N, Hawkey CJ, Swannell AJ, Trye P, Cottrell J. Famotidine for the prevention of gastric and duodenal ulcers caused by non-steroidal anti-inflammatory drugs. *N Engl J Med.* 1996;334:1435–9.

105. Hudson N, Taha AS, Russell RI, Sturrock RG, Trye P, Cottrell J et al. Famotidine for healing and maintenance in non-steroidal anti-inflammatory drug-associated gastroduodenal ulceration. *Gastroenterology.* 1997;112:1817–22.

106. Yeomans ND, Tulassay Z, Juhasz L, Racz I, Howard JM, van Rensburg CJ et al. for the ASTRONAUT Study Group. A comparison of omeprazole and ranitidine for treating and preventing ulcers associated with non-steroidal anti-inflammatory drugs. *N Engl J Med.* 1998;338:719–26.

107. Hawkey CJ, Karrasch JA, Szcepanski L, Walker DG, Barkun A, Swannell AJ et al. for the Omeprazole vs Misoprostol for NSAID-Induced Ulcer Management (OMNIUM) Study Group. Omeprazole compared with misoprostol for ulcers associated with non steroidal anti inflammatory drugs. *N Engl J Med.* 1998;338:727–34.

108. Hawkey CJ, Tulassay Z, Szczepanski L, van Rensburg CJ, Filipowicz-Sosnowska A, Lanas A et al. *Helicobacter pylori* eradication in patients taking non-steroidal, anti-inflammatory drugs: the HELP NSAIDs study. *Lancet.* 1998;352:1016–21.

109. Cullen D, Bardhan KD, Eisner M, Kogut DG, Peacock RA, Thomas JM et al. Primary gastroduodenal prophylaxis with omeprazole for non-steroidal anti-inflammatory drug users. *Aliment Pharmacol Ther.* 1998;12:135–40.

110. Ekstrom P, Carling L, Wetterhus S, Wingren PE, Anker-Hansen O, Lundergardh G. Prevention of peptic ulcer and dyspeptic symptoms with omeprazole in patients receiving continuous non-steroidal anti-inflammatory drug therapy. A Nordic multicentre study. *Scand J Gastroenterol.* 1996;31:753–8.

111. Laine L, Harper S, Simon T, Bath R, Johanson J, Schwartz H et al. A randomized trial comparing the effect of rofecoxib, a cyclooxygenase-2 specific inhibitor, with that of ibuprofen on the gastroduodenal mucosa of patients with osteoarthritis. *Gastroenterology.* 1999;117:776–83.

112. Hawkey CJ, Laine I, Simon T, Beaulieu A, Maldonado-Cocco J, Acevedo E et al. for the Rofecoxib Osteoarthritis Endoscopy Multinational Study Group. Comparison of the effect of rofecoxib (a cyclooxygenase 2 inhibitor), ibuprofen and placebo on the gastroduodenal mucosa of patients with osteoarthritis. *Arthritis Rheum.* 2000;43:370–7.

113. Chan FKL, Sung JJY, Chung SCS, To KF, Yung MY, Leung VKS et al. Randomized trial of eradication of *Helicobacter pylori* before non-steroidal anti-inflammatory drug therapy to prevent peptic ulcer. *Lancet.* 1997;350:975–9.

114. Huang JQ, Lad RJ, Sridhar S, Sumanac K, Hunt RH. *H. pylori* infection increases the risk of non-steroidal anti-inflammatory drug (NSAID)-induced gastro-duodenal ulceration. *Gastroenterology.* 1999;116:A192.

115. Hawkey CJ, Swannell AJ, Naesdal J, Walan A, Yeomans ND. Influence of sex and *Helicobacter pylori* on type and location of lesions in NSAID-users. *Gastroenterology.* 1998;114:A145.

116. Hawkey CJ, Harper S, Quan H, Bolognese J, Mortensen E. for the Rofecoxib Osteoarthritis Endoscopy Multinational Study Group. Effect of rofecoxib on endoscopic ulcers in osteoarthritis patients: analysis of potential risk factors. *Ann Rheum Dis.* 2000;59(Suppl.):POS-290.

117. Hawkey CJ, Swannell AJ, Naesdal J, Walan A, Yeomans ND. Men are from Mars, Women are from Venus: sex-related differences in ulcer disease expression and the influence of *Helicobacter pylori. Gut.* 1998;42(Suppl.1):A112.

118. Hawkey CJ, Kahan A, Steinbruck K, Alegre C, Naumelou E, Begaud B et al. and the International MELISSA Study Group. Gastrointestinal tolerability of the COX-2 inhibitor, meloxicam, in osteoarthritis patients: The Meloxicam Large Scale International Study Safety Assessment (MELISSA). *Br J Rheumatol.* 1998;37:937–45.

119. Dequeker J, Hawkey C, Kahan A, Steinbruck K, Alegre C, Baumelou E et al. on behalf of the SELECT Study Group. Improvement in gastrointestinal tolerability of the selective COX-2 inhibitor, meloxicam, compared with piroxicam: results of the safety and efficacy large scale evaluation of COX inhibiting therapies (SELECT) trial in osteoarthritis. *Br J Rheumatol.* 1998; 37; 946–51.

120. Cryer B, Redfern JS, Goldschmiedt M, Lee E, Feldman M. Effect of aging on gastric and duodenal mucosal prostaglandin concentrations in humans. *Gastroenterology.* 1992;102:1118–23.

121. Fries JF, Williams CA, Bloch DA, Michel BA. Non-steroidal anti-inflammatory drug-associated gastropathy: incidence and risk factor models. *Am J Med.* 1991;91:213–22.

122. Smalley WE, Ray WA, Daugherty JR, Griffin MR. Nonsteroidal anti-inflammatory drugs and the incidence of hospitalizations for peptic ulcer disease in elderly persons. *Am J Epidemiol.* 1995;141:539–45.

123. Moore RA, Phillips CJ. Cost of NSAID adverse effects to the UK National Health Service. *J Med Econom.* 1999;2:45–55.

124. De Pouvourville G. The iatrogenic cost of non-steroidal anti-inflammatory drug therapy. *Br J Rheumatol.* 1995;34:19–24.

125. Bolten WW, Lang B, Wagner AV, Krobot KJ. Konsequenzen und Kosten der NSA-Gastropathie in Deutschland [Consequences and costs of NSAID-gastropathy in Germany]. *Akt Rheumatol.* 1999;24:127–34.

126. Ruigomez A, García Rodríguez LA, Hasselgren G, Johansson S, Wallander MA. Overall mortality among patients surviving an episode of peptic ulcer bleeding. *J Epidemiol Community Health.* 2000;54:130–3.

127. Carson JL, Strom BL, Morse ML, West SL, Soper KA, Stolley PD et al. The relative gastrointestinal toxicity of the nonsteroidal anti-inflammatory drugs. *Arch Intern Med.* 1987;147:1054–9.

128. Bloom BS. Risk and cost of gastrointestinal side effects associated with nonsteroidal anti-inflammatory drugs. *Arch Intern Med.* 1989;149:1019–22.

129. Silverstein FE, Graham DY, Senior JR, Davies HW, Struthers BJ, Bittman RM et al. Misoprostol reduces serious gastrointestinal complications in patients with rheumatoid arthritis receiving nonsteroidal anti-inflammatory drugs. A randomized double-blind placebo-controlled trial. *Ann Intern Med.* 1995;123:241–9. Editorial comment in: *Ann Intern Med.* 1995;123:309–10.

130. Hallas J, Lauritsen J, Dalsgard Villadsen H, Freng Gram L. Nonsteroidal anti-inflammatory drugs and upper gastrointestinal bleeding, identifying high-risk groups by excess risk estimates. *Scand J Gastroenterol.* 1995;30:438–44.

131. Smalley WE, Ray WA, Daugherty JR, Griffin MR. Nonsteroidal anti-inflammatory drugs and the incidence of hospitalizations for peptic ulcer disease in elderly persons. *Am J Epidemiol.* 1995;141:539–45.

132. Tramer MR, Moore RA, Reynolds DJM, McQuay HJ. Quantitative estimation or rare adverse events which follow a biological progression. A new model applied to chronic NSAID use. *Pain.* 2000;85:169–82.

133. Office of Population Census and Surveys. Annual Mortality Statistics. 1999. DHSS, London.

134. Hawkey CJ. Non steroidal anti-inflammatory drugs and peptic ulcers. Facts and figures multiply, but do they add up? *Br Med J.* 1990;300:278–84.

135. Griffin MR, Piper JM, Daugherty JR, Snowden M, Ray WA. Nonsteroidal anti-inflammatory drug use and increased risk for peptic ulcer disease in elderly persons. *Ann Intern Med.* 1991;114:257–63.

136. Somerville K, Faulkner G, Langman MJS. Non-steroidal anti-inflammatory drugs and bleeding peptic ulcer. *Lancet.* 1986;i:462–4.

137. Stack WA, Hawkey GM, Atherton JC, Logan RF, Hawkey CJ. Interactions of risk factors for peptic ulcer bleeding. *Gastroenterology.* 1999;116:A97.

138. Lanas AI, Bajador E, Serrano P, Fuentes J, Carre-o S, Guardia J et al. Nitrovasodilators, low-dose aspirin, nonsteroidal anti-inflammatory drugs, and the risk of upper gastrointestinal bleeding. *N Engl J Med.* 2000;343:834–9.

139. Gabriel SE, Jaakkimainen L, Bombardier C. Risk for serious gastrointestinal complications related to use of nonsteroidal anti-inflammatory drugs: a meta-analysis. *Ann Intern Med.* 1991;115:787–96.

140. García Rodríguez LA, Jick H. Risk of upper gastrointestinal bleeding and perforation associated with individual non-steroidal anti-inflammatory drugs. *Lancet.* 1994;343:769–72.

141. Langman MJS, Weil J, Wainwright P, Lawson DH, Rawlins MD, Logan RF et al. Risk of bleeding peptic ulcer associated with individual non-steroidal anti-inflammatory drugs. *Lancet.* 1994; 343:1075–8.

142. Holvoet J, Terriere L, Van Hee W, Verbist L, Fierens E, Hautekeete ML. Relation of upper gastrointestinal bleeding to non-steroidal anti-inflammatory drugs and aspirin: a case-control study. *Gut.* 1991;32:730–4.

143. Hochain P, Berkelmans I, Czernichow P, Duhamel C, Tranvouez JL, Lerebours E et al. Which patients taking non-aspirin non-steroidal anti-inflammatory drugs bleed? A case-control study. *Eur J Gastroenterol Hepatol.* 1995;7:419–26.

144. Weil J, Langman MJS, Wainwright P, Lawson DH, Rawlins M, Logan RFA et al. Peptic ulcer bleeding: accessory risk factors and interactions with non-steroidal anti-inflammatory drugs. *Gut.* 2000;46:27–31.

145. Piper JM, Ray WA, Daugherty JR, Griffin MR. Corticosteroid use and peptic ulcer disease: role of nonsteroidal anti-inflammatory drugs. *Ann Intern Med.* 1991;114:735–40.

146. Shorr RI, Ray WA, Daugherty JR, Griffin MR. Concurrent use of nonsteroidal anti-inflammatory drugs and oral anticoagulants places elderly persons at high risk for hemorrhagic peptic ulcer disease. *Arch Intern Med.* 1993;153:1665–70.

147. Henry D, Lim LL, Garcia Rodríguez LA, Perez Gutthann S, Carson JL, Griffin M et al. Variability in risk of gastrointestinal complications with individual non-

steroidal anti-inflammatory drugs: results of a collaborative meta-analysis. *Br Med J*. 1996;312:1563–6.

148. Perez-Gutthann S, García Rodríguez LA, Raiford DS. Individual nonsteroidal antiinflammatory drugs and other risk factors for upper gastrointestinal bleeding and perforation. *Epidemiology*. 1997;8:18–24.

149. Brooks PM. Day RO. Nonsteroidal anti-inflammatory drugs-differences and similarities. *N Engl J Med*. 1991;324:1716–25.

150. Hudson N, Balsitis M, Filipowicz B, Hawkey CJ. Effect of *Helicobacter pylori* colonization on gastric mucosal eicosanoid synthesis in patients taking non-steroidal anti-inflammatory drugs. *Gut*. 1993;34:748–51.

151. Labenz J, Tillenburg B, Peitz U, Verdu E, Stolte M, Borsch G et al. Effect of curing *Helicobacter pylori* infection on intragastric acidity during treatment with ranitidine in patients with duodenal ulcer. *Gut*. 1997;41:33–6.

152. Aalykke C, Lauritsen JM, Hallas J, Reinholdt S, Krogfelt K, Lauritsen K. *Helicobacter pylori* and risk of ulcer bleeding among users of non steroidal anti-inflammatory drugs: A case control study. *Gastroenterology*. 1999;116:1305–9.

153. Cullen DJE, Hawkey GM, Greenwood DC, Humphries H, Shepherd V, Logan RFA et al. Peptic ulcer bleeding: relative roles of *Helicobacter pylori* and nonsteroidal and anti-inflammatory drugs. *Gut*. 1997;41:459–62.

154. Wu CY, Poon SK, Chen GH, Chang CS, Yeh HZ. Interaction between *Helicobacter pylori* and non-steroidal anti-inflammatory drugs in peptic ulcer bleeding. *Scand J Gastroenterol*. 1999;34:234–7.

155. Labenz J, Peitz U, Kohl H, Kaiser J, Malfertheiner P, Hackelsberger A et al. *Helicobacter pylori* increases the risk of peptic ulcer bleeding: a case-control study. *Ital J Gastroenterol Hepatol*. 1999;31:110–4.

156. Pilotto A, Leandro G, Di Mario F, Franceschi M, Bozzola L, Valerio G. Role of *Helicobacter pylori* infection on upper gastrointestinal bleeding in the elderly: a case-control study. *Dig Dis Sci*. 1997;42:586–91.

157. Santolaria S, Lanas A, Benito R, Perez-Aisa MA, Montoro M, Sainz R. *Helicobacter pylori* infection is a protective factor for bleeding gastric ulcers but not for bleeding duodenal ulcers in NSAID users. *Aliment Pharmacol Ther*. 1999;13:1511–8.

158. Lanas AI, Remacha B, Esteva F, Sainz R. Risk factors associated with refractory peptic ulcers. *Gastroenterology*. 1995;109:1124–33.

159. Piper DW, McIntosh JH, Ariotti DE, Fenton BH, MacLennan R. Analgesic ingestion and chronic peptic ulcer. *Gastroenterology*. 1981;80:427–32.

160. McIntosh JH, Fung CS, Berry G, Piper DW. Smoking, nonsteroidal anti-inflammatory drugs, and acetaminophen in gastric ulcer. A study of associations and of the effects of previous diagnosis on exposure patterns. *Am J Epidemiol*. 1988;128:761–70.

161. Roth SH, Agrawal N, Mahowald M, Montoya H, Robbins D, Miller S et al. Misopostol heals gastroduodenal injury in patients with rheumatoid arthritis receiving aspirin. *Arch Intern Med*. 1989;149:775–9.

162. Ten Wolde S, Dijkmans BA, Janssen M, Hermans J, Lamers CB. High-dose ranitidine for the prevention of recurrent peptic ulcer disease in rheumatoid arthritis patients taking NSAIDs. *Aliment Pharmacol Ther*. 1996;10:347–51.

163. Bianchi Porro G, Parente F, Imbesi V, Montrone F, Caruso I. Role of *Helicobacter pylori* in ulcer healing and recurrence of gastric and duodenal ulcers in longterm NSAID users. Response to omeprazole dual therapy. *Gut*. 1996;39:22–7.

164. Chan FK, Sung JJ, Suen R, Lee YT, Wu JC, Leung WK et al. Does eradication

of *Helicobacter pylori* impair healing of nonsteroidal anti-inflammatory drug associated bleeding peptic ulcers? A prospective randomized study. *Aliment Pharmacol Ther.* 1998;12:1201–5.

165. Agrawal N, Safdi M, Wrible L, Karvois D, Greski-Rose P, Huang B. Effectiveness of lansoprazole in the healing of NSAID-induced gastric ulcer in patients continuing to take NSAIDs. *Gastroenterology.* 1998;114:A52.

166. Hudson N, Murray FE, Cole AT, Filipowicz B, Hawkey CJ. Effect of sucralfate on aspirin-induced mucosal injury and impaired haemostasis in humans. *Gut.* 1997;41:19–23.

167. Hudson N, Murray FE, Cole AT, Turnbull GM, Lettis S, Hawkey CJ. Ranitidine bismuth citrate and aspirin-induced gastric mucosal injury. *Aliment Pharmacol Ther.* 1993; 7: 515–21.

168. Koch M, Capurso L, Dezi A, Ferrario F, Scarpignato C. Prevention of NSAID-induced gastroduodenal mucosal injury: meta-analysis of clinical trials with misoprostol and H_2-receptor antagonists. *Dig Dis.* 1995;1:62–74.

169. Rostrum A, Wells G, Tugwell P, Welch V, Dube C, McGowan J. Prevention of chronic NSAID induced upper gastrointestinal toxicity. *Cochrane Database Syst Rev.* 2000;CD002296.

170. Raskin JB, White RH, Jackson JE, Weaver AL, Tindall EA, Lies RB et al. Misoprostol dosage in the prevention of nonsteroidal anti-inflammatory drug-induced gastric and duodenal ulcers: a comparison of three regimens. *Ann Intern Med.* 1995;123:344–50.

171. Wight NJ, Hawkey CJ. Peptic Ulcer Disease: NSAID Related. In: Irvine EJ, Hunt RH, editors. *Evidence Based Gastroenterology: A Framework for Clinical Practice.* Hamilton, Ontario, Canada: BC Becker Inc. 2001: in press.

172. Raskin JB, White RH, Jaszewski R, Korsten MA, Schubert TT, Fort JG. Misoprostol and ranitidine in the prevention of NSAID-induced ulcers: a prospective, double-blind, multicenter study. *Am J Gastroenterol.* 1996;91:223–7.

173. Silverstein FE, Graham DY, Senior JR, Davies HW, Struthers BJ, Bittman RM et al. Misoprostol reduces serious gastrointestinal complications in patients with arthritis receiving non-steroidal antiinflammatory drugs – a randomized double blind placebo controlled study. *Ann Int Med.* 1995;123:241–9.

174. Sung JJ. Management of nonsteroidal anti-inflammatory drug-related peptice ulcer bleeding. *Am J Med.* 2001;110(Suppl 1):S29–S32.

175. Chan FKL, Sung JYJ, Ching JYL, Wu CY, Lee YT, Chan WK et al. Prospective randomized trial of misoprostol plus naproxen versus nabumetone to prevent recurrent ulcer hemorrhage in high-risk NSAID users. *Gastroenterology.* 1999;116:A134.

176. Walt RP. Misoprostol for the treatment of peptic ulcer and anti inflammatory-drug-induced gastroduodenal ulceration. *N Engl J Med.* 1992;327:1575–80.

177. Singh G, Ramey DR, Morfeld D, Shi H, Hatoum HT, Fries JF. Gastrointestinal tract complications of non-steroidal anti-inflammatory drug treatment in rheumatoid arthritis: a prospective observational cohort study. *Arch Intern Med.* 1996;156:1530–6.

178. Rose P, Huang B, Lukasik N, Collis C. Evidence that lansoprazole is effective in preventing NSAID induced ulcers. *Gastroenterology.* 1999;116:A295.

179. Chan FKL, Sung JY, Suen R, Lee YT, Leung WK, Leung VKS et al. Eradication of *H. pylori* versus maintenance acid suppression to prevent recurrent ulcer hem-

orrhage in high risk NSAID users: a prospective randomized study. *Gastroenterology.* 1998;114:A87.

180. Slattery J, Warlow CP, Shorrock CJ, Langman MJS. Risks of gastrointestinal bleeding during secondary prevention of vascular events with aspirin – analysis of gastrointestinal bleeding during UK-TIA trial. *Gut.* 1995;37:509–11.

181. Weil J, Colin-Jones D, Langman M, Lawson D, Logan R, Murphy M et al. Prophylactic aspirin and risk of peptic ulcer bleeding. *Br Med J.* 1995;310:827–30.

182. Patrono C, Coller B, Dalen JE, Fuster V, Gent M, Harker LA et al. Platelet-active drugs: the relationships among dose, effectiveness, and side effects. *Chest.* 1998;114:470S–488S.

183. Serrano P, Lanas A, Arroya MT, Casanovas JA. Risk stratification of upper gastrointestinal bleeding in cardiovascular patients on low dose aspirin: a cohort study. *Gastroenterology.* 2000;118:A862.

184. Lanas A, Fuentes J, Benito R, Bajador E, Serrano P, Sainz R. *Helicobacter pylori* increases the risk of gastrointestinal bleeding in patients taking low dose aspirin. *Gastroenterology.* 2000;118:A252.

185. Daneshmend TK, Stein AG, Bhaskar NK, Hawkey CJ. Abolition by omeprazole of aspirin-induced gastric mucosal injury in man. *Gut.* 1990;31:514–17.

186. Donnelly MT, Goddard AF, Filipowicz B, Morant S, Shield MJ, Hawkey CJ. Low dose misoprostol for the prevention of low dose-aspirin induced gastroduodenal injury. *Aliment Pharmacol Ther.* 2000;14:543–9.

187. Morris AJ, Wasson LA, MacKenzie JF. Small bowel enteroscopy in undiagnosed gastrointestinal blood loss. *Gut.* 1992;33:887–9.

188. Allison MC, Howatson AG, Torrance CJ, Lee FD, Russell RI. Gastrointestinal damage associated with the use of nonsteroidal antiinflammatory drugs. *N Engl J Med.* 1992;327:749–54.

189. Bjarnason I, Williams P, So A, Zaneli GD, Levi AJ, Gumpel JM et al. Intestinal permeability and inflammation in rheumatoid arthritis: effects of non-steroidal anti-inflammatory drugs. *Lancet.* 1984;ii:1171–4.

190. Bjarnason I, Zanelli G, Prouse P, Smethurst P, Smith T, Levi S et al. Blood and protein loss via small-intestinal inflammation induced by non-steroidal anti-inflammatory drugs. *Lancet.* 1987;ii:711–4.

191. Morris AJ, Murray L, Sturrock RD, Madhok R, Capell HA, Mackenzie JF. Short report: the effect of misoprostol on the anaemia of NSAID enteropathy. *Aliment Pharmacol Ther.* 1994;8:343–6.

192. Collins AJ, Du Toit JA. Upper gastrointestinal findings and faecal occult blood in patients with rheumatic diseases taking nonsteroidal anti-inflammatory drugs. *Br J Rheumatol.* 1987;26:295–8.

193. Hedenbro JL, Wetterberg P, Vallgren S, Bergqvist L. Lack of correlation between fecal blood loss and drug-induced gastric mucosal lesions. *Gastrointest Endosc.* 1988;34:247–51.

194. Levi S, de Lacey G, Price AB, Gumpel MJ, Levi AJ, Bjarnason I. 'Diaphragm-like' strictures of the small bowel in patients treated with non-steroidal anti-inflammatory drugs. *Br J Radiol.* 1990;63:186–9.

195. Kwo PY, Tremaine WJ. Nonsteroidal anti-inflammatory drug-induced enteropathy: case discussion and review of the literature. *Mayo Clin Proc.* 1995;70:55–61.

196. Langman MJ, Morgan L, Worrall A. Use of anti-inflammatory drugs by patients admitted with small or large bowel perforations and haemorrhage. *Br Med J Clin Res Ed.* 1985;290:347–9.

197. Morris AJ, MacKenzie JF. Small-bowel enteroscopy and NSAID ulceration. *Lancet.* 1991;337:1550.

198. Zalev AH, Gardiner GW, Warren FE. NSAID injury in the small intestine. *Abdominal Imaging.* 1998;23:40–4.

199. Satoh H, Guth PH, Grossman MI. Role of bacteria in gastric ulceration produced by indomethacin in the rat: cytoprotective action of antibiotics. *Gastroenterology.* 1983;84:483–9.

200. Khazaeinia T, Jamali F. Evaluation of gastrointestinal toxicity of ibuprofen using surrogate markers in rats: effect of formulation and route of administration. *Clin Experiment Rheumatol.* 2000;18:187–92.

201. Morris AJ, Murray L, Sturrock RD, Madhok R, Capell HA, Mackenzie JF. Short report: the effect of misoprostol on the anaemia of NSAID enteropathy. *Aliment Pharmacol Ther.* 1994;8:343–6.

202. Bjarnason I, Hopkinson N, Zanelli G, Prouse P, Smethurst P, Gumpel JM et al. Treatment of non-steroidal anti-inflammatory drug induced enteropathy. *Gut.* 1990;31:777–80.

203. Cole AT, Hyman-Taylor P, Hawkey CJ. Low dose aspirin: Selective inhibition of rectal dialysis thromboxane B_2 in healthy volunteers. *Aliment Pharmacol Ther.* 1994;8:521–6.

204. Dominitz JA, Koepsell TD, Boyko EJ. Association between analgesic use and inflammatory bowel disease (IBD) flares: a retrospective cohort study. *Gastroenterology.* 2000;118:A581.

205. Faucheron JL. Toxicity of non-steroidal anti-inflammatory drugs in the large bowel. *Eur J Gastroenterol Hepatol.* 1999;11:389–92.

206. Hawkey CJ. COX-2 inhibitors. *Lancet.* 1999;353:307–14.

207. Bombardier C, Laine L, Reicin A, Shapiro D, Burgos-Vargas R, Davis B et al. A double-blind comparison of rofecoxib and naproxen on the incidence of clincially important upper gastrointestinal events in the VIGOR Trial. *N Engl J Med.* 2000;343:1520–8.

208. Silverstein FE, Faich G, Goldstein JL, Simon LS, Pincus T, Whelton A et al. Gastrointestinal toxicity with celecoxib vs non-steroidal anti-inflammatory drugs for osteoarthritis and rheumatoid arthritis. The CLASS study: a randomized controlled trial. *J Am Med Assoc.* 2000;284:1247–55.

209. Scott LJ, Lamb HM. Rofecoxib. *Drugs.* 1999;58:499–505.

210. Boyce EG, Breen GA. Celecoxib: a COX-2 inhibitor for the treatment of osteoarthritis and rheumatoid arthritis. *Hosp Formul.* 1999;34:405–17.

211. Luong C, Miller A, Barnett J Chow J, Ramesha C, Browner MF. Flexibility of the NSAID binding site in the structure of cyclooxygenase-2. *Nature Struct Biol.* 1996;3:927–33.

212. Furst DE. Meloxicam: selective COX-2 inhibition in clinical practice. *Semin Arthritis Rheum.* 1997;26:21–7.

213. Lipscomb GR, Wallis N, Armstrong G, Rees WD. Gastrointestinal tolerability of meloxicam and piroxicam: a double-blind placebo-controlled study. *Br J Clin Pharmacol.* 1998;46:33–7.

214. Dvornik DM. Tissue selective inhibition of prostaglandins biosynthesis by etodolac. *J Rheumatol.* 1997;47:40–7.

215. Laine L, Sloane R, Ferretti M, Cominelli F. A randomized double-blind comparison of placebo, etodolac and naproxen on gastrointestinal injury and prostaglandin production. *Gastrointest Endosc.* 1995;42:428–33.

216. Bennett A. Overview of nimesulide. *Rheumatol.* 1999;38:1–3.

217. Shah AA, Murray FE, Fitzgerald DJ. The *in vivo* assessment of nimesulide cyclo-oxygenase-2 selectivity. *Rheumatol.* 1999;38:19–23.

218. Warner TD, Giuliano F, Vojnovic I, Bukasa A, Mitchell JA, Vane JR. Non-steroidal drug selectivities for cyclooxygenase-1 rather than cyclooxygenase-2 are associated with human gastrointestinal toxicity: a full *in vitro* analysis. *Proc Natl Acad Sci USA.* 1999;96:7563–8.

219. Ehrich EW, Dallob A, De Lepeleire I, Van Hecken A, Riendeau D, Yuan W et al. Characterization of rofecoxib as a cyclooxygenase-2 isoform inhibitor and demonstration of analgesia in the dental pain model. *Clin Pharmacol Ther.* 1999;65:336–47.

220. McAdam BF, Catella-Lawson F, Mardini IA, Kapoor S, Lawson JA, FitzGerald GA. Systemic biosynthesis of prostacyclin by cyclooxygenase (COX)-2: the human pharmacology of a selective inhibitor of COX-2. *Proc Natl Acad Sci USA.* 1999;96:272–7. (Published erratum appears in *Proc Natl Acad Sci USA.* May 11, 1999;96:5890.)

221. Panara MR, Renda G, Sciulli MG, Santini G, Di Giamberardino M, Rotondo MT et al. Dose-dependent inhibition of platelet cyclooxygenase-1 and monocyte cyclooxygenase-2 by meloxicam in healthy subjects. *J Pharmacol Exp Ther.* 1999;290:276–80.

222. Lanza FL, Rack MF, Simon TJ, Quan H, Bolognese JA, Hoover ME et al. Specific inhibition of cyclooxygenase-2 with MK-0966 is associated with less gastro-duodenal damage than either aspirin or ibuprofen. *Aliment Pharmacol Ther.* 1999;13:761–7.

223. Simon LS, Lanza FL, Lipsky PE, Hubbard RC, Talwalker S, Schwartz BD et al. Preliminary study of the safety and efficacy of SC-58635, a novel cyclooxygenase-2 inhibitor: efficacy and safety in two placebo-controlled trials in osteoarthritis and rheumatoid arthritis, and studies of gastrointestinal and platelet effects. *Arthritis Rheum.* 1998;41:1591–602.

224. Porto A, Almeida H, Cunha MJ, Macciocchi A. Double-blind study evaluating by endoscopy the tolerability of nimesulide and diclofenac on the gastric mucosa in osteoarthritic patients. *Eur J Rheumatol Inflammation.* 1994;14:33–8.

225. Laine L, Harper S, Simon T, Bath R, Johanson J, Schwartz H et al. A randomized trial comparing the effect of rofecoxib, a cyclooxygenase-2 specific inhibitor, with that of ibuprofen on the gastroduodenal mucosa of patients with osteoarthritis. *Gastroenterology.* 1999;117:776–83.

226. Hawkey C, Laine L, Simon T, Beaulieu A, Maldonado-Cocco J, Acevedo E et al. Comparison of the effect of rofecoxib (a cyclooxygenase 2 inhibitor), ibuprofen, and placebo on the gastroduodenal mucosa of patients with osteoarthritis: a randomized, double-blind, placebo-controlled trial. The Rofecoxib Osteoarthritis Endoscopy Multinational Study Group. *Arthritis Rheum.* 2000;43:370–7.

227. Simon LS, Weaver AL, Graham DY, Kivitz AJ, Lipsky PE, Hubbard RC et al. Anti-inflammatory and upper gastrointestinal effects of celecoxib in rheumatoid arthritis: a randomized controlled trial. *J Am Med Assoc.* 1999;282:1921–8.

228. Emery P, Zeidler H, Kvien TK, Guslandi M, Naudin R, Stead H et al. Celecoxib versus diclofenac in long-term management of rheumatoid arthritis: randomized double-blind comparison. *Lancet.* 1999;354:2106–11.

229. Langman MJ, Jensen DM, Watson DJ, Harper SE, Xhao P-L, Quan H. Incidence of upper gastrointestinal perforations, symptomatic ulcers and bleeding (PUBS).

Rofecoxib compared to NSAIDs. *J Am Med Assoc.* 1999;282:1929–33.

230. Goldstein JL, Silverstein FE, Agrawal NM, Hubbard RC, Kaiser J, Maurath CJ et al. Reduced risk of upper gastrointestinal ulcer complications with celecoxib, a novel COX-2 inhibitor. *Am J Gastroenterol.* 2000;95:1681–90.

231. Daniels B, Seidenberg B. Cardiovascular safety profile of rofecoxib in controlled clinical trials. *Arthritis Rheum.* 1999;42:S143.

232. Wallace JL. Inhibition of both cyclooxygenase (COX)-1 and COX-2 is required for NSAID-induced erosion formation. *Gastroenterology.* 2000;118:A19.

233. Mizuno H, Sakamoto C, Matsuda K, Wada K, Uchida T, Noguchi H et al. Induction of cyclooxygenase 2 in gastric mucosal lesions and its inhibition by the specific antagonist delays healing in mice. *Gastroenterology.* 1997;112:387–97.

234. Jackson LM, Wu KC, Mahida YR, Jenkins D, Hawkey CJ. Cyclooxygenase (COX)-1 and -2 in normal, inflamed and ulcerated human gastric mucosa. *Gut.* 2000;47:762–70.

235. Schmassmann A, Peskar BM, Stettler C, Netzer P, Stroff T, Flogerzi B et al. Effects of inhibition of prostaglandin endoperoxide synthase-2 in chronic gastro-intestinal ulcer models in rats. *Br J Pharmacol.* 1998;123:795–804.

236. Catella-Lawson F, McAdam B, Morrison BW, Kapoor S, Kujubu D, Antes L et al. Effects of specific inhibition of cyclooxygenase-2 on sodium balance, hemo-dynamics, and vasoactive eicosanoids. *J Pharmacol Exp Ther.* 1999;289:735–41.

237. Rossat J, Mailard M, Nussberger J, Brunner HR, Burnier M. Renal effects of selec-tive cyclooxygenase-2 inhibition in normotensive salt-depleted subjects. *Clin Pharmacol Ther.* 1999;66:76–84.

238. Hawkey CJ. Non-steroidal anti-inflammatory drug-associated ulcers. In: Olbe L, editor. *Proton Pump Inhibitors.* Basle, Boston, Berlin: Berhauser Verlag; 1999;193–204.

17 | Epidemiology of upper gastrointestinal side effects of non-steroid anti-inflammatory drugs

[1]LUIS ALBERTO GARCÍA RODRÍGUEZ AND
[2]SONIA HERNÁNDEZ-DÍAZ

[1]*Spanish Centre for Pharmacoepidemiologic Research (CEIFE),
Madrid, Spain and* [2]*Department of Epidemiology, Harvard School
of Public Health, Boston, USA.*

Gastrointestinal side effects associated with use of non-steroid anti-inflammatory drugs (NSAIDs) can range from mild dyspepsia to severe complications that lead to hospitalization and, in some instances, may be fatal. In this chapter we shall review the epidemiological evidence accumulated during the past decades on the risk of serious upper gastrointestinal complications (UGIC) in users of one of the most widely used drug class, NSAIDs. We will focus on UGIC defined as bleeding, perforation, or other serious upper gastrointestinal tract event resulting in hospitalization or visit to a specialist.

EPIDEMIOLOGICAL TERMS

We will start by briefly translating the epidemiological terms used in this chapter. Readers familiar with them may want to skip this section. Those wishing to achieve a comprehensive understanding of epidemiological methods should consider this section an oversimplification and will want to refer to the references[1-3].

Measures of frequency

In order to measure the frequency of a given disease, one can count prevalent cases or incident cases (new diagnoses). In this review, only incident cases will be considered. The most common measures of frequency, using incident cases, are the incidence risk and the incidence rate. The former measures the proportion of individuals that develop the disease in a determined period of time (e.g. 1% in 5 years). The second measures the number of new cases per unit of time (e.g. 0.01 cases per year or, the equivalent, 10 cases per 1000 persons per year). We will be using the unit person-years when reporting incidence rates.

Measures of association

We will use the incidence rate difference between persons exposed versus non-exposed to NSAIDs to estimate the absolute number of extra cases among NSAID users per unit of person-time. We will use the incidence rate ratio to estimate how many times higher the incidence rate is among exposed as compared with non-exposed. Although risk ratio and rate ratio are not exactly the same thing, for simplicity we will consider them similar enough and will use the term relative risk (RR) to refer to either of them.

Study design

Cohorts and case-controls are the two major epidemiological designs that have been used to study the association between NSAIDs and UGIC. In a cohort, persons are enrolled and followed for a period of time after which we can count the events and calculate incidence rates (among other measures). Exposed and non-exposed groups can be defined and compared with respect to the disease incidence. Case-control studies are an efficient way of estimating measures of association. After ascertaining the cases and defining their source population (i.e. all the persons that would be counted as cases if they had the event), the researcher takes a sample of controls. Controls will give an estimate of the exposure distribution in the source population. The frequency of exposure among controls can be compared with the frequency of exposure among cases. With case-control studies we will not have direct measures of disease frequency as we can have in cohort studies.

Bias

Bias is the difference between a reported and the true finding. Together with chance, a bias might always be an alternative explanation for an association or lack of association in epidemiological studies.

Pharmacoepidemiological studies have one major advantage: they are not performed in an experimental setting. They study the effect of drugs in the general population, with their real pattern of drug use and in real 'non-ideal' patients. On the other hand, pharmacoepidemiological studies have one major disadvantage: they are not performed in an experimental setting. They do not have random allocation of treatments, nor a placebo control group, nor blinding precautions. Patients using NSAIDs in the real world may not be comparable with patients that are not using them. They may differ not only in their exposure to the drug, but also in their age, sex, disease history, etc. One guaranteed difference between users and non-users of a medication is normally the indication for that medication. These sociodemographic or health related characteristics may have an independent effect on the risk of UGIC. If that happens, the groups we want to compare (exposed versus non-exposed to a drug) may not be comparable. This scenario of non-comparability is what we call confounding, and the unbalanced characteristics between exposed and unexposed groups that affect the risk of UGIC are candidates for confounders. To diminish confounding, researchers can randomize the exposure (a luxury limited to clinical trials), restrict the study to subgroups without room for confounding, use matching on risk factors to make groups comparable, and use stratified analysis or control for the potential confounders in multivariate statistical models.

Other than confounding, bias can arise from the way researchers select their comparison groups (selection bias) or from the way they collect the information (information bias).

Data sources

Adequate data resources for the estimation of incidence rates for rare diseases such as UGIC are mostly limited to large-scale claims databases such as large Health Maintenance Organizations or Health Departments; and to computerized medical records such as the General Practice Research Database (GPRD) in the United Kingdom. As a by-product of the computerized medical and pharmacy claims processing and management system, a large volume of information is accumulated and provides a valuable source for performing pharmacoepidemiological studies.

On other occasions, studies are designed *ad hoc*, where information on NSAID use and gastrointestinal events will come from questionnaires, interviews or medical records (field-based studies).

FREQUENCY OF GASTROINTESTINAL SIDE EFFECTS

To evaluate the impact of the upper gastrointestinal toxicity associated with NSAIDs, public health authorities often want to know the excess number of cases attributable to NSAID use. To answer this question we first need to know the baseline incidence of UGIC among non-users. Further, it will be important to identify persons at particularly high risk for UGIC. The following paragraphs are devoted to the incidence of UGIC in the general population and in persons with particular risks.

Overall incidence rate of UGIC

Epidemiological studies in Western countries have reported an incidence of hospitalization for complicated peptic ulcer disease among non-users of

NSAIDs of approximately 1 case per 1000 persons per year[4-7]. However, even within complicated gastrointestinal events, there is still place for variability in outcome definition. Such definition will affect the incidence rate estimate. For instance, severe uncomplicated gastrointestinal ulcer (requiring hospitalization) occurs more frequently than bleeding; and bleeding occurs more frequently than ulcer perforation. Studies reported 1 case of bleeding for every 1 or 2 cases of non-bleeding ulcer[8], and 1 case of perforation per 6 or 7 cases of bleeding[4,7,9-11]. Within outcome definitions, incidence rate estimates decrease when hospitalization (surrogate for severity) or dead for a given event is required. One study showed an incidence rate of 0.05 per 1000 person-years for fatal gastrointestinal complications, that would translate to a 5% case fatality[8]. In addition, exclusion of UGIC events potentially attributable to causes other than NSAIDs (such as cirrhosis, chronic liver disease, alcoholism, Mallory–Weiss syndrome, cancer, oesophageal varices or haematological disorders) tends to reduce the incidence rate estimates, as shown when studies present data with and without exclusions[4,5,8].

Factors affecting the risk of UGIC

The incidence of UGIC is strongly dependent on age and to a lesser extent on gender[14]. Incidence rates have been shown consistently to increase exponentially with age[5-7,10,12,15,16]. After age 75 years, the incidence of UGIC is over 5 cases per 1000 person-years. Men present a twofold greater risk of developing UGIC than women all along the age range[5,7,12,15,16] (Figure 1).

After age, the second most important independent risk factor for UGIC is

Figure 1 Age- and sex-specific rates of UGIC among users and non-users of NSAIDs (Saskatchewan 1982–86: ref. 5).

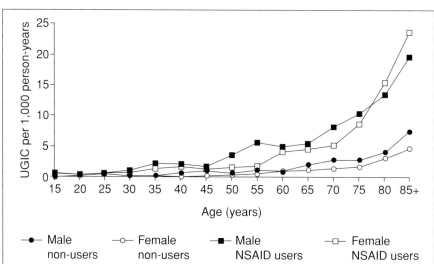

having had a previous episode of UGIC. Compared with individuals without a prior history, persons with a previous complicated ulcer have a risk of UGIC more than 10 times higher[5,7,15–18]. Hence, if for individuals with no prior history of UGIC the baseline incidence rate is about 1 case per 1000 persons per year, for patients with a history of UGIC the baseline incidence rate would be greater than 10 cases per 1000 persons per year (Figure 2).

Both tobacco and alcohol have been shown to be moderate risk factors for UGIC, with up to twofold increases in risk for both smokers and heavy drinkers[17,19–22]. It has been suggested that smoking is preferentially associated with gastroduodenal perforation and high alcohol intake with bleeding[23].

The use of certain medications other than NSAIDs has also been associated with a greater risk of UGIC. Epidemiological studies have shown that steroids roughly double the risk of having a new episode of UGIC[5,7,15,16,18,24]. Paracetamol at high doses may also increase the risk of UGIC (reference 21 and unpublished observation). Finally, it is well known that oral anti-coagulants more than double the risk of UGIC[16,26,27].

NSAIDS AND THE RISK OF UGIC

Current intake of NSAIDs, studied as a therapeutic class, has been consis-tently associated with an average fourfold increase in UGIC (Figure 3)[14,27–29].

Figure 2 Specific rates of UGIB per 1000 person-years according to severity of prior history and use of NSAIDs (GPRD 1993–1997). (Assuming a baseline incidence rate of 1 case per 1000 person-years.)

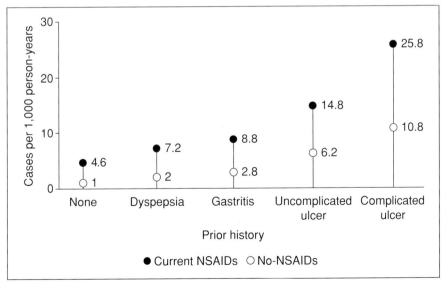

Figure 3 Relative risk (RR) and 95% confidence intervals (CIs) of UGIC associated with non-aspirin NSAID use (epidemiological studies from 1990 to 1999).

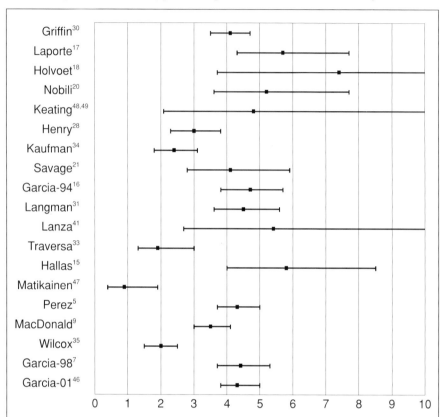

Effect of dose

The risk of developing UGIC increases proportionally with NSAID dose. Users of low daily doses experience a two- to threefold increase in risk, whereas users of medium and high daily doses have between a four- and sixfold increase in risk, respectively[5,7,16,19,30,31].

Effect of duration

Conflicting results exist concerning the risk during the first month of therapy. Some studies suggest that the RR of UGIC is higher among persons who had just started treatment; other studies have shown that the RR associated with current NSAID use is maintained relatively constant even after many months of continuous treatment. In summary, it seems that NSAID use increases the risk of UGIC among new users and among those already on therapy for several months, although the RR may be slightly greater for new users[5,7,16,19,30,31].

A biological explanation has been proposed to explain a lower gastrotoxic NSAID effect for patients on treatment for a long time: the gastric mucosa tends to adapt to continuous insults[32]. However, methodological pitfalls such as self-selection of patients resistant to NSAID gastrotoxicity (i.e. only patients who can tolerate NSAIDs will remain on treatment) might also explain the apparent effect modification over the period of treatment. In any case, this translates into an ever-increasing cumulative risk during NSAID treatment.

On the other hand, it is well accepted that the risk of UGIC typically drops quickly once NSAID treatment is stopped. On average, 1–2 months after the end of therapy the risk returns to the baseline incidence found among persons not using NSAIDs[5,7,12,16,30,33].

Effect of pharmacokinetics

NSAIDs with a long half-life or NSAIDs with a short half-life in slow release formulations are associated with a greater risk of UGIC than NSAIDs with a short half-life in regular formulations[19]. We found that even after allowing for daily dose, NSAIDs with a long half-life or slow-release formulation were still associated with a greater risk than NSAIDs with a short half-life (unpublished observation).

Effect of multiple NSAIDs use

Users of multiple NSAIDs simultaneously had over a tenfold increase in the risk of developing UGIC, compared with non-users[5,7,16]. This finding may be attributable, in part, to an augmentation of the total resulting dose. The same studies showed that patients who had recently switched NSAIDs also presented a greater risk of UGIB when compared with patients who remained on a single NSAID. This could reflect, in part, an increased risk among patients on NSAIDs who switched therapy due to early NSAID-related adverse effects.

Effect of individual NSAIDs

When individual NSAIDs are compared, ibuprofen is consistently associated with the lowest risk of gastrotoxicity, followed by diclofenac, sulindac, naproxen, indomethacin and ketoprofen, whereas azapropazone and ketorolac are the most gastrotoxic. Of the other widely used conventional NSAIDs, only piroxicam presents an above-average increase in risk. However, most individual NSAIDs are associated with a RR between 2 and 4 when administrated at low to medium doses, and all present a greater risk with increasing dose (Figure 4). At doses resulting in an anti-inflammatory effect (i.e. high doses), users of ibuprofen have a similar UGIC risk to users of other NSAIDs at high doses[28,29].

Figure 4 Pooled relative risk (RR) and 95% confidence intervals (CIs) of UGIC associated with individual non-aspirin NSAID use (epidemiological studies from 1990 to 1999). Circle, RR for low doses; squares, RR for high doses.

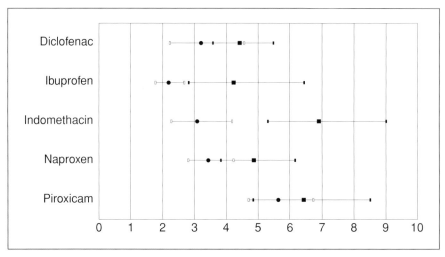

Site and type of UGIC

The relative risk for NSAID users compared with non-users tends to be higher for perforations (RR around 7) than for bleeding lesions (RR around 4). However, the risk associated with NSAIDs is similar for lesions located in the stomach and duodenum[5,7,15–19,21,30,31,33–35].

Absolute risks

If one wants to know the excess number of UGIC attributable to NSAID use, we will need to do a minor calculation and a major assumption. The expected incidence rate is about 1 per 1000 person-years for persons non-exposed to NSAIDs. Persons using NSAIDs will have about four times this figure: 4 cases per 1000 person-years. The number of cases extra 'caused' by NSAIDs would be 3 per 1000 persons using NSAIDs per year. We have assumed implicitly that persons using NSAIDs are otherwise identical to non-users in their risk of UGIC and that, were they not exposed, their risk would be the one calculated for non-exposed persons. The total number of cases attributable to NSAID use in a general population (i.e. with users and non-users) will depend on the frequency of NSAID use in that population.

CONCURRENCE OF NSAIDS AND OTHER GASTROTOXIC FACTORS

Up to this point we have considered several factors related with UGIC individually. Now, we will appraise what would happen to persons with more than one risk factor simultaneously. Should we sum the risks inherent to each individual characteristic? Should we multiply them? Will they cancel each other out? Specifically, if we focus on NSAIDs, we would like to know whether NSAIDs have the same gastrotoxic effect in different groups of patients and which would be the absolute risk for an NSAID user with additional risk factors. The following paragraphs summarize the main combinations studied so far in epidemiological studies.

Age and gender

Non-steroid anti-inflammatory drug use is associated with about fourfold increased risk across all age groups[4,15,17,19–21,30,31]. Therefore, patients over 75 years taking NSAIDs would present an absolute incidence rate around 20 UGIC cases per 1000 person-years[5]. The impact of NSAIDs on the risk of UGIC is somewhat stronger in women than in men, especially at very advanced ages (Figure 1)[5,15–19,30].

Prior history

Exposure to NSAIDs causes an almost fivefold increase in the risk of UGIC for patients without prior history (from 1 to 5 cases per 1000 persons per year), and a greater than twofold increase in patients with a history of peptic ulcer disease (from 10 to 25 cases per 1000 persons per year)[5,7,15–17,19]. Hence, the NSAID effect on the risk of UGIC decreases proportionally with the severity of the prior gastrointestinal condition. However, patients with a history of complicated ulcer disease present the greatest absolute risk of UGIC when taking NSAIDs (about 25 cases per 1000 person-years) and would result in around 15 cases per 1000 persons per year that could be attributable to NSAID treatment (Figure 2).

Tobacco and alcohol

No interaction with NSAIDs has been reported for these two factors.

Concomitant medication

The use of steroids has been found to reinforce the risk associated with NSAIDs[14,36]. Piper et al. found a relative risk of 1.1 among patients taking only steroids and of 14.6 among patients taking steroids and NSAIDs concurrently, as compared with users of none[24]. Perez-Gutthann et al. found an effect of 2.2 and 12.5 for users of steroids only and for concomitant users of both steroids and NSAIDs, respectively, compared with non-users of either drug[5]. We also observed a potentiation of the risk associated with NSAIDs among persons taking concomitant steroids in the GPRD, especially among users of high doses of NSAIDs. Concomitant use of systemic steroids with high doses of NSAIDs was associated with a twelvefold increased risk of UGIC[37].

Concurrent use of both warfarin and NSAIDs has been associated with more than a tenfold increase in the risk of UGIC[26]. We found a substantial interaction between NSAIDs and high dose paracetamol in the GPRD data; the risk associated with concomitant use of these two drugs was higher than the sum of the risks estimated for each of them individually (unpublished observation).

ASPIRIN AND THE RISK OF UGIC

Epidemiological studies have reported risks of UGIC from 1 to 10 times higher among aspirin users, with an estimated pooled relative risk between 2 and 3[14,27,28]. The risk associated with aspirin is dose-dependent but is still present at low doses (below 300 mg/day)[19,21,38,39].

Although endoscopic studies showed a reduction in gastric and duodenal injury with the use of enteric-coated aspirin[40–43], observational studies have not shown a clear difference in UGIC risk between enteric-coated or buffered formulations and plain aspirin[38,39].

The risk of UGIC is higher during the first weeks of treatment (fourfold increased risk), and is higher for patients using aspirin regularly than for patients using aspirin occasionally[19,38,39]. Finally, the risk associated with simultaneous use of aspirin and NSAIDs is only slightly higher than the sum of their individual risks[19].

PROBLEMS ENCOUNTERED IN EPIDEMIOLOGICAL STUDIES OF NSAIDS AND UGIC

Confounding

Elderly persons tend to use more medications than young persons. Non-steroid anti-inflammatory drugs are not an exception. Since advanced age is associated with a higher risk of UGIC, NSAID users would have a higher risk of UGIC than non-users, even if NSAIDs were innocuous. On the other hand, patients with prior history of gastrointestinal complications, especially if they were related to NSAIDs, will tend to avoid medications with gastrointestinal side effects. Hence, on average, there will be fewer persons with prior history of gastrointestinal events among NSAID users than among non-users. Since prior ulcer history is associated with a higher risk of UGIC, NSAID users would tend to have a lower risk of UGIC. To control for these confounders, researchers have often adjusted their relative risk estimates for antecedents of upper gastrointestinal disorders, age, sex and several other risk factors. In addition, since NSAIDs are prescribed to patients with certain diseases, illnesses themselves and not the drugs might be responsible for the UGIC (confounding by indication). However, the drop in risk after treatment is stopped and the dose–response found, point clearly to a drug effect rather than a disease effect. Moreover, once NSAID dose is accounted for, no difference in risk of UGIC between the various NSAID indications has been shown.

Selection bias

Selection bias appears in case-control studies when the reason for a control being selected is related somehow to the use of NSAIDs or other gastrotoxic factors. That would result in underestimation or overestimation of relative risks for NSAIDs, depending on the exact factors associated with the selection of controls.

Information bias

Interviews, questionnaires and registries are subject to errors in the information they provide. Recall of past exposure may be incomplete when interviews or self-administered questionnaires are used as the source of data. However, carefully designed questionnaires, administered within a short period of time after exposure, may substantially reduce information errors. If recall of past exposure were better among UGIC cases than among controls (differential misclassification of exposure), a higher proportion of exposed cases will report NSAID use than exposed controls. That would lead to an overestimation of the relative risk.

Use of claims database codes for diagnoses may be subject to a substantial degree of misclassification which is inherent in billing records. However, chart review and confirmation of diagnosis can diminish diagnosis errors. Computerized prescription data may also underestimate over the counter drug use and overestimate exposure when compliance with the drug supplied is incomplete. However, misclassification of NSAID exposure is expected to be small as usually only ibuprofen is purchased over the counter. In addition, misclassification of NSAID exposure is probably similar for cases and non-cases in registry-based studies and thus would tend to result in conservative relative risk estimates.

FUTURE DIRECTIONS

Future research will show whether newer NSAIDs, and especially new selective COX-2 inhibitors, are clinically safer and more cost-effective than other therapeutic approaches to reduce the toxicity associated with conventional NSAIDs. Epidemiological data regarding these new alternatives are still sparse. *Helicobacter pylori* has been identified in the past few years as a factor in the development of gastrointestinal ulcer, but whether there is an interaction between *H. pylori* infection and NSAIDs is still being discussed[44]. Similarly, there are still limited data regarding the association between NSAIDs and small and large lower gastrointestinal tract complications[35,45].

CONCLUSIONS

In summary, the incidence of UGIC is in the order of 1 case per 1000 persons per year, is slightly higher in men than in women, and increases substantially with age and with the severity of a prior history of peptic ulcer. Non-aspirin NSAID use is associated with around a fourfold increased risk of UGIC. The risk associated with NSAID use is dose dependent and is common to all individual NSAIDs. Although ibuprofen has been found to present the lowest overall relative risk, in the vast majority of epidemiological studies most NSAIDs are associated with similar increases in risk when administrated at comparable daily doses. The increased risk is maintained during the duration of treatment and drops quickly once treatment is stopped. Individuals of advanced age, history of complicated peptic ulcer disease, and concomitant use of anticoagulants and steroids are at an especially high risk of developing UGIC when treated with NSAIDs.

Address all correspondence to: Dr Luis Alberto García Rodríguez, CEIFE, Almirante, 28-2, 28004 Madrid, Spain.

REFERENCES

1. Rothman KJ, Greenland S. *Modern Epidemiology.* Philadelphia: Lippincott-Raven; 1998.
2. Walker AM. *Observation and Inference. An Introduction to the Methods of Epidemiology.* Newton Lower Falls: Epidemiology Resources Inc.; 1991.
3. Jick H, García Rodríguez LA, Pérez-Guthann S. Principles of epidemiological research on adverse and beneficial drug effects. *Lancet.* 1998;352:1767–70.
4. García Rodríguez LA, Walker AM, Pérez-Gutthann S. Nonsteroidal antiinflammatory drugs and gastrointestinal hospitalizations in Saskatchewan: A cohort study. *Epidemiology.* 1992;3:337–42.
5. Pérez-Gutthann S, Garcia Rodriguez LA, Raiford DS. Individual nonsteroidal antiinflammatory drugs and other risk factors for upper gastrointestinal bleeding and perforation. *Epidemiology.* 1997;8:18–24.
6. Menniti-Ippolito F, Maggini M, Raschetti R, Da Cas R, Traversa G, Walker AM. Ketorolac use in outpatients and gastrointestinal hospitalization: a comparison with other non-steroidal anti-inflammatory drugs in Italy. *Eur J Clin Pharmacol.* 1998;54:393–7.
7. García Rodríguez LA, Cattaruzzi C, Troncon MG, Agostinis L. Risk of hospitalization for upper gastrointestinal tract bleeding associated with ketorolac, other nonsteroidal anti-inflammatory drugs, calcium antagonists, and other antihypertensive drugs. *Arch Intern Med.* 1998;158:33–9.
8. Guess HA, West R, Strand LM, Helstom D, Lydick EG, Bergman U et al. Fatal upper gastrointestinal hemorrage or perforation among users and nonusers of nonsteroidal anti-inflammatory drugs in Saskatchewan, Canada 1983. *J Clin Epidemiol.* 1988;41:35–45.
9. MacDonald TM, Morant SV, Robinson GC, Shield MJ, McGilchrist MM, Murray FE et al. Association of upper gastrointestinal toxicity of non-steroidal

anti-inflammatory drugs with continued exposure: cohort study. *BMJ.* 1997;315:1333–7.

10. Smalley WE, Ray WA, Daugherty JR, Griffin MR. Nonsteroidal anti-inflammatory drugs and the incidence of hospitalizations for peptic ulcer disease in elderly persons. *Am J Epidemiol.* 1995;141:539–45.

11. Schoon I-M, Mellstrom D, Oden A, Yfferberg B-O. Incidence of peptic ulcer disease in Gothenburg, 1985. *BMJ.* 1989;299:1131–4.

12. Lanza LL, Walker AM, Bortnichack EA, Dreyer NA. Peptic ulcer and gastrointestinal hemorrhage associated with nonsteroidal anti-inflammatory drug use in patients younger than 65 years. A large health maintenance organization cohort study. *Arch Intern Med.* 1995;155:1371–7.

13. Bloom BS. Risk and cost of gastrointestinal side effects associated with nonsteroidal anti-inflammatory drugs. *Arch Intern Med.* 1989;149:1019–22.

14. Gabriel SE, Jaakkimainen L, Bombardier C. Risk for serious gastrointestinal complications related to use of nonsteroidal anti-inflammatory drugs. *Ann Med.* 1991;115:787–96.

15. Hallas J, Lauritsen J, Dalsgard Villadsen H, Freng Gram L. Nonsteroidal anti-inflammatory drugs and upper gastrointestinal bleeding, identifying high-risk groups by excess risk estimates. *Scand J Gastroenterol.* 1995;30:438–44.

16. García Rodríguez LA, Jick H. Risk of upper gastrointestinal bleeding and perforation associated with individual non-steroidal anti-inflammatory drugs. *Lancet.* 1994;343:769–72.

17. Laporte J-R, Carné X, Vidal X, Moreno V, Juan J. Upper gastrointestinal bleeding in relation to previous use of analgesics and non-steroidal antiinflammatory drugs. *Lancet.* 1991;337:85–9.

18. Holvoet J, Terriere L, Van Hee W, Verbist L, Fierens E, Hautekeete M. Relation of upper gastrointestinal bleeding to non-steroidal anti-inflammatory drugs and aspirin: a case-control study. *Gut.* 1991;32:730–4.

19. Henry D, Dobson A, Turner C. Variability in the risk of major gastrointestinal complications from nonaspirin nonsteroidal anti-inflammatory drugs. *Gastroenterology.* 1993;105:1078–88.

20. Nobili A, Mosconi P, Franzosi MG, Tognoni G. Non-steroidal anti-inflammatory drugs and upper gastrointestinal bleeding, a post-marketing surveillance case-control study. *Pharmacoepidemiol Drug Safety.* 1992;1:65–72.

21. Savage R, Moller P, Ballantyne C, Wells J. Variation in the risk of peptic ulcer complications with nonsteroidal antiinflammatory drug therapy. *Arthritis Rheum.* 1993;36:84–90.

22. Kelly JP, Kaufman DW, Koff RS, Laszlo A, Wiholm B-E, Shapiro S. Alcohol consumption and the risk of major upper gastrointestinal bleeding. *Am J Gastroenterol.* 1995;90:1058–64.

23. Andersen IB, Jorgensen T, Bonnevie O, Gronbaek M, Sorensen TI. Smoking and alcohol intake as risk factors for bleeding and perforated peptic ulcers: A population based cohort study. *Epidemiology.* 2000;11:434–9.

24. Piper JM, Ray WA, Daugherty JR, Griffin MR. Corticosteroid use and peptic ulcer disease: Role of nonsteroidal anti-inflammatory drugs. *Ann Intern Med.* 1991;114:735–40.

25. Carson J, Strom B, Soper K, West S, Morse M. The association of non-steroidal anti-inflammatory drugs with upper gastrointestinal tract bleeding. *Arch Intern Med.* 1987;147:85–8.

26. Shorr RI, Ray WA, Daugherty JR, Griffin MR. Concurrent use of nonsteroidal anti-inflammatory drugs and oral anticoagulants places elderly persons at high risk for hemorrhagic peptic ulcer disease. *Arch Intern Med.* 1993;153:1665–70.

27. Bollini P, Garcia Rodriguez LA, Perez Gutthann S, Walker AM. The impact of research quality and study design on epidemiologic estimates of the effect of non-steroidal anti-inflammatory drugs on upper gastrointestinal tract disease. *Arch Intern Med.* 1992;152:1289–95.

28. Henry D, Lim LL, García Rodríguez LA, Gutthann SP, Carson JL, Griffin M et al. Variability in risk of gastrointestinal complications with individual non-steroidal anti-inflammatory drugs: results of a collaborative meta-analysis. *BMJ.* 1996;312:1563–6.

29. Hernández-Díaz S, García Rodríguez LA. Overview of epidemiological studies published in the nineties on the association between non-steroidal anti-inflammatory drugs and upper gastrointestinal bleed/perforation. *Arch Intern Med.* 2001, in press.

30. Griffin MR, Piper JM, Daugherty JR, Snowden M, Ray WA. Nonsteroidal anti-inflammatory drug use and increased risk for peptic ulcer disease in elderly persons. *Ann Intern Med.* 1991;114:257–63.

31. Langman JS, Weil J, Wainwright P, Lawson DH, Rawlins MD, Logan RFA et al. Risks of bleeding peptic ulcer associated with individual non-steroidal anti-inflammatory drugs. *Lancet.* 1994;343:1075–8.

32. Olivero J, Graham D. Gastric adaptation to nonsteroidal anti-inflammatory drugs in man. *Scand J Gastroenterol.* 1992;27(suppl 193):53–8.

33. Traversa G, Walker AM, Ippolito FM, Caffari B, Capurso L, Dezi A et al. Gastroduodenal toxicity of different nonsteroidal antiinflammatory drugs. *Epidemiology.* 1995;6:49–54

34. Kaufman DW, Kelly JP, Sheehan JE, Laszlo A, Wiholm BE, Alfredsson L et al. Nonsteroidal anti-inflammatory drug use in relation to major upper gastrointestinal bleeding. *Clin Pharmacol Ther.* 1993;53:485–94.

35. Wilcox CM, Alexander LN, Cotsonis GA, Clark WS. Nonsteroidal antiinflammatory drugs are associated with both upper and lower gastrointestinal bleeding. *Dig Dis Sci.* 1997;42:990–7.

36. Hansen JM, Hallas J, Lauritsen JM, Bytzer P. Non-steroidal anti-inflammatory drugs and ulcer complications: a risk factor analysis for clinical decision-making. *Scand J Gastroenterol.* 1996;31:126–30.

37. Hernández-Díaz S, García Rodríguez L. Steroids and risk of upper gastrointestinal bleeding/perforation. *Am J Epidemiol.* 2001, in press.

38. Weil J, Colin-Jones D, Langman M, Lawson D, Logan R, Murphy M et al. Prophylactic aspirin and risk of peptic ulcer bleeding *BMJ.* 1995;310:827–30.

39. Kelly JP, Kaufman DW, Jugelon JM, Sheehan JE, Koff RS, Shapiro S. Risk of aspirin-associated major upper-gastrointestinal bleeding with enteric-coated or buffered product. *Lancet.* 1996;348:1414–16.

40. Hotiezer JW, Silvoso GR, Burks M, Ivey KJ. Comparison of the effects of regular and enteric-coated aspirin on gastroduodenal mucosa of man. *Lancet.* 1980;2:609–12.

41. Lanza FL, Royer GL, Nelson RS. Endoscopic evaluation of the effects of aspirin, buffered aspirin, and enteric-coated aspirin on gastric and duodenal mucosa. *N Engl J Med.* 1980;304:136–7.

42. Hawthorne AB, Mahida YR, Cole AT, Hawkey CJ. Aspirin-induced gastric mucosal damage: prevention by enteric coating and relation to prostaglandin synthesis. *Br J Clin Pharmacol.* 1991;32:77–83.

43. Petroski D. Endoscopic comparison of three aspirin preparations and placebo. *Clin Ther.* 1993;15:314–20.

44. Wolfe MM, Lichtenstein DR, Singh G. Gastrointestinal toxicity of nonsteroidal antiinflammatory drugs. *N Engl J Med.* 1999;340:1888–99.

45. Lanas A. Objective evidence of aspirin use in both ulcer and nonulcer upper and lower gastrointestinal bleeding. *Gastroenterology.* 1992;103:862–9.

46. Hernández-Díaz S, García Rodríguez L. Epidemiologic assessment of the safety of conventional nonsteroidal anti-inflammatory drugs. *Am J Med.* 2001, in press.

47. Matikainen M, Kangas E. Is there a relationship between the use of analgesics and non-steroidal anti-inflammatory drugs and acute upper gastrointestinal bleeding? A Finnish case-control prospective study. *Scand J Gastroenterol.* 1996;31:912–6.

48. Keating J, Chandran H. Antiinflammatory drugs and emergency surgery for peptic ulcers in the Waikato. *NZ Med J.* 1992;105:127–9.

49. Keating JP, McIlwaine J. Simultaneous small and large bowel ulceration associated with short term NSAID use. *NZ Med J.* 1993;106:438.

18 | Cyclooxygenase-2: a target for prevention of colorectal cancer

RAYMOND N. DUBOIS

Departments of Medicine and Cell Biology, MCN C-2104, Vanderbilt University Medical Center, The Vanderbilt-Ingram Cancer Center, Veteran Affairs Medical Center, Nashville, TN 37232-2279, USA.

Colorectal cancer is the second leading cause of cancer deaths in the United States, resulting in about 55000 deaths per year[1]. There have been several observational studies of the effects of exposure to non-steroid anti-inflammatory drugs (NSAIDs) and subsequent development of colorectal cancer[2]. These studies have been carried out in a variety of settings around the world, utilizing the outcomes of both colorectal cancer occurrence and mortality. Similar studies have revealed a reduction in the occurrence of adenomatous polyps in NSAID users[2]. Recently, a case control study also found a significant risk reduction with use of non-aspirin NSAIDs[3]. Therefore, the effect of NSAID use on colorectal cancer risk appears to be associated with the whole class of NSAIDs and not just one specific drug.

The side effects of any agent used for cancer prevention must be low to ensure compliance and to achieve the desired result, since the absolute risk of colorectal cancer in the general population is quite low. However, if high risk populations can be identified readily by genetic screening or by other testing, then the use of chemoprotective agents in those populations may be reasonable, due to a favourable risk:benefit ratio.

NSAID USE AND REDUCTION OF ADENOMA SIZE AND NUMBER IN FAMILIAL ADENOMATOUS POLYPOSIS PATIENTS

Familial adenomatous polyposis (FAP) is a rare inherited disease with variable phenotypic expression. It is associated with an increased risk of colorectal cancer at a young age. FAP is only responsible for about 1% of colorectal carcinomas in the general population. The genetic mutation responsible for this disease resides in the adenomatous polyposis coli (*APC*) gene located on chromosome 5. Somatic mutations in the *APC* gene have been reported in over 50% of sporadic colorectal cancer cases[4]. Colorectal cancer develops in most instances due to a series of histopathological and molecular changes in colonic epithelial cells (Figure 1). Genes that are affected during colorectal carcinogenesis include those that function as tumour suppressors (*APC, p53*), oncogenes (*Ras*) and DNA repair genes[5]. Waddell and Loughry first reported that regular use of the NSAID sulindac led to regression of rectal adenomas in four patients with FAP[6]. Following Waddell's initial account, several cases were reported describing adenoma resolution in FAP patients taking sulindac[2]. The first randomized placebo-controlled double-blind study of sulindac use in FAP patients was reported by Labayle et al.[7]. Sulindac treatment resulted in a complete or nearly complete regression of polyps in all patients. Giardiello et al. conducted another randomized double-blind controlled trial evaluating sulindac use in 40 patients with FAP[8]. The sulindac treated group were found to have a 44% decrease in polyp number and a 35% decrease in polyp size. However, no patient was found to have complete resolution of adenomas. Recently, a trial reporting the use of celecoxib, a selective COX-2 inhibitor, in FAP patients demonstrated a 30% reduction in polyp burden[9]. These results indicate that inhibition of COX-2 results in antineoplastic effects in humans.

POTENTIAL MECHANISMS FOR CHEMOPREVENTION OF INTESTINAL TUMOURS BY ASPIRIN AND OTHER NSAIDS

The anti-inflammatory and analgesic properties of NSAIDs are probably due to their inhibition of cyclooxygenase (COX) enzymes. These enzymes catalyse

Figure 1 Scheme for development of colorectal cancer. Colorectal cancer arises from a series of mutations in key genes which regulate cell growth and programmed cell death. COX-2 levels are increased in about 50% of adenomas and 80% of colorectal cancers.

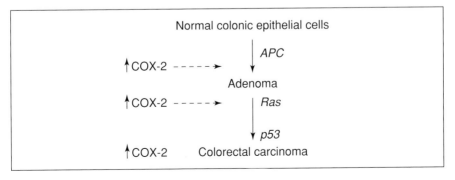

the conversion of arachidonic acid to endoperoxide (PGH_2), which is a substrate for a variety of prostaglandin (PG) synthases leading to formation of PGs and other eicosanoids. Two isoforms of COX have been reported, each possessing similar activities, but differing in expression patterns and sensitivity to inhibition by NSAIDs. COX-1, discovered first, is expressed constitutively in many tissues but can be regulated under certain circumstances[10]. A second inducible isoform of COX, referred to as COX-2, is induced by many factors[11]. The formation of COX-2 protein parallels the increase in PG production following stimulation with mitogens or tumour promoters in a wide variety of cell types[12].

Does COX-2 play a causal role in the development of gastrointestinal (GI) malignancy? We have found increased COX-2 expression in ~80% of human colorectal adenocarcinomas when compared with normal adjacent colonic mucosa[13] and this has been reported by other investigators using different techniques and patient populations[14–16]. Additionally, COX-2 mRNA and protein levels are increased in intestinal tumours that develop in rodents following carcinogen treatment[17] and in adenomas which develop in multiple intestinal neoplasia (*Min*) mice[18]. When intestinal epithelial cells are forced to express COX-2 constitutively they develop phenotypic changes, which include increased adhesion to extracellular matrix (ECM) and resistance to undergo programmed cell death[19]. Importantly, treatment with selective COX-2 inhibitors leads to a marked reduction in tumour burden in several different animal models[20–22].

Our observation of elevated COX-2 expression in three different models of colorectal cancer has led us to consider the possibility that COX-2 expression is related to colorectal carcinogenesis in a causal way. One study has provided compelling evidence that directly links COX-2 expression to intestinal tumour promotion[21]. This report shows that $APC^{\Delta716}$ mice, which develop hundreds of intestinal adenomas, bred with COX-2 null mice have an 80–90% reduction in tumour multiplicity in the homozygous COX-2 null offspring. These results suggest that COX-2 acts as a tumour promoter in the intestine and increased levels of COX-2 expression may result directly or indirectly from disruption of the *APC* gene. Interestingly, overexpression of *Wnt-1* or *Wnt-3A*, known modulators of the APC signalling pathway, causes a significant increase in COX-2 expression[23,24].

MECHANISMS FOR ANTI-NEOPLASTIC EFFECTS OF NSAIDS

Epidemiological data strongly support the chemoprotective effects of NSAIDs against gastrointestinal malignancies, while the data evaluating their benefit in other types of cancers is only emerging at this point. The precise mechanism by which NSAIDs prevent and/or cause regression of colorectal

tumours is not known. Despite different chemical structures, inhibition profiles, and drug half-lives, all NSAIDs in clinical use inhibit COX activity. Some
investigators have reported effects of NSAIDs which are not likely to be
due to their inhibition of COX activity. For example, some NSAIDs induce
apoptosis and alter gene expression in cultured cells given relatively high
concentrations (200–1000 µM)[25]. Some of these studies use COX-deficient
cell lines or drug metabolites lacking COX-inhibitory activity to rule out
the involvement of the COX pathway. The specific mechanisms for these
COX-independent effects and their therapeutic implications are not yet well
understood. However, work with the sulindac sulphone derivative implicates
signalling pathways not related to COX inhibition[26].

Prostaglandins are bioactive lipids that can affect the biological behaviour
of intestinal epithelial cells[27]. They usually act within the local environment
in which they are produced. In general, there are two classes of PG receptors
which can transduce signals upon ligand binding. The G-coupled seven transmembrane spanning receptors[28] and the nuclear peroxisome proliferation-
activated responses (PPAR)[29] are activated by binding of PGs to each respective receptor. Figure 2 schematically depicts some of the ligands which activate
the nuclear PPAR. PPARs are normally bound to a *cis* element located in the
promoter region as a heterodimer with retinoid X receptor (RXR). Activation
of gene transcription occurs only after ligand binding to each component of the
heterodimer (Figure 2). Several groups have demonstrated that PGs can serve
as activating ligands for PPARγ and PPARδ nuclear hormone receptors[29,30].
Mice lacking the PG EP$_1$ receptor developed fewer tumours following
carcinogen treatment than wild-type mice[31,32]. Figure 3 demonstrates hypothetical interactions in which PGs could modulate interactions with the *APC*
gene pathway. Future work aimed at obtaining a better understanding of how

Figure 2 The role of PPAR nuclear receptors in gene regulation.

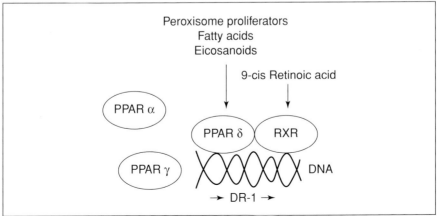

Figure 3 Hypothetical modulation of neoplastic pathways by PGE_2 signalling. PGE_2 receptors (EP_1–EP_4) are coupled to G protein signalling pathways which can activate intracellular calcium mobilization. Calcium is known to inhibit glycogen synthase kinase-3β (GSK3β) activity which could then lead to accumulation of β-catenin (b-cat) in the cytoplasm. This leads to nuclear localization of β-catenin and activation of transcription of the peroxisome proliferator activated receptor δ (PPARδ) via binding to T cell factor/lymphocyte enhancer factor (Tcf/LEF) *cis* regulatory elements.

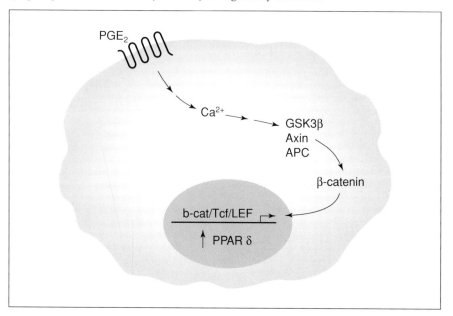

modulation of these PG-mediated signal transduction pathways affects the biology of carcinoma cells is essential to obtain a clear understanding of the role of COX in carcinogenesis.

SUMMARY

Prevention of colorectal cancer would have a significant impact on our society and is an important goal to achieve. Hopefully, advances in the discovery and testing of colorectal cancer genes will make the identification of cohorts at high risk for developing cancer more likely. Additionally, if agents such as the selective COX-2 inhibitors prove to be effective and have fewer adverse effects than non-selective NSAIDs, the risk:benefit ratio would be favourable. The next advance in this area of research will come from an improved understanding of the PG signalling pathways involved in the promotion of carcinogenesis. It is likely that targeting of more than one signalling pathway with combinations of agents will be more effective for cancer prevention than one agent alone. Human clinical trials evaluating the antineoplastic effects of selective COX-2 inhibitors are underway to determine if there is a role for these agents in cancer prevention and/or treatment.

ACKNOWLEDGEMENTS

This work was supported in part from the United States Public Health Services Grants DK 47297 (RND), P01CA77839 (RND), P30CA-68485 (RND). RND is a recipient of a VA Research Merit Grant. The author thanks the T. J. Martell Foundation and Katie Couric for their generous support.

Address all correspondence to: Raymond N. DuBois, M.D., Ph.D., Department of Medicine/GI; MCN C-2104, Vanderbilt University Medical Center, Nashville, TN 37232-2279, USA.

REFERENCES

1. Landis SH, Murray T, Bolden S, Wingo PA. Cancer statistics. *CA Cancer J Clin.* 1999;49:8–31.
2. Smalley W, DuBois RN. Colorectal cancer and non steroidal anti-inflammatory drugs. *Advances in Pharmacology.* 1997;39:1–20.
3. Smalley W, Ray WA, Daugherty J, Griffin MR. Use of nonsteroidal anti-inflammatory drugs and incidence of colorectal cancer: a population-based study. *Arch Int Med.* 1999;159:161–9.
4. Powell SM, Zilz N, Beazer-Barclay Y, Bryan TM, Hamilton SR, Thibodeau SN et al. APC mutations occur early during colorectal tumorigenesis. *Nature.* 1992;359:235–7.
5. Janne PA, Mayer RJ. Chemoprevention of colorectal cancer. *N Engl J Med.* 2000;342:1960–8.
6. Waddell WR, Loughry RW. Sulindac for polyposis of the colon. *J Surg Oncol.* 1983;24:83–7.
7. Labayle D, Fischer D, Vielh P, Drouhin F, Pariente A, Bories C et al. Sulindac causes regression of rectal polyps in familial adenomatous polyposis. *Gastroenterology.* 1991;101:635–9.
8. Giardiello FM, Hamilton SR, Krush AJ, Piantadosi S, Hylind LM, Celano P et al. Treatment of colonic and rectal adenomas with sulindac in familial adenomatous polyposis. *N Engl J Med.* 1993;328:1313–6.
9. Steinbach G, Lynch PM, Phillips RKS, Wallace MH, Hawk E, Gordon GB et al. The effect of celecoxib, a cyclooxygenase-2 inhibitor, in familial adenomatous polyposis. *N Engl J Med.* 2000;342:1946–52.
10. Smith CJ, Morrow JD, Roberts LJ, Marnett LJ. Differentiation of monocytoid THP-1 cells with phorbol ester induces expression of prostaglandin endoperoxide synthase-1 (COX-1). *Bioch Biophys Res Commun.* 1993;192:787–93.
11. Williams CW, DuBois RN. Prostaglandin endoperoxide synthase: why two isoforms? *Am J Physiol.* 1996;270:G393–400.
12. Williams CS, Mann M, DuBois RN. The role of cyclooxygenases in inflammation, cancer and development. *Oncogene.* 1999;18:7908–16.

13. Eberhart CE, Coffey RJ, Radhika A, Giardiello FM, Ferrenbach S, DuBois RN. Up-regulation of cyclooxygenase-2 gene expression in human colorectal adenomas and adenocarcinomas. *Gastroenterology.* 1994;107:1183–88.

14. Kargman S, O'Neill G, Vickers P, Evans J, Mancini J, Jothy S. Expression of prostaglandin G/H synthase-1 and -2 protein in human colon cancer. *Cancer Res.* 1995;55:2556–9.

15. Sano H, Kawahito Y, Wilder RL, Hashiramoto A, Mukai S, Asai K et al. Expression of cyclooxygenase-1 and -2 in human colorectal cancer. *Cancer Res.* 1995;55:3785–9.

16. Chapple KS, Cartwright EJ, Hawcroft G, Tisbury A, Bonifer C, Scott N et al. Localization of Cyclooxygenase-2 in human sporadic colorectal adenoma. *Am J Pathol.* 2000;156:545–53.

17. DuBois RN, Radhika A, Reddy BS, Entingh AJ. Increased cyclooxygenase-2 levels in carcinogen-induced rat colonic tumors. *Gastroenterology.* 1996;110:1259–62.

18. Williams CW, Luongo C, Radhika A, Zhang T, Lamps LW, Nanney LB et al. Elevated cyclooxygenase-2 levels in *Min* mouse adenomas. *Gastroenterology.* 1996;111:1134–40.

19. Tsujii M, DuBois RN. Alterations in cellular adhesion and apoptosis in epithelial cells overexpressing prostaglandin endoperoxide synthase-2. *Cell.* 1995;83:493–501.

20. Kawamori T, Rao CV, Seibert K, Reddy BS. Chemopreventive activity of celecoxib, a specific cyclooxygenase-2 inhibitor, against colon carcinogenesis. *Cancer Res.* 1998;58:409–12.

21. Oshima M, Dinchuk JE, Kargman SL, Oshima H, Hancock B, Kwong E et al. Suppression of intestinal polyposis in APC$^{\Delta716}$ knockout mice by inhibition of prostaglandin endoperoxide synthase-2 (COX-2). *Cell.* 1996;87:803–9.

22. Sheng H, Shao J, Kirkland SC, Isakson P, Coffey R, Morrow J et al. Inhibition of human colon cancer cell growth by selective inhibition of cyclooxygenase-2. *J Clin Invest.* 1997;99:2254–9.

23. Howe LR, Subbaramaiah K, Chung WJ, Dannenberg AJ, Brown AM. Transcriptional activation of cyclooxygenase-2 in *Wnt-1*-transformed mouse mammary epithelial cells. *Cancer Res.* 1999;59:1572–7.

24. Haertel-Wiesmann M, Liang Y, Fantl WJ, Williams LT. Regulation of cyclo-oxygenase-2 and periostin by *wnt-3* in mouse mammary epithelial cells. *J Biol Chem.* 2000;275:32046–51.

25. Williams CS, Smalley W, DuBois RN. Aspirin use and potential mechanisms for colorectal cancer prevention. *J Clin Invest.* 1997;100:1–5.

26. Goluboff ET, Shabsigh A, Saidi JA, Weinstein IB, Mitra N, Heitjan D et al. Exisulind (sulindac sulfone) suppresses growth of human prostate cancer in a nude mouse xenograft model by increasing apoptosis. *Urology.* 1999;53:440–5.

27. DuBois RN, Abramson SB, Crofford L, Gupta RA, Simon LS, Van De Putte LB et al. Cyclooxygenase in biology and disease. *FASEB J.* 1998;12:1063–73.

28. Breyer MD, Breyer RM. Prostaglandin receptors: their role in regulating renal function. *Curr Opin Nephrol Hypertens.* 2000;9:23–9.

29. Kliewer SA, Lehmann JM, Milburn MV, Willson TM. The PPARs and PXRs: nuclear xenobiotic receptors that define novel hormone signaling pathways. *Recent Prog Horm Res.* 1999;54:345–67.

30. Gupta RA, Tan J, Krause WF, Geraci MW, Willson TM, Dey SK et al. Prostacyclin-mediated activation of peroxisome proliferation-activated receptor δ in colorectal cancer. *Proc Natl Acad Sci USA.* 2000;97:13275–80.

31. Watanabe K, Kawamori T, Nakatsugi S, Ohta T, Ohuchida S, Yamamoto H et al. Role of the prostaglandin E receptor subtype EP1 in colon carcinogenesis. *Cancer Res.* 1999;59:5093–6.
32. Watanabe K, Kawamori T, Nakatsugi S, Ohta T, Ohuchida S, Yamamoto H et al. Inhibitory effect of a prostaglandin E receptor subtype EP(1) selective antagonist, ONO-8713, on development of azoxymethane-induced aberrant crypt foci in mice. *Cancer Lett.* 2000;156:57–61.

19 | Role of cyclooxygenase-2 in carcinogenesis other than colorectal cancer

ARI RISTIMÄKI,[1,3] KIRSI NARKO,[1] OUTI NIEMINEN[2] AND KIRSI SAUKKONEN[1]

[1]*Department of Obstetrics and Gynaecology,* [2]*Department of Surgery, and* [3]*Department of Pathology, Helsinki University Central Hospital and the Haartman Institute, University of Helsinki, Finland.*

Record linkage studies in Finland and Sweden have demonstrated a lower incidence of stomach and colorectal cancers among patients with rheumatoid arthritis when compared with the general population[1-3]. Since these patients use extensive amounts of non-steroid anti-inflammatory drugs (NSAIDs), it was suggested that the use of NSAIDs could be responsible for reduced cancer incidence. Subsequently, several population-based observational and controlled epidemiological studies have shown that prolonged use of aspirin and other NSAIDs is associated with a 40–50% reduction in the risk of colorectal cancer[4-6]. Furthermore, sulindac, another NSAID, causes regression of colorectal adenomatous polyps in patients with familial adenomatous polyposis (FAP), and several NSAIDs inhibit carcinogenesis in experimental animal models[5,6]. Interestingly, the effect of NSAIDs does not seem to be restricted to colorectal cancer, since the use of aspirin has been associated with reduced incidence of both cancer of the oesophagus and the stomach[7-11], and possibly with that of lung and breast cancers[12,13].

The best known target of NSAIDs is cyclooxygenase (COX), the rate-limiting enzyme in the conversion of arachidonic acid to prostanoids (see Chapter 1). Two COX genes have been cloned (COX-1 and COX-2); encoding proteins that share over 60% identity at the amino acid level and have similar enzymatic activities[14-16]. The most striking difference between the COX genes is in the regulation of their expression. While COX-1 is constitutively expressed and the expression is not usually regulated, expression of COX-2 is low or not detectable in most tissues, but can be highly induced in response to cell activation by hormones, proinflammatory cytokines, growth factors and tumour promoters. Thus, COX-1 is considered as a housekeeping gene, and prostanoids synthesized via the COX-1 pathway are thought to be responsible for cytoprotection of the stomach, for vasodilatation in the kidney, and for production of a proaggregatory prostanoid, thromboxane, by the platelets. In contrast, COX-2 is an inducible immediate-early gene, and its pathophysiological role has been connected to inflammation, reproduction and carcinogenesis[14,17]. However, it is important to bear in mind that this model may be too simplistic, since expression of COX-2 has been linked to physiological function and development of the kidney, and since, at least in some instances, prostanoids produced by COX-2 act as anti-inflammatory and/or immunosuppressive agents[18–20]. It should also be recognized that NSAIDs may have other cellular targets than COX enzymes[21]. Importantly, however, recent studies suggest that COX-2 is one of the targets of NSAIDs in the prevention of intestinal carcinogenesis. First, elevated levels of COX-2 mRNA and protein, but not those of COX-1, have been detected in human colorectal cancer[14,17]. Second, selective COX-2 inhibitors suppress neoplasia formation in rodent models of intestinal carcinogenesis, and genetic disruption of COX-2 suppresses the polyp formation in APC$^{\Delta716}$-knockout (adenomatous polyposis coli gene mutation) and in *Min* (multiple intestinal neoplasia) mice, which are models for FAP[17,22,23]. In addition to colorectal cancer, expression of COX-2 is elevated in several human malignancies and in animal models of carcinogenesis. This review concentrates on the expression and relevance of COX-2 in carcinogenesis other than colorectal cancer, (for colorectal cancer see chapter 18).

ANALYSIS OF COX-2 GENE EXPRESSION IN CANCER SPECIMENS

COX-2 gene products can be measured in tissue samples by analysing either mRNA, by using Northern blot analysis or reverse transcriptase–polymerase chain reaction (RT-PCR), or protein by using Western blotting or immunoprecipitation. The advantage of these techniques is that they deliver relatively quantitative data, although this can be difficult in the case of RT-PCR, especially when studying small tissue samples. Levels of COX-2 mRNA and protein correlate relatively well in cancer specimens, but it should be emphasized that, at least in reproductive tissues, the level of the mRNA may correlate better with the biologically active COX-2 protein than the amount of the immunoreactive protein. Furthermore, these techniques do not identify the cellular location of the gene products, and thus optimally one should combine them with either *in situ* hybridization or immunohistochemistry. Both of these techniques should deliver similar data since COX-2 is an intracellular enzyme.

It is important to recognize that COX-2 gene products, especially mRNA, are relatively labile and thus the tissue collection needs to be planned carefully to minimize delays and variability in tissue handling. When analysing gene expression from whole-tissue specimens, one should still examine the histological section of the sample in order to confirm the type of the tumour and percentage of tumour cells within the specimen. Special care should be taken in collection of control material, since COX-2 expression may be elevated in adjacent non-neoplastic mucosa next to the tumour. Thus, optimally, one should use material obtained from subjects who do not suffer from malignancies or chronic inflammatory diseases. However, this can be especially problematic when, for example, deciding on the 'right' control tissue for metaplastic tissue (adaptive substitution of one type of differentiated cell for another type of adult cell) or when studying carcinomas that originate from a very thin layer of epithelium, as is the case for the ovaries.

Specificity of reagents (probes and antibodies) can be tested by using known control tissues or cell lines that express only one of the COX isoforms, or by using recombinant proteins. However, even an antibody that has been confirmed to be COX-2-specific in immunoblotting does not necessarily perform well in immunohistochemistry. In our experience, simple omission of the primary antibody or its replacement with a non-immune control serum are not sufficient control experiments. More adequately one should perform preadsorption with either antigenic peptide or recombinant protein. In addition, several specimens need to be examined, since some antibodies give both specific and unspecific signals. In fact, in our experience, all non-affinity purified polyclonal antibody preparations tested suffer from either poor sensitivity or poor specificity in immunohistochemistry. In contrast, all cancer cell staining of a monoclonal antibody (160112, Cayman Chemical Co., Ann Arbor, MI, USA) was blocked by antigenic peptide or recombinant COX-2 protein but not by COX-1 protein or a non-COX-2 peptide. The pattern of the COX-2 staining is diffuse or of a slightly granular cytoplasmic type with occasional perinuclear positivity, especially in strongly staining cells. Interestingly, the staining of an individual cancer specimen can be quite heterogeneous, ranging from strong to none within a single sample. However, optimally one should confirm the immunohistochemistry data even with this antibody by using an unrelated COX-2 antibody or by detecting mRNA using *in situ* hybridization.

GASTRIC CANCER

Cancer of the stomach is one of the most frequent and lethal malignancies in the world[24]. The aetiopathogenesis of gastric cancer is complex and incompletely understood, but diet, infections and genetic factors are involved. More than 90% of gastric cancers are adenocarcinomas, which are divided into two histological types (intestinal and diffuse) by the Laurén classification[25]. Pathogenesis of the intestinal type cancer has been connected to precursor changes, such as chronic atrophic gastritis, intestinal metaplasia and dysplasia, while the diffuse type lacks well-recognized premalignant lesions.

Normal human stomach mucosa expresses almost exclusively the COX-1 isoform of the two known COX enzymes[26–28]. Elevated levels of COX-2 mRNA and protein, but not those of COX-1, have been detected in 67–100% of gastric adenocarcinoma specimens when compared with paired non-neoplastic mucosa and measured by Northern and Western blot analyses[27–32] (Table 1). A limited number of immunohistochemical observations have been made about the expression of COX-2 in gastric cancer. These data show quite variable frequency and diversity in cellular distribution of immunoreactive COX-2 protein[27,29,33,34]. Our unpublished data indicate that the frequency of COX-2-positive intestinal type gastric adenocarcinomas is approximately 60% and that only a few diffuse-type tumours (6%) stain for COX-2 as detected by immunohistochemistry (Figure 1a). In agreement with our data, colorectal tumours with a histological pattern of signet ring cells, a typical feature of diffuse type gastric cancer[24,25], contain low levels of COX-2 immuno-reactivity[35]. In addition to different histological patterns, recent reports indicate that tumours with certain genotypic features (defective mismatch repair) express reduced amounts of COX-2 in both gastric and colorectal cancers[31,35]. It is important to note that in our experience gastric adenocarcinoma specimens have a high frequency (up to 50%) of COX-2-positive erosions and ulcerations. This injury-associated COX-2 expression localizes to the connective tissue cells and inflammatory cells. Thus, the frequency of COX-2-positive tumours may be overestimated when analysing mRNA or protein from whole-tissue preparations, since a proportion of the signal may originate from non-neoplastic cells at sites of mucosal injury. This is especially important in regard to tumours that express low or non-detectable levels of COX-2 (diffuse-

Table 1 COX-2 expression in gastric, oesophageal and lung adenocarcinomas

COX-2 *gene product*	*Gastric*	*Oesophageal*	*Lung*
mRNA	73% (*n* = 11)[a]	100% (*n* = 5)[b]	75% (*n* = 4)[a]
Protein	73% (*n* = 186)[c] (range 67–100%)	78% (*n* = 27)[d]	79% (*n* = 192)[c] (range 72–100%)

Method of detection:
[a] Northern blot
[b] Reverse transcriptase polymerase chain reaction
[c] Western blot
[d] Immunohistochemistry
The following references were used: gastric[27–32], oesophagus[68,70] and lung[76,77,79–81].

Figure 1 COX-2 immunoreactivity localized almost exclusively to the neoplastic epithelial cells in human gastric (a, b), oesophageal (c, d) and lung (e, f) premalignant and malignant lesions, as detected by immunohistochemistry using a COX-2-specific monoclonal antibody (160112, Cayman Chemical Co., Ann Arbor, MI, USA). (a) Intestinal type gastric adenocarcinoma (insert shows preadsorption control with the antigenic peptide). (b) Definitive dysplasia of the stomach that showed no evidence for invasion (insert shows the preadsorption control). (c) Oesophageal adenocarcinoma. (d) Oesophageal squamous cell carcinoma. Note the non-neoplastic epithelium on the left and strongly staining cancer cells on the right. (e) Bronchiolo-alveolar type of lung adenocarcinoma (insert shows the preadsorption control). (f) Squamous cell carcinoma of the lung (insert shows the preadsorption control). Original magnification for a–c, e and f, ×400. Magnification for d, ×200.

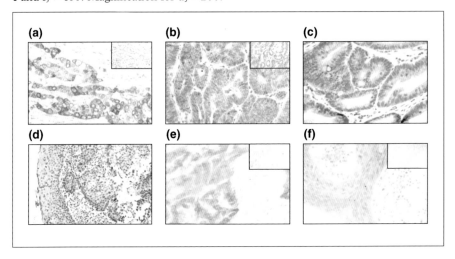

type gastric adenocarcinoma) but are frequently associated with mucosal injuries.

Helicobacter pylori has been classified as a Group 1 carcinogen for gastric cancer by WHO[24]. Although factors released by *H. pylori*-induced expression of COX-2 in a gastric carcinoma cell line[36], it is unlikely that the infection itself is a major cause for COX-2 expression in carcinoma cells *in vivo*. We would like to propose that elevated COX-2 expression in gastric cancer is more likely to depend on intrinsic events within the carcinoma cell, such as activation of oncogenes or inactivation of anti-oncogenes, and/or paracrine interaction of the tumour cells with the stromal compartment. In support of this, it is the carcinoma cells rather than the stroma that express COX-2 in gastric cancer[27,29,33,34], while in *H. pylori* gastritis COX-2 expression is localized to the connective tissue cells and inflammatory mononuclear cells rather than to the epithelial cells[37–40]. Interestingly, our results suggest that COX-2 is expressed in dysplastic epithelium of the stomach (Figure 1b), This indicates that overexpression of COX-2 in the epithelial cells is not restricted to the invasive cancer, but is also present in precarcinogenic lesions (Figure 2). However, it is possible that chronic inflammation-induced expression of COX-2 in fibroblasts and in macrophages contributes to the sequence leading to neoplastic transformation.

COX-2 expression has been reported to correlate with invasion of the lymphatic vessels, lymph node metastasis, and advanced tumour stage in gastric cancer[30,31]. Furthermore, it was recently reported that COX-2 expression correlates with density of CD34-positive microvascular endothelial cells, which may imply that COX-2 overexpression is associated with angiogenesis in gastric cancer[32]. This is supported by experimental animal studies, in which a COX-2-selective inhibitor suppressed angiogenesis and tumour growth of a COX-2-expressing gastric cancer cell line in nude mice[41]. Interestingly, a non-selective COX inhibitor reduced angiogenesis in xenografts of a non-COX-2 expressing cell line, indicating that inhibition of vascular endothelial COX-1 may be an anti-angiogenic target. These data are consistent with *in vitro* experiments on angiogenesis[42,43].

In animal models, inhibition of COX-2 delayed ulcer healing of the stomach[44–46] and exacerbated inflammation-associated colonic injury[47,48].

Figure 2 Chronic irritation and inflammation, which may lead to neoplastic transformation, seem to induce COX-2 expression mainly in non-epithelial cells such as fibroblasts and mononuclear inflammatory cells. COX-2 is expressed in preneoplastic lesions, especially in dysplasias, predominantly in the neoplastic epithelium. In adenocarcinomas COX-2 is expressed almost exclusively by the cancer cells.

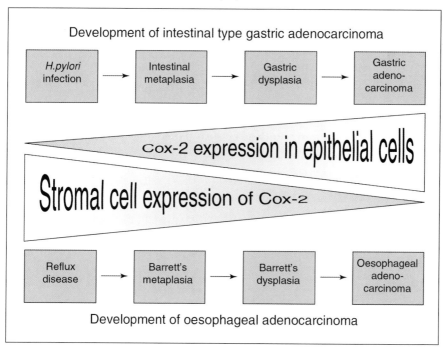

Thus, although selective COX-2 inhibitors spare normal gastrointestinal prostanoid synthesis, and therefore are safer than the non-selective drugs, they may reduce healing processes of the gastrointestinal mucosa. However, it is not known whether these animal models are applicable to humans. Pro-inflammatory cytokines (IL-1 and TNF-α) upregulate COX-2 expression during ulcer healing in the rat[49]. There may also exist an amplifying loop between hepatocyte growth factor (HGF) and COX-2-derived prostanoids, since, on the one hand, prostaglandins (PGs) induce production of HGF by gastric fibroblasts[50,51] and, on the other hand, HGF can trigger COX-2 expression in gastric epithelial cells[52,53]. Interestingly, HGF also stimulates PG production by gastric carcinoma cells[54]. It is not known, whether stromal cell-derived growth factors or cytokines stimulate expression of COX-2 in adenocarcinoma cells *in vivo*.

In contrast to several other animal models of carcinogenesis[5,6], NSAIDs (aspirin and flurbiprofen) enhance chemically-induced gastric carcinogenesis in the rat[55-57]. This may indicate that prostanoids produced by the gastric mucosa protect against the action of carcinogens in this rodent model. In contrast to the rat, chemically-induced gastric tumour multiplicity and incidence were reduced by sulindac and ibuprofen in mice[58]. PGs inhibit the growth of human gastric adenocarcinoma cell lines *in vitro* and *in vivo*[59-61]. It is unclear, which, if any, of these experimental models are relevant to human carcinogenesis. Indeed, epidemiological studies suggest that the use of NSAIDs is associated with a reduced risk of gastric cancer[1,2,7,9-11], and that administration of PGE_1 or PGE_2 induces hyperplasia, but not atypia, of the gastric mucosa[62,63]. Furthermore, a COX-2-selective inhibitor reduced the growth of a COX-2-expressing human gastric carcinoma cell line, but not that of non-expressing cell lines[64,65]. Inhibition of COX-2 also reduces growth of the COX-2 expressing gastric cancer cell line in nude mice, mainly by inducing apoptosis[66]. It remains to be studied whether inhibition of COX-2 suppresses chemically or genetically induced gastric neoplasias in rodents, and whether COX-2 inhibitors can be used in the treatment of patients who have preneoplastic gastric lesions or suffer from gastric cancer.

OESOPHAGEAL CANCER

Barrett's oesophagus is the replacement of normal squamous oesophageal epithelium by a metaplastic specialized columnar lining in response to chronic reflux of acid, gastric contents and bile to the oesophagus[67]. Development of Barrett's oesophagus has been connected to the Western life style, especially obesity, and it predisposes to oesophageal adenocarcinoma. Adenocarcinoma in Barrett's oesophagus follows a sequence of events during which this meta-plastic epithelium develops to a dysplasia, followed by early adenocarcinoma, and eventually an invasive carcinoma. Incidence of oesophageal adenocarcinoma has increased during the past decades and it accounts for up to one half of the oesophageal carcinomas. Squamous cell carcinoma of the oesophagus has been connected with tobacco and alcohol consumption, and this condition is preceded by squamous dysplasia, followed by *in situ* carcinoma, which then transforms to an invasive carcinoma.

COX-2 mRNA levels were found to be elevated in 80% of Barrett's meta-plasia tissues when compared with gastric body control samples, as detected by RT-PCR[68]. COX-2 protein expression was elevated by 1.6–2.2-fold in Barrett's metaplasia when compared with either squamous epithelium of the oesophagus or columnar epithelium of the duodenum, as detected by immunoblotting[69]. However, COX-2 immunoreactivity shows variable local-ization in Barrett's metaplasia, and it is unclear to what extent the positivity is in the lamina propria connective tissue cells and inflammatory cells versus the epithelial cells[68–70]. This discrepancy may partially depend on specificity and sensitivity issues related to different COX-2 antibodies and staining protocols or, alternatively, on tissue collection and handling procedures. In contrast, COX-2 protein has been localized consistently to the epithelial cells of Barrett's dysplasia and oesophageal adenocarcinoma[68,69] (Table 1 and Figure 1c), which is consistent with our data on dysplasia and intestinal type adenocarcinoma of the stomach (see above). Bile acids have been shown to induce COX-2 expression in an oesophageal adenocarcinoma cell line[71] and in organ cultures of Barrett's epithelium[69]. Reflux of bile salts and acid may thus account for the early expression of COX-2 during the development of Barrett's metaplasia, but it is uncertain to what extent this external stimu-lation is responsible for expression of COX-2 in dysplastic and adenocarci-noma cells arising from the Barrett's oesophagus. An alternative hypothesis is that neoplastic cells are either intrinsically more active in expressing COX-2 than non-neoplastic cells, or that stromal cells stimulate COX-2 expression in the cancer cells. COX-2 expression is also elevated in a considerable pro-portion (70–100%) of squamous cell carcinomas of the oesophagus and by precursor lesions leading to this disease[70,72,73] (Figure 1d). A COX-2-selective inhibitor, probably due to increased apoptosis, inhibited prolifera-tion of a COX-2-expressing human squamous carcinoma cell line of the oesophagus, but not that of a non-expressing cell line[70]. Finally, indomethacin has been shown to reduce the number of chemically-induced oesophageal tumours in mice[74].

LUNG CANCER

Lung cancer is the most prevalent malignancy in the world[75]. The role of external factors is particularly important in the pathogenesis of lung cancer, the single most important causal agent being cigarette smoke. Other important factors include exposure to radiation and a number of occupational-related factors, of which asbestos is the best-known example. Lung cancer is divided into different histopathological entities, of which adenocarcinoma and squamous cell carcinoma are the most frequent (25–40% each) followed by small cell lung cancer (20–25%) and large cell carcinoma (10–15%). Certain precursor changes have been associated with lung carcinoma; squamous cell carcinoma is thought to arise from a progressive dysplasia of metaplastic squamous epithelium, while atypia of alveolar lining epithelium is thought to represent a precursor lesion for bronchioloalveolar carcinoma, which is a subtype of lung adenocarcinoma[75].

Normal human lung epithelium expresses only low and scattered or non-detectable levels of COX-2 mRNA and protein[76–78]. Elevated levels of COX-2 mRNA and protein, but not those of COX-1, have been consistently detected in adenocarcinomas of the lung as measured by Northern blot, RT-PCR, and *in situ* hybridization techniques and by Western blot analysis[76–79] (Table 1). Immunohistochemical staining of COX-2 protein shows positivity in 72–100% of adenocarcinomas and in 31–100% of squamous cell carcinomas[76,77,79–81] (Figures 1e and 1f). However, stronger signals of COX-2 gene products have consistently been observed in adenocarcinomas when compared with squamous cell carcinomas[76,77–79]. We reported recently that COX-2 expression is especially high in the bronchioloalveolar adenocarcinoma[77]. All tumours of this type (9/9) were positive for COX-2 and 6/9 (67%) expressed COX-2 with strong intensity. Interestingly, recent reports indicate that inhaled indomethacin reduces bronchorrhoea (airway obstruction caused by sputum excretion that can lead to respiratory failure and even death) in patients with bronchioloalveolar carcinoma[82], which may be mediated via inhibition of COX-2[83].

COX-2 immunoreactivity was localized primarily to the carcinoma cells when compared with the stromal compartment, with the possible exception of inflammatory mononuclear cells[77,79,80,84]. COX-1 staining was weak, and comparable amounts of immunoreactivity were found in the stroma and in the tumour cells[79,84]. COX-2 expression has also been detected in either comparable or even elevated levels in lymph node metastasis when compared with the primary tumours[76,78]. This could indicate a role for COX-2 in acquisition of an invasive and metastatic phenotype. Small cell lung cancer and large cell lung cancer seem to express only low levels of COX-2, although the number of specimens studied is quite low[76,77].

We found elevated levels of COX-2 mRNA and immunoreactivity especially in the well-differentiated lung carcinomas[77]. In support of our finding, well-differentiated adenocarcinomas of the lung have been reported to be the most active producers of PGs[85], and expression of COX-2 correlates positively with the differentiated phenotype in colorectal adenocarcinoma cell lines[86]. However, this is in contrast to other reports that have indicated a stronger expression of COX-2 in poorly differentiated than in well- or moderately differentiated lung adenocarcinomas[76,78]. It is worth mentioning that we detected expression of COX-2 close to necrotic areas of poorly-differentiated adenocarcinomas that were otherwise negative for COX-2[77]. Perhaps hypoxia, which has been shown to induce COX-2 expression in vascular endothelium[87], or hypoxia-induced factors can stimulate COX-2 expression of lung cancer cells. Since K-*ras* oncogene is activated in about one third of lung adeno-carcinomas[88], and activation of *ras* oncogene has been associated with elevated expression of COX-2 in cell culture experiments[89–91], this particular mechanism may also explain part of the COX-2 expression found in lung carcinomas. It is important to recognize that *ras*-induced transformation does not require functional COX enzymes in fibroblasts[92], and that, at least in pancreatic tumours, K-*ras* mutations do not correlate with COX-2 expression[93].

We have also detected COX-2 expression in atypical alveolar epithelium in lung specimens obtained from lung cancer patients, who suffered from asbestosis or fibrosing alveolitis[77]. Fibrosing alveolitis, which is morphologically similar to asbestosis, is associated with atypia of alveolar epithelium and with an increased risk for bronchioloalveolar carcinoma[94]. Similarly, Hida et al.[76] have detected expression of COX-2 in premalignant lesions of the lung. It was recently reported that COX-2 expression correlates with survival in stage I adenocarcinomas of the lung, but not in more advanced lung tumours[81]. Similarly, an association of COX-2 expression and survival has been suggested for colorectal cancer[95]. All this indicates that precursor lesions that can lead to lung adenocarcinoma express COX-2, and that increased COX-2 expression could serve as a prognostic marker for patients undergoing surgical resection of early stage lung adenocarcinomas.

Both non-selective and COX-2-selective NSAIDs reduce nicotine-derived N-nitrosamine-induced lung tumours in rodents[58,96,97]. These tobacco-derived carcinogens also induce COX-2 expression in animal models of lung carcinogenesis[98–100]. There are at least two hypotheses of how COX-2 could promote tumour formation in these models. First, COX can enzymatically activate carcinogens and in this respect COX-2 seems to be the more potent of the two isoenzymes[97]. Second, carcinogen-induced immunosuppression may be partially mediated by COX-2-derived prostanoids, since it has been demonstrated that PGE_2 stimulates production of immunosupressive cytokines (IL-10) and inhibits that of antitumour immunomodulators (IL-12)[80,101]. In agreement with human data (as described earlier), COX-2 expression was not evident or very low in normal lung tissues, with some positivity in macrophage-like cells, but it was highly elevated in adenomas and adeno-carcinomas, and again less induced in hyperplasias or squamous cell carci-nomas of the rat lung[98,100,102]. Interestingly, both COX-1 and COX-2 were induced in mouse lung adenomas and adenocarcinomas, and COX-2 content of normal Clara cells, a putative precursor cell of lung adenocarcinoma, was equal to that of the neoplasms[99]. Finally, NSAIDs reduce proliferation of lung cancer cells *in vitro*[97,103], possibly by inducing apoptosis[104], and by inhibiting their invasive potential *in vivo*[105].

OTHER CANCERS

Squamous cell carcinoma of the skin

COX-2 expression is elevated in actinic keratosis and in squamous cell carcinoma of the human skin, but not in basal cell carcinoma or in melanoma[106,107]. Expression of COX-2 has also been connected to tumour promotion in a multistage carcinogenesis model of the mouse skin (reviewed in ref. 108). As this model so elegantly demonstrates, it is the COX-2-derived $PGF_{2\alpha}$ that can overcome the tumour-inhibitory effect of NSAIDs rather than PGE_2, which is most commonly connected to the pathogenesis of carcinomas[109]. It is also of interest that genetic deletion of COX-2, or its inhibition with selective drugs, reduced tumour formation in this mouse model[110,111]. Interestingly, skin tumour formation is also suppressed in COX-1 knockout animals, although the mechanism of action seems to be independent of $PGF_{2\alpha}$[108,111]. Ultraviolet light (UV) exposure increases COX-2 expression in cultured human keratinocytes and in intact human skin, and celecoxib has been shown to reduce UV-induced skin tumours in mice[112–115].

Squamous cell carcinoma of the head and neck

COX-2 expression is elevated in squamous cell carcinoma of the head and neck and in the adjacent normal-appearing epithelium when compared with oral mucosa from healthy subjects[116]. A selective COX-2 inhibitor (JTE-522) suppressed growth of a human head and neck squamous carcinoma cell line in nude mice[117].

Breast carcinoma

Normal breast tissue does not express COX-2 mRNA, but all breast cancer specimens contained variable amounts of COX-2 transcript that correlated with tumour cell density as detected by RT-PCR[118,119]. In addition, COX-1 mRNA and protein are elevated in breast cancer[119,120]. In fact, data obtained by immunoblotting and immunohistochemistry indicate that overexpression of COX-1 exceeds that of COX-2 in breast cancer[120]. While the expression of COX-2 was localized to the tumour cells, COX-1 was expressed by the stromal cells adjacent to the tumour[120]. Interestingly, the sum of COX-1 and COX-2 mRNA expression correlated with the aromatase activity in the breast cancer specimens[119]. In breast cancer cell lines, mutation of *ras* correlates with high COX-2 expression[121], and *ras* seems to mediate COX-2 expression induced by other oncogenes, such as *src*[122]. Cell culture experiments also suggest that COX-derived prostanoids induce matrix metalloproteinase expression in the tumour cells and production of growth factors (HGF) by the stromal cells, both of which can lead to higher invasive potential[123,124]. Recently celecoxib, as well as ibuprofen, reduced incidence, multiplicity and volume of chemically-induced breast cancers in the rat[125,126].

Pancreatic carcinoma

COX-2 expression has been detected in normal pancreatic islet cells, but not in ductal epithelium or acinar cells[127–130]. Elevated levels of COX-2 mRNA and protein have been detected in 54–100% of pancreatic carcinomas[93,128–131]. No significant correlation between COX-2 expression and prognosis or clinico-pathological factors was evident [131]. However, stronger and more frequent COX-2 expression was detected in invasive ductal adenocarcinomas (72%) than in intraductal papillary–mucinous adenocarcinomas (31%) or in intra-ductal papillary–mucinous adenomas (0%)[131]. Constitutive expression of COX-2 has been found in some pancreatic carcinoma cell lines, and the level of COX-2 expression correlated with the degree of differentiation of the tumours from which the cell lines originated[128]. Sulindac sulphide, indomethacin, and NS-398 inhibited cell proliferation of pancreatic cancer cell lines, but this was evident for both COX-2 expressing and non-expressing cell lines[93,128].

Hepatocellular carcinoma

COX-2 is expressed in liver cirrhosis, precancerous dysplasias of the liver and in hepatocellular carcinoma[132–134]. Expression of COX-2 was higher in well-differentiated tumours than in the less differentiated ones[132–134]. Although COX-2 expression did not correlate with prognosis of hepatocellular carci-noma, it predicted the disease-free survival of patients who suffered from chronic hepatitis or cirrhosis[133].

Transitional cell carcinoma of the urinary bladder

COX-2 is expressed in both non-invasive and invasive transitional cell carci-noma of the urinary bladder[135,161]. Recent animal studies suggest that COX-2 expression, but not that of COX-1, is elevated in bladder cancer[136,137], and that a COX-2-selective NSAID, nimesulide, inhibits chemically-induced bladder carcinoma in the rat[138].

Prostate carcinoma

Elevated levels of COX-2 were found in human and canine prostate adeno-carcinoma[139,140]. However, benign human specimens expressed significant amounts of COX-2 mRNA and protein and the expression of COX-2 in cancerous tissues was elevated only by 1.8–3.4-fold[139]. The biological activity of COX-2 protein in non-neoplastic versus malignant prostatic epithelium is not known. Sulindac, NS-398 and celecoxib can induce apoptosis in human prostate cancer cell lines, but it is unclear to what extent this effect is depen-dent on COX-2[141–143].

Cervical carcinoma

COX-2 expression correlated with lymph node metastasis and to parametrial invasion in stage 1B cervical carcinoma[144].

Ovarian carcinoma

Only COX-1 mRNA and protein have been detected in ovarian adenocarcinoma[27,145].

Other cancers

Studies on COX-2 expression in cancer have largely concentrated on adeno- and squamous cell carcinomas. However, two reports suggest that at least gliomas and retinoblastomas express COX-2[146,147]. Interestingly, in agreement with our data on poorly differentiated lung cancer specimens[77], COX-2 expression was present in glioma cells in the immediate vicinity of necroses[147].

CONCLUSIONS

Is there a connection between epidemiological data and expression of cyclooxygenase-2?

Epidemiological studies indicate that NSAIDs reduce the incidence of cancer especially in the gastrointestinal tract[1-12]. However, the only randomized trial on the effect of aspirin on colorectal cancer risk did not show a protective effect, which may be due to the low dose of the drug and/or short follow-up period[148]. COX-2 gene products have been shown to be consistently expressed with strong intensity and high frequency, especially in gastrointestinal and lung adenocarcinomas (Table 1 and Figure 1). It is interesting to note that while the use of NSAIDs has been associated with lower risk of gastric cancer in the distal part of the stomach (corpus and antrum), the effect of NSAIDs was not apparent in the proximal part (cardia) of the stomach[9,10]. To this end, it is especially intriguing that expression of COX-2 is less prominent in cardia cancer when compared with carcinoma of the distal stomach (ref. 33 and our unpublished data). Similarly, no association between NSAID use and incidence of ovarian cancer was found[149]; again COX-2 expression in ovarian cancer is low or non-existent[27,145]. Thus, there seems to be some correlation between the epidemiological data and the expression of COX-2 in human carcinomas.

The COX-2–tumour hypothesis is further supported by experiments in which non-selective NSAIDs, COX-2-selective drugs, and disruption of the COX-2 gene suppress tumour formation in various experimental animal models. However, this does not rule out the possibility that COX-1 plays a role in carcinogenesis. It should also be recognized that, in addition to tumour cells, expression of COX-1 and/or COX-2 by the tumour stroma (connective tissue cells, inflammatory cells and vascular endothelium) may contribute to tumorigenesis[150,151]. Finally, NSAIDs facilitate effects that are either independent of prostanoids, but still dependent on COX enzymes, or totally COX-independent[21]. However, most of these studies have been performed only *in vitro* and in most cases NSAID concentrations (>100 μM) exceed the pharmacologically relevant *in vivo* doses.

What is the mechanism of cyclooxygenase-2 overexpression in tumours?

The COX-2 gene itself does not seem to mutate during carcinogenesis[152]. Thus, activation of oncogenes or inactivation of anti-oncogenes could enhance COX-2 expression in transformed cells, which has been shown to be the case in cell culture conditions[17,89–91,121,153–155]. However, it is poorly known which (anti)oncogenes are responsible for COX-2 expression in human malignancies. Furthermore, COX enzymes do not seem to be necessary for malignant transformation[92]. In addition to intracrine regulation of COX-2 expression, cytokines and growth factors could induce COX-2 expression in malignant cells via autocrine (tumour cell) or paracrine (stromal) pathways. In fact, it seems that during chronic irritation and inflammation, which may lead to formation of premalignant lesions, it is the stromal compartment that expresses COX-2, but that the expression shifts progressively to the neoplastic epithelial cells as the lesion progresses in the direction of invasive cancer (Figure 2). It is also becoming more apparent that both phenotypic and genotypic subclasses of adenocarcinomas may express COX-2 with quite contrasting frequency and intensity.

What is the mechanism and significance of cyclooxygenase-2-induced tumorigenesis?

It is not well known whether COX-2 contributes to carcinogenesis by removing excess arachidonic acid, by producing prostanoids or by metabolizing other compounds. It has, however, been demonstrated that many effects of COX-2 can be facilitated by either PGE_2 or $PGF_{2\alpha}$, including stimulation of proliferation (in many cases by inhibition of apoptosis), enhanced production of matrix metalloproteinases, promotion of angiogenesis and induction of immunosuppression. It will be of great interest to follow the COX-2 field in future years, and to see whether COX-2 can be used as a prognostic marker in neoplastic conditions. It will also be important to recognize whether expression of either COX-2 and/or COX-1 has a predictive value for the treatment of patients with NSAIDs. Clinically, it is important to determine whether selective COX-2 inhibitors will deliver safer and at least as effective anticancer properties as non-selective NSAIDs. In addition, subtypes of premalignant lesions or advanced cancers (histology, stage and/or genotype) that are especially sensitive to NSAIDs should be recognized. Finally, it will be important to integrate NSAIDs into already existing radio- and/or chemotherapy protocols[156–158] and at the same time continue research on alternative, and hopefully less toxic, combination treatments of cancer[159,160].

ACKNOWLEDGEMENTS

The Helsinki University Central Hospital Research Funds and the Finnish Cancer Foundation supported our original studies. The Helsinki University Biomedical Graduate School supported K.S. We thank Tuija Hallikainen for helping with the preparation of the manuscript.

Address all correspondence to: Dr Ari Ristimäki, Department of Obstetrics and Gynecology, Helsinki University Central Hospital, PO Box 140, FIN-00029 Helsinki, Finland.

REFERENCES

1. Isomäki HA, Hakulinen T, Joutsenlahti U. Excess risk of lymphomas, leukemia and myeloma in patients with rheumatoid arthritis. *J Chron Dis.* 1978;31:691–6.
2. Laakso M, Mutru O, Isomäki H, Koota K. Cancer mortality in patients with rheumatoid arthritis. *J Rheumatol.* 1986;13:522–6.
3. Gridley G, McLaughlin JK, Ekbom A, Klareskog L, Adami HO, Hacker DG et al. Incidence of cancer among patients with rheumatoid arthritis. *J Natl Cancer Inst.* 1993;85:307–11.
4. Thun MJ. Aspirin, NSAIDs, and digestive tract cancers. *Cancer Metastasis Rev.* 1994;13:269–77.
5. Giardiello FM, Offerhaus GJA, DuBois RN. The role of nonsteroidal anti-inflammatory drugs in colorectal cancer prevention. *Eur J Cancer.* 1995;31A:1071–6.
6. International Agency for Research on Cancer. Aspirin. In: *IARC Handbooks on Cancer Prevention*, Vol. 1: *Non-steroidal anti-inflammatory drugs.* Lyon: International Agency for Research on Cancer; 1997:43–90.
7. Thun MJ, Namboodiri MM, Calle EE, Flanders WD, Heath CW Jr. Aspirin use and risk of fatal cancer. *Cancer Res.* 1993;53:1322–7.
8. Funkhouser EM, Sharp GB. Aspirin and reduced risk of esophageal carcinoma. *Cancer.* 1995;76:1116–19.
9. Farrow DC, Vaughan TL, Hansten PD, Stanford JL, Risch HA, Gammon MD et al. Use of aspirin and other nonsteroidal anti-inflammatory drugs and risk of esophageal and gastric cancer. *Cancer Epidemiol Biomarkers Prev.* 1998;7:97–102.
10. Zaridze D, Borisova E, Maximovitch D, Chkhikvadze V. Aspirin protects against gastric cancer: results of a case-control study from Moscow, Russia. *Int J Cancer.* 1999;82:473–6.
11. Coogan PF, Rosenberg L, Palmer JR, Strom BL, Zauber AG, Stolley PD et al. Nonsteroidal anti-inflammatory drugs and risk of digestive cancers at sites other than the large bowel. *Cancer Epidemiol Biomarkers Prev.* 2000;9:119–23.
12. Schreinemachers DM, Everson RB. Aspirin use and lung, colon, and breast cancer incidence in a prospective study. *Epidemiology.* 1994;5:138–46.
13. Harris RE, Namboodiri KK, Farrar WB. Nonsteroidal anti-inflammatory drugs and breast cancer. *Epidemiology.* 1996;7:203–5.

14. Dubois RN, Abramson SB, Crofford L, Gupta RA, Simon LS, van de Putte LBA et al. Cyclooxygenase in biology and disease. *FASEB J.* 1998;12:1063–73.

15. Taketo MM. Cyclooxygenase-2 inhibitors in tumorigenesis (Part I). *J Natl Cancer Inst.* 1998;90:1529–36.

16. Vane JR, Bakhle YS, Botting RM. Cyclooxygenases 1 and 2. *Annu Rev Pharmacol Toxicol.* 1998;38:97–120.

17. Taketo MM. Cyclooxygenase-2 inhibitors in tumorigenesis (Part II). *J Natl Cancer Inst.* 1998;90:1609–20.

18. Gilroy DW, Colville-Nash PR, Willis D, Chivers J, Paul-Clark MJ, Willoughby DA. Inducible cyclooxygenase may have anti-inflammatory properties. *Nat Med.* 1999;5:698–701.

19. Newberry RD, Stenson WF, Lorenz RG. Cyclooxygenase-2-dependent arachidonic acid metabolites are essential modulators of the intestinal immune response to dietary antigen. *Nat Med.* 1999;5:900–6.

20. Lipsky PE, Brooks P, Crofford LJ, DuBois R, Graham D, Simon LS et al. Unresolved issues in the role of cyclooxygenase-2 in normal physiologic processes and disease. *Arch Intern Med.* 2000;160:913–20.

21. Shiff SJ, Rigas B. The role of cyclooxygenase inhibition in the antineoplastic effects of nonsteroidal antiinflammatory drugs. *J Exp Med.* 1999;190:445–50.

22. Langenbach R, Loftin C, Lee C, Tiano H. Cyclooxygenase knockout mice: models for elucidating isoform-specific functions. *Biochem Pharmacol.* 1999;58:1237–46.

23. Reddy BS. The Fourth DeWitt S. Goodman Lecture. Novel approaches to the prevention of colon cancer by nutritional manipulation and chemoprevention. *Cancer Epidemiol Biomarkers Prev.* 2000;9:239–47.

24. Stadtländer CTK, Waterbor JW. Molecular epidemiology, pathogenesis and prevention of gastric cancer. *Carcinogenesis.* 1999;20:2195–207.

25. Laurén P. The two histological main types of gastric carcinoma: diffuse and so-called intestinal-type carcinoma. *Acta Path Microbiol Scand.* 1965;64:31–49.

26. Kargman S, Charleson S, Cartwright M, Frank J, Riendeau D, Mancini J et al. Characterization of prostaglandin G/H synthase 1 and 2 in rat, dog, monkey, and human gastrointestinal tracts. *Gastroenterology.* 1996;111:445–54.

27. Ristimäki A, Honkanen N, Jänkälä H, Sipponen P, Härkönen M. Expression of cyclooxygenase-2 in human gastric carcinoma. *Cancer Res.* 1997;57:1276–80.

28. Soydan AS, Gaffen JD, Weech PK, Tremblay NM, Kargman S, O'Neill G et al. Cytosolic phospholipase A$_2$, cyclo-oxygenases and arachidonate in human stomach tumours. *Eur J Cancer.* 1997;33:1508–12.

29. Uefuji K, Ichikura T, Mochizuki H, Shinomiya N. Expression of cyclooxygenase-2 protein in gastric adenocarcinoma. *J Surg Oncol.* 1998;69:168–72.

30. Murata H, Kawano S, Tsuji S, Tsuji M, Sawaoka H, Kimura Y et al. Cyclooxygenase-2 overexpression enhances lymphatic invasion and metastasis in human gastric carcinoma. *Am J Gastroenterol.* 1999;94:451–5.

31. Yamamoto H, Itoh F, Fukushima H, Hinoda Y, Imai K. Overexpression of cyclooxygenase-2 protein is less frequent in gastric cancers with microsatellite instability. *Int J Cancer.* 1999;84:400–3.

32. Uefuji K, Ichikura T, Mochizuki H. Cyclooxygenase-2 expression is related to prostaglandin biosynthesis and angiogenesis in human gastric cancer. *Clin Cancer Res.* 2000;6:135–8.

33. Ratnasinghe D, Tangrea JA, Roth MJ, Dawsey SM, Anver M, Kasprzak BA et al.

Expression of cyclooxygenase-2 in human adenocarcinomas of the gastric cardia and corpus. *Oncol Rep.* 1999;6:965–8.

34. Lim HY, Joo HJ, Choi JH, Yi JW, Yang MS, Cho DY et al. Increased expression of cyclooxygenase-2 protein in human gastric carcinoma. *Clin Cancer Res.* 2000;6:519–25.

35. Karnes WE Jr, Shattuck-Brandt R, Burgart LJ, DuBois RN, Tester DJ, Cunningham JM et al. Reduced COX-2 protein in colorectal cancer with defective mismatch repair. *Cancer Res.* 1998;58:5473–7.

36. Romano M, Ricci V, Memoli A, Tuccillo C, Di Popolo A, Sommi P et al. *Helicobacter pylori* up-regulates cyclooxygenase-2 mRNA expression and prostaglandin E$_2$ synthesis in MKN 28 gastric mucosal cells *in vitro*. *J Biol Chem.* 1998;273:28560–3.

37. Sawaoka H, Kawano S, Tsuji S, Tsuji M, Sun W, Gunawan ES et al. *Helicobacter pylori* infection induces cyclooxygenase-2 expression in human gastric mucosa. *Prostaglandins Leukot Essent Fatty Acids.* 1998;59:313–16.

38. Fu S, Ramanujam KS, Wong A, Fantry GT, Drachenberg CB, James SP et al. Increased expression and cellular localization of inducible nitric oxide synthase and cyclooxygenase 2 in *Helicobacter pylori* gastritis. *Gastroenterology.* 1999;116:1319–29.

39. McCarthy CJ, Crofford LJ, Greenson J, Scheiman JM. Cyclooxygenase-2 expression in gastric antral mucosa before and after eradication of *Helicobacter pylori* infection. *Am J Gastroenterol.* 1999;94:1218–23.

40. Tatsuguchi A, Sakamoto C, Wada K, Akamatsu T, Tsukui T, Miyake K et al. Localisation of cyclooxygenase 1 and cyclooxygenase 2 in *Helicobacter pylori* related gastritis and gastric ulcer tissues in humans. *Gut.* 2000;46:782–9.

41. Sawaoka H, Tsuji S, Tsujii M, Gunawan ES, Sasaki Y, Kawano S et al. Cyclooxygenase inhibitors suppress angiogenesis and reduce tumour growth *in vivo*. *Lab Invest.* 1999;79:1469–77.

42. Tsujii M, Kawano S, Tsuji S, Sawaoka H, Hori M, DuBois RN. Cyclooxygenase regulates angiogenesis induced by colon cancer cells. *Cell.* 1998;93:705–16.

43. Jones MK, Wang H, Peskar BM, Levin E, Itani RM, Sarfeh IJ et al. Inhibition of angiogenesis by nonsteroidal anti-inflammatory drugs: insight into mechanisms and implications for cancer growth and ulcer healing. *Nat Med.* 1999;5:1418–23.

44. Mizuno H, Sakamoto C, Matsuda K, Wada K, Uchida T, Noguchi H et al. Induction of cyclooxygenase 2 in gastric mucosal lesions and its inhibition by the specific antagonist delays healing in mice. *Gastroenterology.* 1997;112:387–97.

45. Schmassmann A, Peskar BM, Stettler C, Netzer P, Stroff T, Flogerzi B et al. Effects of inhibition of prostaglandin endoperoxide synthase-2 in chronic gastro-intestinal ulcer models in rats. *Br J Pharmacol.* 1998;123:795–804.

46. Shigeta J, Takahashi S, Okabe S. Role of cyclooxygenase-2 in the healing of gastric ulcers in rats. *J Pharmacol Exp Ther.* 1998;286:1383–90.

47. Reuter BK, Asfaha S, Buret A, Sharkey KA, Wallace JL. Exacerbation of inflammation-associated colonic injury in rat through inhibition of cyclooxygenase-2. *J Clin Invest.* 1996;98:2076–85.

48. Morteau O, Morham SG, Sellon R, Dieleman LA, Langenbach R, Smithies O et al. Impaired mucosal defense to acute colonic injury in mice lacking cyclooxygenase-1 or cyclooxygenase-2. *J Clin Invest.* 2000;105:469–78.

49. Takahashi S, Shigeta J, Inoue H, Tanabe T, Okabe S. Localization of cyclooxygenase-2 and regulation of its mRNA expression in gastric ulcers in rats. *Am J Physiol.* 1998;275:G1137–45.

50. Takahashi M, Ota S, Hata Y, Mikami Y, Azuma N, Nakamura T et al. Hepatocyte

growth factor as a key to modulate anti-ulcer action of prostaglandins in stomach. *J Clin Invest.* 1996;98:2604–11.

51. Bamba H, Ota S, Kato A, Matsuzaki F. Nonsteroidal anti-inflammatory drugs may delay the repair of gastric mucosa by suppressing prostaglandin-mediated increase of hepatocyte growth factor production. *Biochem Biophys Res Commun.* 1998;245:567–71.

52. Horie-Sakata K, Shimada T, Hiraishi H, Terano A. Role of cyclooxygenase 2 in hepatocyte growth factor-mediated gastric epithelial restitution. *J Clin Gastroenterol.* 1998;27 (Suppl. 1):S40–6.

53. Jones MK, Sasaki E, Halter F, Pai R, Nakamura T, Arakawa T et al. HGF triggers activation of the COX-2 gene in rat gastric epithelial cells: action mediated through the ERK2 signaling pathway. *FASEB J.* 1999;13:2186–94.

54. Hori T, Shibamoto S, Hayakawa M, Takeuchi K, Oku N, Miyazawa K et al. Stimulation of prostaglandin production by hepatocyte growth factor in human gastric carcinoma cells. *FEBS Lett.* 1993;334:331–4.

55. Murasaki G, Zenser TV, Davis BB, Cohen SM. Inhibition by aspirin of N-[4-(5-nitro-2-furyl)-2-thiazolyl] formamide-induced bladder carcinogenesis and enhancement of forestomach carcinogenesis. *Carcinogenesis.* 1984;5:53–5.

56. Newberne PM, Charnley G, Adams K, Cantor M, Suphakarn V, Roth D et al. Gastric carcinogenesis: a model for the identification of risk factors. *Cancer Lett.* 1987;38:149–63.

57. Lehnert T, Deschner EE, Karmali RA, DeCosse JJ. Effect of flurbiprofen and 16,16-dimethyl prostaglandin E_2 on gastrointestinal tumorigenesis induced by N-methyl-N'-nitro-N-nitrosoguanidine in rats: glandular epithelium of stomach and duodenum. *Cancer Res.* 1990;50:381–4.

58. Jalbert G, Castonguay A. Effects of NSAIDs on NNK-induced pulmonary and gastric tumorigenesis in A/J mice. *Cancer Lett.* 1992;66:21–8.

59. Nakamura A, Chiba T, Yamatani T, Yamaguchi A, Inui T, Morishita T et al. Prostaglandin E_2 and $F_{2\alpha}$ inhibit growth of human gastric carcinoma cell line KATO III with simultaneous stimulation of cyclic AMP production. *Life Sci.* 1989;44:75–80.

60. Watson SA, Durrant LG, Morris DL. The effect of the E_2 prostaglandin enprostil, and the somatostatin analogue SMS 201 995, on the growth of a human gastric cell line, MKN 45G. *Int J Cancer.* 1990;45:90–4.

61. Shimakura S, Boland CR. Eicosanoid production by the human gastric cancer cell line AGS and its relation to cell growth. *Cancer Res.* 1992;52:1744–9.

62. Tytgat GN, Offerhaus GJ, van Minnen AJ, Everts V, Hensen-Logmans SC, Samson G. Influence of oral 15(R)-15-methyl prostaglandin E_2 on human gastric mucosa. A light microscopic, cell kinetic, and ultrastructural study. *Gastroenterology.* 1986;90:1111–20.

63. Peled N, Dagan O, Babyn P, Silver MM, Barker G, Hellmann J et al. Gastric-outlet obstruction induced by prostaglandin therapy in neonates. *N Engl J Med.* 1992;327:505–10.

64. Tsuji S, Kawano S, Sawaoka H, Takei Y, Kobayashi I, Nagano K et al. Evidences for involvement of cyclooxygenase-2 in proliferation of two gastrointestinal cancer cell lines. *Prostaglandins Leukot Essent Fatty Acids.* 1996;55:179–83.

65. Sawaoka H, Kawano S, Tsuji S, Tsujii M, Murata H, Hori M. Effects of NSAIDs on proliferation of gastric cancer cells *in vitro*: possible implication of cyclooxygenase-2 in cancer development. *J Clin Gastroenterol.* 1998;27(Suppl. 1):S47–52.

66. Sawaoka H, Kawano S, Tsuji S, Tsujii M, Gunawan ES, Takei Y et al. Cyclooxygenase-2 inhibitors suppress the growth of gastric cancer xenografts via induction of apoptosis in nude mice. *Am J Physiol*. 1998;274:G1061–7.

67. Jankowski JA, Wright NA, Meltzer SJ, Triadafilopoulos G, Geboes K, Casson AG et al. Molecular evolution of the metaplasia–dysplasia–adenocarcinoma sequence in the esophagus. *Am J Pathol*. 1999;154:965–73.

68. Wilson KT, Fu S, Ramanujam KS, Meltzer SJ. Increased expression of inducible nitric oxide synthase and cyclooxygenase-2 in Barrett's esophagus and associated adenocarcinomas. *Cancer Res*. 1998;58:2929–34.

69. Shirvani VN, Ouatu-Lascar R, Kaur BS, Omary MB, Triadafilopoulos G. Cyclooxygenase 2 expression in Barrett's esophagus and adenocarcinoma: *Ex vivo* induction by bile salts and acid exposure. *Gastroenterology*. 2000;118:487–96.

70. Zimmermann KC, Sarbia M, Weber AA, Borchard F, Gabbert HE, Schrör K. Cyclooxygenase-2 expression in human esophageal carcinoma. *Cancer Res*. 1999;59:198–204.

71. Zhang F, Subbaramaiah K, Altorki N, Dannenberg AJ. Dihydroxy bile acids activate the transcription of cyclooxygenase-2. *J Biol Chem*. 1998;273:2424–8.

72. Ratnasinghe D, Tangrea J, Roth MJ, Dawsey S, Hu N, Anver M et al. Expression of cyclooxygenase-2 in human squamous cell carcinoma of the esophagus; an immunohistochemical survey. *Anticancer Res*. 1999;19:171–4.

73. Shamma A, Yamamoto H, Doki Y, Okami J, Kondo M, Fujiwara Y et al. Upregulation of cyclooxygenase-2 in squamous carcinogenesis of the esophagus. *Clin Cancer Res*. 2000;6:1229–38.

74. Rubio CA. Further studies on the therapeutic effect of indomethacin on esophageal tumours. *Cancer*. 1986;58:1029–31.

75. Hammar S. Common neoplasms. In: Dail DH, Hammar SP, editors. *Pulmonary Pathology*, 2nd edition. New York: Springer-Verlag; 1994:1123–78.

76. Hida T, Yatabe Y, Achiwa H, Muramatsu H, Kozaki K, Nakamura S et al. Increased expression of cyclooxygenase 2 occurs frequently in human lung cancers, specifically in adenocarcinomas. *Cancer Res*. 1998;58:3761–4.

77. Wolff H, Saukkonen K, Anttila S, Karjalainen A, Vainio H, Ristimäki A. Expression of cyclooxygenase-2 in human lung carcinoma. *Cancer Res*. 1998;58:4997–5001.

78. Ochiai M, Oguri T, Isobe T, Ishioka S, Yamakido M. Cyclooxygenase-2 (COX-2) mRNA expression levels in normal lung tissues and non-small cell lung cancers. *Jpn J Cancer Res*. 1999;90:1338–43.

79. Watkins DN, Lenzo JC, Segal A, Garlepp MJ, Thompson PJ. Expression and localization of cyclo-oxygenase isoforms in non-small cell lung cancer. *Eur Respir J*. 1999;14:412–18.

80. Huang M, Stolina M, Sharma S, Mao JT, Zhu L, Miller PW et al. Non-small cell lung cancer cyclooxygenase-2-dependent regulation of cytokine balance in lymphocytes and macrophages: up-regulation of interleukin 10 and down-regulation of interleukin 12 production. *Cancer Res*. 1998;58:1208–16.

81. Achiwa H, Yatabe Y, Hida T, Kuroishi T, Kozaki K, Nakamura S et al. Prognostic significance of elevated cyclooxygenase 2 expression in primary, resected lung adenocarcinomas. *Clin Cancer Res*. 1999;5:1001–5.

82. Homma S, Kawabata M, Kishi K, Tsuboi E, Narui K, Nakatani T et al. Successful treatment of refractory bronchorrhea by inhaled indomethacin in two patients with bronchioloalveolar carcinoma. *Chest*. 1999;115:1465–8.

83. Tamaoki J, Kohri K, Isono K, Nagai A. Inhaled indomethacin in bronchorrhea in bronchioalveolar carcinoma: Role of cyclooxygenase. *Chest*. 2000;117:1213–14.

84. Hida T, Leyton J, Makheja AN, Ben-Av P, Hla T, Martinez A et al. Non-small cell lung cancer cycloxygenase activity and proliferation are inhibited by non-steroidal antiinflammatory drugs. *Anticancer Res*. 1998;18:775–82.

85. Bennett A, Carroll MA, Stamford IF, Whimster WF, Williams F. Prostaglandins and human lung carcinomas. *Br J Cancer*. 1982;46:888–93.

86. Parker J, Kaplon MK, Alvarez CJ, Krishnaswamy G. Prostaglandin H synthase expression is variable in human colorectal adenocarcinoma cell lines. *Exp Cell Res*. 1997;236:321–9.

87. Schmedtje JF Jr, Ji YS, Liu WL, DuBois RN, Runge MS. Hypoxia induces cyclooxygenase-2 via the NF-κB p65 transcription factor in human vascular endothelial cells. *J Biol Chem*. 1997;272:601–8.

88. Rodenhuis S, Slebos RJ. Clinical significance of *ras* oncogene activation in human lung cancer. *Cancer Res*. 1992;52(Suppl.):2665s–9s.

89. Subbaramaiah K, Telang N, Ramonetti JT, Araki R, DeVito B, Weksler BB et al. Transcription of cyclooxygenase-2 is enhanced in transformed mammary epithelial cells. *Cancer Res*. 1996;56:4424–9.

90. Heasley LE, Thaler S, Nicks M, Price B, Skorecki K, Nemenoff RA. Induction of cytosolic phospholipase A2 by oncogenic Ras in human non-small cell lung cancer. *J Biol Chem*. 1997;272:14501–4.

91. Sheng GG, Shao J, Sheng H, Hooton EB, Isakson PC, Morrow JD et al. A selective cyclooxygenase 2 inhibitor suppresses the growth of H-*ras*-transformed rat intestinal epithelial cells. *Gastroenterology*. 1997;113:1883–91.

92. Zhang X, Morham SG, Langenbach R, Young DA. Malignant transformation and antineoplastic actions of nonsteroidal antiinflammatory drugs (NSAIDs) on cyclooxygenase-null embryo fibroblasts. *J Exp Med*. 1999;190:451–9.

93. Yip-Schneider MT, Barnard DS, Billings SD, Cheng L, Heilman DK, Lin A et al. Cyclooxygenase-2 expression in human pancreatic adenocarcinomas. *Carcinogenesis*. 2000;21:139–46.

94. Fox B, Ridson RA. Carcinoma of the lung and diffuse interstitial pulmonary fibrosis. *J Clin Pathol*. 1968;21:486–91.

95. Sheehan KM, Sheahan K, O'Donoghue DP, MacSweeney F, Conroy RM, Fitzgerald DJ et al. The relationship between cyclooxygenase-2 expression and colorectal cancer. *JAMA*. 1999;282:1254–7.

96. Duperron C, Castonguay A. Chemopreventive efficacies of aspirin and sulindac against lung tumorigenesis in A/J mice. *Carcinogenesis*. 1997;18:1001–6.

97. Rioux N, Castonguay A. Prevention of NNK-induced lung tumorigenesis in A/J mice by acetylsalicylic acid and NS-398. *Cancer Res*. 1998;58:5354–60.

98. El-Bayoumy K, Iatropoulos M, Amin S, Hoffmann D, Wynder EL. Increased expression of cyclooxygenase-2 in rat lung tumours induced by the tobacco-specific nitrosamine 4-(methylnitrosamino)-4-(3-pyridyl)-1-butanone: the impact of a high-fat diet. *Cancer Res*. 1999;59:1400–3.

99. Bauer AK, Dwyer-Nield LD, Malkinson AM. High cyclooxygenase 1 (COX-1) and cyclooxygenase 2 (COX-2) contents in mouse lung tumours. *Carcinogenesis*. 2000;21:543–50.

100. Kitayama W, Denda A, Yoshida J, Sasaki Y, Takahama M, Murakawa K et al. Increased expression of cyclooxygenase-2 protein in rat lung tumours induced by *N*-nitrosobis(2-hydroxypropyl)amine. *Cancer Lett*. 2000;148:145–52.

101. Stolina M, Sharma S, Lin Y, Dohadwala M, Gardner B, Luo J et al. Specific inhibition of cyclooxygenase 2 restores antitumour reactivity by altering the balance of IL-10 and IL-12 synthesis. *J Immunol*. 2000;164:361–70.

102. Ermert L, Ermert M, Goppelt-Struebe M, Walmrath D, Grimminger F, Steudel W et al. Cyclooxygenase isoenzyme localization and mRNA expression in rat lungs. *Am J Respir Cell Mol Biol*. 1998;18:479–88.

103. Soriano AF, Helfrich B, Chan DC, Heasley LE, Bunn PA Jr, Chou TC. Synergistic effects of new chemopreventive agents and conventional cytotoxic agents against human lung cancer cell lines. *Cancer Res*. 1999;59:6178–84.

104. Hida T, Kozaki K, Muramatsu H, Masuda A, Shimizu S, Mitsudomi T et al. Cyclooxygenase-2 inhibitor induces apoptosis and enhances cytotoxicity of various anticancer agents in non-small cell lung cancer cell lines. *Clin Cancer Res*. 2000;6:2006–11.

105. Kozaki K, Miyaishi O, Tsukamoto T, Tatematsu Y, Hida T, Takahashi T et al. Establishment and characterization of a human lung cancer cell line NCI-H460-LNM35 with consistent lymphogenous metastasis via both subcutaneous and orthotopic propagation. *Cancer Res*. 2000;60:2535–40.

106. Leong J, Hughes-Fulford M, Rakhlin N, Habib A, Maclouf J, Goldyne ME. Cyclooxygenases in human and mouse skin and cultured human keratinocytes: association of COX-2 expression with human keratinocyte differentiation. *Exp Cell Res*. 1996;224:79–87.

107. Müller-Decker K, Reinerth G, Krieg P, Zimmermann R, Heise H, Bayerl C et al. Prostaglandin-H-synthase isozyme expression in normal and neoplastic human skin. *Int J Cancer*. 1999;82:648–56.

108. Marks F, Fürstenberger G. Cancer chemoprevention through interruption of multistage carcinogenesis. The lessons learnt by comparing mouse skin carcinogenesis and human large bowel cancer. *Eur J Cancer*. 2000;36:314–29.

109. Müller-Decker K, Scholz K, Marks F, Fürstenberger G. Differential expression of prostaglandin H synthase isozymes during multistage carcinogenesis in mouse epidermis. *Mol Carcinog*. 1995;12:31–41.

110. Müller-Decker K, Kopp-Schneider A, Marks F, Seibert K, Fürstenberger G. Localization of prostaglandin H synthase isoenzymes in murine epidermal tumours: suppression of skin tumour promotion by inhibition of prostaglandin H synthase-2. *Mol Carcinog*. 1998;23:36–44.

111. Langenbach R, Loftin CD, Lee C, Tiano H. Cyclooxygenase-deficient mice. A summary of their characteristics and susceptibilities to inflammation and carcinogenesis. *Ann NY Acad Sci*. 1999;889:52–61.

112. Buckman SY, Gresham A, Hale P, Hruza G, Anast J, Masferrer J et al. COX-2 expression is induced by UVB exposure in human skin: implications for the development of skin cancer. *Carcinogenesis*. 1998;19:723–9.

113. Fischer SM, Lo HH, Gordon GB, Seibert K, Kelloff G, Lubet RA et al. Chemopreventive activity of celecoxib, a specific cyclooxygenase-2 inhibitor, and indomethacin against ultraviolet light-induced skin carcinogenesis. *Mol Carcinog*. 1999;25:231–40.

114. Isoherranen K, Punnonen K, Jansen C, Uotila P. Ultraviolet irradiation induces cyclooxygenase-2 expression in keratinocytes. *Br J Dermatol*. 1999;140:1017–22.

115. Pentland AP, Schoggins JW, Scott GA, Khan KN, Han R. Reduction of UV-induced skin tumours in hairless mice by selective COX-2 inhibition. *Carcinogenesis*. 1999;20:1939–44.

116. Chan G, Boyle JO, Yang EK, Zhang F, Sacks PG, Shah JP et al. Cyclooxygenase-2 expression is up-regulated in squamous cell carcinoma of the head and neck. *Cancer Res.* 1999;59:991–4.

117. Nishimura G, Yanoma S, Mizuno H, Kawakami K, Tsukuda M. A selective cyclooxygenase-2 inhibitor suppresses tumour growth in nude mouse xenografted with human head and neck squamous carcinoma cells. *Jpn J Cancer Res.* 1999;90:1152–62.

118. Parret ML, Harris RE, Joarder FS, Ross MS, Clausen KP, Robertson FM. Cyclooxygenase-2 gene expression in human breast cancer. *Int J Oncol.* 1997;10:503–7.

119. Brueggemeier RW, Quinn AL, Parrett ML, Joarder FS, Harris RE, Robertson FM. Correlation of aromatase and cyclooxygenase gene expression in human breast cancer specimens. *Cancer Lett.* 1999;140:27–35.

120. Hwang D, Scollard D, Byrne J, Levine E. Expression of cyclooxygenase-1 and cyclooxygenase-2 in human breast cancer. *J Natl Cancer Inst.* 1998;90:455–60.

121. Gilhooly EM, Rose DP. The association between a mutated *ras* gene and cyclooxygenase-2 expression in human breast cancer cell lines. *Int J Oncol.* 1999;15:267–70.

122. Subbaramaiah K, Telang N, Ramonetti JT, Araki R, DeVito B, Weksler BB et al. Transcription of cyclooxygenase-2 is enhanced in transformed mammary epithelial cells. *Cancer Res.* 1996;56:4424–9.

123. Matsumoto-Taniura N, Matsumoto K, Nakamura T. Prostaglandin production in mouse mammary tumour cells confers invasive growth potential by inducing hepatocyte growth factor in stromal fibroblasts. *Br J Cancer.* 1999;81:194–202.

124. Takahashi Y, Kawahara F, Noguchi M, Miwa K, Sato H, Seiki M et al. Activation of matrix metalloproteinase-2 in human breast cancer cells overexpressing cyclooxygenase-1 or -2. *FEBS Lett.* 1999;460:145–8.

125. Parrett ML, Abou-Issa HM, Alshafie G, Ross MS, Harris RE, Robertson FM. Comparative ability of ibuprofen and N-(4-hydroxyphenyl)retinamide to inhibit development of rat mammary adenocarcinomas associated with differential inhibition of gene expression of cyclooxygenase isoforms. *Anticancer Res.* 1999;19:5079–85.

126. Harris RE, Alshafie GA, Abou-Issa H, Seibert K. Chemoprevention of breast cancer in rats by celecoxib, a cyclooxygenase 2 inhibitor. *Cancer Res.* 2000;60:2101–3.

127. Sorli CH, Zhang HJ, Armstrong MB, Rajotte RV, Maclouf J, Robertson RP. Basal expression of cyclooxygenase-2 and nuclear factor-interleukin 6 are dominant and coordinately regulated by interleukin 1 in the pancreatic islet. *Proc Natl Acad Sci USA.* 1998;95:1788–93.

128. Molina MA, Sitja-Arnau M, Lemoine MG, Frazier ML, Sinicrope FA. Increased cyclooxygenase-2 expression in human pancreatic carcinomas and cell lines: growth inhibition by nonsteroidal anti-inflammatory drugs. *Cancer Res.* 1999;59:4356–62.

129. Okami J, Yamamoto H, Fujiwara Y, Tsujie M, Kondo M, Noura S et al. Overexpression of cyclooxygenase-2 in carcinoma of the pancreas. *Clin Cancer Res.* 1999;5:2018–24.

130. Tucker ON, Dannenberg AJ, Yang EK, Zhang F, Teng L, Daly JM et al. Cyclooxygenase-2 expression is up-regulated in human pancreatic cancer. *Cancer Res.* 1999;59:987–90.

131. Koshiba T, Hosotani R, Miyamoto Y, Wada M, Lee JU, Fujimoto K et al. Immunohistochemical analysis of cyclooxygenase-2 expression in pancreatic tumours. *Int J Pancreatol.* 1999;26:69–76.

132. Koga H, Sakisaka S, Ohishi M, Kawaguchi T, Taniguchi E, Sasatomi K et al. Expression of cyclooxygenase-2 in human hepatocellular carcinoma: relevance to tumour dedifferentiation. *Hepatology*. 1999;29:688–96.

133. Kondo M, Yamamoto H, Nagano H, Okami J, Ito Y, Shimizu J et al. Increased expression of COX-2 in nontumour liver tissue is associated with shorter disease-free survival in patients with hepatocellular carcinoma. *Clin Cancer Res*. 1999;5:4005–12.

134. Shiota G, Okubo M, Noumi T, Noguchi N, Oyama K, Takano Y et al. Cyclo-oxygenase-2 expression in hepatocellular carcinoma. *Hepatogastroenterology*. 1999;46:407–12.

135. Mohammed SI, Knapp DW, Bostwick DG, Foster RS, Khan KN, Masferrer JL et al. Expression of cyclooxygenase-2 (COX-2) in human invasive transitional cell carcinoma (TCC) of the urinary bladder. *Cancer Res*. 1999;59:5647–50.

136. Kitayama W, Denda A, Okajima E, Tsujiuchi T, Konishi Y. Increased expression of cyclooxygenase-2 protein in rat urinary bladder tumours induced by *N*-butyl-*N*-(4 hydroxybutyl) nitrosamine. *Carcinogenesis*. 1999;20:2305–10.

137. Khan KN, Knapp DW, Denicola DB, Harris RK. Expression of cyclooxygenase-2 in transitional cell carcinoma of the urinary bladder in dogs. *Am J Vet Res*. 2000;61:478–81.

138. Okajima E, Denda A, Ozono S, Takahama M, Akai H, Sasaki Y et al. Chemopreventive effects of nimesulide, a selective cyclooxygenase-2 inhibitor, on the development of rat urinary bladder carcinomas initiated by *N*-butyl-*N*-(4-hydroxybutyl)nitrosamine. *Cancer Res*. 1998;58:3028–31.

139. Gupta S, Srivastava M, Ahmad N, Bostwick DG, Mukhtar H. Over-expression of cyclooxygenase-2 in human prostate adenocarcinoma. *Prostate*. 2000;42:73–8.

140. Tremblay C, Dore M, Bochsler PN, Sirois J. Induction of prostaglandin G/H synthase-2 in a canine model of spontaneous prostatic adenocarcinoma. *J Natl Cancer Inst*. 1999;91:1398–403.

141. Liu XH, Yao S, Kirschenbaum A, Levine AC. NS398, a selective cyclooxygenase-2 inhibitor, induces apoptosis and down-regulates *bcl-2* expression in LNCaP cells. *Cancer Res*. 1998;58:4245–9.

142. Lim JT, Piazza GA, Han EK, Delohery TM, Li H, Finn TS et al. Sulindac derivatives inhibit growth and induce apoptosis in human prostate cancer cell lines. *Biochem Pharmacol*. 1999;58:1097–107.

143. Hsu AL, Ching TT, Wang DS, Song X, Rangnekar VM, Chen CS. The cyclooxygenase-2 inhibitor celecoxib induces apoptosis by blocking Akt activation in human prostate cancer cells independently of *bcl-2*. *J Biol Chem*. 2000;275:11397–403.

144. Ryu HS, Chang KH, Yang HW, Kim MS, Kwon HC, Oh KS. High cyclooxygenase-2 expression in stage IB cervical cancer with lymph node metastasis or parametrial invasion. *Gynecol Oncol*. 2000;76:320–5.

145. Doré M, Coté LC, Mitchell A, Sirois J. Expression of prostaglandin G/H synthase type 1, but not type 2, in human ovarian adenocarcinomas. *J Histochem Cytochem*. 1998;46:77–84.

146. Deininger MH, Weller M, Streffer J, Mittelbronn M, Meyermann R. Patterns of cyclooxygenase-1 and -2 expression in human gliomas *in vivo*. *Acta Neuropathol*. 1999;98:240–4.

147. Karim MM, Hayashi Y, Inoue M, Imai Y, Ito H, Yamamoto M. COX-2 expression in retinoblastoma. *Am J Ophthalmol*. 2000;129:398–401.

148. Sturmer T, Glynn RJ, Lee IM, Manson JE, Buring JE, Hennekens CH. Aspirin

use and colorectal cancer: post-trial follow-up data from the Physicians' Health Study. *Ann Intern Med.* 1998;128:713–20.

149. Cramer DW, Harlow BL, Titus-Ernstoff L, Bohlke K, Welch WR, Greenberg ER. Over-the-counter analgesics and risk of ovarian cancer. *Lancet.* 1998;351:104–7.

150. Masferrer JL, Leahy KM, Koki AT, Zweifel BS, Settle SL, Woerner BM et al. Antiangiogenic and antitumour activities of cyclooxygenase-2 inhibitors. *Cancer Res.* 2000;60:1306–11.

151. Williams CS, Tsujii M, Reese J, Dey SK, DuBois RN. Host cyclooxygenase-2 modulates carcinoma growth. *J Clin Invest.* 2000;105:1589–94.

152. Spirio LN, Dixon DA, Robertson J, Robertson M, Barrows J, Traer E et al. The inducible prostaglandin biosynthetic enzyme, cyclooxygenase 2, is not mutated in patients with attenuated adenomatous polyposis coli. *Cancer Res.* 1998;58:4909–12.

153. Howe LR, Subbaramaiah K, Chung WJ, Dannenberg AJ, Brown AM. Transcriptional activation of cyclooxygenase-2 in Wnt-1-transformed mouse mammary epithelial cells. *Cancer Res.* 1999;59:1572–7.

154. Subbaramaiah K, Altorki N, Chung WJ, Mestre JR, Sampat A, Dannenberg AJ. Inhibition of cyclooxygenase-2 gene expression by p53. *J Biol Chem.* 1999;274:10911–15.

155. Vadlamudi R, Mandal M, Adam L, Steinbach G, Mendelsohn J, Kumar R. Regulation of cyclooxygenase-2 pathway by HER2 receptor. *Oncogene.* 1999;18:305–14.

156. Milas L, Kishi K, Hunter N, Mason K, Masferrer JL, Tofilon PJ. Enhancement of tumour response to gamma-radiation by an inhibitor of cyclooxygenase-2 enzyme. *J Natl Cancer Inst.* 1999;91:1501–4.

157. Soriano AF, Helfrich B, Chan DC, Heasley LE, Bunn PA Jr, Chou TC. Synergistic effects of new chemopreventive agents and conventional cytotoxic agents against human lung cancer cell lines. *Cancer Res.* 1999;59:6178–84.

158. Kishi K, Petersen S, Petersen C, Hunter N, Mason K, Masferrer JL et al. Preferential enhancement of tumour radioresponse by a cyclooxygenase-2 inhibitor. *Cancer Res.* 2000;60:1326–31.

159. Mestre JR, Subbaramaiah K, Sacks PG, Schantz SP, Tanabe T, Inoue H et al. Retinoids suppress epidermal growth factor-induced transcription of cyclooxygenase-2 in human oral squamous carcinoma cells. *Cancer Res.* 1997;57:2890–5.

160. Jacoby RF, Cole CE, Tutsch K, Newton MA, Kelloff G, Hawk ET et al. Chemopreventive efficacy of combined piroxicam and difluoromethylornithine treatment of Apc mutant Min mouse adenomas, and selective toxicity against Apc mutant embryos. *Cancer Res.* 2000;60:1864–70.

161. Ristimäki A, Nieminen O, Saukkonen K, Hotakainen K, Nordling S, Haglund C. Expression of cyclooxygenase-2 in human transitional cell carcinoma of the urinary bladder. *Am J Pathol.* 2001; in press.

20 | The human pharmacology of the coxibs: inhibitors of cyclooxygenase-2

GARRET A. FITZGERALD[1] AND CARLO PATRONO[2]

[1]*Center for Experimental Therapeutics, University of Pennsylvania, USA and* [2]*Department of Medicine and Aging, University of Chieti, Italy.*

The crystallization of both COX isoforms identified a structural basis for the rational design of selective inhibitors of COX-2[1–3]. The rationale which underlay their development was configured on the observation that this isoform was readily induced by inflammatory cytokines and mitogens, whereas COX-1 was the isoform expressed predominantly in gut epithelium. This prompted the hypothesis that COX-2 was the source of prostanoid formation in settings such as arthritis and, perhaps, cancer, whereas inhibition of COX-1 dependent cytoprotective prostanoids accounted for the gastrointestinal (GI) side effects of traditional non-steroid anti-inflammatory drugs (NSAIDs). These drugs are rather non-selective inhibitors in *in vitro* screening systems.

Aside from the actual structural preference of a compound for inhibiting either isozyme, many factors will contribute to the ultimate expression of clinical selectivity in an individual. Thus, interindividual differences in absorption, distribution, metabolism and excretion (ADME) can influence the extent and duration of enzyme inhibition. Consumption of other drugs or behaviours such as cigarette smoking or drinking alcohol can potentially influence these pharmacokinetic variables, as may coincidental disease. For example, the likelihood of an NSAID-induced GI bleed is highly dependent on the extent of underlying GI pathology[4]. Finally, there is the possibility that genetic variability in proteins relevant to ADME of such drugs, or indeed, in the COX enzymes themselves, may interact with environmental variables to modify drug response.

In the short period of a decade since the discovery of COX-2[5–8], two rationally designed inhibitors – chemically classified by WHO as the 'coxibs', celecoxib and rofecoxib (Figure 1) – have gained regulatory approval in the United States and other countries. While approval was based on a favourable profile of surrogate GI endpoints, such as pain and endoscopic visualization of ulcers, the first controlled studies of their impact versus conventional NSAIDs on actual clinical outcomes – both efficacy and adverse effects – have recently been reported. These results permit the first evaluation of the therapeutic ratio of these compounds as even more selective inhibitors enter human development.

SELECTIVE AND NON-SELECTIVE INHIBITION OF CYCLOOXYGENASE ISOFORMS

This chapter will focus on the clinical pharmacology of the coxibs. In this regard, it is worth considering the biochemical basis for assessing selectivity of any such compound in humans. A variety of assay systems has been employed to determine COX-2 selectivity[9,10]. Amongst existing inhibitors, the hierarchies of the concentrations necessary for 50% inhibition (the $IC_{50}s$) of COX-1:COX-2 vary according to the assay and/or measurement system employed. While estimates vary from roughly 0.5 (favouring COX-1 as the target) to 10 (favouring COX-2) for traditional NSAIDs, rofecoxib, but

Figure 1 Chemical structures of the two coxibs approved for clinical use by the FDA.

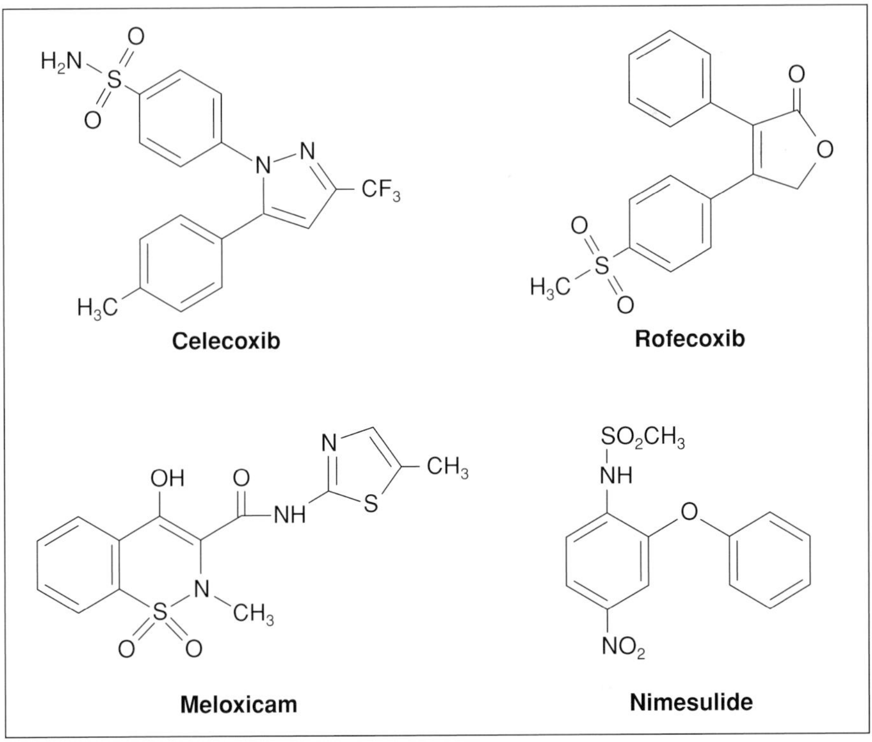

Celecoxib

Rofecoxib

Meloxicam

Nimesulide

not celecoxib, shows a ratio of greater than 50[9–12]. It is unknown whether the relatively small differences in selectivity ratios amongst traditional NSAIDs translate into similar differences in humans and whether they accord with true clinical differences in drug efficacy and/or adverse effect profile. Attempts to discriminate between such compounds with terms such as COX-2 or COX-1 'preferential' is, in our view, misleading.

The biochemical selectivity of a compound can be assessed *ex vivo* in humans by using whole blood assays of isoform capacity[9–14], expressing the ratio of the IC_{50}s. All selective inhibitors ultimately become non-selective as a function of concentration. Rofecoxib[15–17] is the most biochemically selective of presently available compounds. Interestingly, the selectivity of celecoxib[10,18,19] approximates that of two older compounds, meloxicam and nimesulide (Figure 1). Meloxicam has, for some time, been reported to have a lower incidence of GI side effects than other conventional NSAIDs[20,21]. Nimesulide is another COX-2-selective NSAID in use before the discovery of COX-2[22].

CYCLOOXYGENASE INHIBITORS IN ARTHRITIS AND PAIN

Clinical pharmacology

The first of the coxibs to be approved in the USA was celecoxib. Although absolute bioavailability studies have not been published, it appears to be well absorbed, with peak plasma levels around 3 h after dosing. It is widely distributed and highly protein bound and is eliminated mainly by cytochrome P450 2C9 (CYP 2C9) dependent metabolism in the liver[23]. The short pharmacodynamic half-life of celecoxib necessitates twice-daily dosing. Plasma levels of rofecoxib also peak roughly 3 h after dosing and is also highly protein bound. Like celecoxib, it is also biotransformed to inactive metabolites, mainly in the liver, but CYP isozymes play a minor role. The mean effective half-life has been estimated at 17 h, permitting once-daily dosing.

One might anticipate that either renal or hepatic dysfunction might modify the dose-related responses to either drugs. Similarly, they are susceptible to interaction with other highly protein bound drugs. In the case of celecoxib, drugs that affect the expression and/or function of CYP 2C9 might interact; drug interactions with both fluconazole and lithium have been reported[24]. Although predicted, interactions with warfarin seem unlikely[18]. Little information is available on pharmacokinetic variability amongst ethnic groups or pharmacogenetic variables of potential relevance to drug response.

Clinical trials in arthritis

As already mentioned, the first approach to clinical evaluation of the coxibs was to determine if equieffective doses of coxibs and NSAID comparators differed in their impact on surrogate GI variables. The rationale was that although serious GI adverse effects are not frequent, the number of people taking NSAIDs makes this is a large problem. Between 10 and 20% of patients taking NSAIDs experience dyspepsia[25] and 5–15% of patients with rheumatoid arthritis (RA) discontinue taking NSAIDs for this reason[26]. Mortality from GI adverse effects of NSAIDs has been estimated at 0.22% per year, with an annual relative risk of 4.21[27].

Simon et al. randomized 1149 patients to receive celecoxib 100 mg, 200 mg or 400 mg per day, naproxen 500 mg twice daily or placebo for 12 weeks. Signs and symptoms were assessed[28] and endoscopy was performed before and within 7 days of completion of the study. All doses of celecoxib and naproxen appeared to be similarly efficacious, as assessed by the number of tender or painful joints, the number of swollen joints or when the number of responders were assigned by American College of Rheumatology criteria. All were superior to placebo. By contrast, the incidence of GI ulcers was 4% in the placebo group, 6%, 4% and 6% at the three doses of celecoxib and 26% with naproxen. The failure to discriminate a dose-dependent effect with celecoxib would accord with studies of its inhibitory effects on COX-2 *ex vivo*, which suggest that all of these doses are at the top of the dose–response curve[29]. A second study of celecoxib in RA was reported by Emery and colleagues[30]. In this case, 655 patients with adult onset RA were randomly assigned to 200 mg twice daily of celecoxib or diclofenac SR 75 mg twice daily for 24 weeks. This study was not placebo controlled. Again, endoscopy was performed before and within 7 days of completion of the study. Efficacy of the two active treatments was similar. GI ulcers were detected in 15% of the diclofenac group and in 4% of the celecoxib group. Although these studies are consistent with celecoxib exhibiting clinical selectivity, they are not sized to detect small differences in efficacy, such as might be expected if COX-1 played a minor role in prostaglandin (PG) formation in inflammation.

An attempt to estimate the impact of selective COX-2 inhibitors on GI clinical endpoints was reported recently[31]. Analysis of eight double-blind randomized trials of osteoarthritis (OA) assessed the effects of rofecoxib at 12.5, 25 or 50 mg/day in 1209, 1603 and 545 patients, versus ibuprofen 800 mg three times a day, diclofenac 50 mg three times per day or nabumetone 1500 mg per day in 847, 590 and 127 patients, respectively. The cumulative incidence of upper GI perforations, symptomatic gastroduodenal ulcers and upper GI bleeding (PUBs) was significantly lower in the rofecoxib group (1.3% versus 1.8%; $P = 0.046$) than with the NSAIDs as a whole, and the overall relative risk for rofecoxib over 12 months was 0.51 (95% CI 0.26–1.00). The cumulative incidence of dyspepsia was also slightly lower for rofecoxib versus all NSAIDs over 6 months (23.5 % versus 25.5%; p< 0.02), but thereafter, the incidence rates converged. A relatively modest reduction in the low incidence of PUBs on NSAIDs is likely to be important, given the large number of patients taking NSAIDs. The effect on symptoms was less impressive.

However, the relationship between GI symptoms, visualization of ulcers on endoscopy and actual PUBs is recognized to be tenuous[32,33], so it was encouraging to see a pattern consistent with what had been seen with COX-2 inhibitors using surrogate GI endpoints.

A prospective trial of rofecoxib 50 mg daily versus naproxen 500 mg twice per day on the incidence of PUBs in 8076 RA patients – the VIGOR study (Table 1) – has recently been reported[34]. The mean age of the patients included was 58 years and 80% were females. Almost 60% were taking chronic steroids and 8% had a prior history of a PUB. Confirming the suggestion from the overview analysis in OA, this study established that the incidence of confirmed PUBs is significantly reduced from 4.5% per year to 2.1% per year (a decline of 54%; $P < 0.001$) by rofecoxib. Two prospective studies of celecoxib (400 mg twice daily), each of 4000 patients, with diclofenac (75 mg twice daily) or ibuprofen (800 mg three times a day) as respective comparators, were designed to be combined in the CLASS study[35]. In this case, 72% of the patients had OA. While the study lasted 13 months, data from only 6 months has been presented. Unlike VIGOR, patients were permitted to take low dose aspirin and there was no significant difference in the incidence of the primary endpoint – complicated ulcers – between the groups (0.7% on celecoxib versus 1.5% on either NSAID; $P = 0.09$). However, the incidence of PUBs, a prespecified secondary endpoint, was significantly lower (2% versus 3.5%; $P = 0.03$) on celecoxib.

Despite verification of the 'COX-2 hypothesis' in two prospective trials, there are some caveats. First, the likelihood of suffering a PUB on an NSAID is markedly conditioned by pre-existing risk factors, including age and a history of ulcer and GI bleeding. Such patients have a risk of a complicated ulcer on an NSAID of about 5%, in contrast to an incidence of 0.4% in RA patients with no risk factors[36]. It has been estimated that switching to a selective COX-2 inhibitor would halve the risk of a PUB. Thus, 500 low risk,

Table 1 Comparison of the VIGOR and CLASS surveys

	VIGOR (n = 8076)	*CLASS (n = 7982)*
Drug	Rofecoxib 50 mg q.d.s. (2 max. chronic dose)	Celecoxib 400 mg b.i.d. (2 max. chronic dose)
Patients	RA	OA (72%), RA (28%)
Comparators	Naproxen 500 mg b.i.d.	Ibuprofen 800 mg t.i.d.; diclofenac 75 mg b.i.d.
Low-dose aspirin	No	Yes (21%)
Duration	Median 9 months; maximum 13 months	Median 9 months; maximum 13 months
Analysis	Intent to treat	Excludes events 0–2; >6 months
1° endpoint	Clinical UGI events	Complicated ulcers
2° endpoint	Complicated UGI events	Symptomatic/complicated ulcers

but only 40 high risk patients would have to be switched to prevent one complicated ulcer. This translates into estimated incremental costs of roughly US$400 000 and US$30 000, respectively, to prevent a PUB in the two populations[37]. Secondly, patients with symptomatic or recognized GI ulceration were excluded from entry into the VIGOR study. The distinct roles of the two COX enzymes in the setting of an established ulcer is unknown. For example, COX-2, as well as COX-1, has been detected in apparently normal GI epithelium, raising the possibility that it makes some contribution to the generation of cytoprotective prostaglandins[38]. However, the VIGOR study suggests that COX-1 plays the major cytoprotective role. Of more concern is that GI epithelial COX-2 is upregulated by a range of insults[39], including *H. pylori*[40]. Expression is increased in the margin of healing ulcers and COX-2 inhibitors impair ulcer healing in mice[41]. This may reflect an impact on angiogenesis and/or the restoration of epithelial integrity[42–44]. Thirdly, we still have much to learn about the potential risks of COX-2 inhibition in the GI tract. For example, COX-2-dependent products influence the intestinal response to antigen, perhaps via modulation of T cell function and COX-2 inhibitors impair tolerance of dietary antigens in a mouse model[45]. Deletion of either COX isoform exacerbates dextran-induced colonic inflammation in mice and blockade of COX-2 exacerbates the response to dextran in COX-1-deleted mice[46]. COX-2 inhibition also exacerbates experimental colitis in rats[47].

Thus, in summary, the results of the VIGOR study establish rofecoxib as a clinically selective COX-2 inhibitor. The cost-effectiveness of the intervention and its applicability to the general population is being debated.

COX-2 INHIBITORS AND CARDIOVASCULAR DISEASE

COX-1 is expressed constitutively in endothelial and vascular smooth muscle cells. COX-2 is upregulated by cytokines, growth factors, phorbol esters and lipopolysaccharide (LPS) in both cell types[48–50] and by injury to smooth muscle cells *in vitro*[51]. These observations would be consistent with COX-2 playing an important role in the increased prostacyclin formation observed in syndromes of platelet activation[52,53]. Both COX-2 and COX-1 are upregulated in the foam cells and smooth muscle cells of the human atherosclerotic plaque[54]. However, COX-2 is important under physiological conditions also. Thus, structurally distinct selective COX-2 inhibitors all depress urinary prostacyclin metabolites[55] in healthy individuals[29,56,57]. Also, physiological rates of shear upregulate COX-2 expression in endothelial cells *in vitro*[58]. Prostacyclin is thought to be part of a homeostatic defence mechanism that limits the consequences of platelet activation *in vivo*[59–61]. Deletion of the prostacyclin receptor has resulted in mice that exhibit increased sensitivity to thrombotic stimuli, but do not develop spontaneous thrombosis[62].

What are the implications of these observations for selective COX-2 inhibitors? First, if there is a risk of thrombosis, one would expect it to be small, as there are several defence mechanisms, including nitric oxide (NO) and ecto-ADPase (ecto-adenosine diphosphatase). Secondly, one would expect a risk to emerge initially as case reports in patients at particular risk. Interestingly, thrombosis has occurred on celecoxib in patients with lupus anticoagulant[63]. However, these are precisely the people who develop spontaneous thrombosis anyway, so such information must be interpreted with caution.

The VIGOR trial included 8076 RA patients, 4% of whom had a prior history of a major vascular event. The use of concomitant low dose aspirin was prohibited and patients were to have discontinued its use to participate in this study. Major vascular events (non-fatal myocardial infarction (MI), non-fatal cerebrovascular accident or vascular death) occurred more frequently (0.8% versus 0.4%; $P < 0.05$) on rofecoxib than on naproxen. This difference was due largely to a difference in MI (0.4% on rofecoxib versus 0.1% on naproxen), with comparable rates of ischaemic cerebrovascular accidents (0.2% versus 0.2%) and vascular deaths (0.2% versus 0.2%). In contrast to VIGOR, roughly 22% of the patients in the CLASS trial took low dose aspirin. There was a non-significant difference in the incidence of any cardiovascular events between the main treatment groups: 1.4% with celecoxib versus 1.0% with NSAIDs. However, *post hoc* analysis suggested that the addition of aspirin abolished the difference in the incidence of PUBs between celecoxib and the NSAID comparators.

The difference in myocardial infarctions in VIGOR may be explained in several ways. First, it could be the play of chance. The number of events is small and, even if real, the estimate of the magnitude of the difference may be fallible. Secondly, although the effect would be surprising in its magnitude, it would be consistent with suppression of prostacyclin. This would be a class-specific effect, but may not have been revealed in the celecoxib study because of the difference in patient substrate and/or the nature of the comparators. There is evidence that patients with RA have an increased risk of thrombotic events[64,65]. This is not true of OA, which was the main focus of the celecoxib study. Finally, naproxen may actually be protective against cardiovascular events. There is no convincing evidence that NSAIDs, including naproxen, protect against cardiovascular events[66]. However, naproxen has an extended half-life and suppresses completely the capacity of platelets to make thromboxane A_2 (TXA_2) throughout its dosing interval[67]. One might expect a similar benefit from ibuprofen, which has a similar half-life, but not from diclofenac, which is much shorter lived. Although the magnitude of such a theoretical benefit is also unknown, it seems unlikely to account for a 45% difference between the groups. Aspirin, which would be expected to work via this mechanism, reduces the primary incidence of important vascular events by roughly 20%[68-70] and their secondary incidence by around 25%[71,72]. Clearly, irrespective of the underlying explanation, these data focus attention on the need for further information on the cardiovascular impact of selective inhibitors of COX-2.

In the interim, what approach might be taken for cardioprotection in patients with arthritis? The benefit:risk ratio established by controlled trials indicates that patients who have suffered a prior cardiovascular event should be on low dose aspirin[73]. Should these individuals need antiarthritic medication, there may be an additional suppressive effect on prostacyclin biosynthesis. However, the impact of being on a COX-2 inhibitor or an NSAID should be indistinguishable, while the GI adverse effect profile is likely to favour a selective COX-2 inhibitor. In patients who have not had a prior cardiovascular event, but do have cardiovascular risk factors, the indication for prophylactic low dose aspirin is more arguable[73]. Many such patients receiving a COX-2 inhibitor for RA will be placed on adjuvant therapy. One option is low dose aspirin. However, this combination may have eroded the GI advantage of celecoxib over NSAIDs in the CLASS study. A possible alternative is a controlled release formulation of low dose aspirin, which has been shown to be cardioprotective and, unlike conventional formulations, preserves prostacyclin[74]. However, the incidence of serious bleeding events – even on this preparation – although rare, is double the placebo rate[69]. Thromboxane antagonists avoid suppression of prostacyclin and are at least as effective as aspirin in the prevention of acute coronary occlusive events[75]. Indeed, they have been shown to protect against NSAID gastropathy in experimental animals[76]. Finally, clopidogrel is roughly as effective and has a GI adverse effect profile which is indistinguishable from that of aspirin[77], but it is much more expensive.

In summary, expression of COX-2 appears to play the predominant role in prostacyclin formation by vascular tissues under both physiological and pathological conditions. Aside from atherothrombotic vascular disease, COX-2 may have relevance to other aspects of cardiovascular biology. For example, suppression of COX-2-dependent prostacyclin formation increases the susceptibility of ventricular myocytes to oxidant injury[78]. Suppression of the antiplatelet and vasoconstrictor effects of prostacyclin by selective COX-2 inhibitors poses a theoretical hazard to those at risk of thrombotic disease, and this is consistent with the cardiovascular outcome in the VIGOR trial. However, these results might also be attributable to cardiovascular benefit from naproxen or to the play of chance.

COX-2 INHIBITORS AND RENAL FUNCTION

Given the wide range of potential effects of COX-2 on renal development and function, remarkably little information on the detailed renal pharmacology of COX-2 inhibitors in humans is available. Chronic administration of rofecoxib (50 mg daily) or celecoxib (200 mg or 400 mg, b.i.d.), but not naproxen or indomethacin, causes an early, transient phase of sodium retention, which does not result in detectable oedema or hypertension in healthy subjects[57,79]. After 14 days, the glomerular filtration rate (GFR) declines modestly, but significantly with indomethacin, but not on rofecoxib, implicating COX-1 in the preservation of renal function in this group of elderly (59–80 years) subjects with normal renal function[57]. Meloxicam blunts the renin response to intravenous frusemide in healthy volunteers[80]. A study of rofecoxib in 75 patients aged 60–80 years on a low salt diet reported that GFR is suppressed by both indomethacin and rofecoxib to a similar degree[79]. Thus, in renoprival settings, one might anticipate a similar adverse effect profile with COX-2 inhibitors as observed with conventional NSAIDs. Indeed, an uncontrolled evaluation of the incidence of renal adverse effects in the controlled trials of celecoxib in arthritis accords with this proposal[81]. Thus, one can anticipate the possibility that selective COX-2 inhibitors might indeed precipitate renal failure in individuals critically dependent on vasodilator prostanoids to maintain renal function and, indeed, cases of such complications have been reported[82]. The role of COX-2 in tubular function in humans is poorly understood. While both rofecoxib and celecoxib do result in transient sodium retention, this is mild. However, both drugs elevate blood pressure during chronic administration in normotensive and hypertensive rats[83] and reports of clinical fluid retention are increased over a range of doses of both compounds in the clinical trials database of the Food and Drug Administration (FDA)[84]. Clearly more dose-related information is needed on the effects of these compounds on tubular function and haemodynamics in populations at risk, such as those with compromised renal, hepatic and cardiac function as well as in patients with hypertension.

In summary, we have little detailed information on the renal effects of COX-2 inhibitors, specifically in populations with an activated renin–angiotensin system. Although these compounds are approved for postmenopausal females, off label usage, particularly in juvenile arthritis, is a possibility and the potential effects of selective inhibitors on renal development in humans must be considered carefully.

COX-2 INHIBITORS AND CANCER

A reduction in the incidence of colon cancer in individuals taking aspirin[85] prompted interest in COX in carcinogenesis. This study was followed by many others of aspirin[86–89] and NSAIDs[90], which supported the original observation, although some failed to do so. COX-2 is overexpressed in most colonic cancers and in polyps of patients with familial adenomatous polyposis (FAP)[91,92]. Indeed, the degree of expression appeared to correlate with survival in cancer patients[93]. Subsequently, COX-2 has been found to be expressed in a wide variety of epithelial tumours[94,95].

FAP results from an inactivating mutation in the suppressor adenomatous polyposis coli (APC) gene[96]. Expression of APC in human colorectal cells with inactive endogenous APC alleles induces apoptosis. Overexpression of COX-2 in a rat intestinal line prevents apoptosis, which is restored by a selective COX-2 inhibitor[97]. Irrespective of the mechanisms by which COX-2 might facilitate cellular proliferation, important evidence which compliments the clinical experience derives from mouse models. Mice with an inactivating APC mutation have a FAP phenotype[98]. When crossed into mice deficient in COX-2, the number of their polyps was reduced in a gene dose dependent manner. Furthermore, a selective COX-2 inhibitor also reduced polyp number. It is unclear how suppression of COX-2 expression and/or product formation might restore antitumour reactivity. This may, in part, result from suppression of PGs that directly influence cellular proliferation or modulate cytokine synthesis, acting via membrane receptors or via ligation of peroxisomal proliferator activated receptors (PPARs). PGs may also modulate the nuclear translocation and function of tumour suppressor gene products. It is unclear whether the efficacy of aspirin, NSAIDs or indeed COX-2 inhibitors, may be independent of effects on eicosanoid synthesis. For example, such drugs might regulate COX-2 transcription by ligating PPARs, and aspirin has been postulated to act as an inhibitor of IκB kinase. Clinical experience is limited. Recently, Steinbach et al.[99] reported on a study in 77 patients with FAP. Celecoxib 400 mg b.i.d. significantly reduced the number of polyps by around 30%, while the effects of 100 mg b.i.d. did not differ from those of placebo. This is a potentially important observation, as so many people with FAP progress to develop colon cancer. Unfortunately, the study did not include an aspirin or NSAID control, so it is unknown whether COX-1 inhibition would have a similar effect, at less expense. This would be logical to address, as deletion of COX-1, just like COX-2, reduces both polyp formation in the Min mouse and chemically induced skin carcinogenesis[100].

In summary, COX isozymes appear to play a complex but important role in carcinogenesis. Both a compound which is relatively selective for COX-1 (sulindac)[90] and one which is quite biochemically selective for COX-2 (celecoxib)[99] suppress polyps in patients with FAP. Epidemiological data suggest that the incidence of colonic tumours is reduced in patients taking non-selective inhibitors, such as aspirin. Although the FDA has extended approval for the use of celecoxib in the treatment of FAP, controlled comparisons of biochemically selective COX-2 inhibitors with non-selective inhibitors in larger studies would seem timely.

COX-2 INHIBITORS AND THE BRAIN

Expression of COX-2, but also COX-1, is increased in the senile plaques characteristic of Alzheimer's disease (AD)[101,102]. Epidemiological studies have suggested a delayed rate of progression in patients with AD who are taking aspirin, and a small controlled study suggests a modest effect of an NSAID[103–105]. Hints of areas of additional interest emerge from experimental models. Thus, in the rat, COX-2 is transiently increased via NMDA receptors in neurons at risk of death after focal ischaemia and a COX-2 inhibitor reduces infarction volume in an inducible nitric oxide synthase (iNOS) dependent manner[106]. Perhaps suggesting a role in meningitis, LPS induces leptomeningeal expression of COX-2, and its products mediate cerebral vasodilatation[107]. COX-2 is expressed in the dendritic spines of excitatory neurons[108], suggesting a role in postsynaptic signalling and in synaptic remodeling. Interestingly, pharmacological inhibitors of COX-2 aggravate induced seizure activity and consequent neuronal cell death in the hippocampus[109] in the rat. They also fail to influence brain oedema and may worsen motor functional recovery after head trauma[110]. Despite these observations, we have limited information on the effects of selective COX-2 inhibitors in the brain. Phase II studies in AD are near completion. These will provide some information on tolerability, although they are too small to address the issue of efficacy, hinted at by observational studies of aspirin consumption in this disease.

In summary, the widespread distribution of COX-2 in human brain and its regulated expression in animal models suggest the importance of this isozyme and/or its products in central physiology and pathology. Based on studies that associate use of aspirin and NSAIDs with delayed onset and progression of AD, some modest prospective evidence for the efficacy of an NSAID and upregulation of COX-2 in AD lesions, this is presently the aspect of neurological disease with therapeutic promise for these compounds.

COX-2 INHIBITORS IN REPRODUCTION AND DEVELOPMENT

COX-2 appears to play a pivotal role in reproduction and development. Mice deficient in COX-2, but not COX-1, exhibit multiple defects in ovulation, fertilization, implantation and decidualization[111]. COX-1-derived products appear most important in preparing the uterus for implantation[112], while COX-2 is dramatically upregulated at the site and time of implantation. However, COX-2-dependent PG formation substitutes for COX-1 prior to implantation in COX-1-deleted mice[113]. This occurs coincidentally with co-localized upregulation of prostacyclin synthase and PPARδ, for which prostacyclin may be a ligand. Both PPARδ agonists and prostacyclin analogues restore implantation in COX-2-deficient mice[114]. However, mice deficient in either the membrane receptor for prostacyclin or in PPARδ do not exhibit a reproductive phenotype[57,115]. COX-2 appears to be the predominant source of the increased generation of the $PGF_{2\alpha}$[116] which is critical to initiation of parturition[117].

Little information is available on the impact of COX-2 inhibitors on human pregnancy. However, interest has been expressed in their potential value in the prevention of preterm delivery or conception. Given their potential effects on the fetus, care should be taken to avoid off label usage by women in the reproductive age group.

SUMMARY

In just over a decade, we have moved from discovery of COX-2 to phase III clinical trials demonstrating that selective COX-2 inhibitors cause significantly fewer serious GI adverse events than a traditional NSAID. This remarkable progress has been accompanied by the prospect of additional efficacy in preventing and delaying the progression of cancer and perhaps also AD. It is important to recognize that even more selective inhibitors of COX-2 have entered human development and that we have much yet to learn about the clinical pharmacology, therapeutic potential and hazards of these drugs.

ACKNOWLEDGEMENTS

Supported by grants HL 66376, HL 62250 and HL 54500 from the National Institutes of Health. Dr FitzGerald is the Robinette Foundation Professor of Cardiovascular Medicine.

Address all correspondence to: Dr Garret A. FitzGerald, University of Pennsylvania, Department of Pharmacology, 153 Johnson Pavilion, 3620 Hamilton Walk, Philadelphia, PA 19104-6084, USA.

REFERENCES

1. Loll PJ, Picot D, Garavito RM. The structural basis of aspirin activity inferred from the crystal structure of inactivated prostaglandin H$_2$ synthase. *Nature Struct Biol.* 1995;2:637–43.
2. Luong C, Miller A, Barnett J, Chow J, Ramesha C, Browner MF. Flexibility of the NSAID binding site in the structure of human cyclooxygenase-2. *Nature Struct Biol.* 1996;3:927–33.
3. Kurumbail RG, Stevens AM, Gierse JK, McDonald JJ, Stegeman RA, Pak JY et al. Structural basis for selective inhibition of cyclooxygenase-2 by anti-inflammatory agents. *Nature.* 1996;384:644–8.
4. García Rodríguez LA, Hernández-Díaz S. The risk of upper gastrointestinal complications associated with nonsteroidal anti-inflammatory drugs, glucocorticoids, acetaminophen and combinations of these agents. *Arthritis Res.* 2001;3:98–101.
5. Xie W, Chipman JG, Robertson DL, Erikson RL, Simmons DL. Expression of a mitogen-responsive gene encoding prostaglandin synthase is regulated by mRNA splicing. *Proc Natl Acad Sci USA.* 1991;88:2692–6.

6. Kujubu DA, Herschman HR. Dexamethasone inhibits mitogen induction of the TIS10 prostaglandin synthase/cyclooxygenase gene. *J Biol Chem*. 1992;267:7991–4.
7. O'Banion MK, Winn VD, Young DA. cDNA cloning and functional activity of a glucocorticoid-regulated inflammatory cyclooxygenase. *Proc Natl Acad Sci USA*. 1992;89:4888–92.
8. Lee SH, Soyoola E, Chanmugam P, Hart S, Sun W, Zhong H et al. Selective expression of mitogen-inducible cyclooxygenase in macrophages stimulated with lipopolysaccharide. *J Biol Chem*. 1992;267:25934–8.
9. Patrignani P, Panara MR, Greco A, Fusco O, Natolie Iacobelli S et al. Biochemical and pharmacological characterization of the cyclooxygenase activity of human blood prostaglandin endoperoxide synthases. *J Pharmacol Exp Ther*. 1994;271:1705–12.
10. Warner TD, Giuliano F, Vojnovic I, Bukasa A, Mitchell JA, Vane JR. Nonsteroid drug selectivities for cyclo-oxygenase-1 rather than cyclo-oxygenase-2 are associated with human gastrointestinal toxicity: A full in vitro analysis. *Proc Natl Acad Sci USA*, 1999;96:7563–8.
11. Patrignani P, Panara MR, Sciulli MG, Santini G, Renda G, Patrono C. Differential inhibition of human prostaglandin endoperoxide synthase-1 and -2 by nonsteroidal anti-inflammatory drugs. *J Physiol Pharmacol*. 1997;48:623–31.
12. Chan C-C, Boyce S, Brideau C, Charleson S, Cromlish W, Ethier D et al. Rofecoxib [Vioxx, MK-0966; 4-(4'-Methylsulfonylphenyl)-3-phenyl-2-(5H)-furanone]: A potent and orally active cyclooxygenase-2 inhibitor. Pharmacological and biochemical profiles. *J Pharmacol Exp Ther*. 1999;290:551–60.
13. Patrono C, Ciabattoni G, Pinca E, Pugliese F, Castrucci G, DeSalvo A et al. Low dose aspirin and inhibition of thromboxane B_2 production in healthy subjects. *Thromb Res*. 1980;17:317–27.
14. Cryer B, Feldman M. Cyclooxygenase-1 and cyclooxygenase-2 selectivity of widely used nonsteroidal anti-inflammatory drugs. *Am J Med*. 1998;104:413–21.
15. Malmstrom K, Daniels S, Kotey P, Seidenberg BC, Desjardins PJ. Comparison of rofecoxib and celecoxib, two cyclooxygenase-2 inhibitors, in postoperative dental pain: a randomized, placebo-and active-comparator-controlled clinical trial. *Clin Ther*. 1999;21:1653–63.
16. Day R, Morrison B, Luza A, Castaneda D, Strusberg A, Nahir M et al. A randomized trial of the efficacy and tolerability of the COX-2 inhibitor rofecoxib vs ibuprofen in patients with osteoarthritis. Rofecoxib/Ibuprofen Comparator Study Group. *Arch Intern Med*. 2000;160:1781–7.
17. Cannon GW, Caldwell JR, Holt P, McLean B, Seidenberg B, Bologriese J et al. Rofecoxib, a specific inhibitor of cyclooxygenase 2, with clinical efficacy comparable with that of diclofenac sodium: results of a one-year, randomized, clinical trial in patients with osteoarthritis of the knee and hip. Rofecoxib Phase III Protocol 035 Study Group. *Arthritis Rheum*. 2000;43:978–87.
18. Karim A, Tolbert D, Piergies A, Hubbard RC, Harper K, Wallemark CB et al. Celecoxib does not significantly alter the pharmacokinetics or hypoprothrombinemic effect of warfarin in healthy subjects. *J Clin Pharmacol*. 2000;40:655–63.
19. Clemett D, Goa KL. Celecoxib: a review of its use in osteoarthritis, rheumatoid arthritis and acute pain. *Drugs*. 2000;59:957–80.
20. Dequeker J, Hawkey C, Kahan A, Steinbrück K, Alegre C, Baumelou E et al. Improvement in gastrointestinal tolerablility of the selective cyclooxygenase (COX)-2 inhibitor, meloxicam, compared with piroxicam: results of the Safety and

Efficacy Large-scale Evaluation of COX-2 inhibiting therapies (SELECT) trial in osteoarthritis. *Br J Rheumatol.* 1998;37:946–51.

21. Martin RM, Biswas P, Mann RD. The incidence of adverse events and risk factors for upper gastrointestinal disorders associated with meloxicam use amongst 19 087 patients in general practice in England: cohort study. *Br J Clin Pharmacol.* 2000;50:35–42.

22. Famaey JP. In vitro and in vivo pharmacological evidence of selective cyclo-oxygenase-2 inhibition by nimesulide: an overview. *Inflamm Res.* 1997;46:437–46.

23. Tang C, Shou M, Mei Q, Rushmore TH, Rodrigues AD. Major role of human liver microsomal cytochrome P450 2C9 (CYP 2C9) in the oxidative metabolism of cele-coxib, a novel cyclooxygenase-II inhibitor. *J Pharmacol Exp Ther.* 2000;293:453–9.

24. Davies NM, McLachlan AJ, Day RO, Williams KM. Clinical pharmacokinetics and pharmacodynamics of celecoxib: a selective cyclo-oxygenase-2 inhibitor. *Clin Pharmacokinet.* 2000;38:225–42.

25. Larkai EN, Smith JL, Lidsky MD, Graham DY. Gastroduodenal mucosa and dyspeptic symptoms in arthritic patients during chronic steroidal anti-inflammatory drug use. *Am J Gastroenterol.* 1987;82:1153–8.

26. Wolfe MM, Lichtenstein DR, Singh G. Gastrointestinal toxicity of nonsteroidal antiinflammatory drugs. *N Engl J Med.* 1999;340:1888–99.

27. Singh G, Triadfilopoulus G. Epidemiology of NSAID-induced GI complications. *J Rheumatol.* 1999;26(suppl 26):18–24.

28. Simon LS, Weaver AL, Graham DY, Kivitz AJ, Lipsky PE, Hubbard RC et al. Anti-inflammatory and upper gastrointestinal effects of celecoxib in rheumatoid arthritis: a randomized controlled trial. *JAMA.* 1999;282:1921–8.

29. McAdam BF, Catella-Lawson F, Mardini IA, Kapoor S, Lawson JA, FitzGerald GA. Systemic biosynthesis of prostacyclin by cyclooxygenase (COX)-2: The human pharmacology of a selective inhibitor of COX-2. *Proc Natl Acad Sci USA.* 1999;96:272–7.

30. Emery P, Zeidler H, Kvien TK, Guslandi M, Naudin R, Stead H et al. Celecoxib versus diclofenac in long-term management of rheumatoid arthritis: randomised double-blind comparison. *Lancet.* 1999;354:2106–11.

31. Langman MJ, Jensen DM, Watson DJ, Harper SE, Zhao PL, Quan H et al. Adverse upper gastrointestinal effects of rofecoxib compared with NSAIDs. *JAMA.* 1999;282:1929–33.

32. Shallcross TM, Heatley RV. Effect of non-steroidal anti-inflammatory drugs on dyspeptic symptoms. *BMJ.* 1990;300:368–9.

33. Kimmey MB. Role of endoscopy in nonsteroidal anti-inflammatory drug clinical trials. *Am J Med.* 1998;105:28S–31S.

34. Bombardier C, Laine L, Hochberg M, Day R, Shapiro D, Reicin A. A prospective double-blind GI outcomes study of rofecoxib vs. naproxen. *Digestive Diseases Workshop 2000, San Diego.*

35. Silverstein F, Simon L, Faich J, Lefkowith J. A prospective double-blind GI out-comes trial of celecoxib. *Digestive Diseases Workshop 2000, San Diego.*

36. Silverstein FE, Graham DY, Senior JR, Davies HW, Struthers BJ, Bittman RM et al. Misoprostol reduced serious complications in patients with rheumatoid arthritis receiving nonsteroidal anti-inflammatory drugs. *Ann Intern Med.* 1995;123:241–9.

37. Peterson WL, Cryer B. COX-1-sparing NSAIDs – is the enthusiasm justified? *JAMA.* 1999;282:1961–3.

38. Zimmermann KC, Sarbia M, Schror K, Weber AA. Constitutive cyclooxygenase-2 expression in healthy human and rabbit gastric mucosa. *Mol Pharmacol.* 1998;54:536–40.

39. Sawaoka H, Kawano S, Tsuji S, Tsuji M, Sun W, Gunawan ES et al. *Helicobacter pylori* infection induces cyclooxygenase-2 expression in human gastric mucosa. *Prostaglandins Leukot Essent Fatty Acids.* 1998;59:313–6.

40. McCarthy CJ, Crofford LJ, Greenson J, Scheiman JM. Cyclooxygenase-2 expression in gastric antral mucosa before and after eradication of *Helicobacter pylori* infection. *Am J Gastroenterol.* 1999;94:1218–23.

41. Mizuno H, Sakamoto C, Matsuda K, Wada K, Uchida T, Noguchi H et al. Induction of cyclooxygenase 2 in gastric mucosal lesions and its inhibition by the specific antagonist delays healing in mice. *Gastroenterology.* 1997;112:387–97.

42. Prescott SM. Is COX-2 the alpha and the omega in cancer? *J Clin Invest.* 2000;105:1511–13.

43. Jones MK, Wang H, Peskar BM, Levin E, Itani RM, Sarfeh IJ et al. Inhibition of angiogenesis by nonsteroidal anti-inflammatory drugs: insight into mechanisms and implications for cancer growth and ulcer healing. *Nature Med.* 1999;5:1418–23.

44. Majima M, Hayashi I, Muramatsu M, Katada J, Yamashina S, Katori M. Cyclooxygenase-2 enhances basic fibroblast growth factor-induced angiogenesis through induction of vascular endothelial growth factor in rat sponge implants. *Br J Pharmacol.* 2000;130:641–9.

45. Newberry RD, Stenson WF, Lorenz RG. Cyclooxygenase-2 dependent arachidonic acid metabolites are essential modulators of the intestinal immune response to dietary antigen. *Nature Med.* 1999;5:900–6.

46. Morteau O, Morham SG, Sellon R, Dieleman LA, Langenbach R, Smithies D et al. Impaired mucosal defense to acute colonic injury in mice lacking cyclooxygenase-1 or cyclooxygenase-2. *J Clin Invest.* 2000;105:469–78.

47. Reuter BK, Asfaha S, Buret A, Sharkey KA, Wallace JL. Exacerbation of inflammation-associated colonic inflammation in rats through inhibition of cyclooxygenase-2. *J Clin Invest.* 1996;98:2076–85.

48. Rimarachin JA, Jacobson JA, Szabo P, Maclouf J, Creminon C, Weksler BB. Regulation of cyclooxygenase-2 expression in aortic smooth muscle cells. *Arterioscler Thromb.* 1994;14:1021–31.

49. Cao C, Matsumura K, Yamagata K, Watanabe Y. Endothelial cells of the rat brain vasculature express cyclooxygenase-2 mRNA in response to systemic interleukin-1 beta: a possible site of prostaglandin sythesis responsible for fever. *Brain Res.* 1996;733:263–72.

50. Young W, Mahboubi K, Haider A, Li I, Ferreri NR. Cyclooxygenase-2 is required for tumor necrosis factor-alpha- and angiotensin II-mediated proliferation of vascular smooth muscle cells. *Circ Res.* 2000;86:906–14.

51. Wu KK. Injury-coupled induction of endothelial eNOS and COX-2 genes: a paradigm for thromboresistant gene therapy. *Proc Assoc Am Physicians.* 1998;110:163–70.

52. FitzGerald GA, Smith B, Pedersen AK, Brash AR. Increased prostacyclin biosynthesis is increased in patients with severe atherosclerosis and platelet activation. *N Engl J Med.* 1984;310:1065–8.

53. Fitzgerald DJ, Roy L, Catella F, FitzGerald GA. Platelet activation in unstable coronary disease. *N Engl J Med.* 1986;315:983–9.

54. Schonbeck U, Dukhova GK, Graber P, Coulter S, Libby P. Augmented expression of cyclooxygenase-2 in human atherosclerotic lesions. *Am J Pathol.* 1999;155:1281–91.

55. FitzGerald GA, Pedersen AK, Patrono C. Analysis of prostacyclin and thromboxane biosynthesis in cardiovascular disease. *Circulation*. 1983;67:1174–7.

56. Cullen L, Kelly L, Connor SO, Fitzgerald DJ. Selective cyclooxygenase-2 inhibition by nimesulide in man. *J Pharmacol Exp Ther*. 1998;287:578–82.

57. Catella-Lawson F, McAdam B, Morrisson B, Kapoor S, Kujubu D, Amtes L et al. Effects of specific inhibition of cyclooxygenase-2 on sodium balance, hemodynamics, and vasoactive eicosanoids. *J Pharm Exp Ther*. 1999;289:735–41.

58. Topper JN, Cai J, Falb D, Gimbrone MA Jr. Identification of vascular endothelial genes differentially responsive to fluid mechanical stimuli: cyclooxygenase-2, manganese superoxide dismutase, and endothelial cell nitric oxide synthase are selectively up-regulated by steady laminar shear stress. *Proc Natl Acad Sci USA*. 1996;93:10417–22.

59. Roy L, Knapp HR, Robertson RM, FitzGerald GA. Endogenous biosynthesis of prostacyclin during cardiac catheterization and angiography in man. *Circulation*. 1985;71:434–40.

60. Fitzgerald DJ, Catella F, Roy L, FitzGerald GA. Marked platelet activation in vivo after intravenous streptokinase in patients with acute myocardial infarction. *Circulation*. 1988;77:142–50.

61. Nowak J, Murray JJ, Oates JA, FitzGerald GA. Biochemical evidence of a chronic abnormality in platelet and vascular function in healthy individuals who smoke cigarettes. *Circulation*. 1987;76:6–14.

62. Murata T, Ushikubi F, Matsuoka T et al. Altered pain perception and inflammatory response in mice lacking prostacyclin receptor. *Nature*. 1997;388:678–82.

63. Crofford LJ, Oates JC, McCune WJ, Gupta S, Kaplan MJ, Catella-Lawson F et al. Thrombosis in patients with connective tissue diseases treated with specific cyclooxygenase-2 inhibitors: a report of four cases. *Arthritis Rheum*. 2000;43:1891–6.

64. Wallberg-Jonsson S, Ohman ML, Dahlqvist SR. Cardiovascular morbidity and mortality in patients with seropositive rheumatoid arthritis in Northern Sweden. *J Rheumatol*. 1997;24:445–51.

65. Wallberg-Jonsson S, Cederfelt M, Rantapaa Dahlqvist S. Hemostatic factors and cardiovascular disease in active rheumatoid arthritis: an 8 year followup study. *J Rheumatol*. 2000;27:71–5.

66. García Rodríguez LA, Varas C, Patrono C. Differential effects of aspirin and nonaspirin nonsteroidal antiinflammatory drugs in the primary prevention of myocardial infarction in postmenopausal women. *Epidemiology*. 2000;11:382–7.

67. Van Hecken A, Schwartz JI, Depre M, De Leeleire I, Dallob A, Tanaka W et al. Comparative inhibitory activity of rofecoxib, meloxican, diclofenac, ibuprofen and naproxen on COX-2 versus COX-1 in healthy volunteers. *J Clin Pharmacol*. 2000;40:1109–20.

68. Steering Committee of the Physician's Health Study Research Group. Final reports on the aspirin component of the ongoing Physician's Health Study. *N Engl J Med*. 1989;321:129–35.

69. The Medical Research Council's General Practice Research Framework. Thrombosis prevention trial: randomised trial of low-intensity oral anticoagulation with warfarin and low-dose aspirin in the primary prevention of ischaemic heart disease in men at increased risk. *Lancet*. 1998;351:233–41.

70. Hansson L, Zanchetti A, Carruthers SG, Dahlof B, Elmfeldt D, Julius S et al. Effects of intensive blood-pressure lowering and low-dose aspirin in patients with hypertension: principal results of the Hypertension Optimal Treatment (HOT) randomized trial. *Lancet*. 1998;351:1755–62.

71. Antiplatelet Trialists' Collaboration. Collaborative overview of randomised trials of antiplatelet therapy-I: Prevention of death, myocardial infarction, and stroke by prolonged antiplatelet therapy in various categories of patients. *BMJ*. 1994;308:81–106.

72. Hankey GJ, Warlow CP. Treatment and secondary prevention of stroke: evidence, costs, and effects on individual and populations. *Lancet*. 1999;354:1457–63.

73. Patrono C, Coller B, Dalen JE, Fuster V, Gent M, Harker LA et al. Platelet active drugs. The relationships among dose, effectiveness, and side effects. *Chest*. 1998;114(suppl 5):470S–88S.

74. Clarke RJ, Price P, Mayo G, FitzGerald GA. Preservation of systemic prostacyclin synthesis by controlled release, low dose aspirin: selectivity for thromboxane A$_2$. *N Engl J Med*. 1991;325:1137–41.

75. Savage MP, Goldberg S, Bove AA, Macdonald RG, Bass TA, Margolis JR et al. Multi-hospital eastern Atlantic restenosis trial II: A placebo-controlled trial of thromboxane blockade in the prevention of restenosis following coronary angio-plasty. *Am Heart J*. 1991;122:1239–44.

76. Ogletree ML, O'Keefe EH, Durham SK, Rubin B, Aberg G. Gastroprotective effects of thromboxane receptor antagonists. *J Pharmacol Exp Ther*. 1992;263:374–80.

77. CAPRIE Steering Committee. A randomised, blinded, trial of clopidogrel versus aspirin in patients at risk of ischaemic events (CAPRIE). *Lancet*. 1996;348:1329–39.

78. Adderley SR, Fitzgerald DJ. Oxidative damage of cardiomyocytes is limited by extra-cellular regulated kinases 1/2-mediated induction of cyclooxygenase-2. *J Biol Chem*. 1999;274:5038–46.

79. Swan SK, Rudy DW, Lasseter KC, Ryan CF, Buechel KL, Lambrecht LJ et al. Randomized evaluations of the effects of cyclooxygenase-2 inhibition on renal func-tion of elderly subjects on a low salt diet. A randomized, controlled trial. *Ann Intern Med*. 2000;133:1–9.

80. Stichtenoth DO, Wagner B, Frolich JC. Effect of selective inhibition of the inducible cyclooxygenase on renin release in healthy volunteers. *J Investig Med*. 1998;46:290–6.

81. Whelton A, Brater DC, Sica DA, Verburg KM, Drower EJ, Geis GS. Effects of celecoxib and naproxen on renal function in renal insufficiency patients. *Am J Soc Nephrol*. 1999;10:92A.

82. Perazella MA, Eras J. Are selective COX-2 inhibitors nephrotoxic? *Am J Kidney Dis*. 2000;35:937–40.

83. Muscara MN, Vergnolle N, Lovren F, Triggle CR, Elliott SN, Asfaha S et al. Selective cyclo-oxygenase-2 inhibition with celecoxib elevated blood pressure and promotes leukocyte adherence. *Br J Pharmacol*. 2000;129:1423–30.

84. Lipsky PE. Unresolved issues in the role of cyclooxygenase-2 in normal physiology and disease. In: Velo G, Perucca E, special editors. Abstracts of the Joint Meeting of VII World Conference on Clinical Pharmacology and Therapeutics IUPHAR – Division of Clinical Pharmacology & 4th Congress of the European Association for Clinical Pharmacology and Therapeutics (EACPT). *Br J Clin Pharmacol*. 2000:15.

85. Kune GA, Kune S, Watson LF. Colorectal cancer risk, chronic illnesses, opera-tions, and medications: case control results from the Melbourne Colorectal Cancer Study. *Cancer Res*. 1988;48:4399–404.

86. Thun MJ. Aspirin and gastrointestinal cancer. *Adv Exp Med Biol*. 1997;400A:395–402.

87. Paganini-Hill A, Chao A, Ross RK, Henderson BE. Aspirin use and chronic diseases: a cohort study of the elderly. *BMJ*. 1989;299:1247–50.

88. Greenberg ER, Baron JA, Freeman DH Jr, Mandel JS, Haile R. Reduced risk of large-bowel adenomas among aspirin users. The Polyp Prevention Study Group. *J Natl Cancer Inst*. 1993;85:912–16.

89. Logan RF, Little J, Hawtin PG, Hardcastle JD. Effect of aspirin and non-steroidal anti-inflammatory drugs on colorectal adenomas: case-control study of subjects participating in the Nottingham faecal occult blood screening programme. *BMJ*. 1993;307:285–9.

90. Giardiello FM, Hamilton SR, Krush AJ, Piantadosi S, Hylind LM, Celano P et al. Treatment of colonic and rectal adenomas with sulindac in familial adenomatous polyposis. *N Engl J Med*. 1993;328:1313–16.

91. Eberhart CE, Coffey RJ, Radhika A, Giardiello FM, Ferrenbach S, DuBois RN. Up-regulation of cyclooxygenase 2 gene expression in human colorectal adenomas and adenocarcinomas. *Gastroenterology*. 1994;107:1183–8.

92. Sano H, Kawahito Y, Wilder RL, Hashiramoto A, Mukai S, Asai K et al. Expression of cyclooxygenase-1 and -2 in human colorectal cancer. *Cancer Res*. 1995;55:3785–9.

93. Sheehan KM, Sheahan K, O'Donoghue DP, MacSweeney F, Conroy RM, Fitzgerald DJ et al. The relationship between cyclooxygenase-2 expression and colorectal cancer. *JAMA*. 1999;282:1254–7.

94. Marrogi A, Pass HI, Khan M, Metheny-Barlow LJ, Harris CC, Gerwin BI. Human mesothelioma samples overexpress both cyclooxygenase-2 (COX-2) and inducible nitric oxide synthase (NOS2): in vitro antiproliferative effects of a COX-2 inhibitor. *Cancer Res*. 2000;60:3696–700.

95. Komhoff M, Guan Y, Shappell HW, Davish Jack G, Shyr Y et al. Enhanced expression of cyclooxygenase-2 in high grade human transitional cell bladder carcinomas. *Am J Pathol*. 2000;157:29–35.

96. Shibata H, Toyama K, Shioya H, Ito M, Hirota M, Hasegawa S et al. Rapid colorectal adenoma formation initiated by conditional targeting of the Apc gene. *Science*. 1997;278:120–3.

97. Tsujii M, DuBois RN. Alterations in cellular adhesion and apoptosis in epithelial cells overexpressing prostaglandin endoperoxide synthase 2. *Cell*. 1995;83:493–501.

98. Oshima M, Dinchuk JE, Kargman SL, Oshima H, Hancock B, Kwong E et al. Suppression of intestinal polyposis in ApcΔ716 knockout mice by inhibition of cyclooxygenase 2 (COX-2). *Cell*. 1996;87:803–9.

99. Steinbach G, Lynch PM, Phillips RK, Wallace MH, Hawk E, Gordon GB et al. The effect of celecoxib, a cyclooxygenase-2 inhibitor, in familial adenomatous polyposis. *N Engl J Med*. 2000;342:1946–52.

100. Langenbach R, Loftin C, Lee C, Tiano H. Cyclooxygenase knockout mice: models for elucidating isoform-specific functions. *Biochem Pharmacol*. 1999:58:1237–46.

101. Ho L, Pieroni C, Winger D, Purohit DP, Aisen PS, Pasinetti GM. Regional distribution of cyclooxygenase-2 in the hippocampal formation in Alzheimer's disease. *J Neurosci Res*. 1999;57:295–303.

102. Lukiw WJ, Bazan NG. Cyclooxygenase 2 RNA message abundance, stability, and hypervariability in sporadic Alzheimer neocortex. *J Neurosci Res*. 1997;50:937–45.

103. Breitner JC, Gau BA, Welsh KA, Plassman BL, McDonald WM, Helms MJ et al. Inverse association of anti-inflammatory treatments and Alzheimer's disease: initial results of a co-twin control study. *Neurology*. 1994;44:227–32.

104. Anthony JC, Breitner JC, Zandi PP, Meyer MR, Jurasova I, Norton MC et al.

Reduced prevalence of AD in users of NSAIDs and H_2 receptor antagonists: the Cache County study. *Neurology.* 2000;54:2066–71.

105. Emilien G, Beyreuther K, Masters CL, Maloteaux JM. Prospects for pharmacological intervention in Alzheimer disease. *Arch Neurol.* 2000;57:454–9.

106. Miettinen S, Fusco FR, Yrjänheikki J, Hirvonen T, Roivainen R, Narhi M et al. Spreading depression and focal brain ischemia induce cyclooxygenase-2 in cortical neurons through N-methyl-D-aspartic acid-receptors and phospholipase A_2. *Proc Natl Acad Sci USA.* 1997;94:6500–5.

107. Brian JE Jr, Moore SA, Faraci FM. Expression and vascular effects of cyclooxygenase-2 in brain. *Stroke.* 1998;29:2600–6.

108. Yamagata K, Andreasson KI, Kaufmann WE, Barnes CA, Worley PF. Expression of a mitogen-inducible cyclooxygenase in brain neurons: regulation by synaptic activity and glucocorticoids. *Neuron.* 1993;11:371–86.

109. Marcheselli VL, Bazan NG. Sustained induction of prostaglandin endoperoxide synthase-2 by seizures in hippocampus. *J Biol Chem.* 1996;271:24794–9.

110. Dash PK, Mach SA, Moore AN. Regional expression and role of cyclooxygenase-2 following experimental traumatic brain injury. *J Neurotrauma.* 2000;17:69–81.

111. Lim H, Paria BC, Das SK, Dinchuk JE, Langenbach R, Trzaskos JM et al. Multiple female reproductive failures in cyclooxygenase 2-deficient mice. *Cell.* 1997;91:197–208.

112. Tsuboi K, Sugimoto Y, Iwane A, Yamamoto K, Yamamoto S, Ichikawa A. Uterine expression of prostaglandin H_2 synthase in late pregnancy and during parturition in prostaglandin F receptor-deficient mice. *Endocrinology.* 2000;141:315–24.

113. Reese J, Brown N, Paria BC, Morrow J, Dey SK. COX-2 compensation in the uterus of COX-1 deficient mice during the pre-implantation period. *Mol Cell Endocrinol.* 1999;150:23–31.

114. Lim H, Gupta RA, Ma WG, Paria BC, Moller DE, Morrow JD et al. Cyclooxygenase-2-derived prostacyclin mediates embryo implantation in the mouse via PPARδ. *Genes Dev.* 1999;13:1561–74.

115. Peters JM, Lee SS, Li W, Ward JM, Gavrilova O, Everett C et al. Growth, adipose, brain, and skin alterations resulting from targeted disruption of the mouse peroxisome proliferator-activated receptor beta (delta). *Mol Cell Biol.* 2000;20:5119–28.

116. Muglia LJ. Genetic analysis of fetal development and parturition control in the mouse. *Pediatr Res.* 2000;47:437–43.

117. Sugimoto Y, Yamasaki A, Segi E, Tsubai K, Aze Y, Nishimura T et al. Failure of parturition in mice lacking the prostaglandin F receptor. *Science.* 1997;277:681–3.

21 Clinical experience with celecoxib: a cyclooxygenase-2 specific inhibitor

J.B. LEFKOWITH, K.M. VERBURG AND G.S. GEIS
Pharmacia Clinical Research and Development, Skokie, IL, USA.

THE COX-2 HYPOTHESIS

Non-steroid anti-inflammatory drugs (NSAIDs) are currently the most common agents used in the treatment of the signs and symptoms of arthritis and pain. Their clinical efficacy is mediated via inhibition of the prostaglandin (PG)-production pathway, acting on cyclooxygenase (COX), the enzyme which catalyses the production of prostanoids from arachidonic acid (AA)[1,2]. In addition to their role as autacoids responsible for normal physiological functions in the gastrointestinal (GI) tract, kidney, reproductive system and platelets, PGs (and thromboxane) are key mediators of inflammation and pain[2]. The inhibition by NSAIDs of the production of PGs that mediate inflammation and pain provides their therapeutic effect. However, the mode of action of conventional NSAIDs also results in GI-, renal- and platelet-related side effects due to the concomitant inhibition of the synthesis of PGs involved in normal physiological functions[3–5].

Two distinct COX isoforms have recently been described[2,6–8]. Both isoforms perform the same catalytic reaction, inhibiting the conversion of AA to prostanoids. The COX isoform designated COX-1 is expressed constitutively in most tissues throughout the body, including the GI tract, kidneys and platelets[2,6]. Cyclooxygenase-2, however, is normally expressed at low levels in normal tissue, but it is induced to high expression by inflammatory mediators at sites of inflammation[7–9].

Conventional NSAIDs inhibit both COX-1 and COX-2 with negligible specificity *in vitro*[10]. The therapeutic benefits of NSAIDs are thought to be due to their inhibition of COX-2, which is induced in inflammation and mediates the inflammatory response[11]. The GI and platelet side effects attributed to

461

conventional NSAIDs are probably the result of COX-1 inhibition, since this isoform is the major isoform expressed in these tissues. The cause of renal effects of conventional NSAIDs remains uncertain since both isoforms may be expressed by the kidney in various physiological and pathophysiological states[12].

With the discovery of the two isoforms of COX, it was postulated that specific inhibition of the COX-2 isoform would provide the therapeutic anti-inflammatory and analgesic effects of conventional NSAIDs without the side effects with which they are associated[13]. This hypothesis has been supported by animal models using selective COX-2 inhibitors[11,14].

The development of celecoxib, the first in a new class of agents designed specifically to inhibit COX-2, was based on this hypothesis. *In vitro*, celecoxib is highly selective for COX-2, demonstrating 300–>2000-fold separation in inhibition curves versus COX-1 in a wide range of experimental conditions. This selectivity results from the structure of celecoxib that allows it to occupy space in the active site of COX-2, which is not present in COX-1.

The binding between celecoxib and COX-2 forms a tight enzyme–inhibitor complex that dissociates slowly and is non-competitive with the substrate. In high concentrations, celecoxib inhibits COX-1, but the kinetics of this interaction are conventionally competitive. Celecoxib's *in vitro* kinetics are mirrored *in vivo*. Animal studies have shown that celecoxib doses that inhibit COX-2-derived PG production have little or no effect on COX-1-derived PG production in the GI mucosa, kidneys or platelets.

Prior to the clinical development of celecoxib, the compound underwent extensive toxicological evaluation, including acute, subchronic, chronic, genetic and reproductive toxicology, as well as carcinogenicity testing. The lack of preclinical toxicological findings and the observed substantial safety margins allowed for the clinical development of this compound, focusing on the following goals:

1. elucidation of the pharmacokinetic profile of celecoxib;
2. establishing the therapeutic efficacy of celecoxib as an analgesic and anti-inflammatory agent;
3. evaluating the GI and platelet effects of celecoxib as a means to examine the COX-2 specificity of this agent in humans; and
4. determination of the overall safety and tolerability profile in the target patient population.

HUMAN PHARMACOKINETICS

The human pharmacokinetic profile of celecoxib was determined from 32 studies, in which 1566 subjects/patients received single or multiple oral doses of the agent.

Absorption and distribution

Celecoxib has an apparent plasma clearance of ~500 ml min^{-1} (30 l h^{-1}), adjusted for 70 kg body weight in healthy young adults after single-dose administration (data on file: Pharmacia Corporation). It is extensively bound to plasma proteins (~97%)[15], and this binding remains constant within the wide therapeutic concentration range of the total drug. There is no preferential distribution between red blood cells and plasma[16]. Celecoxib is extensively distributed, with a volume of distribution at steady state of ~500 l/70 kg after a single 200 mg oral dose in healthy young adults. Its plasma elimination half-life is ~10–12 h (data on file: Pharmacia Corporation).

The absorption of celecoxib is increased slightly by food and decreased slightly by antacids (data on file: Pharmacia Corporation). These effects are not clinically important and do not lead to a need for dose adjustment, however.

Metabolism

Celecoxib is extensively metabolized in the liver, via the cytochrome P450 2C9 enzyme pathway[16] – co-administration with fluconazole (an inhibitor of cytochrome P450 2C9) results in an approximately twofold increase in the area under the concentration–time curve of celecoxib (data on file: Pharmacia Corporation). None of the metabolites of celecoxib exhibits COX-inhibiting activity[17].

Celecoxib is excreted via the faeces and urine; the inactive acid metabolite is the major excreted material and constitutes ~54% of the dose in faeces and 19% in urine. In faeces, 2.6% of the dose is unchanged drug[17], while no unchanged drug is recovered from urine.

Drug–drug interactions

Since celecoxib is metabolized by cytochrome P450 2C9[15], it has the potential to interact with other substrates of this enzyme, affecting their pharmacokinetics. As a result, drug–drug interaction studies were conducted with multiple doses of celecoxib and tolbutamide, phenytoin, glyburide (data on file: Pharmacia Corporation) and warfarin[18] (all known substrates of cytochrome P450 2C9 with narrow therapeutic windows). Since some NSAIDs have been reported to decrease the renal clearance of drugs that are eliminated mainly via the kidney[5], the effects of celecoxib on the renal clearance of methotrexate[19] and lithium (data on file: Pharmacia Corporation) were also studied.

Celecoxib 200 mg b.i.d. for 7 days has no clinically important interactions with tolbutamide, phenytoin, glyburide (data on file: Pharmacia Corporation) or S-warfarin[18] (the more pharmacologically active enantiomer, and that thought to be responsible for most warfarin interactions)[20]. This is in contrast to some of the conventional NSAIDs, which have been reported to interact with these cytochrome P450 2C9 substrates. There was no difference in prothrombin time in patients receiving multiple doses of warfarin plus placebo compared with warfarin plus celecoxib. Furthermore, no interactions have been reported from other studies with celecoxib and ketoconazole or methylphenidate (data on file: Pharmacia Corporation). Fluconazole, however, increases the area under the concentration–time curve of celecoxib approximately twofold when the agents are coadministered.

The kinetics of methotrexate were not significantly affected by coadministration of celecoxib 200 mg b.i.d. for 7 days[18]. Serum concentrations of lithium increased by 17% when coadministered with celecoxib (data on file: Pharmacia Corporation). However, the increased lithium concentrations did not exceed the upper limit of its therapeutic range (1.5 mEq l^{-1}) in any subjects who received celecoxib plus lithium, and the interaction was not considered clinically significant.

EFFICACY IN OSTEOARTHRITIS

Osteoarthritis (OA) is the most common form of arthritis, and, as a result, the number of patients receiving treatment with, and experiencing adverse events from, conventional NSAIDs is high.

The extensive celecoxib clinical trial programme has evaluated celecoxib in adults with OA of the knee and hip. Large, randomized, double-blind, controlled studies of up to 12 weeks duration have compared celecoxib 50 to 200 mg b.i.d. with placebo and/or comparator NSAIDs (naproxen 500 mg b.i.d., diclofenac 75 mg b.i.d., ibuprofen 800 mg t.i.d.) in patients with OA[21–25]. These studies have shown that celecoxib is as effective as full therapeutic doses of conventional NSAIDs, and that the maximal effective dose of celecoxib in OA is 200 mg day^{-1}. They also support a once-daily regimen. The patient assessment of arthritis pain (VAS), the Western Ontario and McMaster Universities (WOMAC) OA index and the American Pain Society (APS) patient outcome questionnaire were among the measures used to assess efficacy.

A total of 1093 patients with symptomatic OA of the knee were included in a 12-week study to compare the efficacy and safety of celecoxib at doses of 50, 100 and 200 mg b.i.d. and naproxen 500 mg b.i.d. with placebo[21]. The efficacy of the agents was based on disease assessments using standard and well validated measures such as VAS, patient and physician global assessments, the WOMAC OA index and the APS patient outcome questionnaire.

Celecoxib was as effective as naproxen in relieving the signs and symptoms of OA of the knee, as shown by all measures of efficacy in this study. All arthritis outcome measures of efficacy with celecoxib were significantly better ($P \leq 0.05$) than placebo and at 200 mg, celecoxib and naproxen were equally effective. A dose of 200 mg of celecoxib was the maximally effective dose. Representative results from the study (WOMAC Composite score) are shown in Figure 1.

Figure 1 Improvements from baseline in mean WOMAC Index Composite scores for osteoarthritis patients after 12 weeks of celecoxib or naproxen[21].

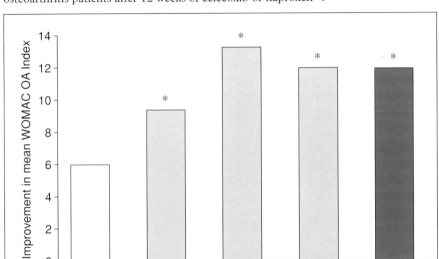

As determined by the APS pain questionnaire, pain relief began within 2 days of the start of therapy, and the maximum analgesic effect was reached within 1 week.

A 6-week, placebo-controlled study in 688 patients with symptomatic OA of the knee indicated that celecoxib 100 mg b.i.d. provides a similar level of pain relief as the full therapeutic dose of diclofenac (50 mg t.i.d.)[22]. Efficacy was assessed as before using standard measures, including WOMAC and APS indices.

The active treatments conferred statistically superior improvements over placebo in all measures of efficacy. Both active treatments were also equivalent in terms of therapeutic effect. In addition, the degree of acute pain experienced by patients was significantly reduced within 24 h of initiating either therapeutic agent (Table 1). Both active treatments were statistically superior to placebo ($P < 0.01$) for all APS measures, and at all time points studied. These effects were maintained for the entire 6-week study period.

Celecoxib was also shown to be as effective as naproxen in managing the signs and symptoms of OA of the hip[23]. A total of 1061 patients with OA of the hip in arthritis flare were studied over a 12-week period while receiving celecoxib 50, 100 or 200 mg b.i.d., naproxen 500 mg b.i.d., or placebo.

Celecoxib significantly reduced the severity of OA symptoms at each dose,

Table 1 APS pain measures: mean change from baseline score on day 1[22]

	Current pain	*Worst pain*	*Average pain*	*Pain interfered*
Placebo	−0.39	−0.7	−0.61	−3.34
Celecoxib	−0.89*	−1.33*	−1.03*	−6.81*
Diclofenac	−0.67*	−1.06*	−0.97*	−5.06*

*P < 0.05 versus placebo

for every efficacy endpoint at each assessment visit compared with placebo. In addition, the 100 mg and 200 mg doses were equivalent, and both were equally as effective as naproxen.

Two 6-week, double-blind, randomized, placebo-controlled studies, including 1404 patients, have also established that celecoxib 100 mg b.i.d. and 200 mg once daily are equally effective and well tolerated in managing the signs and symptoms of OA of the knee[24,25]. These additional data suggest that the pharmacodynamic effects of the drug cannot be simply extrapolated from the half-life and that once-daily dosing is equally effective to divided doses.

EFFICACY IN RHEUMATOID ARTHRITIS

Celecoxib has been evaluated in adults with arthritis flare after discontinuation of NSAID therapy, and in those with active rheumatoid arthritis (RA). Celecoxib demonstrated clinical efficacy for the relief of the signs and symptoms of RA, with efficacy comparable with full therapeutic doses of naproxen and diclofenac in relieving the signs and symptoms of RA. The maximal effective dose of celecoxib is 200 mg b.i.d.[26,27].

A total of 1149 adult patients with symptomatic RA were enrolled in a placebo-controlled study to compare the efficacy and tolerability of celecoxib 100, 200 or 400 mg b.i.d. with naproxen 500 mg b.i.d.[26]. Standard measures of efficacy were taken at 2, 6 and 12 weeks, and included the American College of Rheumatology (ACR)-20 Responders Index.

All celecoxib doses resulted in significant improvements in the signs and symptoms of RA compared with placebo for all efficacy measures. The relief offered by celecoxib reached its maximum within 2 weeks of the start of treatment, and was sustained for the entire 12 weeks of the study period. The results for the ACR-20 Responders Index showed significant improvements ($P < 0.05$) compared with placebo for all celecoxib doses and naproxen.

There was no difference in the number of patients responding according to this composite measure of efficacy between any of the celecoxib doses, or any of the celecoxib doses and naproxen. The total number of swollen joints was also reduced significantly ($P < 0.05$) from baseline compared with placebo, and again all the celecoxib doses were equally effective, and as effective as naproxen. In contrast to naproxen, the number of tender and painful joints was reduced significantly ($P < 0.05$) from baseline for all of the celecoxib doses compared with placebo (Figure 2).

EFFICACY IN PAIN

Cyclooxygenase-2 mediates the production of PGs, which are also associated with pain. Since celecoxib inhibits COX-2, it is expected to exert clinically useful analgesic effects.

The analgesic effects of celecoxib have been confirmed in patients undergoing dental extraction and in post-orthopaedic surgery patients[28,29]. In both of these studies, celecoxib was significantly better than placebo as an analgesic, and single-dose celecoxib was as effective as comparator drugs.

The randomized, controlled, double-blind post-orthopaedic pain study compared celecoxib 200 mg, hydrocodone 10 mg/paracetamol 1000 mg and placebo in 418 patients who had undergone uncomplicated orthopaedic surgery other than total hip or knee replacement[29]. Patients initially received a single dose of study drug (single dose study period). If they had not requested rescue medication, or had received only one dose of rescue medication, at 8 h post-study drug dose they remained in the study, and took up to three doses of study drug daily for a further 5 days (multiple dose study period).

During the single dose study period, there were no significant differences

Figure 2 Change from baseline in number of tender/painful and swollen joints in rheumatoid arthritis patients after 24 weeks of celecoxib or diclofenac[27].

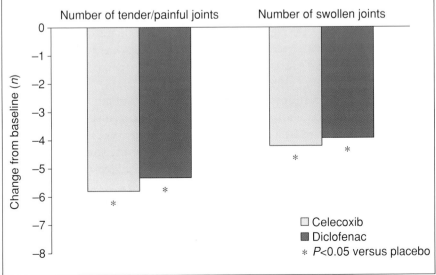

between celecoxib and hydrocodone/paracetamol in relief of pain or time of onset of analgesia. Both active treatments were significantly ($P < 0.05$) more effective than placebo. The analgesic effects of celecoxib were observed after a median of 35 min post-administration. The median time to rescue medication was longer in the celecoxib group (> 8 h) than among the patients taking hydrocodone/paracetamol (7 h 25 min), but this difference failed to reach statistical significance.

In the multiple-dose study period, the mean maximum pain intensity scores were significantly lower ($P < 0.05$) with celecoxib than with hydrocodone/paracetamol, as was the mean total APS Score ($P = 0.001$). This pattern was repeated for all APS daily activity parameters. Furthermore, a consistent trend towards greater efficacy with celecoxib than with hydrocodone/paracetamol was seen in a number of other efficacy endpoints: fewer celecoxib-treated patients required rescue medication; fewer celecoxib doses were required to ease pain; and an increasing number of patients no longer required analgesic medication compared with the hydrocodone/paracetamol group[29].

GASTROINTESTINAL SAFETY

As a specific inhibitor of COX-2, celecoxib was postulated to have anti-inflammatory and analgesic efficacy through COX-2 inhibition, in the absence of deleterious GI effects resulting from COX-1 inhibition. As shown above[29], celecoxib was equally effective as conventional NSAIDs in the treatment of OA, RA and pain. Accordingly, the GI effects of celecoxib were studied in prospective clinical trials[26,27,30,31]. The GI safety assessments focused on the two outcomes that are thought to be the most relevant in determining GI mucosal toxicity: development of endoscopically observed gastroduodenal ulcers and the occurrence of clinically significant upper gastrointestinal (UGI) events. In order to assess GI safety rigorously, doses two and four times the maximum clinically effective doses for RA and OA, respectively, were evaluated.

Endoscopy studies

The incidence of UGI ulceration with celecoxib treatment compared with conventional NSAIDs and placebo has been investigated endoscopically in randomized clinical trials lasting up to 24 weeks among 2089 OA and RA patients[26,27,29]. These studies showed that celecoxib was associated with significantly fewer ulcers than the conventional NSAIDs used as comparators, even at twice the usual dose used for RA and four times the usual dose used for OA. The incidence of ulcers seen with celecoxib was similar to that seen with placebo.

In total, celecoxib 100 mg, 200 mg or 400 mg b.i.d. was administered to 1175 patients who were evaluated endoscopically; 492 patients received naproxen 500 mg b.i.d.[26] and 218 endoscopically evaluated patients received diclofenac 75 mg b.i.d.[27]. The remaining 204 patients received placebo.

In the endoscopy studies comparing the incidence of ulcers with celecoxib and naproxen treatment, naproxen consistently resulted in significantly more GI ulcers[26] than celecoxib (data on file: Pharmacia Corporation). In a 12-week, placebo-controlled study, 1149 adult patients with RA were given celecoxib 100 mg, 200 mg or 400 mg b.i.d., naproxen 500 mg b.i.d. or placebo[26]. The incidence of gastroduodenal ulcers was evaluated endoscopically at the end of treatment compared with baseline, and was found to be significantly higher ($P < 0.001$) in the naproxen 500 mg b.i.d. treatment arm (36/137, 26% patients) than with even the highest dose of celecoxib studied (400 mg b.i.d.; 8/130, 6% patients) (Figure 3). Celecoxib treatment at any of the doses did not result in more gastroduodenal ulcers than placebo.

Single post-treatment endoscopy studies, such as those described above, may underrepresent the true rates of ulceration associated with COX-2 specific inhibitors since subclinical ulcers may arise and resolve during the study period. Therefore, a study using serial endoscopy to assess GI effects was conducted (data on file: Pharmacia Corporation). Celecoxib 200 mg b.i.d. and naproxen 500 mg b.i.d. were compared in patients with either RA ($n = 148$) or OA ($n = 389$), with endoscopies being performed after 4, 8 and 12 weeks of therapy. Overall, 270 patients were treated with celecoxib and 267 with naproxen.

The cumulative incidence of ulcers was significantly higher after 12 weeks

Figure 3 Incidence of gastroduodenal ulcers over 12 weeks of treatment with celecoxib or naproxen[26].

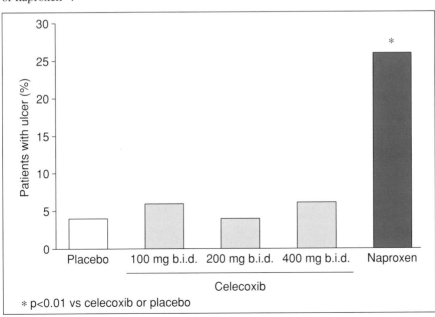

of naproxen treatment than with celecoxib (48% versus 9%, $P < 0.001$, Kaplan–Meier analysis).

A further study was conducted in patients with adult-onset RA, of whom 430 were evaluated endoscopically[27]. Of note in this study was that patients were not prescreened endoscopically prior to study entry and thus may have had asymptomatic ulcers at baseline. Celecoxib 200 mg b.i.d. was compared with diclofenac 75 mg b.i.d. for 24 weeks. Gastroduodenal ulcers were detected in significantly more ($P < 0.001$) patients treated with diclofenac compared with celecoxib: 33/218 (15%) versus 8/212 (4%), respectively. Furthermore, the ulcers were approximately twice the size in diclofenac-treated patients (average 1 cm diameter) compared with those in the celecoxib group (0.5 cm). Significantly more ulcers were detected in the stomach ($P < 0.002$) and duodenum ($P < 0.003$) of patients in the diclofenac-treated group than in those treated with celecoxib.

Upper gastrointestinal complications

Although endoscopically observed ulcers are a marker of GI toxicity, significant UGI ulcer complications are a more clinically relevant endpoint. Such ulcer complications are perforation, bleeding and gastric outlet obstruction. A meta-analysis of serious UGI events in patients with RA or OA enrolled in 15 studies (14 randomized, controlled; one non-comparative) was conducted as part of the celecoxib clinical development programme[30]. The incidence of GI events in these studies was significantly less with celecoxib treatment than with conventional NSAIDs (pooled data).

In the 14 randomized, controlled studies of 2 to 24 weeks' duration, 6376 patients received celecoxib (in doses ranging from 25 to 400 mg b.i.d.), 2768 received a conventional NSAID (naproxen 500 mg b.i.d., diclofenac 50–75 mg b.i.d. or ibuprofen 800 mg t.i.d.) and 1864 received placebo.

A total of 11 serious UGI events (nine bleeding, two outlet obstruction) were judged to be clinically significant, nine among those patients treated with conventional NSAIDs and two among celecoxib-treated patients (none from the placebo group). Expressed as annual incidence, the data show that there is a significantly greater ($P = 0.002$) risk of serious, clinically significant, GI ulcer complications when patients are treated with a conventional NSAID than with celecoxib (Figure 4).

The risk of a conventional NSAID-related GI event was 1.68% greater than if the patient had received celecoxib (95% CI: 0.35% to 2.62%). Celecoxib was not associated with a greater risk of GI events than placebo (95% CI: (–0.08% to 0.47%).

Long-term gastrointestinal safety

A prospective, randomized study (Celecoxib Long-term Arthritis Safety Study, CLASS) was recently completed to determine the incidence of UGI

Figure 4 Annualized incidence of clinically significant adverse upper gastrointestinal events[30].

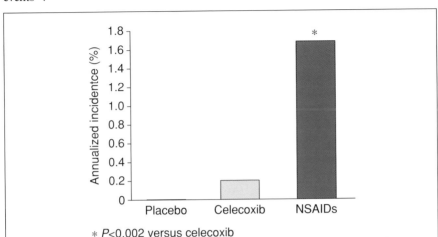

* $P<0.002$ versus celecoxib

ulcer complications alone or combined with symptomatic gastroduodenal ulcers (as distinguished from asymptomatic endoscopic ulcers) among arthritis patients chronically receiving celecoxib or conventional NSAIDs[31]. The study compared supratherapeutic doses of celecoxib (400 mg b.i.d. or two and four times the maximum effective doses for RA and OA, respectively) with commonly used therapeutic doses of conventional NSAIDs (ibuprofen 800 mg t.i.d. and diclofenac 75 mg b.i.d.).

A total of approximately 8000 patients were randomized to either celecoxib or conventional NSAIDs (ibuprofen or diclofenac). Aspirin use for cardiovascular prophylaxis ($\leq$325 mg) was permitted during the study. For patients not taking aspirin, the annualized incidence rates of UGI ulcer complications alone, or combined with symptomatic ulcers, for celecoxib versus conventional NSAIDs were 0.44% versus 1.27% ($P = 0.037$) and 1.40% versus 2.91% ($P = 0.017$). For all patients, the annualized incidence rates of UGI ulcer complications alone, or combined with symptomatic ulcers, for celecoxib compared with conventional NSAIDs were 0.76% versus 1.45% ($P = 0.092$) and 2.08% versus 3.54% ($P = 0.023$), respectively[31]. These data confirm the GI safety of celecoxib relative to conventional NSAIDs and also show the independent ulcerogenicity of low dose aspirin.

PLATELET FUNCTION

Of the two COX isoenzymes, platelets express only the COX-1 variant[32], which is required for platelet aggregation. Thus, the COX-2 hypothesis suggests that celecoxib, as a COX-2-specific inhibitor, would have no platelet-related adverse events, such as prolonged aggregation times, leading to increased bleeding.

Studies have shown that celecoxib has no discernible effect on platelet aggregation[33,34]. A principal feature of these studies was that the celecoxib doses used exceeded the recommended clinical dose range for maximum anti-inflammatory and analgesic effects in patients with OA or RA.

In a randomized, double-blind, placebo-controlled study in 24 healthy adults, the effects on platelet function of celecoxib and naproxen were compared[33]. Trial participants were given a supratherapeutic dose of celecoxib (600 mg b.i.d.), naproxen (500 mg b.i.d.) or placebo, for 10 days. Platelet function was assessed, ex $vivo$, at baseline and on day 10, using aggregation, bleeding time and serum concentrations of the stable thromboxane (TX) A_2 metabolite TXB_2, as parameters.

On all these platelet function parameters, celecoxib treatment was equivalent to placebo. Statistically significant ($P < 0.05$) decreases in platelet aggregation and TXB_2 levels were shown with naproxen treatment. In addition, bleeding time increased significantly ($P < 0.05$), by almost 3 min, at each post-dose time point, following naproxen treatment.

Similarly, no effects on platelet function were reported in a study with 4–6 times the highest recommended dose of celecoxib[34]. Celecoxib 1600 mg day^{-1} or 2400 mg day^{-1} was compared with naproxen 1000 mg day^{-1} in a 12-day, randomized, double-blind, placebo-controlled study in 56 healthy subjects. Platelet aggregation and bleeding times were assessed 1, 3 and 12 days into the study. At these supratherapeutic doses, celecoxib was safe and well tolerated. Furthermore, there were no clinically significant adverse events related to platelet function as a result of celecoxib treatment.

The CLASS study demonstrated the potential clinical relevance of this lack of platelet effects in that fewer haemostasis-related adverse effects were reported with celecoxib compared with conventional NSAIDs[31]. For example, the incidences of anaemia (2.0% versus 4.4%; $P < 0.05$) and haematochezia (0.4% versus 1.0%; $P < 0.05$) were significantly lower in the celecoxib group.

Celecoxib was also associated with a lower incidence ($P < 0.05$) of clinically meaningful reductions in haematocrit ($\geq 10\%$) and haemoglobin (> 2 g dl^{-1}) for the entire patient cohort. In parallel with these findings, serum iron to iron binding capacity ratios increased with celecoxib and decreased with conventional NSAIDs ($+1.4\%$ versus $(-2.3\%, P < 0.05)$[31]. These data suggest that celecoxib may result in less occult GI bleeding than conventional NSAIDs.

RENAL SAFETY

The relative physiological roles of COX-1 and COX-2 in the kidney remain unclear, although the differential expression and localization of COX-1 and

COX-2 suggests that the two isoenzymes may have different physiological functions and may have species-related differences in their functions[12,35-37]. However, numerous experimental findings suggest that the potential for renal toxicity with conventional NSAIDs may result from non-specific inhibition of COX-1 and COX-2[11,38-40]. In the clinical setting, this can be manifested as decreased renal blood flow and glomerular filtration rate, leading to risk of acute renal impairment, salt retention, hypertension and peripheral oedema[41]. Less commonly, but more seriously, acute renal failure, papillary necrosis and complications of nephrotic syndrome have been reported following conventional NSAID treatment[39].

Celecoxib has been shown to have no measurable effects on the glomerular filtration rate in healthy elderly subjects[42]. The elderly are particularly susceptible to adverse renal effects of treatment, since renal function decreases with age. In order to assess the renal safety of celecoxib in this key population, a single-blind, randomized, two-period crossover study was conducted in 29 healthy volunteers aged 65–85 years[42]. Subjects received either celecoxib (200 mg b.i.d. for 5 days followed by 400 mg b.i.d. for 5 days) or naproxen (500 mg b.i.d. for 10 days). Measurements of glomerular filtration rate were used to monitor renal function. The glomerular filtration rate was unchanged from baseline (80.1 ml min^{-1} 1.73m^{-2}) with celecoxib 200 mg b.i.d. on day one and following escalation to 400 mg b.i.d. on day 6. In contrast, the glomerular filtration rate was reduced by 6% on day 1 and 9% on day 6 with naproxen (baseline level 84.3 ml min^{-1} 1.73m^{-2}). The treatment difference achieved statistical significance on day 6 ($P = 0.004$). Both agents were associated with transitory decreases in sodium excretion. The study suggests that celecoxib may have less renal toxicity than conventional NSAIDs.

The CLASS study demonstrated that celecoxib at supratherapeutic doses appears to be associated with less renal toxicity when compared with conventional NSAID therapy. Both hypertension (2.3% versus 1.7%) and increases in serum creatinine levels (1.2% versus 0.7%) were significantly more common in patients on conventional NSAIDs ($P < 0.05$)[31].

CARDIOVASCULAR SAFETY

It has been postulated that specific COX-2 inhibition may be associated with an increased risk of thromboembolic cardiovascular events via unopposed inhibition of vascular prostacyclin (i.e. without a corresponding inhibition of platelet thromboxane)[43]. However, this hypothesis was not substantiated by the findings derived from CLASS[31]. In this trial, celecoxib was associated with similar incidences of thromboembolic cardiovascular events, e.g. cerebrovascular accidents and myocardial infarction, compared with conventional NSAIDs. No treatment-related differences in such events were apparent in the cohort of patients not taking aspirin for cardiovascular prophylaxis who would conjecturally be the most vulnerable to this putative effect.

GENERAL SAFETY

The results from the celecoxib clinical trial programme and specific safety and tolerability studies suggest that celecoxib offers safety advantages over conventional NSAIDs with respect to non-mechanism based toxicities.

Gastrointestinal tolerability

In order to test the overall GI tolerability of celecoxib compared with naproxen, a meta-analysis of five randomized, 12-week, double-blind, placebo-controlled clinical studies in RA and OA patients was conducted[44]. Patients received celecoxib 50 mg b.i.d. ($n = 690$), 100 mg b.i.d. ($n = 1131$), 200 mg b.i.d. ($n = 1125$) or 400 mg b.i.d. ($n = 434$), naproxen 500 mg b.i.d. ($n = 1099$) or placebo ($n = 1136$). The incidence and time of onset of moderate-to-severe abdominal pain, dyspepsia and nausea (combined as a composite end-point) were analysed.

Significantly more ($P < 0.05$) patients withdrew due to naproxen-related GI events than from any of the celecoxib treatment arms or placebo. Celecoxib-related adverse events were similar to placebo (Table 2).

The risk of developing these GI events was also calculated. Naproxen treatment (after controlling for independent predictors) results in a significantly higher risk of developing moderate-to-severe abdominal pain, dyspepsia and nausea than celecoxib. Celecoxib, however, presents no greater risk than placebo for developing these symptoms (Table 3).

Thus, celecoxib has superior GI tolerability compared with conventional NSAIDs. Although the positive predictive value for symptoms leading to clinically significant events is poor, data suggest that GI intolerability is related to more serious outcomes[45].

Hepatic safety

Although the incidence of serious hepatic toxicity with conventional NSAIDs is low, cases of hepatotoxicity have been documented as a result of treatment with diclofenac in particular[46].

A meta-analysis of hepatic safety data undertaken during the clinical development of celecoxib (including over 13 000 patients) indicates that the incidence of adverse hepatic events was significantly higher ($P < 0.05$) among patients treated with conventional NSAIDs (diclofenac, naproxen, ibuprofen) than with celecoxib[47]. The incidence of clinically significant elevations in alanine aminotransferase (ALT) among conventional NSAID-treated patients was significantly higher ($P < 0.05$) than among those treated with celecoxib. The majority of the adverse hepatic events in the controlled studies included in

Table 2 Number of patients (%) withdrawn from treatment with celecoxib compared with naproxen and placebo[44]

	Placebo	Celecoxib				Naproxen
		50 mg b.i.d.	100 mg b.i.d.	200 mg b.i.d.	400 mg b.i.d.	500 mg b.i.d.
Number treated	1136	690	1131	1125	434	1099
Withdrawn	660 (58)	281 (41)	458 (41)	423 (38)	171 (39)	427 (39)
GI-related withdrawal	18 (2)	11 (2)	27 (2)	29 (3)	7 (2)	54 (5)

Table 3 Risk of developing moderate-to-severe upper GI symptoms with celecoxib compared with naproxen and placebo[44]

	Relative risk	P value
Naproxen (500 mg b.i.d.)	1.0	–
Celecoxib (100 mg b.i.d.)	0.60	< 0.001
Celecoxib (200 mg b.i.d.)	0.63	0.001
Celecoxib (400 mg b.i.d.)	0.56	0.015
Placebo	0.63	0.002

this analysis were associated with diclofenac treatment, which resulted in a significantly higher incidence ($P < 0.001$) of clinically important elevations in ALT than celecoxib, and a higher incidence than naproxen or ibuprofen.

The CLASS data confirm that celecoxib has an improved hepatotoxicity profile compared with conventional NSAIDs. In this long-term study, the incidence of serum ALT or aspartate aminotransferase elevations that exceeded three times the upper limit of normal was five- to ten-fold higher ($P < 0.05$) in patients receiving conventional NSAIDs than in the celecoxib group[31].

CELECOXIB IN CHEMOPREVENTION: A POTENTIAL NEW APPLICATION

A number of studies have reported that conventional NSAIDs can lead to complete or almost complete regression of rectal adenomas[48–55]. It is suggested that this effect is mediated by COX-2 rather than COX-1[56–59]. Studies in rodents have provided data to support the involvement of COX-2[60–63], and COX-2 has been shown to be upregulated in colonic neoplasms in humans[64].

These findings led to an interest in the possible role of celecoxib in the management of neoplastic conditions. This potential was first assessed in the human disease, familial adenomatous polyposis (FAP). This is a genetic disorder with a near 100% risk of colon cancer[65]. Although conventional NSAID treatment can lead to regression of colorectal adenomas in FAP patients, the associated GI side effects mean that their use for the long-term prevention of cancer is restricted[66]. The COX-2 isoenzyme is overexpressed in adenomas[64], and thus the specific inhibition of this enzyme may provide a clinically effective method of controlling FAP, with improved safety compared with conventional NSAIDs.

In a 6-month, double-blind, randomized clinical study in 77 patients with FAP (who had five or more endoscopically assessable polyps), celecoxib 100 mg and 400 mg b.i.d. were compared with placebo. Efficacy was assessed at the end of the trial, and based on a reduction in the number and size of baseline polyps; the extent of colorectal polyposis was also assessed by a panel of endoscopists[67].

Celecoxib 400 mg resulted in a significant reduction in both the number ($P = 0.003$) and overall size ($P = 0.001$) of colorectal polyps compared with placebo. The observed changes were a 28% reduction in the number with celecoxib 400 mg compared with 4.5% for placebo (Figure 5).

There was also a 30.7% reduction in overall polyp burden (sum of polyp diameters) compared with 4.9%, respectively. The number of rectal polyps was also significantly reduced ($P = 0.01$) with celecoxib 400 mg compared with placebo (22.5% reduction with celecoxib versus 3.1% increase with placebo). The endoscopy review panel also reported a significant improvement ($P \le 0.02$) in the extent of polyposis with celecoxib 400 mg compared with placebo. No difference in efficacy end-points was observed between celecoxib 100 mg and placebo. Both celecoxib regimens were well tolerated[67].

Figure 5 Colorectal polyps in patients with familial adenomatous polyposis after six months of celecoxib or placebo[67].

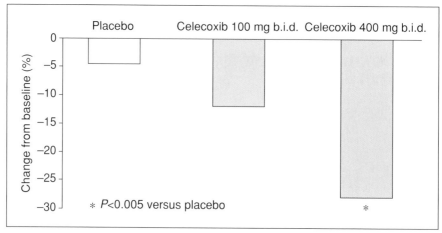

The results from this study have stimulated further research to investigate the potential of celecoxib as a therapy in other areas of oncology, including Barrett's oesophagus and actinic keratosis[67].

SUMMARY

In summary, it can be seen that celecoxib is equally as effective as conventional NSAIDs in relieving the signs and symptoms of OA or RA, and managing pain. It has decreased GI toxicity and platelet effects at doses two- to four-fold or greater above the maximum recommended for a therapeutic effect in RA and OA compared with conventional NSAIDs, validating its COX-2 selectivity. Celecoxib may also have lower renal toxicity than conventional NSAIDs, but further study is required to elucidate the relative roles of COX-1 and COX-2 in the kidney. The data from cardiovascular event analyses do not suggest an increased risk of myocardial infarction or other cardiovascular events with celecoxib compared with conventional NSAIDs, despite theoretical concerns regarding specific COX-2 inhibition and cardiovascular safety. Celecoxib has not demonstrated any cause for substantive safety concerns regarding idiosyncratic toxicities. Its generally positive safety profile and encouraging results in FAP studies suggest that celecoxib may have wide applications in cancer chemoprevention.

Address all correspondence to: J.B. Lefkowith, Pharmacia Clinical Research and Development, Skokie, IL, USA.

REFERENCES

1. Abramson SR, Weissman G. The mechanisms of action of nonsteroidal anti-inflammatory drugs. *Arthritis Rheum.* 1989;32:1–9.
2. Smith WL, DeWitt DL. Prostaglandin endoperoxide H synthases -1 and -2. *Adv Immunol.* 1996;62:167–215.
3. Geis GS, Stead H, Wallemark C-B, Nicholson PA. Prevalence of mucosal lesions in the stomach and duodenum due to chronic use of NSAIDs in patients with rheumatoid arthritis or osteoarthritis, an interim report on prevention by misoprostol of diclofenac associated lesions. *J Rheumatol.* 1991;18 (Suppl 28):11–4.
4. Schafer AI. Effects of nonsteroidal antiinflammatory drugs on platelet function and systemic homeostasis. *J Clin Pharmacol.* 1995;35:209–19.
5. Palmer BF. Renal complications associated with use of nonsteroidal anti-inflammatory agents. *J Invest Med.* 1995;43:516–33.
6. Kargman S, Charleson S, Cartwright M, Frank J, Riendeau D, Mancini J et al. Characterization of prostaglandin G/H synthase 1 and 2 in rat, dog, monkey, and human gastrointestinal tracts. *Gastroenterology.* 1996;111:445–54.
7. Xie W, Chipman JG, Robertson DL, Erikson RL, Simmons DL. Expression of a mitogen-responsive gene encoding prostaglandin synthase is regulated by mRNA splicing. *Proc Natl Acad Sci USA.* 1991;88:2692–6.

8. Kujubu DA, Fletcher BS, Varnum BC, Lim RW, Herschman HR. TIS10, a phorbol ester tumor promoter-inducible mRNA from Swiss 3T3 cells, encodes a novel prostaglandin synthase/cyclooxygenase homologue. *J Biol Chem.* 1991;266:12866–72.

9. Masferrer JL, Zweifel BS, Seibert K, Needleman P. Selective regulation of cellular cyclooxygenase by dexamethasone and endotoxin in mice. *J Clin Invest.* 1990;86:1375–9.

10. Gierse JK, Hauser SD, Creely DP, Koboldt C, Rangwala SH, Isakson PC et al. Expression and selective inhibition of the constitutive and inducible forms of human cyclo-oxygenase. *Biochem J.* 1995;305:479–84.

11. Anderson GD, Hauser SD, McGarity KL, Bremer ME, Isakson PC, Gregory SA. Selective inhibition of cyclooxygenase (COX)-2 reverses inflammation and expression of COX-2 and interleukin 6 in rat adjuvant arthritis. *J Clin Invest.* 1996;97:2672–9.

12. Khan KNM, Venturini CM, Bunch RT, Brassard JA, Koki AT, Morris DL et al. Interspecies differences in renal localization of cyclooxygenase isoforms: implications in nonsteroidal anti-inflammatory drug-related nephrotoxicity. *Toxicol Pathol.* 1998:26:612–20.

13. Verburg KM, Maziasz TJ, Weiner E, Loose L, Geis S, Isakson PC. COX-2-specific inhibitors: definition of a new therapeutic concept. *Am J Ther.* 2001; in press.

14. Penning TD, Talley JJ, Bertenshaw SR, Carter JS, Collins PW, Docter S et al. Synthesis and biological evaluation of the 1,5-diarylpyrazole class of cyclooxygenase-2 inhibitors: identification of 4-[5-(4-methylphenyl)-3-(trifluoromethyl)-1H-pyrazol-1-yl]benzenesulfonamide (SC-28635, celecoxib). *J Med Chem.* 1997;40:1347–79.

15. Paulson SK, Kaprak TA, Gresk CJ. Plasma protein binding of celecoxib in mice, rat, rabbit, dog and human. *Biopharm Drug Dispos.* 1999;20:293–9.

16. Karim A, Tolbert D, Burton E. SC-58635 (Celecoxib): a highly selective inhibitor of cyclooxygenase-2. Disposition kinetics in man and identification of its major CYP450 isoenzyme in its biotransformation [abstract]. *Pharm Res.* 1997;14(Suppl):617.

17. Paulson SK, Hribar JD, Liu NWK. Metabolism and excretion of [^{14}C]celecoxib in healthy male volunteers. *Drug Metab Dispos.* 2000;28:308–14.

18. Haase KK, Rojas-Fernandez CH, Lane L, Frank DA. Potential interaction between celecoxib and warfarin. *Ann Pharmacother.* 2000;34:666–7.

19. Karim A, Tolbert DS, Hunt TL, Hubbard RC, Harper KM, Geis GS. Celecoxib, a specific COX-2 inhibitor, has no significant effect on methotrexate pharmacokinetics in patients with rheumatoid arthritis. *J Rheumatol.* 1999;26:2539–43.

20. Koch-Weser J, Sellers EM. Drug interactions with coumarin anticoagulants. *N Engl J Med.* 1971;285:547–58.

21. Bensen WG, Fiechtner JJ, McMillen JI. Treatment of osteoarthritis with celecoxib a cyclooxygenase-2 inhibitor: a randomised controlled trial. *Mayo Clin Proc.* 1999;74:1095–105.

22. Lefkowith JL, Wendt HL, Burr AM, Zhao WW, Geis GS. A comparative study of efficacy and safety in patients with osteoarthritis of the knee receiving either celecoxib, a COX-2 specific inhibitor, or diclofenac [abstract]. *Ann Rheum Dis.* 2000;59(Suppl 1):296.

23. Geis GS, Hubbard RC, Wood EM, Lefkowith JB, Yu S, Zhao W. Efficacy of

celecoxib, a COX-2 specific inhibitor, in osteoarthritis of the hip [abstract]. *Ann Rheum Dis.* 1999;42(Suppl):144.

24. Williams GW, Ettlinger RE, Ruderman EM, Hubbard RC, Lorien ME, Yu SS et al. Treatment of osteoarthritis with a once-daily dosing regimen of celecoxib: a randomised, controlled trial. *J Clin Rheum.* 2000;6:65–74.

25. Lefkowith JL, Hubbard RC, Zhao WW, Geis GS. A comparison study of the efficacy of two celecoxib dosing regimens – 200 mg QD versus 100 mg BID – in treating the signs and symptoms of osteoarthritis of the knee [abstract]. *Ann Rheum Dis.* 2000;59(Suppl 1):297.

26. Simon LS, Weaver AL, Graham DY, Kivitz AJ, Lipsky PE, Hubbard RC et al. Anti-inflammatory and upper gastrointestinal effects of celecoxib in rheumatoid arthritis: a randomised controlled trial. *JAMA.* 1999;282:1921–8.

27. Emery P, Zeidler H, Kvien TK, Guslandi M, Naudin R, Stead H et al. Celecoxib versus diclofenac in long-term management of rheumatoid arthritis: randomised double-blind comparison. *Lancet.* 1999;354:2106–11.

28. Lefkowith JB. Cyclooxygenase-2 specificity and its clinical implications. *Am J Med.* 1999;106(5B):43S–50S.

29. Brugger A, Richardson ER, Drupka, Cui H, Zhao WW, Verburg KM et al. Comparison of celecoxib, hydrocodone/acetominophen and placebo for relief of postoperative pain [abstract]. *Ann Rheum Dis.* 2000;59(Suppl 1):46.

30. Goldstein JL, Silverstein FE, Agrawal NM, Hubbard RC, Kaiser J, Maurath CJ et al. Reduced risk of upper gastrointestinal ulcer complications with celecoxib, a novel COX-2 inhibitor. *Am J Gastroenterol.* 2000;95;1681–90.

31. Silverstein FE, Faich G, Goldstein JL, Simon LS, Pincus T, Whelton A et al. Gastrointestinal toxicity with celecoxib vs non steroidal anti-inflammatory drugs for osteoarthritis and rheumatoid arthritis. The CLASS study: a randomized controlled trial. *J Am Med Assoc.* 2000;284:1247–99.

32. Patrignani P, Sciulli MG, Manarini S, Santini G, Cerletti C, Evangelista V. COX-2 is not involved in thromboxane biosynthesis by activated human platelets. *J Physiol Pharmacol.* 1999;50:661–7.

33. Leese PT, Hubbard RC, Karim A, Isakson PC, Yu SS, Geis GS. Effects of celecoxib, a novel cyclooxygenase-2 inhibitor, on platelet function in healthy adults: a randomised, controlled trial. *J Clin Pharmacol.* 2000;40:124–32.

34. Geis GS, FitzGerald GA, Karim A, Hubbard RC, Harper K, Yu S. A comparative study of platelet function in subjects receiving celecoxib, a COX-2 specific inhibitor, or ibuprofen, a non-specific inhibitor of cyclooxygenase. Proceedings of the 63rd Annual Scientific Meeting of the American College of Rheumatology, November 13–17, 1999; Boston, MA: American College of Rheumatology; 1999.

35. O'Neill GP, Ford-Hutchinson AW. Expression of mRNA for cyclooxygenase-1 and cyclooxygenase-2 in human tissues. *FEBS Lett.* 1993;330:156–60.

36. Harris RC, McKanna JA, Akai Y, Jacobson HR, Dubois RN, Breyer MD et al. Cyclooxygenase-2 is associated with the macula densa of rat kidney and increases with salt restriction. *J Clin Invest.* 1994;6:2504–10.

37. Kömhoff M, Gröne H-J, Klein T, Seyberth HW, Nüsing RM. Localization of cyclooxygenase-1 and -2 in adult and fetal human kidney; implication for renal function. *Am J Physiol.* 1997;272:F460–8.

38. Masferrer JL, Zweifel BS, Manning PT, Hauser SD, Leahy KM, Smith WG et al. Selective inhibition of inducible cyclooxygenase 2 in vivo is anti-inflammatory and non-ulcerogenic. *Proc Natl Acad Sci USA.* 1994;91:3228–32.

39. Seibert K, Zhang Y, Leahy K, Hauser S, Masferrer J, Perkins W et al. Pharmacological and biochemical demonstration of the role of cyclooxygenase 2 in inflammation and pain. *Proc Natl Acad Sci USA*. 1994;91:12013–7.

40. Chan CC, Boyce S, Brideau C, Ford-Hutchinson AW, Gordon R, Guay D et al. Pharmacology of a selective cyclooxygenase-2 inhibitor, L-745,337: A novel non-steroidal anti-inflammatory agent with an ulcerogenic sparing effect in rat and non-human primate stomach. *J Pharmacol Exp Ther*. 1995;274:1531–7.

41. Whelton A. Nephrotoxicity of nonsteroidal anti-inflammatory drugs: physiologic foundations and clinical implications. *Am J Med*. 1999;106(5B):13S–24S.

42. Whelton A, Schulman G, Wallemark C, Drower EJ, Isakson PC, Verburg KM et al. Effects of celecoxib and naproxen on renal function in the elderly. *Arch Intern Med*. 2000;160:1465–70.

43. McAdam BF, Catella-Lawson F, Mardini IA, Kapoor S, Lawson JA, FitzGerald GA. Systemic biosynthesis of prostacyclin by cyclooxygenase (COX)-2: the human pharmacology of a selective inhibitor of COX-2. *Proc Natl Acad Sci USA*. 1999;96:272–7.

44. Bensen WG, Zhao SZ, Burke TA, Zabinski RA, Makuch RW, Maurath CJ et al. Upper gastrointestinal tolerability of celecoxib, a COX-2 specific inhibitor, compared to naproxen and placebo. *J Rheum*. 2000;27:1876–83.

45. Wolfe F. The epidemiology of NSAID associated gastrointestinal disease. *Eur J Rheumatol Inflamm*. 1991;11:12–28.

46. Banks AT, Zimmerman HJ, Ishak KG, Harter JG. Diclofenac associated hepatotoxicity: analysis of 180 cases reported to the Food and Drug Administration as adverse reactions. *Hepatology*. 1995;22:820–7.

47. Maddrey WC, Maurath CJ, Verburg KM, Geis GS. The hepatic safety and tolerability of the novel cyclooxygenase (COX)-2 inhibitor celecoxib. *Am J Ther*. 2000;7:153–8.

48. Waddell WR, Loughry RW. Sulindac for polyposis of the colon. *J Surg Oncol*. 1983;24:83–7.

49. Rigau J, Pique JM, Rubio E, Tarrech JM, Bordas JM. Effects of long-term sulindac therapy on colonic polyposis. *Ann Intern Med*. 1991;115:952–4.

50. Winde G, Schmid KW, Schlegel W, Fischer R, Osswald H, Bunte H. Complete reversion and prevention of rectal adenomas in colectomized patients with familial adenomatous polyposis by rectal low-dose sulindac maintenance treatment: advantages of a low-dose nonsteroidal anti-inflammatory drug regimen in reversing adenomas exceeding 33 months. *Dis Colon Rectum*. 1995;38:S13–S30.

51. Reddy BS, Rao CV, Rivenson A, Kelloff G. Inhibitory effect of aspirin on azoxymethane-induced colon carcinogenesis in F344 rats. *Carcinogenesis*. 1993;14:1493–7.

52. Kune GA, Kune S, Watson LF. Colorectal cancer risk, chronic illnesses, operations, and medications: case control results from the Melbourne Colorectal Cancer Study. *Cancer Res*. 1988;48:4399–404.

53. Giovannucci E, Rimm EB, Stampfer MJ, Colditz GA, Ascherio A, Willett WC. Aspirin use and the risk for colorectal cancer and adenoma in male health professionals. *Ann Intern Med*. 1994;121:241–6.

54. Giardiello FM, Stanley RH, Krush AJ, Piantadosi S, Hylind LM, Celano P et al. Treatment of colonic and rectal adenomas with sulindac in familial adenomatous polyposis. *N Engl J Med*. 1993;328:1313–6.

55. Nugent KP, Farmer KC, Spiegelman AD, Williams CB, Phillips RK. Randomised

controlled trial of the effect of sulindac on duodenal and rectal polyposis and cell proliferation in patients with familial adenomatous polyposis. *Br J Surg.* 1993;80:1618–9.

56. Taketo MM. Cyclooxygenase-2 inhibitors in tumorigenesis. *J Natl Cancer Inst.* 1998;90:1609–20.

57. Kopp E, Ghosh S. Inhibition of NF-kappa B by sodium salicylate and aspirin. *Science.* 1994;265:956–9.

58. He T-C, Chan TA, Vogelstein B, Kinzler KW. PPARδ is an APC-regulated target of nonsteroidal anti-inflammatory drugs. *Cell.* 1999;99:335–45.

59. Piazza GA, Alberts DS, Hisson LJ, Paramka NS, Li H, Finn T et al. Sulindac sulfone inhibits azoxymethane-induced colon carcinogenesis in rats without reducing prostaglandin levels. *Cancer Res.* 1997;57:2909–15.

60. Oshima M, Dinchuk JE, Kargman SL, Oshima H, Hancock B, Kwong E et al. Suppression of intestinal polyposis in Apc delta716 knockout mice by inhibition of cyclooxygenase 2 (COX-2). *Cell.* 1996;87:803–9.

61. Boolbol SK, Dannengerg AJ, Chadburn A, Martucci C, Guo XJ, Ramonetti JT et al. Cyclooxygenase-2 overexpression and tumor formation are blocked by sulindac in a murine model of familial adenomatous polyposis. *Cancer Res.* 1996;56:2556–60.

62. Reddy BS, Rao CV, Seibert K. Evaluation of cyclooxygenase-2 inhibitior for potential chemopreventive properties in colon carcinogenesis. *Cancer Res.* 1996;56:4566–9.

63. Kawamon T, Rao CV, Seibert K, Reddy BS. Chemopreventive activity of celecoxib, a specific cyclooxygenase-2 inhibitor, against colon carcinogenesis. *Cancer Res.* 1998;58:409–12.

64. Eberhart CE, Coffey RJ, Radhika A, Giardiello FM, Ferrenbach S, DuBois RN. Up-regulation of cyclooxygenase 2 gene expression in human colorectal adenomas and adenocarcinomas. *Gastroenterology.* 1994;107:1183–8.

65. Kinzler KW, Nilbert MC, Su LK, Vogelstein B, Bryan TM, Levy DB et al. Identification of FAP locus genes from chromosome 5q21. *Science.* 1991;253:661–5.

66. Wolfe MM, Lichenstein DR, Singh G. Gastrointestinal toxicity of nonsteroidal anti-inflammatory drugs. *N Engl J Med.* 1999;240:1888–99.

67. Steinbach G, Lynch PM, Phillips RK, Wallace MH, Hawk E, Gordon GB et al. The effect of celecoxib, a cyclooxygenase-2 inhibitor, in familial adenomatous polyposis. *N Engl J Med.* 2000;342:1946–52.

22 | Etodolac: clinical profile of an established selective cyclooxygenase-2 inhibitor

RICHARD A. JONES

Shire Pharmaceuticals Limited, East Anton, Andover, Hampshire SP10 5RG, UK.

Non-steroid anti-inflammatory drugs (NSAIDs), used for the treatment of arthritic conditions, are the most commonly prescribed group of drugs world-wide. They have been shown to induce their therapeutic effects by decreasing biosynthesis of prostaglandins (PGs) and other anti-inflammatory agents. Further work in this area has shown that NSAIDs decrease the production of proinflammatory PGs by the inhibition of cyclooxygenase (COX), which catalyses the conversion of arachidonic acid to PGH_2. Other enzymes then form PGs, prostacyclin and thromboxane from PGH_2.

COX exists in two isoforms: the constitutive isoform, COX-1, and the inducible isoform, COX-2. COX-1 is widely expressed and plays a part in homeostatic functions such as maintaining the integrity of the gastric mucosa, platelet aggregation and regulating gastrointestinal (GI) and renal blood flow. COX-2 has highly restricted expression, although constitutive expression is seen in the kidney and brain, but it is dramatically upregulated at inflammatory sites[1].

It is postulated that the anti-inflammatory efficacy of NSAIDs derives from inhibition of inducible COX-2, whereas the unwanted side effects, such as irritation and ulceration of the stomach lining and renal problems, arise from inhibition of COX-1[2,3]. NSAIDs that selectively inhibit COX-2 and have minimal effects on COX-1 (etodolac, meloxicam, rofecoxib, celecoxib and nimesulide) might be expected to have high anti-inflammatory efficacy and reduced GI and renal toxicity[2,4,5]. Clinical data support this hypothesis[2,3].

CLINICAL DEVELOPMENT OF ETODOLAC

Etodolac was developed in a search for novel NSAIDs with an improved efficacy/side effect balance. Etodolac was derived from a new chemical class of NSAIDs, the pyranocarboxylates, and the chemical nomenclature is 1,8-diethyl-1,3,4,9-tetrahydropyrano-[3,4-b]indole-1-acetic acid (Figure 1). This molecule was selected for clinical development because of its superior therapeutic index between gastric irritation and anti-inflammatory effects in a wide range of preclinical tests.

Although the COX-2 theory of inflammation had not yet been proposed, PGs were recognized as playing an important part in the pathogenesis of pain and inflammation and also in gastric and renal protection[6]. The clinical programme demonstrated that etodolac effectively inhibited PG synthesis at sites of inflammation, but appeared not to affect the levels of PGs in the stomach or duodenum. This was clearly demonstrated in a four-week, double-blind, randomized comparative study of etodolac (600 mg day^{-1}) versus naproxen (1000 mg day^{-1}) in patients with rheumatoid arthritis (RA) that was published in 1990[7,8]. Assays of endoscopic biopsies of gastric and duodenal mucosa revealed that there was no overall suppression of gastric or duodenal PGs in patients receiving etodolac. In contrast, there were marked reductions in gastric and duodenal PGs following treatment with naproxen. A similar study conducted in healthy volunteers has confirmed these observations[9]. Preliminary results of a study comparing etodolac and diclofenac also confirm the lack of suppression of gastric or duodenal PGs in subjects receiving etodolac[10].

The improved safety profile of etodolac when compared with routinely used NSAIDs posed an anomaly during its development and early years of clinical use as there was no explanation available at that time. The advent of the COX-2 theory of inflammation served as the possible rationale for etodolac's improved safety profile.

SELECTIVE COX-2 INHIBITION BY ETODOLAC

Since the formulation of the COX-2 theory, etodolac has been shown to be COX-2 selective in a variety of assay systems[2,4,11-14] which are detailed in

Figure 1 Chemical structure of etodolac (1,8-diethyl-1,3,4,9-tetrahydropyrano-[3,4-b]indole-1-acetic acid).

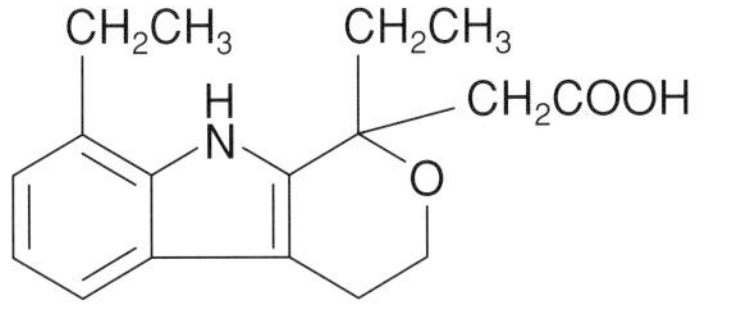

Table 1. These have included *in vitro* systems such as cell lines, isolated enzyme systems and the human whole-blood assay, and *ex vivo* systems such as gastric biopsies.

In general, results using isolated cells or enzyme systems tend to give higher COX-2/COX-1 selectivity ratios than the whole-blood assay, which is becoming the 'gold standard' for measuring the relative activities of drugs on COX-1 and COX-2. The William Harvey modified human whole-blood assay study, in which etodolac has been compared directly with more than 40 NSAIDs, including meloxicam, rofecoxib and celecoxib, is the most recent and comprehensive study[11]. An important aspect of this assay system is that it takes into account the plasma protein binding of the drugs. In the modified human whole-blood assay, etodolac was shown to have more than twice the COX-2 selectivity of meloxicam and celecoxib.

There have been attempts to correlate the results of the assay systems with clinical data. For example, in a human platelet/synovial cell study, the rank order of COX-2 selectivity of the agents investigated was found to correlate with the rank order of their incidence rates of serious GI events derived from the ARAMIS database[15]. Etodolac exhibited a higher COX-2 selectivity, and was associated with a lower risk of serious GI events than aspirin, diclofenac, ibuprofen and indomethacin.

As with any *in vitro/ex vivo* data, there must be some caution in extrapolating the results of these assays to the clinical setting. The trends in COX-2 selectivity observed in comparative studies are more meaningful than absolute values or any attempts to compare such values across studies. There are

Table 1 Studies defining the COX-2 selectivity profile of etodolac

Assay system	NSAIDs under investigation	Etodolac showed COX-2 selectivity?
Isolated recombinant human COX isozymes and human whole blood assay (1995)[4]	Etodolac, and a number of other NSAIDs	✓ tenfold
Chinese hamster ovarian (CHO) cells expressing recombinant human COX isozymes (1997)[14]	Etodolac and a number of other NSAIDs, including meloxicam	✓ 1000-fold
Microsomal COX-1 cells, human platelets, CHO cells expressing COX-1 (1997)[13]	Etodolac and >45 other NSAIDs	Etodolac showed low COX-1 inhibition
Human platelets for assessment of thromboxane B_2 production (COX-1), synovial cells from RA patients (1998)[2]	Etodolac, aspirin, diclofenac, ibuprofen, indomethacin, loxoprofen (active metabolite), NS-398, oxaprozin, zaltoprofen	✓ 179-fold
Modified human whole-blood assay (1999)[11]	Etodolac and >40 other NSAIDs including meloxicam, rofecoxib and celecoxib	✓ 23.46-fold

caveats pertaining to each assay system and a defining and clinically relevant test is not yet available. Although these assay systems are clearly of value, notably during the drug development process, they cannot yet unequivocally predict clinical outcomes, and any benefits of COX-2 selectivity have to be established through randomized clinical trials.

CLINICAL EFFECTIVENESS OF ETODOLAC

The efficacy and safety/tolerability of etodolac in the treatment of osteoarthritis (OA) and RA have been conclusively demonstrated in a large number of comparative, randomized, double-blind, parallel-group clinical trials (>2500 OA patients; >1500 RA patients) and during clinical use. This review of the randomized, double-blind, parallel-group clinical trials with etodolac will concentrate primarily on trials in which etodolac was given at the UK licensed dosage of 600 mg day^{-1}.

Efficacy in osteoarthritis

OA is the most common arthropathy. It is a chronic disease process that is characterized by progressive loss of cartilage integrity, osteophyte and appositional new bone formation, and is associated with stiffness and pain. The prevalence of OA increases with age. Reports suggest that, when bone hypertrophy is used as the diagnostic criterion, evidence of OA can be found in most people over the age of 50, while more than 90% of individuals over the age of 80 years are claimed to show signs of this disease. The pain relief of a chronic condition such as OA requires therapeutic agents that demonstrate long-term safety and tolerability, as well as good efficacy in treating the symptoms of the disease. In both clinical trials and everyday practice, etodolac has been proven to satisfy these criteria.

The efficacy of etodolac versus other NSAIDs has been assessed in a number of randomized, double-blind, parallel-group controlled studies, ranging from six to 12 weeks, in patients with confirmed OA of the knee. In these comparative trials, the efficacy of etodolac 600 mg day^{-1} was shown to be comparable with that of:

- naproxen 1000 mg day^{-1} (refs 16–20)
- piroxicam 20 mg day^{-1} (refs 16,18,20)
- diclofenac 150 mg day^{-1} (refs 16,18)
- indomethacin 150 mg day^{-1} (ref. 21)
- tenoxicam 20 mg day^{-1} (ref. 22)

While the recommended dosage of etodolac in the UK is 600 mg day^{-1}, both lower and higher doses have been evaluated in comparative trials with other NSAIDs. In three four-week, randomized, multicentre, parallel-group, double-blind, placebo-controlled studies, patients with OA were assigned to: etodolac 800 mg day^{-1} ($n = 211$) versus naproxen 1000 mg day^{-1} ($n = 109$); etodolac 800 mg day^{-1} ($n = 86$) versus naproxen 1000 mg day^{-1} ($n = 82$); and etodolac 800 mg day^{-1} ($n = 91$) versus nabumetone 1500 mg day^{-1} ($n = 89$)[23]. The results obtained indicate that, with respect to efficacy in the treatment of OA, etodolac 800 mg is at least comparable with nabumetone 1500 mg and naproxen 1000 mg day^{-1}. An earlier 12-week, double-blind, parallel-group study in patients with OA of the hip[24] reported that etodolac, administered at a mean dosage of just 315 mg day^{-1}, offered greater efficacy than aspirin at its usual anti-arthritic dosage of 3200–4800 mg day^{-1}.

Efficacy in rheumatoid arthritis

Similarly to OA, RA is a chronic disorder that affects a large population. This deforming, potentially debilitating condition is characterized by inflammation of the joints, and disease progression frequently leads to joint destruction and deformity. The primary objectives of therapy for RA, therefore, are to alleviate pain and inflammation of the joints, improve mobility and, ideally, halt progression of the disease.

A long-term, randomized, double-blind, parallel-group study of etodolac versus ibuprofen compared the efficacy and safety of these two NSAIDs in the treatment of active RA[25]. A total of 1446 patients were randomized to three years' treatment with etodolac 300 mg day^{-1}, etodolac 1000 mg day^{-1} or ibuprofen 2400 mg day^{-1}. Both dosages of etodolac were found to be of comparable efficacy to ibuprofen 2400 mg day^{-1} in the treatment of RA, and good levels of tolerability were reported for all three treatment regimens. In comparisons with piroxicam, diclofenac, naproxen, indomethacin and aspirin, etodolac has consistently demonstrated levels of efficacy at least comparable with the other NSAIDs in the treatment of RA.

A 12-week, randomized, double-blind, parallel-group study, in which etodolac 600 mg day^{-1} was compared with piroxicam 20 mg day^{-1}, found comparable efficacies for these two treatment regimens in patients with RA[26]. Comparable efficacies of the active treatments were also reported[27] in a six-week, randomized, double-blind, parallel-group study of etodolac 600 mg day^{-1} versus indomethacin 100 mg day^{-1} and in a four-week, randomized, double-blind, parallel-group comparison of sustained-release (SR) etodolac[28] 600 mg day^{-1} versus piroxicam capsules 20 mg day^{-1}.

Randomized, double-blind trials of etodolac 400 mg day^{-1} have found the efficacy of this lower dosage of etodolac to be comparable with that of:

- piroxicam 20 mg day^{-1} (treatment duration 8–12 weeks) (refs 29,30)
- diclofenac 150 mg day^{-1} (treatment duration 12 weeks) (ref. 31)
- naproxen 1000 mg day^{-1} (treatment duration 12 weeks) (ref. 32)
- aspirin 3600–4800 mg day^{-1} (treatment duration 12 weeks) (ref. 33)

SAFETY/TOLERABILITY PROFILE OF ETODOLAC

The most commonly encountered adverse events associated with the use of NSAIDs relate to the GI tract, the central nervous system and the skin[34]. Very rarely, severe adverse events involving pathological liver changes, renal changes and disruption of haematopoiesis have been associated with NSAID use.

The pivotal studies conducted during the late 1980s and early 1990s used different designs in terms of methodology to the latest NSAID studies, but represented the best study designs and expert opinion, particularly for exploring gastric tolerability. Overall, as befits a drug approved in 1985, the safety/tolerability of etodolac have been evaluated in a large number of clinical trials and post-marketing surveillance studies involving over 60000 patients.

Safety/tolerability of etodolac versus aspirin and placebo

A review of adverse events encountered in randomized, double-blind, placebo-controlled clinical trials of at least four weeks duration comparing etodolac ($\leq$600 mg day^{-1}), aspirin and placebo in patients with OA or RA has been presented by Humber[35]. The data from 1324 patients described in this review are summarized in Table 2. Aspirin was used as a comparator since it may be the initial drug of choice in OA and RA being a well-established and inexpensive NSAID. With the exception of indigestion, the incidences of adverse events with etodolac were similar to those with placebo. There was a significantly higher incidence of GI adverse events observed with aspirin than with etodolac.

SAFETY OF ETODOLAC IN LARGE-SCALE AND LONG-TERM STUDIES.

The strength of evidence supporting etodolac as a safe and effective oral NSAID lies in the breadth of clinical data obtained during the clinical development programme, from open-label observational studies and as a result of over 14 years of use in clinical practice. The safety/tolerability of etodolac have been evaluated in clinical trials and open-label, observational studies involving >60000 patients.

The safety of etodolac has been reviewed by examining data from 2629 etodolac-treated patients enrolled in double-blind and open-label clinical trials and from 8334 patients taking etodolac in post-marketing surveillance studies[34,36]. Among the patients who received daily dosages of 50–1000 mg etodolac in placebo-controlled trials of four weeks to seven year's duration, the only GI adverse events occurring more frequently in patients receiving etodolac (n = 1468) than in patients receiving placebo (n = 680) were abdominal pain (9% versus 5%) ($P \leq 0.05$) and dyspepsia (11% versus 6%) ($P \leq 0.05$). The rate of abdominal pain and dyspepsia observed with etodolac was similar to that observed with several other NSAIDs, but was lower than that of aspirin.

Table 2 Incidence (>2%) of treatment emergent adverse events in randomized double-blind, placebo-controlled trials of etodolac versus aspirin

Body system Adverse event	Incidence of adverse events (%)		
	Etodolac (<600 mg day[1]) (n = 739)	Aspirin (<4800 mg day[1]) (n = 227)	Placebo (n = 358)
Gastrointestinal			
Nausea	8.6	21.1[#+]	6.6
Diarrhoea	5.5	5.4	4.8
Epigastric pain	3.3	9.1[#+]	2.0
Heartburn	5.6	9.5[#+]	3.2
Indigestion	5.1[+]	8.7[#+]	2.0
Flatulence	3.5	4.7[+]	1.5
Abdominal pain	3.0	5.8[+]	2.0
Cramps	2.6	9.1[#+]	2.3
Abdominal bloating	1.9	5.0[#+]	1.4
Constipation	1.7	10.2[#+]	2.1
Vomiting	2.5	4.5	2.0
Dyspepsia	0.4	3.6[#+]	0.6
Skin			
Rash	2.4	1.4	1.8
Pruritus	2.8	0.9	1.7
CNS			
Headaches	5.6	6.7	6.4
Dizziness	3.6	5.1	2.3
Ears/nose/throat			
Tinnitus	1.3	18.3[#+]	1.8
Sore throat	0.0	0.0	0.3
Metabolism			
Increased perspiration	0.4	2.2[#+]	0.3
Anorexia	0.7	0.4	2.0

$P \leq 0.05$:[#] Significantly greater than etodolac; [+] Significantly greater than placebo (Adapted from ref. 35.)

The incidence of GI ulceration or GI bleeding in patients receiving etodolac was 0.42% (11 patients). Five patients (0.19%) had duodenal ulcer, three (0.11%) had gastric ulcer and three (0.11%) had pyloric channel ulcer. Drug-related hepatic, renal and haematological complications were rare. In the post-marketing surveillance studies, GI ulceration was confirmed in only five of the 8334 patients receiving etodolac (0.06%).

Two large-scale, open-label observational studies conducted in France have confirmed the safety/tolerability of etodolac[37]. One study was for six weeks involving 1352 patients with RA and 2610 patients with OA; 985

patients with ankylosing spondylitis were also included. The dosage of etodolac was 400–600 mg day^{-1}. A total of 1276 adverse reactions were reported during the study and these were similar to those usually occurring with NSAIDs (GI reactions, mild skin reactions, dizziness and headache). Less than half of the GI reactions (43%) were considered to be related to treatment with etodolac. Only three patients (0.06%) had confirmed gastro-duodenal ulcers, and only two of these were considered to be treatment related. Only six severe reactions were reported during the study and three of these, which included two deaths, were considered unrelated to etodolac. The second study in France included 51355 patients receiving etodolac 200–600 mg day^{-1} for rheumatic conditions for a period of two weeks to one month. In this study, 5170 patients (10.1%) reported a total of 6236 adverse reactions, and 9% of the study population were withdrawn as a result of adverse reactions. GI haemorrhage was the most serious adverse event and was reported for 22 patients (0.04%); all cases healed with treatment. The safety of etodolac was described as either 'very good' or 'good' by 89% of patients and investigators.

The safety of etodolac and ibuprofen have been compared in a three-year study in patients with active RA[25]. Ibuprofen is frequently chosen as a first-line drug in the treatment of RA because it is regarded as the safest and best tolerated of the routinely used NSAIDs. A total of 1446 patients were randomized to treatment with etodolac 300 mg day^{-1} (150 mg b.i.d.), etodolac 1000 mg day^{-1} (500 mg b.i.d.) or ibuprofen 2400 mg day^{-1} (600 mg q.i.d.). In each treatment group, approximately 50% of patients completed the first year of the study, 30% completed two years and 20% completed three years, which was remarkably low because other medical interventions were not permitted during the study (except for low dose oral corticosteroids). The rate of discontinuation because of adverse events was similar for all treatment groups and the rate was highest during the first 100 days of the study. The incidences of adverse events were comparable in the treatment groups, although dyspepsia and rash occurred less frequently with etodolac 300 mg day^{-1} than with ibuprofen (2400 mg day^{-1}) ($P < 0.05$). Over the three-year study, etodolac was associated with a significantly lower incidence of GI ulcers and GI bleeds than ibuprofen (Figure 2), even at the etodolac dosage of 1000 mg day^{-1} (cumulative incidence: etodolac 300 mg day^{-1}, two patients – 0.43%; etodolac 1000 mg day^{-1}, two patients – 0.67%; ibuprofen 2400 mg day^{-1}, nine patients – 4.74%).

GASTROINTESTINAL SAFETY/TOLERABILITY OF ETODOLAC

An improvement in the GI safety/tolerability profile of etodolac relative to comparator NSAIDs observed in clinical trials has been substantiated by:

Figure 2 Cumulative rate of occurrence of GI ulcers and bleeding with etodolac and ibuprofen[25]: A three-year, double-blind, parallel, multicentre study of 1446 rheumatoid arthritis (RA) patients comparing the long-term efficacy and safety of two doses of etodolac (300 mg and 100 mg day^{-1}) with that of ibuprofen (2400 mg day^{-1}).

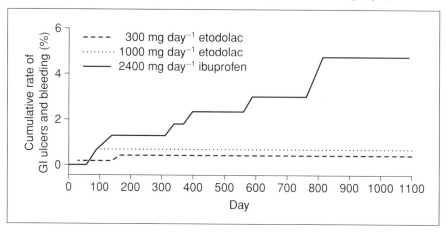

- GI ulcer, perforation and bleed data from clinical practice provided by the Arthritis, Rheumatism and Aging Medical Information System (ARAMIS), the national arthritis database in the USA (ref. 38)
- endoscopic biopsy assays demonstrating no overall suppression of gastric or duodenal PGs with etodolac (refs 7–10)
- gastroscopic studies showing no significant increase in gastric erosion with etodolac compared with placebo (refs 7,39–44)
- microbleeding studies showing significantly less GI blood loss with etodolac than with routinely used NSAIDs (refs 42,45–48)

According to data from ARAMIS, etodolac (data for 88 patient years) and nabumetone (data for 221 patient years) are the only two established NSAIDs that are not associated with serious GI bleeds or other clinically significant events requiring hospitalization[15].

As stated earlier, PGs play not only an important part in the pathogenesis of pain and inflammation but also in gastric protection. Etodolac inhibits the synthesis of PGs at sites of inflammation, but has no marked effect on levels of protective PGs in the stomach or duodenum. This was clearly demonstrated in a four-week, double-blind, randomized comparative study of etodolac (600 mg day^{-1}) versus naproxen (1000 mg day^{-1}) in patients with RA which was supported by other reports[9,10].

During the late 1980s and early 1990s gastroscopic studies in patients with RA[40,42] and OA[7,39,43,44] and in healthy volunteers[41,42,49] demonstrated that etodolac was associated with a significantly lower risk of gastric irritation and injury than some other NSAIDs. The results of some of these studies are summarized in Table 3.

A study by Lanza et al.[41] assessed the effects of various NSAIDs on the GI mucosa by endoscopy. 72 healthy volunteers with a gastroscopy Lanza score of zero were randomly assigned to one of six study groups (12 subjects per group) and received maximal dosages of etodolac, ibuprofen, naproxen, indomethacin or placebo for seven days following an eight-day pre-drug period. The Lanza scale, depending on the severity of GI erosions, expressed the gastroscopy results of all tested NSAIDs. Etodolac showed no significant increase in GI erosion compared with placebo even at the highest dosage of 1000 mg day^{-1}, whereas ibuprofen, naproxen and indomethacin showed significant increases (Figure 3).

Microbleeding studies in healthy volunteers have assessed faecal blood loss associated with the use of etodolac, aspirin, ibuprofen, naproxen and indomethacin[42,45-48]. GI blood loss with conventional formulation etodolac, even at the high dose of 1200 mg day^{-1}, was similar to that seen with placebo. However, GI blood loss was significantly increased with aspirin, ibuprofen, naproxen and indomethacin at their recommended anti-arthritic dosages. In another study in healthy volunteers, etodolac SR at dosages of 600 mg day^{-1} and 1200 mg day^{-1} caused significantly less GI blood loss than naproxen 1000 mg day^{-1} (ref. 46). In patients with OA or RA, treatment with etodolac (300 mg day^{-1} and 1000 mg day^{-1}) has been associated with a significantly lower incidence of GI bleeding than ibuprofen (2400 mg day^{-1}) or piroxicam (20 mg day^{-1})[25,50].

Figure 3 Mean endoscopy scores of various NSAIDs[41]: open-label, analyst-blind, parallel-endoscopy study of 72 healthy subjects following seven days of treatment. The Lanza scale was used to assess gastroscopy scores.

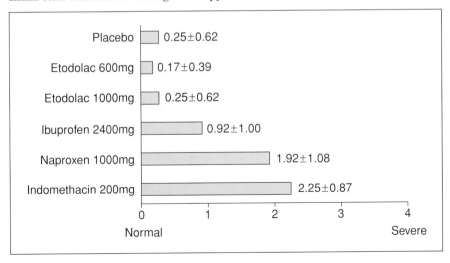

Table 3 Results of gastroscopic studies with etodolac

Author	Comparators	Study population	Study duration	Summary of findings
Lanza et al. (1986)[49]	etodolac (200–600 mg b.i.d.), aspirin (975 mg q.i.d.)	48 normal men	2 weeks	Endoscopy scores were significantly lower for etodolac than aspirin ($P \leq 0.0001$)
Lanza et al. (1987)[41]	etodolac (600 or 1000 mg day^{-1}), indomethacin (150 mg day^{-1}), ibuprofen (2400 mg day^{-1}), naproxen (1000 mg day^{-1}), placebo	72 normal men	1 week	Endoscopy scores similar with etodolac and placebo. Direct gastric scores for etodolac groups were significantly better than for indomethacin, ibuprofen and naproxen groups
Taha et al. (1989)[40]	etodolac (300 mg b.i.d.), naproxen (500 mg b.i.d.)	30 patients with RA	4 weeks	Mucosal lesions in three patients (20%) receiving etodolac (low endoscopy scores) versus eight patients (53%) receiving naproxen (worse endoscopy scores)
Russell (1990)[7]	etodolac (300 mg b.i.d.), naproxen (500 mg b.i.d.)	15 patients with active RA in each of two studies	4 weeks	*Study 1:* three patients receiving etodolac had mucosal lesions at four weeks. One patient receiving naproxen had frank ulceration and six had multiple erosions. *Study 2:* abnormal endoscopy in three patients receiving etodolac (21%) versus nine patients receiving naproxen (64%). Mean endoscopy score lower for etodolac group
Russell et al. (1991)[44]	etodolac (300 mg b.i.d.), naproxen (500 mg b.i.d.)	30 patients with active RA	4 weeks	Upper GI mucosal lesions developed in three of 15 patients receiving etodolac and eight of 15 patients receiving naproxen

USE OF ETODOLAC IN PATIENTS AT HIGH RISK OF SERIOUS NSAID-INDUCED GI EVENTS

Patients at particularly high risk of developing serious NSAID-induced GI adverse events include the elderly (who may have reduced renal function), the more severely disabled, users of corticosteroids, patients with chronic debilitating diseases, smokers, alcoholics and users of anticoagulants[51-53]. Since etodolac appears to have a better safety/tolerability profile than routinely used NSAIDs, it may be particularly useful in these patient groups.

Some NSAIDs have been implicated in various nephrological syndromes, including acute renal failure, papillary necrosis, and disturbances of potassium, sodium and water homeostasis[54]. It has been postulated that these effects may result from inhibition of renal PGs, leading to alterations in renal blood flow with associated renal dysfunction. The effects of etodolac on renal function have been reviewed by examining data obtained from 1382 patients with OA or RA, involving 600 patient-years of active treatment, who participated in 16 double-blind and open-label clinical trials[54]. The trials were of four to 52 weeks duration and involved etodolac dosages of 50–600 mg day^{-1}. The risk of renal function impairment was no greater among patients receiving etodolac than among patients receiving placebo, even in those patients above the age of 65 years. Furthermore, among those patients with abnormal pretreatment renal values, treatment with etodolac did not result in any worsening of renal function.

In a review of the data from 33 double-blind and open-label clinical trials involving etodolac, only 0.27% of 3302 patients receiving etodolac were withdrawn prematurely because of abnormal renal function[36]. None of these renal function abnormalities could be attributed to etodolac alone, since all occurred in patients with previous abnormalities or with co-morbid illnesses. Only 31 patients (0.9%) were withdrawn because of elevated serum levels of liver enzymes or total bilirubin, compared with 18 of 463 patients (4%) receiving aspirin. In only ten of the 31 etodolac-treated patients was etodolac treatment the explanation for the abnormality. In the other 21 cases, other illnesses or complicating factors may have contributed to the abnormal liver function tests. The data review indicated that etodolac therapy posed no greater risk for the elderly than for younger patients. In addition, other trial data have confirmed the efficacy and safety of etodolac (standard formulation 300 mg b.i.d. and sustained-release 600 mg day^{-1}) in patients aged ≥60 years with concomitant diseases and receiving multiple drug therapies[55,56].

The pharmacokinetic profile of etodolac is not significantly different between elderly and younger subjects[35,57]. Consequently, the dosage of etodolac does not usually need to be adjusted for administration to elderly patients. Similarly, in patients with mild to moderate renal impairment and in patients undergoing haemodialysis the pharmacokinetic profile of etodolac does not differ significantly from that in healthy individuals[35,57]. Etodolac may therefore be administered to patients with renal impairment, and even those with end-stage renal disease receiving chronic haemodialysis, without alteration of the dosage regimen. In addition, the pharmacokinetics of etodolac in patients with stable liver cirrhosis does not differ significantly from those in healthy subjects. Although patients with liver disease should be carefully monitored during etodolac therapy, there is no evidence to suggest that the dosage needs to be adjusted in these patients.

CONCLUSION

The recent advent of the COX-2 theory and availability of selective COX-2 inhibitors has stimulated interest in the potential benefits for this class of drug to patients suffering from arthritic conditions. The appropriate use of selective COX-2 inhibitors has been recognized as having an important and positive impact on the reduction of NSAID-induced hospitalization events.

Etodolac was developed in a search for novel NSAIDs with an improved efficacy/side effect balance. Etodolac was derived from a new chemical class of NSAIDs, the pyranocarboxylates, and this molecule was selected for clinical development because of its superior therapeutic index between gastric irritation and anti-inflammatory effects in a wide range of preclinical tests. The improved safety profile of etodolac when compared with existing NSAIDs posed an anomaly for which there was no explanation at that time. The advent of the COX-2 theory served as a possible rationale for etodolac's safety profile. Etodolac has consistently shown COX-2 selectivity in a wide range of *in vitro* and *ex vivo* assay systems, and is recognized as a selective COX-2 inhibitor by regulatory authorities.

A comprehensive safety/tolerability profile of a drug takes many years to establish. Common adverse events will be identified by clinical trials but rarer adverse events are only likely to come to light once a drug is in widespread clinical use. A prime advantage associated with etodolac, when compared with the other COX-2 selective inhibitors, is that it has an efficacy and safety/ tolerability record established through clinical studies extending to seven years duration and over 14 years in clinical practice.

Address all correspondence to: Dr Richard A. Jones, Shire Pharmaceuticals Limited, East Anton, Andover, Hampshire, SP10 5RG, UK.

REFERENCES

1. Vane JR, Bakhle YS, Botting RM. Cyclooxygenases 1 and 2. *Annu Rev Pharmacol Toxicol.* 1998;38:97–120.
2. Kawai S, Nishida S, Kato M, Furumaya Y, Okamoto R, Koshino T et al. Comparison of cyclooxygenase-1 and -2 inhibitory activities of various nonsteroidal

anti-inflammatory drugs using human platelets and synovial cells. *Eur J Pharmacol.* 1998;347:87–94.

3. Vane JR, Botting RM. The future of NSAID therapy: selective COX-2 inhibitors. *Int J Clin Pract.* 2000;54:7–9.

4. Glaser K. Cyclooxygenase selectivity and NSAIDs:cyclooxygenase-2 selectivity of etodolac (Lodine). *Inflammopharmacol.* 1995;3:335–45.

5. Simon LS. The importance of COX 'selectivity'. *J Clin Rheumatol.* 1996;2:135–40.

6. Vane JR. Inhibition of prostaglandin synthesis as a mechanism of action for aspirin-like drugs. *Nature New Biol.* 1971;231:232–5.

7. Russell RI. Endoscopic evaluation of etodolac and naproxen, and their relative effects on gastric and duodenal prostaglandins. *Rheumatol Intl.* 1990;10:17–21.

8. Taha AS, McLaughlin S, Holland PJ, Kelly RW, Sturrock RD, Russell RI. Effect on gastric and duodenal mucosal prostaglandins of repeated intake of therapeutic doses of naproxen and etodolac in rheumatoid arthritis. *Ann Rheum Dis.* 1990;49:354–8.

9. Laine L, Sloane R, Casini-Raggi V, Cominelli F. Randomised, double-blind 1-month trial of placebo, etodolac and naproxen in healthy volunteers: effects on GI injury and prostaglandins. *Esophageal, Gastric and Duodenal Disorders* (April) 1994;A117.

10. Russell RI. COX-2 inhibitors [correspondence]. *Lancet.* 1999;353:1439.

11. Warner TD, Giuliano F, Vojnovic I, Bukasa A, Mitchell JA, Vane JR. Nonsteroid drug selectivities for cyclo-oxygenase-1 rather than cyclo- oxygenase-2 are associated with human gastrointestinal toxicity: a full *in vitro* analysis. *Proc Natl Acad Sci USA.* 1999;96:7563–8.

12. Glaser K, Sung ML, O'Neill K, Belfast M, Hartman D, Carlson R et al. Etodolac selectively inhibits human prostaglandin G/H synthase 2 (PGHS-2) versus human PGHS-1. *Eur J Pharmacol.* 1995;281:107–111.

13. Riendeau D, Charleson S, Cromlish W, Mancini JA, Wong E, Guay J. Comparison of the cyclooxygenase-1 inhibitory properties of nonsteroidal anti-inflammatory drugs (NSAIDs) and selective COX-2 inhibitors, using sensitive microsomal and platelet assays. *Can J Physiol Pharmacol.* 1997;75:1088–95.

14. Riendeau D, Percival MD, Boyce S, Brideau C, Charleson S, Cromlish W et al. Biochemical and pharmacological profile of a tetrasubstituted furanone as a highly selective COX-2 inhibitor. *Br J Pharmacol.* 1997;121:105–17.

15. Singh, G, Terry, R, Ramey, D, Halpern, J, Brown, WB. Comparative GI toxicity of NSAIDs. 19th ILAR Congress, Singapore (June 12th). 1997.

16. Platt PN. Recent clinical experience with etodolac in the treatment of osteoarthritis of the knee. *Clin Rheumatol.* 1989;8:54–62.

17. Palferman T, Struthers G, Williams P. Double-blind parallel comparison of etodolac with naproxen in patients with osteoarthritis of the knee. *Acta Therapeutica.* 1991;17:19–34.

18. Bacon PA. An overview of the efficacy of etodolac in arthritic disorders. *Eur J Rheumatol Inflamm.* 1990;10:22–34.

19. Pena M, Lizarazo H. Double-blind comparison of etodolac and naproxen in patients with osteoarthritis. *Acta Therapeutica.* 1991;17:5–18.

20. Pinals R. Efficacy of etodolac in osteoarthritis: US and European experience. *J Musculoskel Med.* 1991;8:S14–S21.

21. Karbowski A. Double-blind, parallel comparison of etodolac and indomethacin in patients with osteoarthritis of the knee. *Curr Med Res Opin.* 1991;12:309–17.

22. Porzio F. Meta-analysis of three double-blind comparative trials with sustained-release etodolac in the treatment of osteoarthritis of the knee. *Rheumatol Intl.* 1993;13:S19–S24.

23. Schnitzer TJ, Constantine G. Etodolac (Lodine) in the treatment of osteoarthritis: recent studies. *J Rheumatol Suppl.* 1997;47:23–31.

24. Sanda M, Collins S, Mahady J. Three-multicentre study of etodolac (Ultradol) in patients with osteoarthritis of the hip. *Curr Ther Res.* 1983;33:783–92.

25. Neustadt DH. Double blind evaluation of the long-term effects of etodolac versus ibuprofen in patients with rheumatoid arthritis. *J Rheumatol Suppl.* 1997;47:17–22.

26. Lightfoot R. Comparison of the efficacy and safety of etodolac and piroxicam in patients with rheumatoid arthritis. Etodolac Study 326 Rheumatoid Arthritis Investigators Group. *J Rheumatol Suppl.* 1997;47:10–16.

27. Delcambre B. Rheumatoid arthritis: efficacy, safety and therapeutic benefit of etodolac (600mg/daily) versus indomethacin (100mg/daily). *Rheumatologie.* 1990;42:201–6.

28. Jubb RW, Platt PN, Price TR. Double-blind comparison of etodolac sustained-release tablets and piroxicam capsules in patients with rheumatoid arthritis: an interim report. *Curr Ther Res.* 1992;52:769–79.

29. Schattenkirchner M. Double-blind comparison of etodolac and piroxicam in patients with rheumatoid arthritis. *Curr Med Res Opin.* 1991;12:497–506.

30. Briancon D. International experience with etodolac therapy for rheumatoid arthritis: an interim report of comparative efficacy. *Clin Rheumatol.* 1989;8(Suppl 1):63–72.

31. Lonauer G, Tisscher JR, Lim HG, Bijlsma JW. Double-blind comparison of etodolac and diclofenac in patients with rheumatoid arthritis. *Curr Med Res Opin.* 1993;13:70–7.

32. de Queiros MF. Double-blind comparison of etodolac and naproxen in the treatment of rheumatoid arthritis. *Clin Ther.* 1991;13:38–46.

33. Jacob GB, Hart K, Mullane J. Placebo-controlled study of etodolac and aspirin in the treatment of rheumatoid arthritis. *Curr Ther Res.* 1983;33:703–13.

34. Schattenkirchner M. An updated safety profile of etodolac in several thousand patients. *Eur J Rheumatol Inflamm.* 1990;10:56–65.

35. Humber L. Etodolac (Lodine), the first NSAID of the pyranocarboxylic acid class: a review of preclinical and clinical studies through 1992. *Drugs of Today* 1993;29:265–293.

36. Lightfoot R. Safety and pharmacokinetics of etodolac in normal and high-risk populations. *J Musculoskel Med.* 1991;8:S40–S46.

37. Benhamou CL. Large-scale open trials with etodolac (Lodine) in France: an assessment of safety. *Rheumatol Intl.* 1990;10:29–34.

38. Fries J. Toward an understanding of NSAID-related adverse events: the contribution of longitudinal data. *Scand J Rheumatol Suppl.* 1996;102:3–8.

39. Perpignano G, Bogliolo A, Puccetti L. Double-blind comparison of the efficacy and safety of etodolac SR 600 mg u.i.d. and of tenoxicam 20 mg u.i.d. in elderly patients with osteoarthritis of the hip and of the knee. *Int J Clin Pharmacol Res.* 1994;14:203–16.

40. Taha AS, McLaughlin S, Sturrock RD, Russell RI. Evaluation of the efficacy and comparative effects on gastric and duodenal mucosa of etodolac and naproxen in patients with rheumatoid arthritis using endoscopy. *Br J Rheumatol.* 1989;28:329–32.

41. Lanza F, Rack MF, Lynn M, Wolf J, Sanda M. An endoscopic comparison of the

effects of etodolac, indomethacin, ibuprofen, naproxen, and placebo on the gastro-intestinal mucosa. *J Rheumatol.* 1987;14:338–41.

42. Lanza FL, Arnold JD. Etodolac, a new nonsteroidal anti-inflammatory drug: gastro-intestinal microbleeding and endoscopic studies. *Clin Rheumatol.* 1989;8:5–15.

43. Porro G, Caruso I, Petrillo M, Montrone F, Ardizzone S. A double blind gastro-scopic evaluation of the effects of etodolac and naproxen on the gastrointestinal mucosa of rheumatic patients. *J Intern Med.* 1991;229:5–8.

44. Russell RI, Sturrock RD, Taha AS. Upper GI findings parallel minimal GI prostaglandin suppression. Endoscopic studies of patients treated with etodolac. *J Musculoskel Med.* 1991;8:S60–S65.

45. Arnold JD, Salom IL, Berger AE, Meinders JD, Jacob G, Hayden D et al. Comparison of gastrointestinal microbleeding associated with use of etodolac, ibuprofen, indomethacin, and naproxen in normal subjects. *Curr Ther Res.* 1985;37:730–8.

46. Leese P. Comparison of the effects of etodolac SR and naproxen on gastro-intesti-nal blood loss. *Curr Med Res Opin.* 1992;13:13–20.

47. Ryder S, Salom IL, Jacob G, Sanda M, Huth J. Etodolac (Ultradol): the safety profile of a new structurally novel nonsteroidal anti-inflammatory drug. *Curr Ther Res.* 1983;33:946–65.

48. Salom IL, Jacob G, Jallad N, Perdomo CA, Mullane JF, Weidler D. Gastrointestinal microbleeding associated with the use of etodolac, ibuprofen, indomethacin, and naproxen in normal males. *J Clin Pharmacol.* 1984;24:240–6.

49. Lanza F, Panagides J, Salom IL. Etodolac compared with aspirin: an endoscopic study of the gastrointestinal tracts of normal volunteers. *J Rheumatol.* 1986;13:299–303.

50. Jallad NS, Sanda M, Salom IL, Perdomo CS, Garg DC, Mullane JF et al. Gastrointestinal blood loss in arthritic patients receiving chronic dosing with etodolac and piroxicam. *Am J Med Sci.* 1986;292:272–6.

51. Distel M, Mueller C, Bluhmki E. Global analysis of gastrointestinal safety of a new NSAID, meloxicam. *Inflammopharmacol.* 1996;4:71–87.

52. Singh G, Ramey D. NSAID induced gastrointestinal complications: the ARAMIS perspective. *J Rheumatol.* 1998;25:8–16.

53. Russell RI. Defining patients at risk of non-steroidal anti-inflammatory drug gastro-pathy. *Ital J Gastroenterol Hepatol.* 1999;31:S14–S18.

54. Shand DG, Epstein C, Kinberg-Calhoun J, Mullane JF, Sanda M. The effect of etodolac administration on renal function in patients with arthritis. *J Clin Pharmacol.* 1986;26:269–74.

55. Bacon PA. Safety profile of etodolac in the elderly population. *Eur J Rheumatol Inflamm.* 1994;14:19–22.

56. Todesco S, Del Ross T, Marigliano V, Ariani A. Efficacy and tolerability of etodolac in aged patients affected by degenerative joint disease (osteoarthritis) in its active phase. *Int J Clin Pharmacol Res.* 1994;14:11–26.

57. Brater DC, Lasseter KC. Profile of etodolac: pharmacokinetic evaluation in special populations. *Clin Rheumatol.* 1989;8:25–35.

23 | Pharmacological and clinical profile of meloxicam

FRANK DEGNER, STEPHAN LANES, JOANNE VAN RYN
AND RALF SIGMUND

*Boehringer Ingelheim GmbH, Bingerstr. 173, D-55216 Ingelheim,
Germany.*

Arthritic diseases are characterized by inflammation, causing tissue injury, pain and loss of function. Non-steroid anti-inflammatory drugs (NSAIDs) reduce the signs and symptoms of established inflammation within the first days of administration. Although symptoms can be alleviated, chronic inflammatory arthritis is not completely suppressed by NSAIDs and damage to joints usually progresses during drug administration. Although knowledge of their cellular and molecular effects on various aspects of the inflammation process is increasing, NSAID use in the rheumatic diseases is empirical and part of an overall arthritis management approach which is aimed to educate patients about their disease, relieve symptoms and minimize disability and progression of disease[1].

The potential gain of NSAID use is clinically evaluated against potential risks of usage, which may be significant, especially regarding their gastro-intestinal toxicity, their potential for development of functional renal impairment and the precipitation of congestive heart failure in susceptible individuals[2].

The development of prospective longitudinal databases has allowed the study of the epidemiology of the gastrointestinal toxicity of NSAIDs[3–7]. In parallel, new preclinical insights, such as the discovery of multiple cyclo-oxygenase (COX) isoforms[8–10], have been made and modern clinical research methodology has become available, adding evidence-based elements to the empirical approach to arthritis management.

The clinical development of meloxicam has contributed a clinical trial database with more than 30 000 patients, with various rheumatic conditions, studied.

PHARMACOLOGICAL BACKGROUND

Meloxicam was characterized as a potent anti-inflammatory agent in several standard models of inflammation[11,12]. In addition, it was shown to have weak gastric ulcerogenicity in the rat stomach, despite its potent anti-inflammatory activity. When these results were initially obtained, there was no explanation for the improved pharmacological profile of meloxicam in comparison with the standard comparator NSAIDs. At the time, only one COX, the enzyme responsible for the synthesis of prostaglandins, was known, and inhibition of COX activity was thought to be responsible for both the therapeutic effects and side effects of NSAIDs. Inhibition of COX, and thus prevention of the formation of prostaglandins, provided a unifying explanation of the action of NSAIDs, regarding their therapeutic actions as well as their gastrotoxicity, nephrotoxicity and their antithrombotic effects[13].

Since the discovery of a second COX isozyme, COX-2, it has been hypothesized that the anti-inflammatory effects of NSAIDs are achieved through a different mechanism than the often seen side effects of these compounds, including disruption of cytoprotection in the stomach, kidney function and inhibition of platelet aggregation[14–16]. COX-1 is the constitutive isozyme found under physiological conditions in most tissues, a so-called 'house keeping' enzyme, while COX-2 expression is mostly induced, particularly during inflammatory processes[17,18]. However, recent evidence indicates that COX-2 expression is also constitutive in some tissues, such as the central nervous system (CNS) and kidney[19,20]. Most available NSAIDs non-selectively inhibit both enzymes, leading to anti-inflammatory effects (related to COX-2 inhibition) but also to side effects (related to COX-1 inhibition), typically of gastrointestinal nature. It has since been demonstrated that meloxicam inhibits COX-2 more potently than COX-1 at recommended anti-inflammatory doses, thus explaining earlier experimental results.

Meloxicam, in a range of relevant pharmacological models, showed selective inhibition of COX-2 relative to COX-1, and in human *in vivo* studies recommended doses were demonstrated to be COX-1 sparing in a dose-dependent fashion. Thus, at recommended doses of meloxicam, inhibition of platelet aggregation could not be demonstrated[21–23].

CHEMICAL PROPERTIES

Meloxicam, as with all other NSAIDs, including celecoxib and rofecoxib, is classified by the World Health Organization (WHO) according to its chemical structure rather than according to its pharmacological or clinical properties[24]. Meloxicam is an enolcarboxamide, described from 1994 onwards as a selective inhibitor of COX-2 relative to COX-1[25–27]. Minimal changes in its chemical structure can alter the affinity and selectivity for its target enzyme, COX-2[28].

The 5-methyl group on the thiazolyl ring of meloxicam can enter the extra space at the active site of COX-2, accounting for some of its selectivity[29,30]. Effective intracellular access is determined by its unique lipophilic and amphiphilic properties. In its acidic form, meloxicam has membrane solubility 10 times that of piroxicam and comparable with that of other NSAIDs. Meloxicam leaves membranes approximately twice as quickly as diclofenac. Overall, meloxicam transports rapidly across membranes, but within a range that allows it to interact efficiently with its target enzyme[31]. The low water solubility of meloxicam at acidic pH and amphiphilic protonation behaviour are responsible for the tissue kinetics which prevent a high concentration in certain tissues of the gastrointestinal (GI) tract. Thus, meloxicam does not show the typical 'ion trapping' behaviour of the carbonic acid class of NSAID, which may contribute to its clinically observed favourable GI tolerability profile.

COX-2 SELECTIVITY PROFILE *IN VITRO*

Several test models were developed to investigate the COX-2 selectivity of meloxicam relative to COX-1. As with all NSAIDs, depending on the test system used, the concentration that results in 50% inhibition (IC_{50}) and the indices of COX-2 selectivity may differ significantly. COX-2 selectivity is usually expressed as the ratio of the IC_{50} values for COX-2 and for COX-1. As a consequence, comparisons of IC_{50} values and ratios obtained with different compounds should only be performed when the compounds are tested in the same system. Caution should be taken when extrapolating results to predict clinical relevance. However, results obtained in a human whole blood assay are probably more representative than those obtained using animal enzymes in an artificial milieu. In addition, the COX-2 selective profile should only be determined when comparative data are available from several relevant assays. In the different human test systems used, meloxicam consistently showed a selective inhibition of COX-2 relative to COX-1 (Table 1), in contrast to standard NSAIDs such as indomethacin (Table 1), which were either equipotent on COX-1 and COX-2 or which inhibited COX-1 selectively.

The two newer selective COX-2 agents, celecoxib and rofecoxib, were compared with meloxicam using purified human recombinant enzymes. Meloxicam is less potent on COX-1 than celecoxib but more so than rofecoxib. The IC_{50} of meloxicam *in vitro* was 36 μM for COX-1[32], and for celecoxib it was 15 μM[33]. Mean therapeutic concentrations (C_{max}) of around 3 μM for both meloxicam 15 mg[34] and celecoxib 200 mg b.i.d.[35], respectively, have been reported. However, IC_{50} values obtained using isolated human recombinant enzymes are not entirely suited for comparisons with therapeutic plasma or blood concentrations, since drug binding to plasma proteins is not taken into account[36].

Celecoxib and rofecoxib were also compared with meloxicam using the human whole blood assay. In this assay thromboxane A_2 (TXA_2) synthesis in the platelets of clotting whole blood is used to test for COX-1 activity, and prostaglandin E_2 (PGE_2) synthesis in monocytes/macrophages of anticoagulated whole blood stimulated by lipopolysaccharide (LPS) is used to test for COX-2 activity[37]. A comparison of IC_{50} values for COX-1 in the human whole blood assay with therapeutic blood concentrations is given in Table 2 for meloxicam, celecoxib or rofecoxib. Despite variability among experimental conditions, in all four studies with meloxicam[38-40], the IC_{50} for COX-1 inhibition was consistently higher than mean maximal therapeutic blood concentrations[34]. In contrast, in two studies with celecoxib[33,40], IC_{50} values for COX-1 inhibition were found to be lower than the mean maximal therapeutic blood concentration. The IC_{50} for COX-1 inhibition by rofecoxib in the whole blood assay was well above the maximal blood concentration seen therapeutically[40].

Table 1 COX-2 selectivity of meloxicam and indomethacin in human *in vitro* test systems

Test system	IC_{50} COX-1 $\mu mol\ l^{-1}$	IC_{50} COX-2 $\mu mol\ l^{-1}$	Ratio COX-2/-1 Meloxicam	Ratio COX-2/-1 Indomethacin
Human recombinant enzymes (microsomal assay)[14]	36.6	0.49	0.01	3.5
Human recombinant enzymes (whole cell assay)[20]	2.24	0.16	0.07	14.7
Modified human whole blood assay (A549 cells)[40]	5.70	0.23	0.04	10
Human whole blood assay[20]	4.8	0.43	0.09	0.5
Human whole blood assay[12]	3.27	0.25	0.08	0.8

Table 2 Therapeutic blood concentrations and inhibition of COX-1 in the human blood assay *in vitro*

	Meloxicam	Celecoxib	Rofecoxib
Mean maximal recommended blood concentration (C_{max}, ss)	3.1 μM[34] (15 mg q.d.)	2.9 μM[35] (200 mg b.i.d.)	1.0 μM (25 mg q.d.)
IC_{50} COX-1	3.3 μM[28] 4.8 μM[38] 5.5 μM[39] 5.7 μM[40]	1.2 μM[40] 1.6 μM[33] 6.7 μM[33]	63 μM[40]
%TXB_2 inhibition at 80% COX-2 inhibition	~25%[40]	~60%[40]	~15%[40]

ss = steady state

A broad range of non-selective and selective NSAIDs were compared directly using the whole blood assay *in vitro*[40]. In this study it was assumed that an 80% inhibition of COX-2 was required to achieve an anti-inflammatory effect. The level of COX-1 inhibition when COX-2 inhibition was 80% was then determined. The degrees of COX-1 inhibition for celecoxib, meloxicam and rofecoxib were ~60%, ~25% and ~15%, respectively[40].

New assay developments

The human whole blood assay may have the inherent limitation that it is not predictive for target tissues, such as inflamed arthritic joints or the GI tract. Recently developed *in vitro* test systems may overcome this limitation by providing data from these target tissues. In human gastric mucosa pieces[41], interleukin-1 (IL-1) stimulated human chondrocytes[42] and synoviocytes[43] meloxicam demonstrated selective inhibition of COX-2 relative to COX-1 compared with traditional NSAIDs. For meloxicam, the IC_{50} values for inhibition of TXB_2 synthesis in gastric mucosa and platelets were reported to be similar[41].

Experiments using human chondrocyte cultures demonstrated that meloxicam, while effectively inhibiting PGE_2 synthesis in these cells, had no effect on the cellular processes leading to cartilage repair[44]. Radiographically no evidence for cartilage destruction was demonstrated in a 2 year long-term rat model of spontaneous osteoarthritis (OA)[45].

COX-2 SELECTIVITY PROFILE IN ANIMAL STUDIES *IN VIVO*

Meloxicam has potent anti-inflammatory activity, which was demonstrated in several models of acute and subacute inflammation[46,47]. In the carageenan-induced paw oedema model, meloxicam was shown to be as effective as indomethacin, piroxicam and naproxen.

Meloxicam was also active in a model of chronic inflammation, the adjuvant arthritis model[46,47]. Meloxicam inhibited oedema in the inflamed paws in a dose-dependent fashion and achieved maximal efficacy (i.e. defined as >90% inhibition of the day 21 oedema response). Meloxicam was more potent in this model than the comparator substances indomethacin, piroxicam, diclofenac and naproxen. This anti-inflammatory effect was paralleled by a protective effect on bone and cartilage destruction, as well as a reduction in the systemic markers of inflammation[47].

The COX-2 selectivity of meloxicam was also demonstrated by measuring inhibition of PGE_2 synthesis *in vivo*. Meloxicam effectively inhibited PGE_2 production in pleuritic exudate, but had little effect on PGE_2 production in the kidney[46]. This was in contrast to the comparator NSAIDs, which all effectively inhibited the COX-1-dependent PGE_2 production in the kidneys.

The effective analgesic activity of meloxicam was assessed in the inflammatory pain model of Randall-Selitto[38] and confirmed in monoarthritic rats[48] as well as in dog models of acute joint inflammation[49,50]. In addition, meloxicam had analgesic effects in the acetic acid writhing test in mice and the formalin test in rats[51]. The antipyretic effects of meloxicam have been studied after subcutaneous administration of yeast in rat[38] and in a feline endotoxin model[52].

GI side effects are common to all NSAIDs and usually represent the dose-limiting factor for these substances, provided no other toxicity becomes evident during clinical development. The acute ulcerogenic effect of meloxicam in the rat was compared with that of other NSAIDs and also compared with their inhibitory effects in the adjuvant arthritis model. Calculation of the therapeutic index in the rat indicated an approximate tenfold improved benefit to risk ratio for meloxicam over standard comparator NSAIDs[11]. In addition, when comparing the effectiveness of NSAIDs in inhibiting PGE_2 production in gastric juice in the rat *in vivo*, it was demonstrated that meloxicam was the least effective as compared to diclofenac, naproxen and flurbiprofen[46].

COX-2 SELECTIVITY PROFILE IN HUMAN *IN VIVO* STUDIES

The differential inhibition of COX-1 and COX-2 *in vivo* is classically studied by investigating the effects of single or repeated anti-inflammatory doses in humans using the whole blood assay *ex vivo*. As for the *in vitro* assay, TXA_2 synthesis in clotting whole blood and PGE_2 synthesis in anticoagulated whole blood stimulated by LPS are used to test for COX-1 and COX-2 activity, respectively[38].

The effects of therapeutic doses of meloxicam, celecoxib and rofecoxib on COX-1 and COX-2 activity under such conditions, as compared to standard NSAIDs, are summarized in Table 3. It should be noted that this is a summary of different studies, and results may not be directly comparable. Blood samples from volunteers were usually (but not always) taken at peak absorption after drug administration. However, taken together, these data show that both meloxicam and celecoxib inhibit COX-2 to a greater degree than COX-1 when measured as PGE_2 and TXB_2 inhibition, respectively. Both have a similar degree of COX-1 inhibition at their maximal recommended doses of 15 mg daily and 200 mg b.i.d., respectively. Rofecoxib has a smaller effect on COX-1 *ex vivo* when measured as TXB_2 inhibition. In contrast to these agents, comparator substances almost completely inhibited COX-1-dependent TXB_2 production (Table 3).

Platelet aggregation provides a useful functional correlate to more sensitive markers of COX-1 inhibition, such as serum TXB_2 levels. This is illustrated

Table 3 Percentage inhibition of COX-1 versus baseline (measured as TXB$_2$ inhibition in platelets) and COX-2 (measured as PGE$_2$ inhibition) in the human whole blood assay *ex vivo*

Substance	Dose	% Inhibition of		Platelet aggregation	Reference number
		TXB$_2$	PGE$_2$		
Meloxicam	7.5 mg	None	–	None	21
		25%	51% (placebo 10%)	–	39 (sd)
		~47%*	–	–	55 (sd)
	15 mg	35%	70% (placebo 10%)	–	39
		~68%*	–	–	55 (sd)
		~50%*	–	–	55
		66%	–	None	23
		53%	78%	None	22
Rofecoxib	12.5 mg	9%	67%	None	22
	25 mg	5%	69%	None	22
Celecoxib	100 mg	~22%	75% (placebo 36%)	None	56 (sd)
	200 mg	48%	59%	None[35] (100 mg b.i.d., ss)	54 (sd)
	200 mg b.i.d.	29%	77%	–	54
	400 mg	~22%	86% (placebo 36%)	15%	56 (sd)
	400 mg	46%	56%	–	54 (sd)
	600 mg b.i.d.	~55%	–	None	53
Diclofenac	75 mg	~85%*	–	–	55 (sd)
	75 mg b.i.d.	~78%*	–	–	55
	50 mg t.i.d.**	50%	94%	~20%	22
Ibuprofen	800 mg t.i.d.	89%	71%	~80%	22
	800 mg	95%	93% (placebo 36%)	83%	56 (sd)
Naproxen	550 mg t.i.d.	95%	72%	~90%	22
	500 mg b.i.d.	>95%	–	~50%	53
Indomethacin	25 mg t.i.d.	99%	–	87%	21
		95%	–	100%	23

Platelet aggregation to varying stimuli was also measured *ex vivo*. All studies were performed at steady state unless otherwise indicated (sd = single dose, – not performed).
* Estimates at C_{max}.
** Mean over 8h after drug administration and does not represent peak levels.

by the fact that with standard NSAIDs, inhibition of serum TXB$_2$ must be virtually complete (>90%) before platelet aggregation is influenced (Table 3)[57]. Consistent with this, recommended doses of meloxicam (7.5 and 15 mg daily), celecoxib (100 and 200 mg b.i.d.) or rofecoxib (12.5 and 25 mg daily) do not inhibit platelet aggregation. Similar results were also obtained when testing bleeding time[21,22,23].

In conclusion, despite heterogeneity in results obtained from human isolated COX enzymes and TXB_2 measurements in human whole blood assays, meloxicam, celecoxib and rofecoxib share the common characteristics of no effect on platelet aggregation and bleeding time, which may be regarded as functional correlates for selective COX-2 inhibition (Table 3). Meloxicam at recommended doses inhibits COX-2 more than COX-1[20,29] with no significant effects on platelet aggregation or bleeding time.

ABSORPTION, DISTRIBUTION, METABOLISM AND ELIMINATION

Meloxicam allows once a day dosing with a half-life of around 20 h[34]. It is completely absorbed after intramuscular injection and after enteral administration (tablets or suppositories), with an absolute bioavailability of 89–93%. Meloxicam is bound more than 99% to plasma proteins, explaining the relatively small volume of distribution of 10–15 litres[34]. It reaches in the synovial fluid approximately 40–50% of the accompanying total plasma concentrations. Unbound drug concentrations in the synovial fluid are similar to free plasma concentrations, and after a single administration of meloxicam (15 mg) the IC_{50} for COX-2 is exceeded several fold (Figure 1)[36]. The main metabolites of meloxicam are pharmacologically inactive and are excreted equally via the kidneys and the faeces. Total plasma clearance is 7–8 ml min^{-1}

Figure 1 Unbound meloxicam concentrations present in synovial fluid after a single injection of 15 mg. Data are presented as the mean $\pm$ SEM, $n = 40$. IC_{50} of COX-2 inhibition was determined *in vitro* with synoviocytes (dashed line).

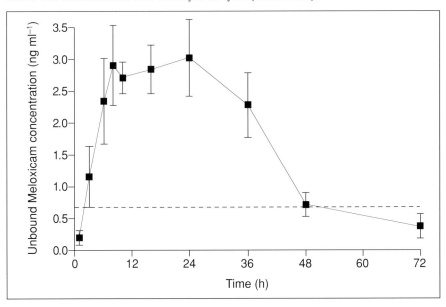

(ref. 34). No pharmacokinetic interaction has been observed in clinical trials between meloxicam and cimetidine[58], β-acetyldigoxin[59], low dose methotrexate[60], frusemide[61,62] or warfarin[63]. Nevertheless appropriate caution is advised when using such co-medications clinically.

THERAPEUTIC EFFICACY

To date, a total of 20 084 patients have been treated with meloxicam in clinical Phase II–IV efficacy and safety trials, as compared with 1397 patients treated with placebo and 13 080 patients treated with active comparators. In Phase I clinical trials 813 subjects were studied. The mean age of all patients treated with meloxicam in Phase II–IV studies was 59 years, 6705 (33%) were older than 65 years and 1956 (10%) were older than 75 years.

Based on this clinical trial programme, meloxicam has been registered since 1995 in 102 countries. Depending on the country, main registered indications refer to the symptomatic management of OA, rheumatoid arthritis (RA) and ankylosing spondylitis. The registered formulations are tablets, capsules, suppositories, an oral suspension and an ampoule for intramuscular injection. In summary, meloxicam at doses of 7.5 or 15 mg daily has been shown clinically to have analgesic and anti-inflammatory activity, leading to beneficial effects in terms of daily life activities and functional outcome measures.

Osteoarthritis

Adequate and well-controlled OA efficacy trials were performed according to a prospective, double-blind, randomized, parallel group and multicentre design following GCP guidelines or guidelines valid at the time of performance of the trials.

Patients with confirmed diagnosis of OA who suffered from at least moderate pain on movement in the target joint at study entry qualified for the trials and were administered single daily doses of meloxicam for up to 6 months.

These trials demonstrated superior efficacy of meloxicam 7.5 mg or 15 mg daily over placebo[64,65] and comparable efficacy in the treatment of OA compared with diclofenac or piroxicam[66–73]. Comparative long-term efficacy was demonstrated for treatment durations of up to six months[68,73].

A 12 week trial[64] performed in the USA investigated, in addition to the recommended doses of 7.5 mg and 15 mg daily, a lower dose (3.75 mg daily) previously not tested in a placebo and active controlled design trial (464 patients treated with meloxicam). Diclofenac, 100 mg daily, was administered as an active control to test for trial and drug sensitivity. OA patients of at least 40 years of age with an acute flare after removal of their previous NSAID and who met the inclusion and exclusion criteria were included in the trial. Meloxicam doses of 7.5 mg and 15 mg were consistently superior to placebo and comparable in efficacy with diclofenac. Meloxicam 3.75 mg was numerically superior to placebo but a significant difference from placebo was observed in only one out of four primary endpoints and three out of six secondary endpoints. Regression analysis indicated increasing efficacy with increasing dose of meloxicam, which had also been shown previously in a placebo-controlled trial for disease activity[65]. Based on the results from these two placebo-controlled trials with meloxicam in OA, the lowest effective dose providing sufficient pain relief and improvement of signs and symptoms is 7.5 mg daily.

Two large-scale trials, MELISSA (Meloxicam Large Scale International Study Safety Assessment) and SELECT (Safety and Efficacy Large scale Evaluation of COX inhibiting Therapies), compared meloxicam 7.5 mg, the recommended starting dose for treatment of OA, with traditional NSAIDs by using their recommended dose for the treatment of OA, i.e. diclofenac 100 mg SR and piroxicam 20 mg[66,67]. Both trials were conducted according to a double-blind, prospective, randomized and parallel group design, reflecting closely the situation under real life prescribing conditions. The aim of these two trials was primarily to assess the tolerability profile of meloxicam in a large international patient population suffering from OA, and secondly, to confirm equivalent efficacy. Patients eligible for inclusion had to suffer from clinically confirmed OA of the hip, knee or hand. In contrast, patients with OA of the spine were eligible only if both clinical and radiological signs and symptoms of OA were present. Pain on active movement had to be greater than 35 mm on a 100 mm horizontal visual analogue scale (VAS). Approximately 20 000 patients altogether, with a mean age of 62 years, were enrolled in the two trials. Of those, 40% of the patients were elderly, i.e. older than 65 years. Overall, meloxicam 7.5 mg once daily was equally effective to both diclofenac 100 mg SR and piroxicam 20 mg in the efficacy endpoints according to the *a priori* defined equivalence ranges of clinical relevance. The incidence of withdrawals due to lack of efficacy was low and comparable for all treatment groups, with withdrawal rates of 1.7 % each in the meloxicam treated groups in both trials and 1.0% and 1.6% in the diclofenac and piroxicam treated groups, respectively.

In summary, clinical trials in OA patients demonstrated the efficacy of meloxicam, in doses of 7.5 or 15 mg day^{-1}, to be comparable with established doses of piroxicam or diclofenac. This was consistent in European and US trials.

Ankylosing spondylitis and rheumatoid arthritis (registered in the European Community)

The efficacy of meloxicam in highly inflammatory rheumatic conditions such as ankylosing spondylitis and RA has been studied in adequately and well-controlled clinical trials[74–77]. In a 1-year placebo and active controlled clinical trial in ankylosing spondylitis, meloxicam 15 mg was effective versus placebo (Figure 2) and comparable versus piroxicam 20 mg. The effect was maintained over 1 year. Dose increase beyond the recommended dose of 15 mg did not provide a clinically meaningful increase in efficacy[74].

In RA, children as well as adults have been studied in clinical trials. An open first Phase I/II clinical trial in 36 children with juvenile RA demonstrated 70% of patients responding to therapy after 12 weeks using established efficacy criteria[78]. In adult patients with RA a European placebo-controlled clinical trial demonstrated efficacy of meloxicam 7.5 mg and 15 mg over placebo[75]. In a US Phase III clinical trial, the efficacy and safety of meloxicam 7.5, 15 and 22.5 mg daily for the treatment of RA was evaluated over 12 weeks, with placebo (negative control) and diclofenac 75 mg b.i.d. (positive control) as comparators. A total of 894 patients over 18 years of age with confirmed RA and who were currently taking NSAIDs were randomized and treated following an NSAID-free period during which a predefined flare had to be demonstrated. Meloxicam efficacy was evident after 2 weeks of treatment and continued to the end of the trial. Meloxicam 7.5 and 22.5 mg was significantly superior to placebo in all five primary efficacy endpoints. Diclofenac 150 mg was superior to placebo for four of five primary efficacy measures, and meloxicam 15 mg was superior for three of five primary endpoints. Overall, this trial demonstrated that meloxicam 7.5 mg, 15 mg or 22.5 mg is effective for the treatment of RA.

As for OA, meloxicam in the dose range from 7.5 mg to 15 mg has been demonstrated to be effective in patients with RA, with a similar efficacy as comparator NSAIDs in established doses[76,77]. Efficacy was maintained for treatment periods of up to 18 months[79].

Figure 2 Long-term functional outcome in ankylosing spondylitis[47].

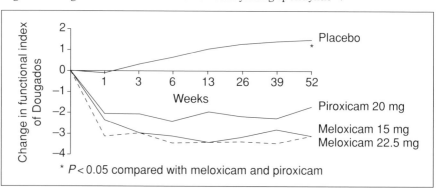

SAFETY AND TOLERABILITY

Meloxicam distinguishes itself from traditional NSAIDs with a reduced risk of GI adverse events consistently demonstrated in randomized clinical trials, large-scale clinical outcome studies, pooled and meta-analyses, as well as in controlled postmarketing experience.

Gastrointestinal tolerability

Overall adverse events, including GI adverse events, of meloxicam have been studied in two large-scale clinical outcome studies[66,67]. These studies demonstrated fewer GI adverse events for meloxicam 7.5 mg than for the comparator NSAIDs diclofenac 100 mg SR ($P < 0.001$) or piroxicam 20 mg ($P < 0.001$). This favourable profile included the GI events dyspepsia, abdominal pain, nausea and vomiting (Figure 3), and was associated with significantly more meloxicam patients completing the studies ($P < 0.001$).

Findings from individual placebo-controlled randomized clinical trials suggest that the favourable GI profile of meloxicam 7.5 mg daily over comparator NSAIDs, observed in the short-term treatment of OA patients[64,66,67], can be extended to meloxicam 15 mg and to RA and ankylosing spondylitis patients[65,74,75]. In these studies, patients on meloxicam experienced consistently fewer GI adverse events over comparator NSAIDs, regardless of time on drug, at the recommended doses of 7.5 mg or 15 mg daily. The cumulative risks for GI adverse events observed in the OA development programme for meloxicam 7.5 mg or 15 mg daily, diclofenac 100 mg or placebo are

Figure 3 Favourable gastrointestinal adverse event profile for meloxicam 7.5 mg over diclofenac 100 mg in a large-scale clinical outcome study[66].

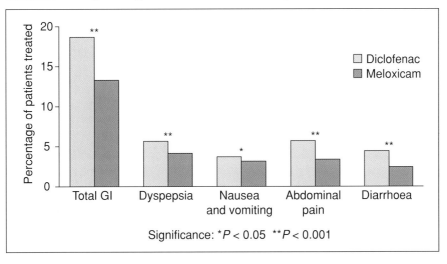

Significance: $^*P < 0.05$ $^{**}P < 0.001$

depicted in Figure 4. While there is a significant difference for both meloxi-cam 7.5 mg and 15 mg daily over diclofenac ($P < 0.001$), the Kaplan–Meier estimates for meloxicam and placebo are similar. After 3 months of treatment the risk estimate for diclofenac for GI adverse events is 27%, whereas the risk estimates for the other three curves are around 22%.

The meloxicam clinical trial database was also analysed beyond OA, regarding the incidence of GI adverse events (Figure 5). The results from these analyses showed consistently fewer GI adverse events for meloxicam versus comparator NSAIDs. For meloxicam in daily doses of 7.5 mg or 15 mg differences in GI adverse events versus comparator NSAIDs were highly significant ($P < 0.0001$ and $P = 0.0004$, respectively). The reduction in risk for gastrointestinal adverse events over comparator NSAIDs was 31% for meloxicam 7.5 mg and 23% for meloxicam 15 mg. These results confirm and further strengthen those from a meta-analysis of published clinical trial experience with meloxicam, which showed statistically significant relative risk reductions in terms of GI adverse events, withdrawals due to GI adverse events, and dyspepsia by 36%, 41% and 27%, respectively for meloxicam over comparator NSAIDs[81]. No clear dose response relationships for meloxicam could be demonstrated, with the overall rate ratio estimates for all GI adverse events for meloxicam 7.5 mg versus placebo being 1.03 ($P = 0.80$), and for meloxicam 15 mg the rate ratio estimate was 1.15 ($P = 0.24$).

Figure 4 Gastrointestinal tolerability of meloxicam 7.5 mg ($n = 10\ 199$) and meloxicam 15 mg ($n = 977$) compared with diclofenac 100 mg ($n = 5396$) and placebo ($n = 294$) in osteoarthritis patients observed in double-blind clinical trials.

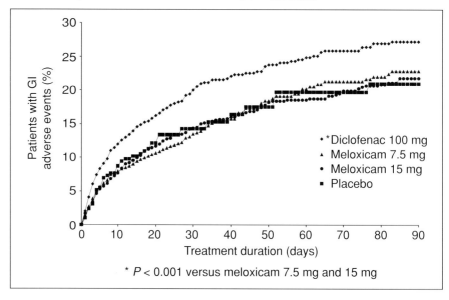

Figure 5 Relative risk (RR) estimates for gastrointestinal adverse events for meloxicam versus placebo (a) and comparator NSAIDs (b). The meloxicam database of all 17 double-blind clinical trials performed in registered indications was analysed by semiparametric survival analysis using the proportional hazards model, i.e. COX regression[80] in a fixed effects analysis. Comparisons were analysed independently according to type of comparator (placebo or active) and according to dose of meloxicam (7.5 mg or 15 mg).

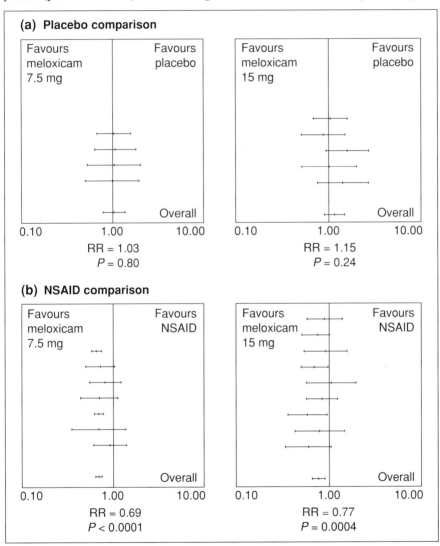

Upper gastrointestinal perforation, ulcer or bleeding

GI effects of NSAIDs include a broad spectrum of events, from small asymptomatic ulcers detected by endoscopic examination to acute, life-threatening bleeding and perforation. The most clinically important events are also the rarest events, and this rarity presents special challenges in assessing risk. The main problem is that most clinical trials are simply too small to measure accurately the risk of the most serious kinds of GI events.

In the two largest clinical trials, namely MELISSA[66] and SELECT[67], fewer cases of upper GI perforation, ulceration or bleeding (PUB) were observed among patients treated with meloxicam 7.5 mg than among those treated with comparator NSAIDs. For meloxicam, upper GI PUB was observed in five and seven cases, whereas for diclofenac 100 mg or piroxicam 20 mg, seven and 16 cases, respectively, were observed[66,67]. No ulcer complications, i.e. ulcer perforation or ulcer bleed, were observed in the meloxicam groups, whereas eight complicated cases were seen in the two comparator groups (four with diclofenac, four with piroxicam). Results on hospitalizations due to GI adverse events (Figure 6) suggested a reduced duration of admission to the hospital for GI complications in the meloxicam-treated group[29,66,67]. Consistent with these results, a meta-analysis based on the published literature revealed for meloxicam a significantly lower odds ratio for upper GI PUB of 0.52 (95% confidence interval from 0.28 to 0.96) versus comparator NSAIDs[81].

Because of the extensive meloxicam development programme, the clinical database is unusually large and thus provides the ability to assess the risk of clinical events of greatest interest using a pooled analysis of all clinical trials performed with meloxicam (Table 4). The recommended starting dose for meloxicam in OA is 7.5 mg day^{-1}, although higher doses are included in the analysis for completeness. Daily doses greater than 15 mg are not approved or recommended.

Figure 6 Number of days in hospital due to GI adverse events for meloxicam 7.5 mg, diclofenac 100 mg SR and piroxicam 20 mg in two large-scale clinical outcome studies[66,67].

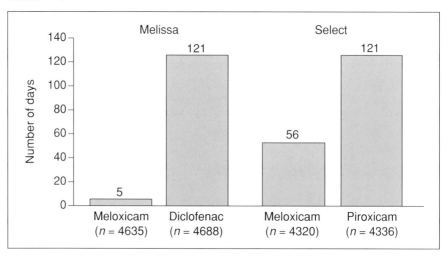

Table 4 Upper GI perforation, ulcer or bleeding (PUB) in all therapeutic Phase II to IV double-blind clinical trials from the meloxicam database

| | | Meloxicam | | |
	Placebo	7.5 mg	15 mg	22.5 mg
Number of patients treated	1397	11 687	3759	515
Number of PUB	0	15	5	3
Mean time on drug (days)	35	31	52	118
Incidence of PUB (%)	0	0.13	0.13	0.58
95% CI for PUB incidence (%)		[0.06–0.19]	[0.02–0.25]	[0.0–1.24]

The upper GI PUB data from all therapeutic randomized double-blind Phase II to IV clinical trials included in the analysis also indicated a low risk for meloxicam at the recommended doses of 7.5 mg or 15 mg daily, with incidences of 0.13% and 0.13%, respectively and the upper 95% confidence interval bounds not exceeding 0.30%; the respective mean times on drug were 1 and 2 months (Table 4). The majority of observed PUBs occurred within the first 4–8 weeks of therapy for all meloxicam treatment groups. Kaplan–Meier estimates for the risk of upper GI PUB events for meloxicam 15 mg daily are given in Figure 7. The risk estimates after 2 and 6 months were low, with 0.25% and 0.45%, respectively. The cumulative risks also tended to increase with dose and duration of treatment. Similar results were obtained in a pooled analysis performed after reviewing clinically serious upper GI perforation, ulceration and bleeding (PUB) in a blinded fashion. The results of this analysis were consistent with the PUB analysis in that the rates were low at daily doses of meloxicam of 7.5 or 15 mg.

In this analysis, data from multiple clinical trials were combined to estimate the risk of clinically serious upper GI PUBs. Therefore these data should be viewed as descriptive.

A strength of this analysis is that it provides direct estimation of the clinical event of interest in a population that was not screened to exclude patients at increased risk of developing the event. Endoscopy studies, for instance, under-estimate the risk of clinical outcomes for at least two reasons. First, patients are screened at the outset so patients with a detectable ulcer are excluded from participation. Secondly, when a patient develops an endoscopic ulcer during the study, therapy is discontinued, so these patients, fortunately, do not have an opportunity to develop a PUB. For these and other reasons endoscopic studies will underestimate the risk of clinical outcomes in an NSAID population. The meloxicam PUB analysis is therefore more representative of risks that might be expected to occur in the general population.

Figure 7 Upper GI perforation, ulcer or bleeding (PUB) for meloxicam 15 mg daily in all therapeutic Phase II to IV double-blind clinical trials. The cumulative Kaplan–Meier estimates after 2 and 6 months are 0.25% and 0.45%, respectively.

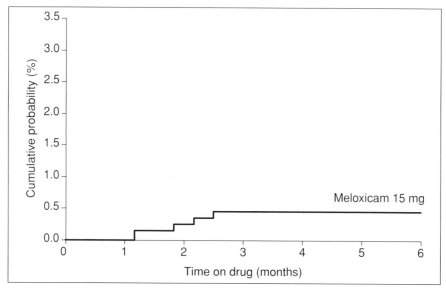

Thromboembolic events

The meloxicam clinical trial database also provides information on safety and tolerability data from system organ classes other than the GI tract. The two large-scale clinical trials MELISSA and SELECT[66,67] provided no evidence for any such additional toxicity risk, including hypertension, oedema or renal adverse events for meloxicam over diclofenac and piroxicam. Theoretically, meloxicam, like other COX-2 inhibitors, could have prothrombotic effects compared to standard NSAIDs[56]. Therefore the meloxicam database for all 59 therapeutic clinical trials, including 32 539 patients treated with either meloxicam or comparators, was analysed for any thromboembolic events (i.e. myocardial infarction and ischaemic stroke according to WHO system organ classes). In the meloxicam clinical trial database overall concomitant low-dose aspirin use was reported in 6.9% of cases, ranging from 4.3% to 8.0% for the different treatment groups.

Forty-five events were coded as myocardial infarctions and 48 events as embolic stroke in the total database. The majority of these 93 thromboembolic events were observed in non-aspirin users (88/93 = 94.6%). The overall fraction of non-aspirin users in the database was 93.1%. The incidence for thromboembolic events in the complete dataset was 0.28%; for the 1397 patients on placebo five such events have been observed (0.36%). There was no evidence of a dose effect relationship for meloxicam for thromboembolic events. Point estimates for thromboembolic events were 1.66, 2.02 and 1.38

per 100 patient-years of exposure for meloxicam 7.5 mg, 15 mg and 22.5 mg, respectively. Point estimates for placebo, diclofenac 100 mg or piroxicam 20 mg were 3.70, 3.05 and 1.19 per 100 patient-years, respectively. The confidence intervals for all treatment groups overlapped due to the rarity of events and size of observed populations. The estimated event rates were similar across treatments. Therefore, current evidence, although limited especially with regard to statistical power, does not support the hypothesis that treatment with meloxicam increases the risk of thromboembolic events.

SYSTEMATIC POST-MARKETING EXPERIENCE

Data obtained from a post-marketing setting experience needs to be interpreted carefully as possible bias can be easily introduced. Three systematic studies of the post-marketing experience with meloxicam have been performed, one of which was using the UK General Practitioners Research Database[82]. In this study the baseline risk of an upper GI event among new users of meloxicam, ibuprofen, diclofenac, naproxen or indomethacin was characterized. The authors selected for analysis a random sample of 5000 meloxicam users, and 5000 users of each of the comparator NSAIDs except indomethacin, for which 2500 subjects were selected. Comparators were matched to meloxicam subjects on age and sex. For each subject, history of certain GI diagnoses and recent use of anti-inflammatory drugs and acid-suppressing drugs were examined. It was found that patients receiving meloxicam were at least twice as likely as patients receiving other NSAIDs to have a recent history of GI diagnoses or treatment. It is concluded that in the UK meloxicam was used more often than other popular NSAIDs among patients who were at increased baseline risk of GI events.

Independently, selective prescription of meloxicam to such high-risk patients was demonstrated in the European controlled pharmacoepidemiological study[83]. In this study meloxicam was prescribed preferentially to patients who had not responded to NSAIDs previously (47% versus 39%), and/or had reported NSAID-induced side effects (19% versus 6%), or had a history of PUB (12% versus 7%) previously. Although selective prescription, and the non-randomized and unblinded nature of this study type limit the conclusions that can be drawn concerning efficacy or tolerability, the results from the European and the Latin American large-scale epidemiological study emphasize the importance of respecting prescribing conditions carefully. In order to minimize the potential risk for an adverse GI event the lowest effective dose should be used for the shortest possible duration. For high-risk patients, alternate therapies that do not involve NSAIDs should be considered.

The European controlled pharmacoepidemiological study[83] assessed the tolerability and efficacy of meloxicam under natural prescribing conditions up to six months in duration. A total of 4526 patients received either meloxicam

($n = 2530$) or a comparator NSAID ($n = 1996$) in a multicentre prospective observational cohort study. Data from randomized centres were analysed in two separate groups: a meloxicam-only group, and a group that was prescribed all comparator NSAIDs. Treatment groups were comparable regarding observed efficacy measures. Moreover, significantly lower rates for meloxicam patients relative to comparator NSAID patients regarding GI adverse drug reactions (1.8% versus 3.2%), including dyspepsia (0.08% versus 0.35%), abdominal pain (0.91% versus 1.9%), gastritis (0.08% versus 0.60%) and bleeding from the GI tract (0.08% versus 0.50%) were reported (Table 5).

Table 5 Summary of patients with GI adverse reactions in a controlled pharmacoepidemiological study[83]

WHO System organ class disorders and preferred term	Meloxicam ($n = 2530$)		NSAID ($n = 1996$)		Relative risk [95% CI]	P value[1]
	n	%	n	%		
Adverse reactions	63	2.5	71	3.6	0.70 [0.50–0.98]	0.04
Gastrointestinal (GI) system in total	45	1.8	63	3.2	0.56 [0.39–0.82]	0.003
Abdominal pain	23	0.91	38	1.90	0.48 [0.29–0.80]	0.006
Gastritis	2	0.08	12	0.60	0.13 [0.03–0.59]	0.002
Nausea	10	0.40	9	0.45	0.88 [0.36–2.15]	ns
Dyspepsia	2	0.08	7	0.35	0.23 [0.05–1.08]	0.049
Diarrhoea	8	0.32	5	0.25	1.26 [0.41–3.86]	ns
Oesophagitis	1	0.04	3	0.15	0.26 [0.03–2.53]	ns
Anorexia	1	0.04	1	0.05	0.79 [0.05–12.6]	ns
Flatulence	0	0	1	0.05	–	ns
Duodenitis	0	0	1	0.05	–	ns
Gastrointestinal disorders not otherwise specified	3	0.12	1	0.05	2.37 [0.25–22.7]	ns
Vomiting	5	0.20	0	0	–	ns
Bleeding from GI tract (i.e. PUB, gastritis haemorrhagic or GI haemorrhage)	2*	0.08	10*	0.50	0.16 [0.04–0.72]	0.007
Any gastric or duodenal ulcer, haematemesis or melaena (PUB)	0	0	6	0.30	–	0.007
Gastric ulcer	0	0	5	0.25	–	ns
Gastric ulcer perforated	0	0	1	0.05	–	ns
Duodenal ulcer	0	0	1	0.05	–	ns
Melaena	0	0	1	0.05	–	ns
Gastritis haemorrhagic	0	0	1	0.05	–	ns
Gastrointestinal haemorrhage	2	0.08	5	0.25	0.32 [0.06–1.63]	ns

*Including one case of serious adverse reaction. CI = confidence interval. Number of patients do not sum up due to the possibility of multiple adverse events per individual. [1]P value (Fisher's exact test) of difference between treatments; ns, not significant.

Table 6 GI tolerability profile of meloxicam (relative risk versus standard comparator NSAIDs) in two prospective controlled large-scale comparative pharmacoepidemiological studies

	European study		Latin American study	
Patients on meloxicam	2530		18356	
Patients on comparator NSAID	1996		3372	
	Relative risk	P value[1]	Relative risk	P value[1]
Adverse reactions	0.70	0.04	0.26	0.001
Dropouts for adverse reactions	0.79	ns	0.07	0.001
Gastrointestinal adverse reactions	0.56	0.003	0.21	0.001
Abdominal pain	0.48	0.006	0.19	0.001
Gastritis	0.13	0.002	0.13	0.001
Nausea	0.88	ns	0.27	0.001
Dyspepsia	0.23	0.049	0.21	0.001
Diarrhoea	1.26	ns	0.31	0.001
Bleeding from GI tract	0.16	0.007	0.06	0.001
Hospitalization for GI bleeding	–	–	0.04	0.001
Upper gastrointestinal endoscopies	–	–	0.22	0.001

[1] P value (Fisher's exact test) of difference between treatments. ns, not significant.

Similar results were obtained in a second prospective controlled large-scale comparative pharmacoepidemiological study comparing Latin American patients on meloxicam ($n = 18\,356$) with those on comparator NSAIDs ($n = 3372$) in a naturalistic setting. Treatment groups were comparable regarding observed efficacy measures. In contrast to the European study, in this study GI risk factors at baseline were comparable among groups. Fewer discontinuations due to adverse events were observed in the meloxicam group (1.1% versus 15.3%, $P < 0.001$). Upper GI endoscopies were performed in 662 patients in total, with 342 patients in the meloxicam group and 298 patients in the comparator group (1.9% versus 8.8%, $P < 0.001$). Eight cases of GI bleeding were observed for meloxicam and 21 such cases for the comparator NSAIDs (0.04% versus 0.62%, $P < 0.001$). Overall, in both the European and the Latin American study the GI tolerability profiles of meloxicam were comparable (Table 6).

The results from these two large-scale comparative studies are consistent with the favourable GI tolerability seen with meloxicam in double-blind comparative clinical trials.

CONCLUSIONS

Selective inhibition of COX-2 relative to COX-1 has been consistently demonstrated for meloxicam in various *in vitro* test systems, in experimental models *in vivo*, and in humans *ex vivo*. Inhibition of thromboxane in human platelets is incomplete and dose dependent; significant inhibition of platelet aggregation has not been observed with meloxicam at recommended daily doses of 7.5 mg and 15 mg. Anti-inflammatory, analgesic activity and anti-pyretic properties have been shown in classical models of inflammation, pain and fever. With once-daily dosing, meloxicam has demonstrated efficacy in OA, RA and ankylosing spondylitis. It has been registered since 1995 in more than 100 countries, has been studied in clinical trials with more than 30 000 patients and has been used by more than 30 million patients worldwide. Clinically, meloxicam offers similar efficacy to existing non-steroid anti-inflammatory drugs in established doses, including diclofenac, piroxicam and naproxen, while associated with fewer GI side effects, as measured by symptoms such as dyspepsia, abdominal pain, diarrhoea, and nausea and vomiting. In large clinical trials meloxicam is associated with lower rates of GI PUBs and their complications than standard NSAIDs, although studies were not powered to detect these differences as statistically significant. Pooled analyses of clinical trials and controlled large-scale comparative pharmaco-epidemiological studies are supportive, indicating a low risk of PUB and serious GI complications at recommended doses.

ACKNOWLEDGEMENTS

We thank S. Senn, Professor of Pharmaceutical and Health Statistics, University College London, UK, for methodological advice and review of the semiparametric survival analysis (COX regression). A full paper on this analysis is in preparation.

REFERENCES

1. Brooks PM, Buckwalter JA. Principles of management of patients with rheumatic disease. In: Klippel JH, Dieppe PA, editors. *Rheumatology*. London: Mosby International; 1998:3:1.1–1.4
2. McGettigan P, Henry D, Page J. Adverse effects of non-steroidal anti-inflammatory drugs on the gastrointestinal tract and kidney: relationship to cyclooxygenase-2 selectivity. In: Vane JR, Botting RM, editors. *Clinical Significance and Potential of Selective COX-2 Inhibitors*. London: William Harvey Press; 1998:149–60.
3. Fries JF, Williams CA, Bloch DA, Michel BA. Nonsteroidal anti-inflammatory drug associated gastropathy: Incidence and risk factor models. *Am J Med.* 1991;91:213–22.
4. Henry D, Dobson A, Turner C. Variability in the risk of major gastrointestinal complications from nonaspirin nonsteroidal anti-inflammatory drugs. *Gastroenterology.* 1993;105:1078–88.
5. Garcia Rodriguez LA, Jick H. Risk of upper gastro-intestinal bleeding and perforation associated with individual non-steroidal anti-inflammatory drugs. *Lancet.* 1994;343:769–72.
6. Langman MJS, Weil J, Wainwright P, Lawson DH, Rawlins MD, Logan RF. Risks

of bleeding peptic ulcer associated with individual non-steroidal anti-inflammatory drugs. *Lancet.* 1994;343:1075–8.

7. Henry D, Lim L, Garcia Rodriguez LA, Perez Gutthann S, Carson JL, Griffin M et al. Variability in risk for gastrointestinal complications with individual non-steroidal anti-inflammatory drugs: results of a collaborative meta-analysis. *BMJ.* 1996;312:1563–6 .

8. O'Banion MK, Sadowski HB, Winn V, Young DA. A serum- and glucocorticoid-regulated 4-kilobase mRNA encodes a cyclooxygenase-related protein. *J Biol Chem.* 1991;266:23261–7.

9. Kujubu DA, Fletcher BS, Varnum BC, Lim RW, Hershman HR. TIS10, a phorbol ester tumor promotor-inducible mRNA from Swiss 3T3 cells, encodes a novel prostaglandin synthase/cyclooxygenase homologue. *J Biol Chem.* 1991;266:12866–72.

10. Xie W, Chipman JG, Robertson DL, Erikson RL, Simmons DL. Expression of a mitogen-responsive gene encoding prostaglandin synthase is regulated by mRNA splicing. *Proc Natl Acad Sci USA.* 1991;88:1692–6.

11. Engelhardt G, Homma D, Schlegel K, Utzmann R, Schnitzler C. Anti-inflammatory, analgesic, antipyretic and related properties of meloxicam, a new non-steroidal anti-inflammatory agent with favourable gastrointestinal tolerance. *Inflamm Res.* 1995;44:423–33.

12. Engelhardt G, Homma D, Schnitzler C. Meloxicam: A potent inhibitor of adjuvant arthritis in the Lewis rat. *Inflamm Res.* 1995;44:548–55.

13. Vane JR, Botting RM. The future of NSAID therapy: selective COX-2 inhibitors. *IJCP.* 2000;54:7–9.

14. Xie W, Robertson DL, Simmons DL. Mitogen-inducible prostaglandin G/H synthase: A new target for nonsteroidal antiinflammatory drugs. *Drug Dev Res.* 1992;25:249–65.

15. Meade EA, Smith WL, DeWitt DL. Differential inhibition of prostaglandin endoperoxide synthase (cyclooxygenase) isozymes by aspirin and other non-steroidal anti-inflammatory drugs. *J Biol Chem.* 1993;268:6610–4.

16. Vane JR. Towards a better aspirin. *Nature.* 1994;367:215–6.

17. Pairet M, Engelhardt G. Distinct isoforms (COX-1 and COX-2) of cyclooxygenase: possible physiological and therapeutic implications. *Fund Clin Pharmacol.* 1996;10:1–15.

18. Pairet M, van Ryn J, Distel M. Overview of COX-2 in inflammation: from the biology to the clinic. In: Willoughby DA, Tomlinson A, editors. *Inducible Enzymes in the Inflammatory Response.* Basel/Switzerland: Birkhauser Verlag; 1999:1–30.

19. Wallace JL. Selective COX-2 inhibitors: is the water becoming muddy? *Trends Pharmacol Sci.* 1999;20:4–6.

20. Wolfe MM, Lichtenstein DR, Singh G. Gastrointestinal toxicity of nonsteroidal antiinflammatory drugs. *N Engl J Med.* 1999;340:1888–99.

21. Stichtenoth DO, Wagner B, Frölich JC. Effects of meloxicam and indomethacin on cyclooxygenase pathways in healthy volunteers. *J Invest Med.* 1997;45:44–9.

22. Schwartz JI, Van Hecken A, De Lepeleire I, Depre M, Wong P, Ebel DL et al. Comparative inhibitory activity of rofecoxib (MK-0966), meloxicam, diclofenac, ibuprofen, and naproxen on COX-2 vs COX-1 in healthy female volunteers. Poster EULAR 1999. *Ann Rheum Dis Abstr.* 1999;857:206.

23. De Meijer A, Vollaard H, de Metz M, Verbruggen B, Thomas C, Novakova I.

Meloxicam 15 mg/day spares platelet function in healthy volunteers. *Clin Pharmacol Ther.* 1999;66:425–30.

24. Guidelines for ATC classification and DDD assignment, WHO Collaborating Centre for Drug Statistics Methodology. http://www.whocc.nmd.no/, 1 June 2000.

25. Engelhardt G. Meloxicam inhibits preferentially COX-2. *Eur J Clin Pharmacol.* 1994;47:A98.

26. Engelhardt G. Meloxicam: a potent inhibitor of COX-2. 9th Int Conf on Prostaglandins and Related Compounds, Florence, 6–10 June 1994.

27. Engelhardt G. Meloxicam inhibits preferably cyclooxygenase-2. *Z Rheumatol.* 1994;53(suppl 1):68.

28. Pairet M, van Ryn J, Schierok H, Mauz A, Trummlitz G, Engelhardt G. Differential inhibition of cyclooxygenases-1 and -2 by meloxicam and its 4'-isomer. *Inflammation Res.* 1998;47:270–6.

29. Hawkey CJ. COX-2 inhibitors. *Lancet.* 1999;353:307–14.

30. Marnett LJ, Kalgutkar AS. Design of selective inhibitors of cyclooxygenase-2 as nonulcerogenic anti-inflammtory agents. *Curr Opin Chem Biol.* 1998;2:482–90.

31. Herbette L, Vecchiarelli M, Trummlitz G. NSAID mechanism of action: the role of intracellular pharmacokinetics. In: Vane J, Botting J, Botting R, editors. *Improved Non-steroid Anti-inflammatory Drugs; COX-2 Enzyme Inhibitors.* London: Kluwer Academic Publishers and William Harvey Press; 1996:85–102.

32. Churchill L, Graham AG, Shih CK, Pauletti D, Farina PR, Grob PM. Selective inhibition of human cyclo-oxygenase-2 by meloxicam. *Inflammopharmacol.* 1996;4:125–35.

33. Celecoxib Summary Basis of Approval, FDA 1999. *Rev Pharmacol Toxicol.* 199;2.

34. Tuerck D, Busch U, Heinzel G, Narjes H. Clinical pharmacokinetics of meloxi-cam. *Drug Res.* 1997;47:253–8.

35. US Prescribing Information celecoxib. 1999

36. Pairet M, van Ryn J. Tests for cyclooxygenase-1 and -2 inhibitioin. In: Vane J, Botting R, editors. *Clinical Significance and Potential of Selective COX-2 Inhibitors.* London: William Harvey Press; 1998:19–30.

37. Brooks P, Emery P, Evans JF, Fenner H, Hawkey CJ, Patrono C et al. Interpreting the clinical significance of the differential inhibition of cyclooxygenase-1 and cyclooxygenase-2. *Rheumatology (Oxford).* 1999;38:779–88.

38. Patrignani P, Panara MR, Sciulli MG, Santini G, Renda G, Patrono C. Differential inhibition of human prostaglandin endoperoxide synthase-1 and -2 by nonsteroidal anti-inflammatory drugs. *J Physiol Pharmacol.* 1997;48:623–31.

39. Panara MR, Renda G, Sciulli MG, Santini G, Di Giamberardino M, Rotondo MT et al. Dose-dependent inhibition of platelet cyclooxygenase-1 and monocyte cyclooxygenase-2 by meloxicam in healthy subjects. *J Pharmacol Exp Ther.* 1999;290:276–80.

40. Warner T, Giuliano F, Vojnovic I, Bukasa A, Mitchell JA, Vane JR. Nonsteroid drug selectivities for cyclo-oxygenase-1 rather than cyclo-oxygenase-2 are associated with human gastrointestinal toxicity: A full in vitro analysis. *Proc Natl Acad Sci USA.* 1999;96:7563–8.

41. Blanco FJ, Guitian R, Moreno J, Hernandez A, Freire M, Atanes A et al. Effect of antiinflammatory drugs on COX-1 and COX-2 activity in human articular chondro-cytes. *J Rheumatol.* 1999;26:1366–73.

42. Kawai S. Cyclooxygenase selectivity and the risk of gastro-intestinal complications

of various non-steroidal anti-inflammatory drugs: a clinical consideration. *Inflamm Res.* 1998:47(suppl 2):S102–6.

43. Tavares IA. The effects of meloxicam, indomethacin or NS-398 on eicosanoid synthesis by fresh human gastric mucosa. *Aliment Pharmacol Ther.* 2000;14:795–9.

44. Bassleer C, Magotteaux Y, Geenan V, Malaise M. Effects of meloxicam compared to acetylsalicylic acid in human articular chondrocytes. *Pharmacology.* 1997;54:49–56.

45. Mohr W, Lehmann H, Engelhardt G. Chondroneutrality of meloxicam in rats with spontaneous osteoarthritis of the ankle joint. *J Rheumatol.* 1997;56:21–30.

46. Engelhardt G. Pharmacology of meloxicam, a new non-steroidal anti-inflammatory drug with an improved safety profile through preferential inhibition of COX-2. *Br J Rheumatol.* 1996;35(suppl. 1):4–12.

47. Engelhardt G, Homma D, Schlegel K, Utzmann R, Schnitzler C. Anti-inflammatory, analgesic, antipyretic and related properties of meloxicam, a new nonsteroidal anti-inflammatory agent with favourable gastrointestinal tolerance. *Inflamm Res.* 1995;44:423–33.

48. Laird JMA, Herrero JF, Garcia de la Rubia P, Cervero F. Analgesic activity of the novel COX-2 preferring NSAID, meloxicam in mono-arthritic rats: Central and peripheral components. *Inflamm Res.* 1997;46:203–10.

49. Cross AR, Budsberg SC, Keefe TJ. Kinetic gait analysis assessment of meloxicam efficacy in a sodium urate-induced synovitis model in dogs. *Am J Vet Res.* 1997;58:626–31.

50. Van Bree H, Justus C, Quirke JF. Preliminary observations on the effects of meloxicam in a new model for acute intraarticular inflammation in dogs. *Vet Res Commun.* 1994;18:217–34.

51. Santos AR, Vedana EM, De Freitas GA. Antinociceptive effect of meloxicam, in neurogenic and inflammatory nociceptive models in mice. *Inflamm Res.* 1998;47:302–7.

52. Justus C, Quirke JF. Dose–response relationship for the antipyretic effect of meloxicam in an endotoxin model in cats. *Vet Res Commun.* 1995;19:321–30.

53. Leese PT, Hubbard RC, Karim A, Isakson PC, Yu SS, Geis GS. Effects of celecoxib, a novel cyclooxygenase-2 inhibitor, on platelet function in healthy adults: A randomized, controlled trial. *J Clin Pharmacol.* 2000;40:124–32.

54. Celecoxib Summary Basis of Approval, FDA 1999. Study 003.

55. Tegeder I, Lötsch J, Krebs S, Muth-Selbach U, Brune K, Geisslinger G. Comparison of inhibitory effects of meloxicam and diclofenac on human thromboxane biosynthesis after single doses and at steady state. *Clin Pharmacol Ther.* 1999;65:533–44.

56. McAdam BF, Catella-Lawson F, Mardini IA, Kapoor S, Lawson JA, Fitzgerald GA. Systemic biosynthesis of prostacyclin by cyclooxygenase (COX)-2: The human pharmacology of a selective inhibitor of COX-2. *Proc Natl Acad Sci USA.* 1999;96:272–7.

57. Reilly IA, FitzGerald GA. Inhibition of thromboxane formation in vivo and ex vivo: implications for therapy with platelet inhibitory drugs. *Blood.* 1987;69:180–6.

58. Busch U, Heinzel G, Narjes H, Nehmiz G. Interaction of meloxicam with cimetidine, Maalox, or aspirin. *J Clin Pharmacol.* 1996;36:79–84.

59. Degner FL, Heinzel G, Narjes H, Tuerck D. The effect of meloxicam on the pharmacokinetics of beta-acetyl-digoxin. *Br J Pharmacol.* 1995;40:486–8.

60. Huebner G, Sander O, Degner FL, Tuerck D, Rau R. Lack of pharmacokinetic

interaction of meloxicam with methotrexate in patients with rheumatoid arthritis. *J Rheumatol.* 1997;24:845–51.

61. Mueller FO, Middle MV, Schall R, Terblanche J, Hundt HKL. An evaluation of the interaction of meloxicam with frusemide in patients with compensated chronic cardiac failure. *Br J Clin Pharmacol.* 1997:44:393–8.

62. Mueller FO, Schall R, de Vaal AC, Groenewoud G, Hundt HKL, Middle MV. Influence of meloxicam on furosemide pharmacokinetics and pharmacodynamics in healthy volunteers. *Eur J Clin Pharmacol.* 1995;48:247–51.

63. Tuerck D, Su CAPF, Heinzel G, Busch U, Bluhmki E. Hoffmann J. Lack of interaction between meloxicam and warfarin in healthy volunteers. *Eur J Clin Pharmacol.* 1997;51:421–5.

64. Yocum DE, Hall DB, Roszko PJ. Efficacy and safety of meloxicam in the treatment of osteoarthritis (OA): results of a phase III double-blind, placebo controlled trial.

65. Lund B, Distel M, Bluhmki E. A double-blind, randomized, placebo-controlled study of efficacy and tolerance of meloxicam treatment in patients with osteoarthritis of the knee. *Scand J Rheumatol.* 1998;27:32–7.

66. Hawkey C, Kahan A, Steinbrück K, Alegre C, Baumelou E, Begaud B et al. Gastrointestinal tolerability of meloxicam compared to diclofenac in osteoarthritis patients. International MELISSA Study Group. Meloxicam Large-scale International Study Safety Assessment. *Br J Rheumatol.* 1998;37:937–45.

67. Dequeker J, Hawkey C, Kahan A, Steinbrück K, Alegre C, Baumelou E et al. Improvement in gastrointestinal tolerability of the selective cyclooxygenase (COX)-2 inhibitor, meloxicam, compared with piroxicam: results of the Safety and Efficacy Large-scale Evaluation of COX-inhibiting Therapies (SELECT) trial in osteoarthritis. *Br J Rheumatol.* 1998;37:946–51.

68. Hosie J, Distel M, Bluhmki E. Meloxicam in osteoarthritis: a 6-month, double-blind comparison with diclofenac sodium. *Br J Rheumatol.* 1996;35(suppl):39–43.

69. Goei The HS, Lund B, Distel MR, Bluhmki E. A double-blind, randomized trial to compare meloxicam 15 mg with diclofenac 100 mg in the treatment of osteoarthritis of the knee. *Osteoarthritis Cartilage.* 1997;5:283–8.

70. Linden B, Distel M, Bluhmki E. A double-blind study to compare the efficacy and safety of meloxicam 15 mg with piroxicam 20 mg in patients with osteoarthritis of the hip. *Br J Rheumatol.* 1996;35(suppl 1):35–8.

71. Carrabba M, Paresce E, Angelini M, Galanti A, Marini MG, Cigarini P. A comparison of the local tolerability, safety and efficacy of meloxicam and piroxicam suppositories in patients with osteoarthritis: a single-blind, randomized, multicentre study. *Curr Med Res Opin.* 1995;13:343–55.

72. Ghozlan PR, Bernhardt M, Velicitat P, Bluhmki E. Tolerability of multiple administration of intramuscular meloxicam: a comparison with intramuscular piroxicam in patients with rheumatoid arthritis or osteoarthritis. *Br J Rheumatol.* 1996;35(suppl 1):51–5.

73. Hosie J, Distel M, Bluhmki E. Efficacy and tolerability of meloxicam versus piroxicam in patients with osteoarthritis of the hip or knee: a six-month double-blind study. *Clin Drug Invest.* 1997;13:175–84.

74. Dougados M, Gueguen A, Nakache JP, Velicitat P, Veys EM, Zeidler H et al. Ankylosing spondylitis: what is the optimum duration of a clinical study? A one year versus a 6 weeks non-steroidal anti-inflammatory drug trial. *Rheumatology (Oxford).* 1999;38:235–44.

75. Lemmel EM, Bolten W, Burgos-Vargas R, Platt P, Missila M, Sahlberg D et al.

Efficacy and safety of meloxicam in patients with rheumatoid arthritis. *J Rheumatol.* 1997;24:282–90.

76. Wojtulewski JA, Schattenkirchner M, Barcelo P, de Loet X, Bevis PJR, Bluhmki E et al. A six-month double-blind trial to compare the efficacy and safety of meloxicam 7.5 mg daily and naproxen 750 mg daily in patients with rheumatoid arthritis. *Br J Rheumatol.* 1996;35(suppl):22–8.

77. Huskisson EC, Narjes H, Bluhmki E. Efficacy and tolerance of meloxicam, a new NSAID, in daily oral doses of 15, 30 and 60 mg in comparison to 20 mg piroxicam in patients with rheumatoid arthritis. *Scand J Rheumatol.* 1994;(suppl 98):115.

78. Foeldvari, I, Burgos-Vargas, R, Thon A. 70% of patients are responders after 12 weeks in the phase I/II study of meloxicam suspension in juvenile rheumatoid arthritis. *Ann Rheumat Dis.* 2000;59(suppl 1):252.

79. Huskisson EC, Ghozlan R, Kurthen R, Degner FL, Bluhmki E. A long-term study to evaluate the safety and efficacy of meloxicam therapy in patients with rheumatoid arthritis. *Br J Rheumatol.* 1996;35(suppl 1):29–34.

80. Cox, DR. Regression models and life tables. *J Roy Stat Soc.* 1972;B34:187–220.

81. Schoenfeld P. Gastrointestinal safety profile of meloxicam: a meta-analysis and systematic review of randomized controlled trials. Proc of a Symp 'Rationalizing Cyclooxygenase Inhibition for Optimization of Efficacy and Safety Profiles'. *Am J Med.* 1999;107(suppl 6A):48S–54S.

82. Lanes SF, Garcia Rodriguez LA, Hwang E.. Baseline risk of gastrointestinal disorders among new users of meloxicam, ibuprofen, diclofenac, naproxen and indomethacin. *Pharmacoepidemiol Drug Safety.* 2000;9:113–7.

83. Degner F, Sigmund R, Zeidler H. Efficacy and tolerability of meloxicam in an observational, controlled cohort study in patients with rheumatic disease. *Clin Ther.* 2000;22:400–10.

24 Nimesulide: a well-established cyclooxygenase-2 inhibitor with many other pharmacological properties relevant to inflammatory diseases

ALAN BENNETT

Academic Department of Surgery, The Rayne Institute, Guy's, King's and St Thomas' School of Medicine, King's College, London SE5 9NU, England.

Nimesulide was developed by Riker 3M in the 1980s. Helsinn Switzerland acquired the worldwide rights for marketing nimesulide, and completed its development and registration. Helsinn Healthcare SA licenses nimesulide to many pharmaceutical companies, including several large multinationals. The drug has been on the market in Italy since 1985, and in over 50 other countries for shorter periods, under various trade names (Ainex, Aulin, Antifloxil, Donulide, Eskaflam, Guaxan, Mesulid, Mutix, Nexen, Nimed, Nimedex, Nisulid, Scaflam, Scaflan, Skaflam). In 1999, nimesulide had the remarkable achievement of being the fifth best-selling non-steroid anti-inflammatory drug (NSAID) worldwide, with a turnover of US$290 million, even though it is not sold in the enormous markets of USA and Japan where no licence has been applied for. In those countries where it is sold, the drug is often in the first or second position for NSAID sales. To date, more than 200 million patients have been treated, including 55 000 in clinical trials. The Hungarian Society for Experimental and Clinical Pharmacology voted nimesulide Drug of the Year in March 2000.

Initial studies on nimesulide preceded the discovery of COX-2, and various mechanisms, not involving inhibition of prostaglandin (PG) synthesis, were examined to determine its anti-inflammatory activity[1]. The explanation of the weak inhibition of rat gastric cyclooxygenase (COX) found in early studies is now known to be due to the preference of nimesulide for COX-2, whereas the gastric enzyme is COX-1. Numerous biochemical investigations, including several human studies, have now shown that nimesulide markedly inhibits COX-2, with substantially less effect on COX-1.

CHEMISTRY

Nimesulide is 4-nitro-phenoxymethane-sulphonanilide (Figure 1), an almost neutral NSAID (pKa about 6.5).

PATHWAYS AFFECTED BY THERAPEUTICALLY RELEVANT LEVELS OF NIMESULIDE

As discussed by Bennett and Villa[2], various investigators have measured nimesulide concentrations in human blood following oral administration of 100 mg. With this dose, the highest mean blood concentration reached is about 6 μg ml^{-1} (~20 μM). NSAIDs bind strongly to plasma proteins, and 99% of nimesulide in blood is bound to albumin[3,4]. Thus the maximum concentration of free (unbound, pharmacologically active) nimesulide is about 100 times less than the total amount. For *in vitro* experiments with no serum proteins present, this 100-fold lower amount is therefore roughly the maximum therapeutically relevant concentration. More can be used if albumin or serum is added, but this has not been determined. With NSAIDs in general, pharmacological studies of clearly excessive concentrations have resulted from ignoring the importance of the extensive protein binding (see later concerning experiments with human gastric mucosal biopsies).

The cut-off point chosen here for therapeutically relevant levels of free nimesulide (0.06 μg ml^{-1}; ~0.2 μM) is realistic but not absolute. Higher levels can occur in blood because:

Figure 1 The chemical structure of nimesulide.

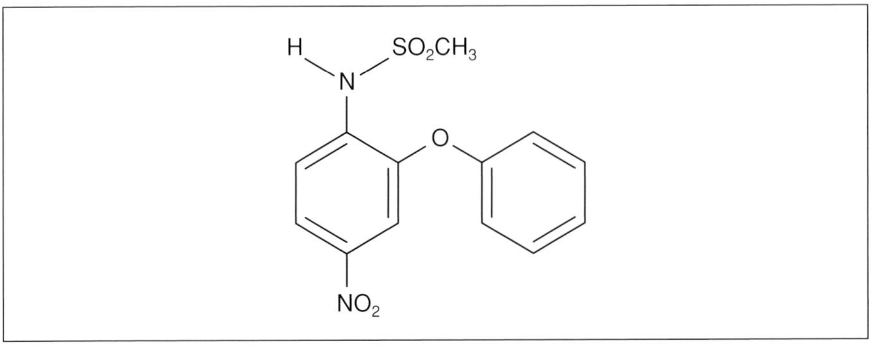

1. doses of 200 mg are sometimes used;
2. mean maximum concentrations above 6 μg ml^{-1} have been reported with 100 mg oral doses;
3. some individual values exceed the mean; and
4. accumulation may occur with repeated administration.

Furthermore, perhaps the amount of free nimesulide increases at inflammatory sites (where the pH is lower), since slightly acid conditions increase levels of free flurbiprofen[5]. It may not matter that amounts above 0.06 μg ml^{-1} of unbound nimesulide can sometimes occur, since there do not appear to be any studies slightly above that level that would be excluded from the present 'therapeutically relevant' classification.

Nimesulide at normal doses *in vivo* or at therapeutically relevant concentrations *in vitro*, as defined in this chapter, has several novel pharmacological actions in addition to preferential inhibition of COX-2 activity (Table 1). Besides studies on prostaglandin (PG) synthesis, nimesulide has been shown in human subjects to affect neutrophil functions and histamine action, but the other candidates for clinical relevance described below have been studied only *in vitro* or in laboratory animals.

Table 1 Actions of nimesulide at normal doses or concentrations, or at therapeutically relevant concentrations *in vitro* (up to 0.06 μg ml^{-1}; ~0.2 μM in the absence of albumin). All the effects listed are inhibitory

Pathway	Man	Lab animals	cells in vitro	Dose/conc	Refs
COX-2 activity	leukocytes *ex vivo*			100 mg b.d.	11,12
			human leukocytes	therapeutic range	8,9,10,13
Superoxide formation	leukocytes *ex vivo*			200 mg	23
Collagenase	synovial fluid *in vitro*			2 μM	26
Histamine action	skin *in vivo*			200 mg	31
Histamine release		guinea-pigs		1.6 μmol kg^{-1}	32
Histamine release		guinea-pigs		0.1–1 mg kg^{-1} i.v.	33
Cytokine action		rats		7 mg kg^{-1}	30
COX -2 formation			human synovocytes	0.03 μg ml^{-1}	22
Metalloprotease formation			human synovocytes	0.03 μg ml^{-1}	25
Chondrocyte apoptosis		rat	chondrocytes	1 pM–1 μM	29

Since the *in vitro* pharmacological activities of its major 4-hydroxy metabolite occur only at relatively high concentrations, most or all of the therapeutic effects are probably due to nimesulide itself. However, this conclusion might have to be modified should protein binding of the metabolite be substantially less than with the parent drug.

Inhibition of prostaglandin synthesis

PGs act in inflammation and pain by augmenting the effects of some other mediators[6]. In general, COX-2 is the main PG-forming COX isoform induced at sites of inflammation, and in the spinal cord due to peripheral pain, whereas constitutive COX-1 forms protective PGs in the gastric mucosa and elsewhere. Numerous studies *in vitro*[7] and on human blood *in vitro* or *ex vivo*[8–13] have now shown that nimesulide preferentially inhibits COX-2, whereas most of the other NSAIDs are more active on COX-1. However, PGs formed by COX-2 at various sites, including gastric ulcers during healing, may be beneficial, and PGs formed by COX-1 may also contribute to inflammation[14]. Indeed, the effectiveness of NSAIDs in alleviating pain correlates better with inhibition of COX-1 than of COX-2, as of course does gastric damage[13].

Nimesulide had no significant effect on COX-1 in human gastric mucosa *ex vivo*[11,12]. Although Cryer and Feldman[10] reported that the concentration of nimesulide causing 50% inhibition of PG formation by human gastric mucosal biopsies was only 8 times lower than the concentration needed to inhibit COX-2 in leukocytes, their conclusion concerning nimesulide and other NSAIDs is flawed. Whereas the leukocytes were studied in blood, the incubates of gastric biopsies did not contain albumin. The potency of the NSAIDs on the gastric mucosa was therefore overestimated, by approximately 100-fold in the case of nimesulide.

Human blood studies with therapeutic levels of nimesulide consistently showed a substantial block of leukocyte COX-2, whereas platelet COX-1 was either not significantly affected[11,12], or reduced slightly[10] or moderately[9,13]. Inhibition of COX-2 is clearly an important part of the therapeutic action of nimesulide, but it is possible that some additional block of COX-1 contributes to its efficacy. The lack of a significant effect on haemostasis[15] might seem to argue against an effect on platelet COX-1, but perhaps the explanation is that nimesulide has a dual effect on platelets[16]. An unanswered question is whether, and to what extent, nimesulide inhibits COX-1 at sites of inflammation and pain.

Preferential COX-2 inhibition by nimesulide was first shown in 1994[17], and subsequently confirmed repeatedly[7]. Our own work in 1995[18] showed:

1. relatively weak inhibition of PG formation by nimesulide in human isolated gastric mucosa/submucosa (COX-1);
2. inhibition of PG formation by human leukocytes (COX-2);

3. pronounced inhibition of sheep pure COX-2; and
4. no inhibition of sheep pure COX-1.

As with all NSAIDs, different experimental conditions (including incubation time, substrate concentration and source of enzymes or cells) can give widely varying COX-2:COX-1 ratios, but all of the numerous studies with nimesulide show a preferential effect on COX-2, and in some studies, including that on sheep enzymes above[18], the inhibition was highly selective[7]. Molecular modelling indicates that block of COX-2 is due to the interaction of nimesulide with the larger channel in COX-2 compared with COX-1[19,20].

There is considerable argument about the degree of COX-2 selectivity shown by celecoxib, rofecoxib and other NSAIDs. Some of this argument is dominated more by marketing than by pharmacology. Because many studies show a small inhibition of COX-1, nimesulide is classified as a preferential COX-2 inhibitor. In any case, moderate selectivity may be better than high selectivity. As discussed again later, inhibition of COX-1 may have therapeutic advantages, provided that it is not sufficient to damage the stomach or kidneys. Furthermore, some inhibition of platelet COX-1[9] might offset the proaggregatory effect of blocking endothelial production of prostacyclin by COX-2, as might occur with rofecoxib. Indeed, use of low-dose aspirin has been suggested in rofecoxib-treated patients who are at risk from thromboembolism[21], but even this dose of aspirin increases gastric damage and so counteracts the value of high COX-2 selectivity.

It is generally assumed that assays based on normal human blood give the most relevant measurements of COX-1/COX-2 selectivity in humans. The ratios at 50% inhibition in these blood experiments show that nimesulide is about 5–59 times more potent on leukocyte COX-2 than on platelet COX-1[9,10,13]. However, it does not necessarily follow that the selectivity is the same at all sites in the body compared with normal blood cells, and that it is not altered by disease. Furthermore, it is probably better to measure NSAID effects on COX-1 at the level that produces 80% inhibition of COX-2[13], which more closely represents the therapeutic blood concentration.

If PGs formed by COX-1 contribute to the pathology, it would presumably be better to inhibit both COX-1 and COX-2 strongly at sites of inflammation, but to spare gastric and renal COX-1. There is probably a pharmacokinetic contribution to the relatively little damage to these organs. The weakly acidic nature of nimesulide, which presumably results in relatively little gastric and renal accumulation, is discussed together with other possible factors in the section on safety and tolerability.

Inhibition of COX-2 formation

Besides inhibiting COX-2 activity, low concentrations of nimesulide have recently been found to reduce the enzyme formation by human synovial fibroblasts in culture[22]. As expected, nimesulide 0.03 μg ml^{-1} or the COX-2 inhibitor NS-398 decreased the fibroblast PGE_2 production induced by inter-leukin-1β, but in addition they suppressed COX-2 mRNA expression and protein synthesis. Thus nimesulide may have a dual inhibitory effect on PG levels, by decreasing both the formation and the activity of COX-2.

Inhibition of neutrophil function: superoxide anions and enzymes

Tissue damage by toxic oxygen species and enzymes can cause inflammation and pain. Nimesulide 200 mg given orally to human volunteers substantially reduced the *ex vivo* production of superoxide anions by phagocytes (neu-trophils plus a few monocytes)[23]. At a concentration that might be therapeu-tically relevant, because some human serum albumin was added, a similar effect occurred with human isolated neutrophils stimulated with fMLP or calcium ionophore, and nimesulide also reduced the release of lysozyme and β-glucuronidase[24]. Other investigators obtained similar results, but at higher concentrations; perhaps this indicates that higher concentrations may some-times be needed *in vitro* to reproduce effects that occur *in vivo*.

Cartilage degradation

The synthesis of stromelysin and collagenase, which cause proteoglycan and collagen degradation, was reduced in human osteoarthritic cartilage stimulated *in vitro* by interleukin-1, and there was a trend for less cartilage breakdown[25]. In human synovial fluid removed from arthritic patients, nimesulide 2 μM (a low concentration in view of the albumin present) inhibited collagenase on average by 63% in the 3/15 samples that showed enzyme activity[26]. Indomethacin can damage joints, as in 'indomethacin hip', but high concen-trations of nimesulide *in vitro* did not affect cartilage proteoglycan synthesis[27], and there was no significant change (either protection or damage) in the articulating cartilage of the tibio-femoral joint of arthritic patients treated with nimesulide or piroxicam for 24 weeks[28]. It therefore seems likely that nimesulide does not damage joints in patients, and this may be important for long-term safety and effectiveness. There is further recent evidence in the following section that is consistent with a beneficial effect of nimesulide on cartilage, but it remains to be seen if chondroprotection occurs in patients.

Chondrocyte survival

Mediators produced in osteoarthritis are thought to play an important role in chondrocyte death. Recent work with a rat immortalized chondrocyte cell line in culture showed that staurosporine caused time- and concentration-dependent apoptosis coincident with increased Bax:Bcl-X mRNA expression, cytochrome C release, and caspase-3 activation[29]. At low concentrations (10^{-12} to 10^{-6} M), nimesulide or the non-selective COX-1/COX-2 inhibitor ibuprofen caused a concentration-dependent protection of the chondrocytes against staurosporine-mediated nuclear damage and cell death. This protection coincided with inhibition of the staurosporine-induced caspase-3 activation. Thus nimesulide or ibuprofen might protect the cartilage in osteoarthritis by inhibiting chondrocyte apoptosis, through a mechanism that does not depend only on COX-2 since there was no protection with NS-398[29]. If this effect occurs in humans, prolongation of chondrocyte survival might be an additional cartilage-protective action of nimesulide.

Cytokines

Tumour necrosis factor-α (TNF-α) governs the release of other hyperalgesic cytokines. In rats, nimesulide 10 mg kg^{-1} (not an exceptionally high dose for rodents but about 7 times the human dose), reduced the hyperalgesic activity of TNF-α by about 70%[30]. Lower doses of nimesulide were not examined. It remains to be seen if this action, and some of the others in this section, occur in patients.

Histamine

In human subjects given nimesulide 200 mg 6 hours previously, the area of the wheal produced by intradermally injected histamine was decreased by about 40%[31]. However, perhaps this involved removal of a PG-induced potentiation of histamine. In anaesthetized guinea-pigs:

1. 1.6 mmol kg^{-1} nimesulide i.v. reduced the anaphylactic release of histamine[32]; and
2. nimesulide 0.1–1 mg kg^{-1} i.v., but not indomethacin 1 mg kg^{-1}, reduced the bronchoconstrictor and histamine-releasing effects of acetaldehyde[33].

The concentration of orally administered nimesulide reaching the gastric mucosa after local absorption is presumably higher than in blood. It may therefore be relevant that in mouse isolated stomach 10 μM nimesulide inhibited the stimulation of gastric acid secretion by histamine[34], and 3 μM inhibited the acid secretion induced by pentagastrin (which acts via histamine release). However, the effect on histamine was not selective, since nimesulide 10 μM also inhibited the response to the acetylcholine analogue methylfurmethide[34]. The mechanism(s) by which nimesulide inhibited acid secretion are not clear, and it remains to be seen if a similar effect contributes to the relatively good gastric tolerability of nimesulide in humans.

NIMESULIDE ACTIONS AT HIGHER CONCENTRATIONS

As discussed earlier, concentrations of nimesulide above 0.06 mg ml^{-1} (~0.2 μM) *in vitro* without added albumin, or above 6 mg ml^{-1} (~20 μM) in blood or the equivalent amount of serum proteins, would usually exceed the therapeutic maximum levels of the free drug in humans. Nimesulide has several other actions *in vitro* at concentrations above this range[2], and the investigators may have overestimated their clinical relevance because they overlooked the importance of using lower concentrations in the absence of albumin. Effects at supratherapeutic blood concentrations may relate to higher amounts occurring at sites of absorption. It may be that future research will show that some of these actions do occur at appropriately low concentrations of nimesulide.

Effects of extremely high concentrations probably relate just to toxicology and pharmacological curiosity. They are listed in reference 2, and are not discussed here. Table 2 shows results with a moderately high nimesulide concentration (the lowest amount tested was either 0.3 μg ml^{-1} or 1 μM in the presence of 1% or 0% serum) on urokinase[35], plasminogen activator inhibitor[35], interleukin-6[35] and cyclic AMP[36]. It is not clear if the novel and potentially important aspect of enhancing the phosphorylation and transcriptional activity of glucocorticoid receptors in human synovial fibroblasts[37] falls into this moderately supratherapeutic category. It would be worth testing all of these effects at lower concentrations of free nimesulide.

THERAPEUTIC USES

Numerous clinical studies over many years have shown the good anti-inflammatory, analgesic and antipyretic activities of nimesulide in a wide range of conditions. These include arthritis, musculoskeletal inflammation, headache, gynaecological and urological problems, postsurgical and cancer pain, vascular diseases, ear nose and throat (ENT) diseases and airways inflammation. Accounts of just a small percentage of the available studies are presented in reference 38.

Table 2 Actions of nimesulide *in vitro* at a moderately high concentration

Pathway	Cells/tissue	Nimesulide	Serum %	Effect %	Ref.
Urokinase synthesis	Synovial fibroblasts	0.3 μg ml^{-1}	1	−50	35
Interleukin-6 synthesis	Synovial fibroblasts	0.3 μg ml^{-1}	1	−50	35
Plasminogen activator inhibitor	Synovial fibroblasts	0.3 μg ml^{-1}	1	+50	35
Histamine action	Bronchial muscle	0.3 μg ml^{-1}	0	−20	36
Cyclic AMP	PMN leukocytes	1 μM	0	+40	33

Experiments are required with lower concentrations *in vitro* or in human subjects with therapeutic doses, to investigate whether the above effects can be put into the 'therapeutically relevant' class as defined in this chapter.

CLINICAL EFFICACY

The effectiveness of nimesulide for the treatment of fever, inflammation and pain at least match those of several other established drugs. Apart from reference 38, which is now several years old, there is substantial more recent evidence of efficacy that has resulted from the continuing development of nimesulide. The drug is at least comparable with various other NSAIDs, including diclofenac, which is one of the world's best-selling NSAIDs (see the section below on safety and tolerability).

ANALGESIA AND ITS SPEED OF ONSET

Nimesulide is clearly a good analgesic, and may well be better than the new selective COX-2 inhibitors. Although rofecoxib and celecoxib are mainly equivalent to other NSAIDs in the treatment of osteoarthritis[39], they seem to be rather poor in dental analgesia, despite claims to the contrary. In the study by Morrison et al.[40] the authors compared a single high dose of rofecoxib (50 mg, the maximum daily dose) with just a 400 mg single dose of ibuprofen (maximum daily dose 1.8–2.4 g), and assessed the postoperative dental pain over 24 hours. The maximum analgesic effect was modest, and was almost identical with both drugs. Furthermore, by 3 h one-third of the rofecoxib group had taken rescue medication (paracetamol plus hydrocodone), and this figure reached 50% at 8 hours. As expected from its fairly long half-life, rofecoxib gave longer lasting analgesia than ibuprofen, which has a half-life of around only 2 hours. In a similar single dose study, rofecoxib 50 mg and ibuprofen 400 mg showed equivalent activity, but 200 mg of celecoxib was less effective[41]. Comparative trials with nimesulide have not yet been performed. If nimesulide has greater analgesic efficacy in dental pain, it will raise interesting questions about the mechanism(s) of action of nimesulide compared with the coxibs. The onset of analgesia is also likely to be quicker with nimesulide, which acts within 20–30 min for pain of oral surgery[42] or dysmenorrhoea[43,44]. Speed of relief is particularly important for treating pains of sudden onset, such as these and headache (reference 45 and other papers in reference 38).

SAFETY AND TOLERABILITY

Adverse drug reactions with nimesulide are typical of those found with other NSAIDs, but gastric and renal tolerance are relatively good. During its 15+ years on the market, nimesulide has been given to many millions of patients, so that its safety and tolerability are well known and there are unlikely to be any unpleasant surprises. Several studies, mainly of short duration, report that the gastric tolerability of nimesulide is superior to that of various other

NSAIDs. Some of these appear in reference 38, but more recently a 24-week study in osteoarthritis found that nimesulide was as efficacious as diclofenac but had a superior gastric safety profile[46]. In a meta-analysis, nimesulide 100 mg twice daily for 2 weeks was at least as efficacious as other NSAIDs in treating osteoarthritis, but the benefit–risk ratio was more favourable since nimesulide was about equal to placebo in safety and tolerability, especially regarding gastrointestinal adverse events[47].

Post-marketing surveillance has shown that since its introduction in 1985, there have been only 1212 reported adverse events (in 845 patients) attributed to nimesulide[48]. Of these, 397 (in 279 subjects) were classified as serious. However, the total incidence is low in relation to the cumulative 2.9 billion days of therapy. In those countries (e.g. Italy, Portugal, Ireland, Greece, Finland, Turkey) where nimesulide is amongst the most frequently prescribed NSAIDs, the number of adverse reactions ascribed to the drug is also relatively low.

In various studies, the incidence of gastric damage with nimesulide was either similar to that with placebo[49], better than various other NSAIDs[46,47], including diclofenac (one of the safest NSAIDs regarding gastric damage), or at least comparable with diclofenac[50]. In the paper by Garcia Rodriguez et al.[51] the crude relative risk for diclofenac and nimesulide was identical (4.2) but the adjusted relative risk was higher for nimesulide. In a personal communication, Garcia Rodriguez said this was because of age differences in the groups, and he does not consider that the findings allow the conclusion of a significant difference in gastric mucosal damage by diclofenac and nimesulide.

The very weakly acidic nature of nimesulide (pKa 6.5) probably contributes to its relatively good gastric tolerability. Most NSAIDs are considerably more acidic than nimesulide, and they can accumulate in high concentrations within the cells of the gastric mucosa/submucosa. This is because the drugs are absorbed substantially in the stomach, and because blood-borne NSAIDs also accumulate within gastric mucosal cells where the extracellular pH is low[52,53]. Under acidic conditions, the extracellular NSAIDs become unionized, enter cells, and ionize at the higher intracellular pH, so that they tend to be retained. Similarly, sites of low pH in the kidney may lead to renal accumulation of NSAIDs, and therefore increase the potential for renal damage. Inhibition of superoxide anion formation by neutrophils[23] and lack of uncoupling of oxidative phosphorylation by nimesulide in patients may be another factor in helping to avoid mucosal damage[54].

Nevertheless some gastric damage can occur with nimesulide, and therefore peptic ulceration is a contraindication (as with the coxibs in gastric bleeding or active peptic ulceration). Part of the explanation might be that COX-2 activation occurs at sites of peptic ulcer repair[14], so that inhibition of the enzyme may be undesirable. As we discussed previously[55,56], important questions also include the amounts of COX-1 and COX-2 normally present in human gastrointestinal mucosa, and the extent of COX inhibition needed to damage the mucosa or hinder its repair. Furthermore, if there is an analogy to the hyperalgesia that persists for several hours after an intradermal injection of PGE_1 or PGE_2 into human skin[6], prostaglandins might exert a protective action long after their synthesis has been inhibited and they have disappeared from the tissues. If so, gastric and renal PG synthesis may need to be inhibited for several hours before substantial tissue damage occurs, and, if the drug half-life is sufficiently short, PG synthesis might resume before the protective effect has worn off. This might help to explain why ibuprofen (half-life $\sim$2 h) can cause less gastric mucosal damage than piroxicam, which is a weaker inhibitor of PG synthesis in human isolated gastric mucosa[55] but has a half-life of up to 3 days. Nimesulide has a moderately short half-life (see Pharmacokinetics, below).

Nimesulide is generally well tolerated in all patients, including the elderly, who are often treated concomitantly with several medicaments. In addition to the upper gastrointestinal tract, damage to the small intestine also occurs with most NSAIDs, but nimesulide treatment seems to be free of this problem[54].

As discussed in the pharmacokinetics section, nimesulide undergoes extensive hepatic metabolism, and hepatic adverse reactions can occur[57], so particular caution is advised in patients with liver problems. During long-term administration, it is advisable to monitor blood levels of hepatic enzymes regularly. When patients experience symptoms compatible with hepatic injury, they should stop taking nimesulide. Nevertheless, severe liver damage by nimesulide is rare, and its incidence is no more than with other commonly used NSAIDs[57]. Kidney damage can also occur with nimesulide, but it is rarely serious. Because nimesulide is metabolized mainly in the liver, renal impairment does not usually cause a problem with the drug. However, for the sake of caution its use is contraindicated in severe, but not moderate, renal impairment. Most of the adverse events relate to skin reactions, and their profile and severity are mainly comparable with those caused by other NSAIDs[58].

Of particular interest, nimesulide can be taken safely by most patients who are intolerant of aspirin or other NSAIDs, for example by developing asthma[38,59]. It remains to be seen if this is due to sparing of COX-1, and if other actions of nimesulide listed in Table 1 are contributory factors.

PHARMACEUTICAL FORMULATIONS AND DOSES

Nimesulide is available as 100 mg tablets or granules (sachets) for oral administration twice daily, or as 200 mg rectal suppositories. In some countries a suspension of nimesulide is also available, and a topical gel has recently been introduced. Accounts of some pharmaceutical aspects are included in a recent overview[60].

PHARMACOKINETICS

Bernareggi[4] wrote an excellent account of this subject. Nimesulide, 100 mg, administered orally to healthy volunteers is rapidly and extensively absorbed, regardless of the presence of food, and distributed rapidly throughout most of the body. The apparent volume of distribution is $0.18–0.39 \, l \, kg^{-1}$, and nimesulide in blood is 99% bound to albumin at two sites (I and II).

Concentrations of approximately 25–80% of the C_{max} appeared in blood at the first sampling time (30 min after administration), consistent with an onset of analgesia within 20–30 minutes. The mean peak blood concentrations of $2.86–6.5 \, \mu g \, ml^{-1}$, which occur within about 70–170 min of oral administration, decline mono-exponentially. With suppositories, peak plasma concentrations are lower and occur somewhat later. In synovial fluid, the therapeutic maximum concentration of free nimesulide seems to be similar to that in blood, since the total reached was about $2.4 \, \mu g \, ml^{-1}$ (ref 61), and the quantity of protein in synovial fluid is somewhat less than in blood.

Nimesulide shows linear pharmacokinetics after oral administration of 25–100 mg, but the plasma level does not increase proportionately with 200 mg. A steady state is achieved within 24–48 h (2–4 administrations) with twice-daily oral or rectal administration, and there is only a modest accumulation of nimesulide and its major 4-hydroxy metabolite. The estimated mean terminal half-life of nimesulide varies from about 1.8 to 4.7 h[4], but although this is only a moderate value, twice-daily administration gives sustained relief, and leukocyte COX-2 remains markedly inhibited for at least 8 hours[13]. Furthermore, nimesulide is apparently retained in the synovial fluid: 12 h after 100 mg orally twice daily for a week, about $1.4 \, \mu g \, ml^{-1}$ remained in the synovial fluid of patients with rheumatoid arthritis[61]. Elimination is mostly by metabolic transformation, with negligible excretion of the unchanged drug in urine and faeces. In addition to the major 4-hydroxy-nimesulide, four minor metabolites have been identified[62].

There is a similar pharmacokinetic profile in children, healthy young subjects and the elderly, and gender has little influence. Similar pharmacokinetics also occur in patients with moderate renal impairment (creatinine clearance $30–80 \, ml \, min^{-1}$), in whom there is no need to reduce the dose, but nimesulide is contraindicated in hepatic impairment or severe renal impairment (see the section on safety and tolerability).

The binding of nimesulide to albumin is not saturable at therapeutic doses, and pharmacokinetic interactions are unlikely except with drugs that are extensively albumin-bound[3,4]. Nimesulide may moderately increase the effect of warfarin, so that it is prudent to measure the clotting time. No clinically important pharmacokinetic interactions occur between nimesulide and glibenclamide, cimetidine, antacids, frusemide, theophylline, digoxin or warfarin. Although nimesulide can displace frusemide, methotrexate, valproic acid and salicylic acid from plasma proteins, and nimesulide may be displaced from plasma protein binding sites by tolbutamide, salicylic acid or valproic acid, these *in vitro* effects are generally considered to be of little or no clinical significance[3,4]. However, the unbound fraction of nimesulide in blood increases up to fourfold in patients with severe renal or hepatic insufficiency[63,64].

CONCLUSIONS

Nimesulide is a very effective NSAID with good anti-inflammatory, analgesic and antipyretic activity in a wide range of conditions. It has a fast onset of analgesia, few drug interactions (which in any case are almost always of minor clinical significance); it is generally safe in patients with respiratory problems, possibly because it spares COX-1, and it produces relatively little gastric or renal damage. The weak acidity of nimesulide may play a part in its gastric and renal tolerability. Side effects with nimesulide are typical of the NSAID class of drugs, but involve mostly skin reactions and usually fewer gastrointestinal adverse events than classical NSAIDs. Nimesulide has a range of other pharmacological effects, including inhibition of various mediators of inflammation and cartilage degradation. It seems likely, but not yet proven, that at least some of these actions not involved with PG synthesis contribute to the clinical effectiveness of nimesulide, and it would be interesting to see if this depends on the type of inflammation and mediators involved.

Address all correspondence to: Alan Bennett, Department of Surgery, The Rayne Institute, Guy's, King's and St Thomas' Medical School, London SE5 9NU, England.

REFERENCES

1. Magni E. The effect of nimesulide on prostanoid formation. *Drugs.* 1993;46(suppl.1):10–14.
2. Bennett A, Villa G. Nimesulide: an NSAID that preferentially inhibits COX-2, and has various unique pharmacological activities. *Exp Opinion Pharmacother.* 2000;1:277–86.
3. Bree F, Nguyen P, Urien S, Albengres E, Macciocchi A, Tillement JP. Nimesulide binding to components within blood. *Drugs.* 1993;46(suppl.1):83–90.
4. Bernareggi A. Clinical pharmacokinetics of nimesulide. *Clin Pharmacokinet.* 1998;35:247–74.
5. Bunczak-Reeh MA, Hargreaves KM. Effect of inflammation on the delivery of drugs to dental pulp. *J Endodontics.* 1998;24:822–4.
6. Ferreira SH, Moncada S, Vane JR. Prostaglandins and the mechanism of analgesia produced by aspirin-like drugs. *Br J Pharmacol.* 1973;49:86–97.
7. Famaey J-P. *In vitro* and *in vivo* pharmacological evidence of selective cyclo-oxygenase-2 inhibition by nimesulide: an overview. *Inflamm Res.* 1997;46:437–46.

8. Patrignani P, Panara MR, Sciulli MG, Santini G, Renda G, Patrono C. Differential inhibition of human prostaglandin endoperoxide synthase-1 and -2 by nonsteroidal anti-inflammatory drugs. *J Physiol Pharmacol.* 1997;48:263–31.

9. Panara MR, Padovano R, Sciulli M, Santini G, Renda G, Rotondo MT et al. Effects of nimesulide on constitutive and inducible prostanoid biosynthesis in human beings. *Clin Pharmacol Ther.* 1998;63:672–81.

10. Cryer B, Feldman M. Cyclooxygenase-1 and cyclooxygenase-2 selectivity of widely used nonsteroidal anti-inflammatory drugs. *Am J Med.* 1998;104:413–21.

11. Cullen L, Kelley L, Connor SO, Fitzgerald DJ. Selective cyclooxygenase-2 inhibition by nimesulide in man. *J Pharm Exp Ther.* 1998;287:578–82.

12. Shah AA, Murray FE, Fitzgerald DJ. The *in vivo* assessment of nimesulide cyclooxygenase-2 selectivity. *Rheumatology.* 1999;38(suppl.1):19–23.

13. Warner TD, Giuliano F, Vojnovic I, Bukasa A, Mitchell JA, Vane JR. Nonsteroid drug selectivities for cyclooxygenase-1 rather than cyclooxygenase-2 are associated with human gastrointestinal toxicity: a full *in vitro* analysis. *Proc Natl Acad Sci USA.* 1999;96:7563–8.

14. Wallace JL. Selective COX-2 inhibitors: is the water becoming muddy? *TIPS.* 1999;20:4–6.

15. Marbet GA, Yasikoff Strub ML, Macciocchi A, Tsakiris DA. The effect of nimesulide versus placebo on hemostasis in healthy volunteers. *Eur J Clin Pharmacol.* 1998;54:383–7.

16. Saeed SA, Afzal MN, Shah BH. Dual effects of nimesulide, a COX-2 inhibitor, in human platelets. *Life Sci.* 1998;63:1835–41.

17. Barnett J, Chow J, Ives D, Chiou M, Mackenzie R, Osen E et al. Purification, characterization and selective inhibition of human prostaglandin G/H synthase 1 and 2 expressed in the baculovirus system. *Biochim Biophys Acta.* 1994;1209:130–9.

18. Tavares IA, Bishai PM, Bennett A. Activity of nimesulide on constitutive and inducible cyclo-oxygenases. *Arzneim-Forsch/Drug Res.* 1995;45:1093–6.

19. Fabiola GF, Pattabhi V, Nagarajan K. Structural basis for selective inhibition of COX-2 by nimesulide. *Bioorg Med Chem.* 1998;6:2337–44.

20. Garcia-Nieto R, Perez C, Checa A, Gago F. Molecular model of the interaction between nimesulide and human cyclooxygenase-2. *Rheumatology.* 1999;38(suppl.1):14–18.

21. Merck informs investigators of preliminary results of gastrointestinal outcomes study with Vioxx R. http:/biz.yahoo.com/prnews/000327/pa_merck_v_1.html

22. Di Battista JA, Fahmi H, He Y, Zhang M, Martel-Pelletier J, Pelletier J-P. Modulation of interleukin-1 induced cyclooxygenase-2 gene expression in human synovial fibroblasts by nimesulide. *Clin Exp Rheumatol.* 2001, in press.

23. Ottonello L, Dapino P, Pastorino G, Dallegri F. Inhibition of the neutrophil oxidative response induced by the oral administration of nimesulide in normal volunteers. *J Clin Lab Immunol.* 1992;37:91–6.

24. Capecchi PL, Ceccatelli L, Beermann U, Laghi Pasini F, Di Perri F. Inhibition of neutrophil function *in vitro* by nimesulide. Preliminary evidence of an adenosine-mediated mechanism. *Arzneim-Forsch/Drug Res.* 1993;43:992–6.

25. Pelletier JP, Martel-Pelletier J. Effects of nimesulide and naproxen on the degradation and metalloprotease synthesis of human osteoarthritic cartilage. *Drugs.* 1993;46(suppl.1):34–9.

26. Barracchini A, Franceschini N, Amicosante G, Oratore A, Minisola G, Pantaleoni G et al. Can non-steroidal anti-inflammatory drugs act as metalloproteinase

modulators? An in-vitro study of inhibition of collagenase activity. *J Pharm Pharmacol*. 1998;50:1417–23.

27. Henrotin YE, Labasse AH, Simonis PE, Zheng SX, Deby GP, Famaey JP et al. Effects of nimesulide and sodium diclofenac on interleukin-6, interleukin-8, proteoglycans and prostaglandin E_2 production by human articular chondrocytes *in vitro*. *Clin Exp Rheumatol*. 1999;17:151–60.

28. Sharma S, Rastogi S, Gupta V, Rohtagi D, Gulati P. Comparative efficacy and safety of nimesulide versus piroxicam in osteoarthritis with special reference to chondroprotection. *Am J Therap*. 1999;6:191–7.

29. Rachita C, Mukherje P, Aisen P, Pasinetti GM. The role of nimesulide in chondrocyte apoptotic death: its role beyond cyclooxygenase COX-2 specific inhibition. *Clin Exp Rheumatol*. 2001, in press.

30. Ferreira SH. The role of interleukins and nitric oxide in the mediation of inflammatory pain and its control by peripheral analgesics. *Drugs*. 1993;46(suppl.1):1–9.

31. Senna GF, Betteli C, Givanni S, Scaricabarozzi I, Andri LG. Antihistaminic activity of nimesulide, a nonsteroidal anti-inflammatory drug. *Allergy Clin Immunol*. 1993;9(part 2):241 [abstract].

32. Berti F, Rossoni G, Buschi A, Robuschi M, Villa LM. Antianaphylactic and antihistaminic activity of the non-steroidal anti-inflammatory compound nimesulide in guinea-pig. *Arzneim-Forsch/Drug Res*. 1990;40:1011–16.

33. Rossoni G, Berti F, Buschi A, Villa LM, Della Bella D. New data concerning the antianaphylactic and antihistaminic activity of nimesulide. *Drugs*. 1993;46(suppl.1):22–8.

34. Tavares IA, Borrelli F, Welsh NJ. Inhibition of gastric acid secretion by nimesulide: a possible factor in its gastric tolerability. *Clin Exp Rheumatol*. in press.

35. Pelletier JP, Mineau F, Fernandes J, Kiansa K, Ranger P, Martel-Pelletier J. Two NSAIDs, nimesulide and naproxen, can reduce the synthesis of urokinase and IL-6 while increasing PAI-I, in human OA synovial fibroblasts. *Clin Exp Rheumatol*. 1997;15:393–8.

36. Bevilacqua M, Vago T, Baldi G, Renesto E, Dallegri F, Norbiato G. Nimesulide decreases superoxide production by inhibiting phosphodiesterase type IV. *Eur J Pharmacol, Molecular Pharmacol Section*. 1994;268:415–23.

37. Di Battista JA, Zhang M, Martell-Pelletier J, Fernandes J, Alaaeddine N, Pelletier JP. Enhancement of phosphorylation and transcriptional activity of the glucocorticoid receptor in human synovial fibroblasts by nimesulide, a preferential cyclooxygenase 2 inhibitor. *Arthritis Rheum*. 1999;42:157–66.

38. Bennett A, Berti F, Ferreira SH (editors). Nimesulide: a multifactorial therapeutic approach to the inflammatory process? A 7-year clinical experience. *Drugs Suppl*. 1993;46(suppl.1):1–283.

39. Cannon GW, Caldwell JR, Holt P, McLean B, Seidenberg B, Bolognese J et al. Rofecoxib, a specific inhibitor of cyclooxygenase 2, with clinical efficacy comparable with that of diclofenac sodium. *Arthritis Rheum*. 2000;43:978–87.

40. Morrison BW, Christensen S, Yuan W, Brown J, Amlani S, Seidenberg B. Analgesic efficacy of the cyclooxygenase-2-specific inhibitor rofecoxib in post-dental surgery pain: a randomised, controlled trial. *Clin Therap*. 1999;21:943–53.

41. Malmstrom K, Daniels S, Kotey P, Seidengerg BC, Desjardins PJ. Comparison of rofecoxib and celecoxib, two cyclooxygenase-2 inhibitors, in postoperative dental pain: a randomized, placebo- and active-comparator-controlled clinical trial. *Clin Ther*. 1999;21:1653–63.

42. Ragot JP, Monti T, Macciocchi A. Controlled clinical investigation of acute analgesic activity of nimesulide in pain after oral surgery. *Drugs.* 1993;46(suppl.1):162–7.

43. Pulkkinen MO. The effect of nimesulide on intrauterine pressure in dysmenorrhoeic women. *Drugs Exptl Clin Res.* 1984;10:599–606.

44. Pulkkinen MO. Nimesulide in dysmenorrhoea. *Drugs.* 1993;46(suppl.1):129–33.

45. Giacovazzo M, Gallo MF, Guidi V, Rico R, Scaricabarozzi I. Nimesulide in the treatment of menstrual migraine. *Drugs.* 1993;46(suppl.1):140–3.

46. Huskisson EC, Macciocchi A, Rahlfs, VW, Bernstein M, Bremner AD, Doyle DV et al. Nimesulide versus diclofenac in the treatment of osteoarthritis of the hip or knee: an active controlled equivalence study. *Curr Therap Res.* 1999;60:253–65.

47. Wober W. Comparative efficacy and safety of nimesulide and diclofenac in patients with acute shoulder, and a meta-analysis of controlled studies with nimesulide. *Rheumatology.* 1999;38(suppl.1):33–8.

48. Helsinn Healthcare SA, data on file.

49. Marini U, Spotti D, Magni E, Monti T. Double-blind endoscopic study comparing the effect of nimesulide and placebo on gastric mucosa of dyspeptic subjects. *Drug Invest.* 1990;2:162–6.

50. Porto A, Reis C, Perdigoto R, Goncalves M, Freitas P, Macciocchi A. Gastroduodenal tolerability of nimesulide and diclofenac in patients with osteoarthritis. *Curr Ther Res.* 1998;59:654–65.

51. Garcia Rodriguez LA, Cattaruzzi C, Troncon MG, Agostinis L. Risk of hospitalisation for upper gastrointestinal tract bleeding associated with ketorolac, other non-steroidal anti-inflammatory drugs, calcium antagonists, and other antihypertensive drugs. *Arch Intern Med.* 1998;158:33–9.

52. Brune K, Graf P. Non-steroidal anti-inflammatory drugs: influence of extra-cellular pH on biodistribution and pharmacological effects. *Biochem Pharmacol.* 1978;27:525–30.

53. Rainsford KD, Schweitzer A, Brune K. Autoradiographic and biochemical observations on the distribution of non-steroidal anti-inflammatory drugs. *Arch Int Pharmacodyn Therap.* 1991;250:180–94 .

54. Bjarnason I, Thjodleifsson B. Gastrointestinal toxicity of nonsteroidal anti-inflammatory drugs: the effect of nimesulide compared with naproxen on the human gastrointestinal tract. *Rheumatology.* 1999;38(suppl.1):24–32.

55. Tavares IA, Collins PO, Bennett A. Inhibition of prostanoid synthesis by human gastric mucosa. *Aliment Pharmacol Therap.* 1987;1:617–26.

56. Bennett A, Tavares IA. NSAIDs, COX-2 inhibitors and the gut. *Lancet.* 1995;346:1105.

57. Rainsford KD. An analysis from clinico-epidemiological data of the principal adverse events from the COX-2-selective NSAID, nimesulide, with particular reference to hepatic injury. *Inflammopharmacology,* 1998;6:203–21.

58. Rainsford KD. Relationship of nimesulide safety to its pharmacokinetics: assessment of adverse reactions. *Rheumatology.* 1999;38(suppl.1):4–10.

59. Bennett A. The importance of COX-2 inhibition for aspirin-induced asthma. *Thorax.* 2000;(suppl. 2):S54–S56.

60. Singla AK, Chawla M, Singh A. Nimesulide: some pharmaceutical and pharmacological aspects – an update. *J Pharm Pharmacol.* 2000;52:467–86.

61. Cherie-Lignere G, Tombolini U, Panarace G, Abbiati G, Montegnani G. La

nimesulide nel liquido sinoviale di pazienti con artrite reumatoide. *Farmaci e Terapia.* 1990;7:173–6.

62. Carini M, Aldini G, Stefani R, Marinello C, Facino RM. Mass spectrometric characterisation and HPLC determination of the main urinary metabolites of nimesulide in man. *J Pharm Biomed Anal.* 1998;18:201–11.

63. Olive G, Rey E. Effect of age and disease on the pharmacokinetics of nimesulide. *Drugs.* 1993;46(suppl.1):73–8.

64. Helsinn Healthcare SA, data on file.

25 | Rofecoxib: clinical studies

BRIGGS MORRISON, THOMAS J. SIMON,
LISA DETORA AND RHODA SPERLING
Merck & Co. Inc., Box 2000, Rahway, NJ 07065, USA.

The discovery of two different isoforms of cyclooxygenase (COX), COX-1 and COX-2, led to intense interest in developing a new generation of therapeutic agents that preserved the efficacy of traditional non-steroid anti-inflammatory agents (NSAIDs) but eliminated some of their untoward side effects. Rofecoxib is one of two new highly selective COX-2 inhibitors that were introduced into the marketplace in 1999. Rofecoxib (Vioxx®, MK-0966) selectively inhibits COX-2 but has no effect on COX-1 at doses well over its clinical dose range[1,2] (Figure 1). In an extensive clinical trials programme, rofecoxib has been shown to provide equivalent anti-inflammatory and analgesic efficacy to non-selective NSAIDs[3–6] but with a significant improvement in gastrointestinal (GI) safety and tolerability[7–13]. This chapter highlights the results from many pivotal studies in the rofecoxib clinical trials programme.

ANTIPYRETIC ACTIVITY

Prostaglandins (PG) mediate the physiological processes that produce febrile symptoms. Although the role of COX-2 in fever had been studied previously, until COX-2 inhibitors were available for study, there was no meaningful evidence to show that COX-2 inhibition alone was sufficient to counteract naturally occurring fever in humans. The antipyretic activity of rofecoxib was assessed in a trial of 94 patients with fever caused by a viral-type illness. Febrile patients experienced a reduction in fever while taking rofecoxib, which was consistent with the hypothesis that fever is primarily mediated by COX-2 induction[14].

CLINICAL STUDIES IN ACUTE ANALGESIA

Clinically, pain is defined as the unpleasant sensory and emotional experience associated with actual or potential tissue damage[15]. Pain is the most commonly

Figure 1 Single dose study in normal volunteers. COX-2 selectivity at supratherapeutic doses. Decreasing values represent decreased inhibition of thromboxane B_2, a measure of COX-1 activity, or of PGE_2, a measure of COX-2 activity.

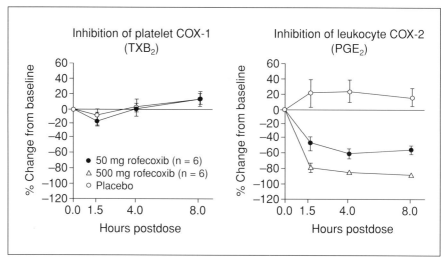

reported symptom of disease – approximately half of all patients report pain as the primary reason for visiting a physician[16,17]. Patients require analgesic treatment for varied lengths of time, depending upon the disease process or injury causing symptoms to appear. The pain that arises as a result of oral surgery, orthopaedic surgery, or primary dysmenorrhoea provide accepted models for the clinical evaluation of acute analgesic medications. The duration of pain can range from one to several days in these various models, and patient responses to treatments provide reliable estimates of the analgesic efficacy of medications[18–21]. These models can be used to evaluate single- or multiple-dose efficacy and to determine appropriate dosing regimens.

Rofecoxib in the oral surgery model

Current data support the hypothesis that the acute pain experienced after oral surgery is caused by increased PG synthesis, and the increase of PGE_2 within the oral surgical site correlates with increased pain after extraction of impacted third molars[22].

Several studies of rofecoxib in the setting of dental pain were conducted. Pain symptoms were evaluated by the patients at specified time points and recorded in the patient diary using established rating scales. The primary end point in each study was the total pain relief over the 8 h post-dose period (TOPAR8), a frequently employed end-point in the assessment of analgesic therapies[23]. Additional end-points were used to characterize the onset of action and peak analgesic effect.

In a pilot study, results indicated that patients with dental pain treated with rofecoxib (50, 250 or 500 mg) experienced symptomatic relief of pain over a prespecified 6 h period[1]. In this study, the degree of pain relief with each dose of rofecoxib was similar to that of ibuprofen (400 mg), the typical dose used to treat dental pain[19,20].

In a follow-up study with measurements taken over a 24 h period, rofecoxib (50 mg) exhibited onset and peak effects which were similar to ibuprofen (400 mg) and significantly different from placebo. However, rofecoxib had a longer duration of efficacy than ibuprofen. The analgesic efficacy of rofecoxib was sustained for up to 24 h after a single dose of medication[4].

A dose-ranging study was conducted to identify the optimal dose of rofecoxib for clinical use in this setting. In a trial comparing rofecoxib (12.5 mg, 25 mg, and 50 mg), naproxen (550 mg) and placebo, all active doses were more effective than placebo as assessed by end-points including onset of action, peak efficacy and duration of effect. The results, however, showed a clear dose-related response. Rofecoxib (50 mg) was identified as the maximum effective dose and gave overall analgesic efficacy comparable with naproxen sodium (550 mg)[4].

In a study comparing rofecoxib (50 mg), celecoxib (200 mg), ibuprofen (400 mg) and placebo, all active agents were more effective than placebo. Results indicated that both rofecoxib (50 mg) and ibuprofen (400 mg) were superior to celecoxib (200 mg) in terms of overall analgesic effect, time to onset of analgesia and peak analgesic effect. In addition, rofecoxib had a longer duration of action than either ibuprofen (400 mg) or celecoxib (200 mg)[24].

Rofecoxib in the dysmenorrhoea model

Dysmenorrhoea is a common gynaecological disorder, affecting over 50% of all menstruating women. Primary dysmenorrhoea appears to be a PG-mediated disorder. It is generally characterized by painful symptoms with menses in patients without any clinically evident pelvic abnormalities[25]. Compared with women without painful symptoms during menstruation, those with primary dysmenorrhoea have been shown to have significantly higher concentrations of PGs in their endometrium and menstrual fluid[25–27]. Primary dysmenorrhoea can be characterized by an increased production of endometrial PG. However, until recently it was unclear whether this increased PG production is mediated by COX-1 and/or COX-2[5].

In a dose-ranging trial of rofecoxib in 127 patients aged 18–44 years with a history of primary dysmenorrhoea, rofecoxib (25 mg and 50 mg) exhibited peak efficacy and onset of analgesia similar to naproxen (550 mg). As in the trials in post-dental surgery, pain symptoms were evaluated by patients at specified time points and recorded in patient diaries using established rating scales[23,28]. The primary end-point was total pain relief over the 8 h post-dose period, and additional end-points characterized the onset and peak analgesic effect[5]. In this study, patients could take additional doses of study medication at 12 h intervals over 3 days, but few patients in any active treatment group used more than the indicated dose[5]. The results of this study demonstrated that COX-2 inhibition alone provided analgesic efficacy in patients with primary dysmenorrhoea.

Rofecoxib in the post-orthopaedic surgical pain model

Post-orthopaedic surgery, like oral surgery, results in pain that is probably mediated by COX-2 dependent PG synthesis[16]. In a study in patients with post-orthopaedic surgical pain, following total hip or total knee replacement, or fracture repair with open reduction and internal fixation, rofecoxib (50 mg) provided clinical efficacy for overall pain relief, time to onset, and peak effect similar to those provided by naproxen (550 mg). Study methods and end-points were similar to those in the post-dental surgery and primary dysmenorrhoea trials. Rofecoxib showed a significantly longer duration of efficacy than naproxen in this trial. Efficacy was sustained for up to 5 days, with additional daily dosing[29].

CLINICAL STUDIES OF ROFECOXIB IN OSTEOARTHRITIS: OVERVIEW

Osteoarthritis (OA) is the most prevalent musculoskeletal disorder worldwide. OA is actually a heterogeneous group of conditions sharing common patho-genetic and radiological features, and is best characterized as an age-related dynamic reaction to joint insult or injury which results in focal loss of articular cartilage over time. This process is accompanied by inflammation and a hypertrophic response in the subchondral bone and the margin of the joint. The principal signs and symptoms of OA include pain, joint stiffness following inactivity, and joint tenderness and swelling[30]. Progressive signs include bony swelling, decreased range of motion, crepitus and muscle weakness. OA ultimately manifests as decreased physical function, or disability, and is associated with a decline in overall health-related quality of life[31].

NSAIDs are frequently prescribed for symptomatic relief of OA and are the eighth most commonly prescribed drug class for patients over age 65 years[32]. Half of all NSAID prescriptions in this age group are given for OA[33]. Although frequently used, NSAIDs are associated with substantial toxicity, most notably of the GI tract[34].

Clinical studies conducted in patients with osteoarthritis

The rofecoxib OA clinical trials programme was designed to evaluate both the short-term and long-term effectiveness of rofecoxib as well as its comparability (both safety and efficacy) with the non-selective NSAIDs that have traditionally been used to treat OA[35,36]. The clinical programme employed end-points consistent with the Outcome Measures in Rheumatology Clinical

Trials (OMERACT) worldwide consensus group. OMERACT's members include clinicians, researchers, regulatory agency officials and health policy experts. The recommended 'core' outcome measures for OA clinical trials include assessments of pain and physical function, and a patient global assessment.

The efficacy profile of rofecoxib has been established in both short-term and long-term placebo and active comparator controlled studies. Over 5500 patients (of which over 3000 patients received rofecoxib) were enrolled into OA studies performed worldwide. Patients were ≥ 40 years of age with knee or hip pain on motion or weight bearing, radiographic evidence of joint space narrowing and/or osteophytes.

The results of a pilot study in patients with knee OA comparing rofecoxib (25 mg and 125 mg) with placebo indicated that rofecoxib was a suitable agent for treating OA[37]. A dose-ranging study was then conducted to identify appropriate doses for further studies against active comparators and in a special patient population: the elderly. When considered together, data from the pilot study and the dose-ranging study indicated that the dose of rofecoxib was generally related to the degree of clinical improvement. The 5 mg dose of rofecoxib was considered to be less effective than higher doses of rofecoxib. The 12.5 and 25 mg doses were identified as providing optimal efficacy with treatment assessed at 6 weeks[37–40].

Three 6-week placebo- and active-comparator-controlled OA studies were conducted. Two of these studies compared the efficacy of rofecoxib with ibuprofen, and the remaining study evaluated the clinical efficacy and safety of rofecoxib exclusively in OA patients aged 80 years and older. The results of all three studies indicated that rofecoxib had an improved efficacy profile relative to placebo[3,41,42].

Rofecoxib was compared with diclofenac, a widely used NSAID, in two identical studies over 1 year of treatment. These two 1-year active-comparator-controlled OA studies were intended to demonstrate clinical efficacy, including maintenance of clinical efficacy with chronic administration of rofecoxib in OA patients requiring extended therapy. This efficacy was durable; treatment effects were maintained for a full year of therapy[6,41].

In phase III trials, treatment with rofecoxib (12.5 or 25 mg o.d.) showed comparable efficacy with the NSAID comparators ibuprofen (2400 mg: 800 mg t.i.d.) and diclofenac (150 mg: 50 mg t.i.d.). Comparisons between active treatments were based on predefined comparability criteria that were satisfied in two independent studies versus each comparator. Rofecoxib provided a prompt onset of clinical efficacy. This efficacy was durable – treatment effects were maintained for a full year of therapy[6,41] (Figure 2).

Figure 2 One year phase III studies in OA patients. Primary end-point was pain walking on a flat surface measured on a Western Ontario and McMaster Universities OA index (WOMAC) 100 mm patient assessment of arthritis pain. Data presented from a combined analysis of two identical trials in patients with OA of the knee or hip, comparing rofecoxib (12.5 and 25 mg) with diclofenac. Overlapping error bars indicate that values were comparable between groups. S = saline; R = rofecoxib (data from ref. 6).

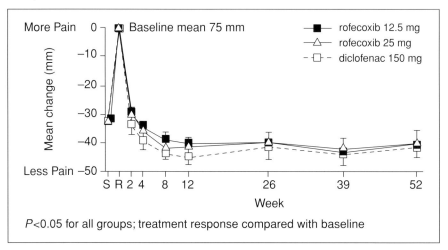

CLINICAL STUDIES IN RHEUMATOID ARTHRITIS: OVERVIEW

Rheumatoid arthritis (RA), a disease characterized by symmetrical erosive synovitis, is generally considered to be an autoimmune disorder of unknown aetiology[43]. The disease course, if left untreated, frequently results in progressive joint destruction, deformity, disability and premature death[49]. Unlike OA, which affects a majority of adults over the age of 50 years, RA occurs infrequently, affecting only 1% of the adult population[44]. The relative rarity of RA creates challenges for both physicians and patients attempting to manage the disease. Recommendations for treating RA emphasize the role of disease modifying agents in conjunction with agents intended to reduce symptoms, especially pain and physical impairment. First-line pharmacological therapy for RA usually involves the use of NSAIDs to reduce joint pain and swelling and improve function. While NSAIDs have analgesic and anti-inflammatory properties, they do not prevent joint destruction. Salicylates and NSAIDs generally provide a prompt onset of analgesic effect, but the signs of inflammation may persist for 1–2 weeks after initiation of treatment[45].

Preliminary clinical trial data in rheumatoid arthritis

Only preliminary data about the efficacy of rofecoxib in patients with RA are available from our clinical trials programme. A long-term efficacy trial is currently underway. A 6-week dose-ranging study comparing placebo and rofecoxib (5 mg, 25 mg and 50 mg) has been reported. In this preliminary study, efficacy was assessed by the ACR20 responder index, a validated measure of clinical efficacy in RA[46,47]. Treatment response was evaluated by the proportion of patients in each group who met the criteria for an ACR20 response (who had a 20% improvement in tender and swollen joint counts and a 20% improvement in three of the five remaining ACR core measures)[48]. The individual ACR core efficacy measurements used as end-points in this trial were: swollen joint count (66 joints); tender joint count (68 joints); patient global assessment of disease activity; investigator global assessment of disease activity; Stanford HAQ disability score; patient global assessment of pain; and C-reactive protein level[47].

In this 6-week trial, the percentage of patients who both completed the treatment period and achieved an ACR20 response were 43.8% with the 25 mg dose of rofecoxib ($P = 0.025$ versus placebo) and 49.7% with the 50 mg dose of rofecoxib ($P = 0.001$ versus placebo). The 5 mg dose of rofecoxib was not significantly different from placebo (rates 33.5% and 31.7%, respectively)[48].

GENERAL SAFETY AND TOLERABILITY PROFILE OF ROFECOXIB

Much of the currently available data about the clinical safety of rofecoxib in patients with RA, OA and acute pain are derived from clinical trials. As described above, clinical trials were conducted to determine the therapeutic properties and the safety profile of rofecoxib in models of pain, inflammation and fever. In the initial clinical programme, rofecoxib was evaluated for safety in approximately 5400 subjects/patients in blinded, controlled clinical trials at various doses ranging from 5 to 1000 mg. In general, treatment with rofecoxib was well tolerated in these studies[49].

Table 1 shows the most common adverse effects in OA patients receiving rofecoxib for up to 6 months[3,6,41].

In 1000 patients in the analgesia studies, the general safety profile was similar to that seen in patients in the OA trials.

GASTROINTESTINAL SAFETY PROFILE OF ROFECOXIB: OVERVIEW

NSAID toxicity is considered to be among the most common serious drug-related adverse events[50]. In the USA, NSAID-induced GI morbidity results in at least 100 000 hospitalizations and 15000 deaths annually[34,51]. Furthermore, chronic NSAID users suffer a 1–4% annual incidence of gastroduodenal perforations, ulcers or bleeds (PUB)[52]. In patients > 65 years, nearly a third of

Table 1 Adverse experiences in patients with osteoarthritis

	Placebo (n = 783) (%)	Rofecoxib (12.5 or 25 mg o.d., n = 2829) (%)	Ibuprofen (2400 mg o.d., n = 847) (%)	Diclofenac (150 mg o.d., n = 498) (%)
Body as a whole/site unspecified				
Abdominal pain	4.1	3.4	4.6	5.8
Asthenia/fatigue	1.0	2.2	2.0	2.6
Dizziness	2.2	3.0	2.7	3.4
Influenza-like disease	3.1	2.9	1.5	3.2
Lower extremity oedema	1.1	3.7	3.8	3.4
Upper respiratory infection	7.8	8.5	5.8	8.2
Cardiovascular system				
Hypertension	1.3	3.5	3.0	1.6
Digestive system				
Diarrhoea	6.8	6.5	7.1	10.6
Dyspepsia	2.7	3.5	4.7	4.0
Epigastric discomfort	2.8	3.8	9.2	5.4
Heartburn	3.6	4.2	5.2	4.6
Nausea	2.9	5.2	7.1	7.4
Eyes, ears, nose and throat				
Sinusitis	2.0	2.7	1.8	2.4
Musculoskeletal system				
Back pain	1.9	2.5	1.4	2.8
Nervous system				
Headache	7.5	4.7	6.1	8.0
Respiratory system				
Bronchitis	0.8	2.0	1.4	3.2
Urogenital system				
Urinary tract infection	2.7	2.8	2.5	3.6

all PUB-related morbidity and mortality is thought to be due to NSAID use[53].

Preliminary data indicated that rofecoxib would have a favourable GI safety profile as compared with traditional non-selective NSAIDs. In healthy human subjects rofecoxib (25 mg and 50 mg daily) did not inhibit the COX-1 mediated synthesis of gastroprotective PGs measured *ex vivo* in gastric mucosal tissue[54]. Furthermore, rofecoxib did not induce gastric ulceration in animal models that are highly sensitive to gastric toxicity induced by NSAIDs[55]. Initial clinical studies were conducted to assess the GI safety of rofecoxib in healthy volunteers.

Trials to assess gastrointestinal safety
The pathogenic process involved in NSAID-induced enteropathy (such as low-grade intestinal inflammation, GI bleeding and intestinal protein loss) may

be initiated by increased intestinal permeability. This increased permeability can be evaluated by comparing the urinary excretion of orally administered markers which would (e.g. L-rhamnose) or would not (e.g. ^{51}Cr EDTA) permeate the intestine under normal conditions[56,57]. In a study where rofecoxib (25 and 50 mg o.d.), indomethacin (50 mg t.i.d.) and placebo were administered to healthy subjects, rofecoxib produced significantly less change in intestinal permeability compared with indomethacin, and met predefined criteria for similarity to placebo[13].

Intestinal microbleeding can be measured by faecal blood loss[58]. This microbleeding may be an indicator of risk for serious upper GI mucosal injury. In a controlled trial, healthy subjects received rofecoxib (25 or 50 mg o.d.), ibuprofen (800 mg t.i.d.) or placebo for 4 weeks[9]. In this study, red blood cell loss with rofecoxib (25 mg and 50 mg) was significantly less than with ibuprofen (2400 mg), but met predefined criteria for similarity to placebo.

Endoscopy studies are a validated method of assessing the incidence of GI erosions[59]. Endoscopy studies conducted in patients receiving rofecoxib required baseline and periodic, prespecified endoscopies. A study compared rofecoxib (250 mg o.d.), ibuprofen (800 mg t.i.d.), aspirin (650 mg q.i.d.) and placebo for 7 days in 170 healthy subjects[12]. Results of the study indicated that rofecoxib (250 mg o.d.) produced significantly fewer endoscopically evident gastroduodenal mucosal injuries than either ibuprofen (2400 mg) or aspirin (2600 mg) and was not statistically different from placebo (Figure 3).

Studies of GI safety were also conducted in a target patient population: OA patients requiring chronic treatment. Two identical studies compared the incidence of gastric and duodenal ulcers detected by fibreoptic endoscopy in OA patients treated with rofecoxib (25 mg or 50 mg), ibuprofen (2400 mg) or placebo over 6 months. Patients 50 years and older with OA involving any joint (hip, knee, spine, etc.) were enrolled; there was no minimum disease activity criteria required for patient eligibility. The incidence of gastroduodenal ulcers ≥ 3 mm (primary end-point) or (5 mm (secondary end-point) in diameter with chronic administration of therapy was evaluated at 12 weeks[8,10]. After an endoscopy, patients received rofecoxib (25 or 50 mg) or ibuprofen (2400 mg) for 12 additional weeks. In each study, patients receiving rofecoxib (25 or 50 mg) demonstrated significantly lower incidence rates of gastroduodenal ulcers ≥ 3 mm or ≥ 5 mm at 12 and 24 weeks compared with those receiving ibuprofen (2400 mg).

GASTROINTESTINAL SAFETY IN EFFICACY TRIALS IN PATIENTS WITH OSTEOARTHRITIS

The most clinically significant GI side effects caused by NSAIDs are often categorized as significant gastromucosal injuries, which include perforations, obstructions, ulcerations and upper GI bleeding (PUB). In addition to gastro-

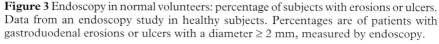

Figure 3 Endoscopy in normal volunteers: percentage of subjects with erosions or ulcers. Data from an endoscopy study in healthy subjects. Percentages are of patients with gastroduodenal erosions or ulcers with a diameter ≥ 2 mm, measured by endoscopy.

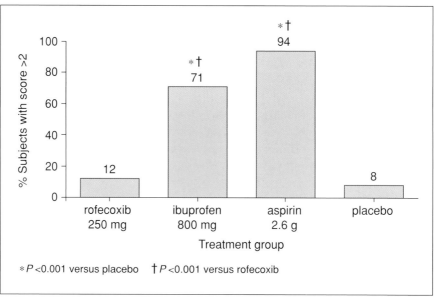

mucosal injuries, NSAIDs are associated with dyspepsia. Dyspeptic symptoms such as acid reflux, epigastric discomfort, heartburn, nausea and vomiting have generally not been a good predictor of mucosal injury, but may reduce drug tolerability.

PUB events are rare and occurred too infrequently in any individual trial to make comparisons between individual treatment groups meaningful. In order to evaluate the relative rate of gastromucosal injury among OA patients in the clinical programme, a prespecified combined analysis of PUBs in eight clinical trials was performed[11]. These trials were the dose ranging study in OA, three 6-week placebo and active comparator controlled studies in patients with OA, two 1-year active comparator-controlled studies in OA, and two 6-month endoscopy studies in patients with OA. The results of these individual trials were discussed above, and elsewhere. Even after combining the data, due to the relative infrequency of PUB events in the clinical programme, sample sizes in this analysis were still too small to make comparisons between individual treatments. Therefore, a comparison of patients who received any clinically effective dose of rofecoxib (12.5 mg, 25 mg or 50 mg) with patients who received any NSAID comparator (ibuprofen, diclofenac and nabumetone) was prespecified and contained enough patient-years of exposure to detect a difference between groups (Figure 4).

The analysis included data from 5435 patients. All PUB events were reported by the investigator and submitted to a blinded committee for adjudication. The 12 month cumulative incidence of clinically evident upper gastrointestinal PUBs, confirmed by an independent adjudication committee, was significantly lower in the rofecoxib group than in the group treated with NSAIDs, with a relative risk of 0.45 ($P < 0.01$)[11] (Figure 5).

An analysis of discontinuations due to GI adverse clinical events and of the incidence of upper GI symptoms (prespecified as acid reflux, dyspepsia, epigastric discomfort, heartburn, nausea and vomiting) was performed in the same pooled population of 5435 OA patients used for the PUB analysis. The results of these analyses showed that significantly fewer patients discontinued rofecoxib due to a GI adverse event compared with the comparator NSAID.

In VIGOR (the VIOXX™ Gastrointestinal Outcomes Research Study), approximately 8000 patients with rheumatoid arthritis were randomly assigned to receive either rofecoxib 50 mg daily or naproxen 500 mg twice daily. The primary analyses in this study were the rates of clinical upper GI events (perforation, ulcer, GI bleeding, or obstruction), complicated events (perforations, obstructions and 'significant' predefined GI bleeds). All events were verified by a blinded independent adjudication committee. The results demonstrated that rofecoxib is associated with a significantly reduced risk of clinical upper GI events (54% reduction), complicated upper GI events (57% reduction), and GI bleeds (62% reduction), compared with naproxen[72].

Figure 4 Prespecified primary comparison versus placebo: combined endoscopy studies. Cumulated gastric/duodenal ulcer role (≥ 3 mm), life table estimate, intent to treat population, in patients with OA. Data from a combined database of two endoscopy studies conducted in patients with OA.

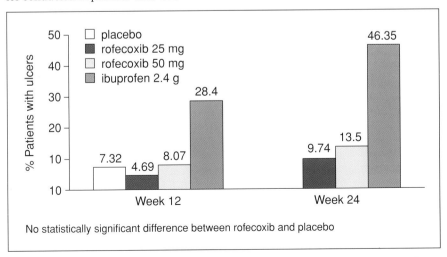

No statistically significant difference between rofecoxib and placebo

Figure 5 Rofecoxib: significantly lower PUB rate than NSAIDs. Data from a combined database, including data from eight clinical trials in patients with OA.

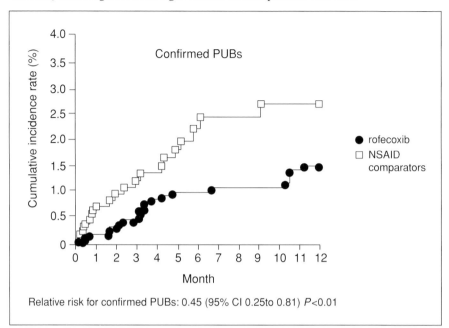

Relative risk for confirmed PUBs: 0.45 (95% CI 0.25to 0.81) *P*<0.01

RENAL SAFETY PROFILE IN CLINICAL TRIALS

NSAIDs have long been known to have mechanism-based effects on renal function. Common effects of NSAIDs on renal function include reductions in glomerular filtration rate (GFR), renal blood flow, and sodium and potassium excretion. Identifiable clinical results of these effects include fluid retention, hypertension, oedema and hyperkalaemia[60,61]. However, as previously noted, COX-2 is constitutively expressed in the kidney and researchers were uncertain whether undesirable renal effects caused by NSAIDs were the result of COX-1 or COX-2 inhibition, or a combination of the two[62]. Preclinical data indicated that rofecoxib was not likely to have a drastically improved renal safety profile in humans[55,63].

Preliminary studies indicate that COX-2 inhibitors have effects on renal function similar to those of traditional non-selective NSAIDs, particularly with respect to sodium homeostasis. In a placebo-controlled study in subjects with normal sodium intake, both rofecoxib (50 mg q.i.d.) and indomethacin (50 mg t.i.d.) were associated with a transient but significant decline in urinary sodium excretion during the first 72 h of treatment. Blood pressure and body weight did not change significantly in any group. However, the GFR was decreased by indomethacin but was not changed significantly by rofecoxib[64].

Selective COX-2 inhibitors were also studied in patients with diminished renal function. In a study of elderly patients with creatinine clearances of 30–80 ml min[-1], both rofecoxib and indomethacin (a non-selective NSAID) reduced the GFR by about 10%[65].

In a placebo-controlled trial comparing rofecoxib (250 mg) and indomethacin (75 mg), elderly subjects were administered a sodium restricted diet in order to enhance renal dependence on PG production. In this study, patients exhibited decreased GFR after receiving single or multiple doses of rofecoxib or indomethacin. Overall, changes in creatinine clearance, serum and urinary sodium, and potassium were less evident in the study population[60]. These data suggest that under certain circumstances COX-2 inhibition may produce effects on renal function similar to those observed with non-selective NSAIDs. Further study is required to establish definitively the renal safety profile of rofecoxib, and to evaluate this hypothesis.

ONGOING SAFETY AND EFFICACY RESEARCH

Cancer

Cancer sites, specifically in lung and colorectal cancers, have been shown to have elevated levels of PGs[66–69]. PG levels in benign adenomatous polyps are also elevated compared with normal mucosal tissue[66]. Further research has suggested that COX-2 plays an important role in colorectal cancer[70,71]. Currently, studies are ongoing to evaluate the effects of rofecoxib in the prevention of preneoplastic lesions.

Alzheimer's disease

COX-2 seems to play an essential role in neural development and adaptation[72]. Inflammatory mechanisms are active in the brains of patients with Alzheimer's disease (AD). The formation of amyloid plaques appears to involve the production and release of inflammatory cytokines, which are known to induce COX-2 activity[73]. The impact of non-specific COX inhibitors on cognitive decline in the elderly is therefore of interest. It has been suggested that the use of anti-inflammatory drugs, such as NSAIDs, is appropriate for investigation since the suppression of the physiological mechanisms of inflammation may act to impede, although not remit, the rate of progression of AD[73]. Currently, patients are being enrolled and data gathered in two large-scale trials in patients with or at risk for AD. One study is designed to assess the efficacy and safety of rofecoxib in the treatment of mild cognitive impairment (MCI)/prevention of conversion to AD. The other is to assess the effects of rofecoxib in slowing the progression of the symptoms of AD[73–75].

CONCLUSION

Rofecoxib has demonstrated clinical efficacy in a number of studies in the areas of acute pain, primary dysmenorrhoea and arthritis[49,76]. In these studies, rofecoxib also demonstrated general safety and tolerability. Analyses conducted to establish further the GI safety profile of rofecoxib have indicated a reduced rate of gastric mucosal injury in a large, combined database from clinical trials in patients with osteoarthritis. Ongoing research will focus on expanding information about the safety and efficacy profiles of rofecoxib in different disease processes and patient populations.

ACKNOWLEDGEMENTS

The authors would like to thank Dr Chris Lines for help with and comments on this manuscript.

REFERENCES

1. Ehrich EW, Dallob A, De Lepeleire I, Van Hecken A, Riendeau D, Yuan W et al. Characterization of rofecoxib as a cyclooxygenase-2 isoform inhibitor and demonstration of analgesia in the dental pain model. *Clin Pharmacol Ther.* 1999;65:336–47.
2. Brooks P, Emery P, Evans JF, Fenner H, Hawkey CJ, Patrono C et al. Interpreting the clinical significance of the differential inhibition of cyclooxygenase-1 and cyclooxgenase-2. *Rheumatol.* 1999;38:779–88.
3. Day R, Morrison B, Luza A, Castaneda O, Strusberg A, Nahir M et al. A randomized trial of the efficacy and tolerability of the COX-2 inhibitor rofecoxib vs ibuprofen in patients with osteoarthritis. *Arch Intern Med.* 2000;160:1781–7.
4. Morrison BW, Christensen S, Yuan W, Brown J, Amlani S, Seidenberg B. Analgesic efficacy of the cyclooxygenase-2-specific inhibitor rofecoxib in post-dental surgery pain: a randomized, controlled trial. *Clin Ther.* 1999;21:943–53.
5. Morrison BW, Daniels SE, Kotey P, Cantu N, Seidenberg B. Rofecoxib, a specific cyclooxygenase-2 inhibitor, in primary dysmenorrhea: a randomized controlled trial. *Obstet Gynecol.* 1999;94:504–8.
6. Cannon GW, Caldwell JR, Holt P, McLean B, Seidenberg B, Bolognese J et al. Rofecoxib, a specific inhibitor of cyclooxygenase 2, with clinical efficacy comparable with that of diclofenac sodium: results of a one-year, randomized, clinical trial in patients with osteoarthritis of the knee and hip. Rofecoxib Phase III Protocol 035 Study Group. *Arthritis Rheum.* 2000;43:978–87.
7. Hawkey C, Laine L, Mortensen E, Harper S, Beaulieu A, Quan H et al. Treatment of osteoarthritis with rofecoxib, a cyclooxygenase-2 (COX-2) specific inhibitor, was associated with a lower incidence of gastroduodenal ulcers compared to ibuprofen and was comparable to placebo treatment. Proceedings of the European League Against Rheumatism 14th Congress. 1999; 207 [Abstract].
8. Hawkey C, Laine L, Simon T, Beaulieu A, Maldonado-Cocco J, Acevedo E et al. Comparison of the effect of rofecoxib (a cyclooxygenase 2 inhibitor), ibuprofen, and placebo on the gastroduodenal mucosa of patients with osteoarthritis: a randomized, double-blind, placebo-controlled trial. *Arthritis Rheum.* 2000;43:370–7.

9. Hunt RH, Bowen B, Mortensen ER, Simon TJ, James C, Cagliola A et al. A randomized trial measuring fecal blood loss after treatment with rofecoxib, ibuprofen or placebo in healthy subjects. *Am J Med.* 2000;109:201–6.

10. Laine L, Harper S, Simon T, Bath R, Johanson J, Schwartz H et al. A randomized trial comparing the effect of rofecoxib, a cyclooxygenase 2-specific inhibitor, with that of ibuprofen on the gastroduodenal mucosa of patients with osteoarthritis. Rofecoxib Osteoarthritis Endoscopy Study Group. *Gastroenterology.* 1999;117:776–83.

11. Langman MJ, Jensen DM, Watson DJ, Harper SE, Zhao PL, Quan H et al. Adverse upper gastrointestinal effects of rofecoxib compared with NSAIDS. *J Am Med Assoc.* 1999;282:1929–33.

12. Lanza FL, Rack MF, Simon TJ, Quan H, Bolognese JA, Hoover ME et al. Specific inhibition of cycloxygenase-2 with MK-0966 is associated with less gastroduodenal damage that either aspirin or ibuprofen. *Aliment Pharmacol Ther.* 1999;13:761–7.

13. Sigthorsson G, Crane R, Simon T, Hoover M, Quan H, Bolognese J et al. COX-2 inhibition with rofecoxib does not increase intestinal permeability in healthy subjects: a double-blind, crossover study comparing rofecoxib with placebo and indomethacin. *Gut.* 2000;47:527-32.

14. Schwartz JI, Chan C-C, Mukhopadhyay S, McBride KJ, Jones TM, Adcock S et al. Cyclooxygenase-2 inhibition by rofecoxib reverses naturally occurring fever in humans. *Clin Pharmacol Ther.* 1999;65:653–60.

15. Pain terms: a current list with definitions and notes on usage. *Pain.* 1986;S216–21.

16. Maciewicz R, Martin JB. Pain: pathophysiology and management. In: Braunwald E, Isselbacher KJ, Petersdorf RG, Wilson JD, Martin JB, Fauci AS, editors. *Harrison's Principles of Internal Medicine*, 11th edn. New York: McGraw-Hill; 1987:13–7.

17. Adams RD, Victor M, Ropper AH. Pain. In: Wonsiewicz MJ, Navrozov M, editors. *Principles of Neurology*, 6th edn. New York: McGraw-Hill; 1997:127–47.

18. Benedetti C. The pathogenic effects of postoperative pain. In: Lipton S, Tunks E, Zoppi M, editors. *Advances in Pain Research and Therapy: the Pain Clinic*, Volume 13. New York: Raven Press; 1990:279–85.

19. Forbes JA. Oral surgery. In: Max MB, Portenoy RK, Laska EM, editors. *Advances in Pain Research and Therapy: the Design of Analgesic Clinical Trials*. New York: Raven Press; 1991:347–74.

20. Stewart PE. Multidose short-term analgesic studies. In: Max MB, Portenoy RK, Laska EM, editors. *Advances in Pain Research and Therapy: the Design of Analgesic Clinical Trials*, Volume 18. New York: Raven Press; 1991:137–49.

21. Dawood MY. Dysmenorrhea. In: Max MB, Portenoy RK, Laska EM, editors. *Advances in Pain Research and Therapy: the Design of Analgesic Clinical Trials*, Volume 18. New York: Raven Press; 1991:429–43.

22. Roszkowski MT, Swift JQ, Hargreaves KM. Effect of NSAID administration on tissue levels of immunoreactive prostaglandin E_2, leukotriene B_4, and (s)-flurbiprofen following extraction of impacted third molars. *Pain.* 1997;3:339–45.

23. Mehlisch DR, Hubbard RC, Isakson P, Karim A, Weaver M, Mills S. Analgesic efficacy and plasma levels of a highly selective inhibitor of COX-2 (SC-58635; SC) in patients with post-surgical dental pain. *Clin Pharmacol Ther.* 1997;61:195 [Abstract].

24. Malmstrom K, Daniels S, Kotey P, Seidenberg BC, Desjardins PJ. Comparison of rofecoxib and celecoxib, two cyclooxygenase-2 inhibitors, in postoperative dental

pain: a randomized, placebo- and active-comparator-controlled clinical trial. *Clin Ther.* 1999;21:1653–63.

25. Dawood MY. Nonsteroidal antiinflammatory drugs and reproduction. *Am J Obstet Gynecol.* 1993;169:1255–65.

26. Bieglmayer C, Hofer G, Kainz C, Reinthaller A, Kopp B, Janisch H. Concentrations of various arachidonic acid metabolites in menstrual fluid are associated with menstrual pain and are influenced by hormonal contraceptives. *Gynecol Endocrinol.* 1995;9:307–12.

27. Nigam S, Benedetto C, Zonca M, Leo-Rossberg I, Lubbert H, Hammerstein J. Increased concentrations of eicosanoids and platelet-activating factor in menstrual blood from women with primary dysmenorrhea. *Eicosanoids.* 1991;4:137–41.

28. Ehrich E, Mehlisch D, Perkins S, Brown P, Wittreich J, Lipschutz K et al. Efficacy of MK 966 a highly selective inhibitor of COX-2 in the treatment of postoperative dental pain. *Arthritis Rheum.* 1996;39(Supp 9):S81(Abs329).

29. Reicin A, Brown J, Jove M, de Andrade JR, Bourne M, Krupa D et al. Rofecoxib in post-orthopedic surgery pain. *Am J Orthop.* 2001;30:40–8.

30. Dieppe P, Lim K. Osteoarthritis and related disorders – clinical features and diagnostic problems. In: Klippel JH, Dieppe PA, Arnett FC, Brooks PM, Canoso JJ et al., editors. *Rheumatology*, 2 edn. London: Mosby; 1998:Chapter 8:3.10–3.16.

31. Cooper C. Osteoarthritis and related disorders – epidemiology. In: Klippel JH, Dieppe PA, Arnett FC, Carette S et al., editors. *Rheumatology*, 2 edn. London: Mosby; 1998:Chapter 8:2.10–2.80.

32. Baum C, Kennedy DL, Forbes MB. Utilization of nonsteroidal antiinflammatory drugs. *Arthritis Rheum.* 1985;28:686–92.

33. Murray MD, Brater DC. Nonsteroidal anti-inflammatory drugs. *Clin Geriatr Med.* 1990;6:365–441.

34. Wolfe MM, Lichtenstein DR, Singh G. Gastrointestinal toxicity of nonsteroidal antiinflammatory drugs. *N Engl J Med.* 1999;340:1888–99.

35. Bellamy N, Kirwan J, Boers M, Brooks P, Straud V, Tugwell P et al. Recommendations for a core set of outcome measures for future phase III clinical trials in knee, hip, and hand osteoarthritis. Consensus development at OMERACT III. *J Rheumatol.* 1997;24:799–802.

36. Bellamy N, Carette S, Ford PM, Kean WF, Le Riche NG, Lussier A et al. Osteoarthritis antirheumatic drug trials. III. Setting the delta for clinical trials – results of a consensus development (Delphi) exercise. *J Rheumatol.* 1992;19:451–7.

37. Ehrich EW, Schnitzer TJ, McIlwain H, Levy R, Wolfe F, Weisman M et al. Effect of specific COX-2 inhibition in osteoarthritis of the knee: a 6 week double blind, placebo controlled pilot study of rofecoxib. Rofecoxib Osteoarthritis Pilot Study Group. *J Rheumatol.* 1999;26:2438–47.

38. Ehrich E, Schnitzer T, McIlwain H, Levy R, Wolfe F, Weisman M et al. MK-966, a highly selective COX-2 inhibitor, is effective in the treatment of osteoarthritis in a 6-week pilot study. *Osteoarthritis Cartilage.* 1997;5:66 [Abstract].

39. Ehrich E, Schnitzer T, Kivitz A, Weaver A, Wolfe F, Morrison B et al. MK-966, a highly selective COX-2 inhibitor, was effective in the treatment of osteoarthritis (OA) of the knee and hip in a 6-week placebo controlled study. *Arthritis Rheum.* 1997;40:(Suppl 9), S85 [Abs 330].

40. Ehrich E, Schnitzer T, Weaver A, Bradham AM, Schiff M, Ko A et al. Treatment with MK-966 (VIOXX™), a specific COX-2 inhibitor, resulted in clinical improve-

ment in osteoarthritis (OA) of the knee and hip, that was sustained over six months. *Rheumatol Eur.* 1998;27:119 [Abstract].

41. Saag K, van der Heijde D, Fisher C, Samara A, De Torai L, Bolognese J et al. Rofecoxib, a new cyclooxygenase 2 inhibitor, shows sustained efficacy, comparable with other nonsteroidal anti-inflammatory drugs: a 6-week and a 1-year trial in patients with osteoarthritis. *Arch Fam Med.* 2000;9:1124–34.

42. Truitt, K, Ettinger Jr, W, Schnitzer T, Greenwald M, Daniels B, Zeng Q et al. Rofecoxib, a COX-2 specific inhibitor, had clinical efficacy and overall safety in treating osteoarthritis patients aged 80 years and older [Abstract]. 206, 859. 1999. Annals Rheumatic Diseases XIV European League Against Rheumatism Congress.

43. Arnett FC, Edworthy SM, Bloch DA. The American Rheumatism Association 1987 revised criteria for the classification of rheumatiod arthritis. *Arthritis Rheum.* 1996;38:727–35.

44. Hochberg MC. Adult and juvenile rheumatoid arthritis: current epidemiologic concepts. *Epidemiol Rev.* 1981;3:27–44.

45. ACR Ad Hoc Committee on clinical guidelines. Guidelines for the management of rheumatoid arthritis. *Arthritis Rheum.* 1996;39:713–22.

46. Felson DT, Anderson JJ, Boers M, Bombardier C, Furst D, Goldsmith C et al. American College of Rheumatology. Preliminary definition of improvement in rheumatoid arthritis. *Arthritis Rheum.* 1995;38:727–35.

47. Hochberg MC, Chang RW, Dwosh I, Lindsey S, Pincus T, Wolfe F. The American College of Rheumatology 1991 revised criteria for the classification of global functional status in rheumatoid arthritis. *Arthritis Rheum.* 1992;35:498–502.

48. Schnitzer TJ, Truitt K, Fleischmann R, Dalgin P, Block J, Zeng Q et al. The safety profile, tolerability, and effective dose range of rofecoxib in the treatment of rheumatoid arthritis. Phase II Rofecoxib Rheumatoid Arthritis Study Group. *Clin Ther.* 1999;21:1688–702.

49. Scott LJ, Lamb MH. Rofecoxib. *Drugs.* 1999;58:499–504.

50. Fries JF, Miller SR, Spitz PW, Williams CA, Hubert HB, Bloch DA. Toward an epidemiology of gastropathy associated with nonsteroidal antiinflammatory drug use. *Gastroenterology.* 1989;96:647–55.

51. Wolfe MM. NSAIDS and the gastrointestinal mucosa. *Hosp Pract.* 1996;37–48.

52. Singh G. Recent considerations in nonsteroidal anti-inflammatory drug gastropathy. *Am J Med.* 1998;105:31S–8S.

53. Griffin MR, Piper JM, Daugherty JR, Snowden M, Ray WA. Nonsteroidal anti-inflammatory drug use and increased risk for peptic ulcer disease in elderly persons. *Ann Intern Med.* 1991;114:257–63.

54. Cryer B, Gottesdiener K, Gertz B, Hsieh P, Dallob A, Feldman M. Effects of a novel cyclooxygenase (COX2) inhibitor on gastric mucosal prostaglandin synthesis in healthy humans. *Am J Gastroenterol.* 1999;57:6:341–6.

55. Chan C-C, Boyce S, Brideau C, Charleson S, Gromlish W, Ethier D et al. Rofecoxib [Vioxx, MK-0966; 4-(4′-methylsulfonylphenyl)-3-phenyl-2-(5H)-furanone]: a potent and orally active cyclooxygenase-2 inhibitor. Pharmacological and biochemical profiles. *J Pharmacol Exp Ther.* 1999;290:551–60.

56. Bjarnason I, Macpherson A, Hollander D. Intestinal permeability: an overview. *Gastroenterology.* 1995;108:1566–81.

57. Bjarnason I, Macpherson A, Rotman H, Schupp J, Hayllar J. A randomized, double-blind, crossover comparative endoscopy study on the gastroduodenal

tolerabilty of a highly specific cyclooxygenase-2 inhibitor, flosulide, and naproxen. *Scand J Gastroenterol.* 1997;32:126–30.

58. Loebl DH, Craig RM, Culic DD, Ridolfo AS, Falk J, Schmid FR. Gastrointestinal blood loss – effect of aspirin, fenoprofen, and acetaminophen in rheumatoid arthritis as determined by sequential gastroscopy and radioactive fecal markers. *J Am Med Assoc.* 1977;237:976–81.

59. Lanza FL. Endoscopic studies of gastric and duodenal injury after the use of ibuprofen, aspirin, and other nonsteroidal anti-inflammatory agents. *Am J Med.* 1984;77(1A):19–24.

60. Swan SK, Rudy DW, Lasseter KC, Ryan CF, Buechel KL, Lambrecht LJ et al. Effect of cyclo-oxygenase inhibition on renal function in elderly persons receiving a low-salt diet. A randomised controlled trial. *Ann Intern Med.* 2000;133:1–9.

61. Harris RC, McKanna JA, Akai Y, Jacobson HR, Dubois RN, Breyer MD. Cyclooxygenase-2 is associated with the macula densa of rat kidney and increases with salt restriction. *J Clin Invest.* 1994;94:2504–10.

62. Kömhoff M, Gröne H-J, Klein T, Seyberth HW, Nüsing RM. Localization of cyclooxygenase-1 and -2 in adult and fetal human kidney: implication for renal function. *Am J Physiol.* 1997;272:F460–8.

63. Chan C-C, Boyce S, Brideau C, Ford-Hutchinson AW, Gordon R, Guay D et al. Pharmacology of a selective cyclooxygenase-2 inhibitor, L-745,337: a novel non-steroidal anti-inflammatory agent with an ulcerogenic sparing effect in rat and nonhuman primate stomach. *J Pharmacol Exp Ther.* 1995;274:1531–7.

64. Catella-Lawson F, McAdam B, Morrison BW, Kapoor S, Kujubu D, Antes L et al. Effects of specific inhibition of cyclooxygenase-2 on sodium balance, hemo-dynamics, and vasoactive eicosanoids. *J Pharmacol Exp Ther.* 1999;289:735–41.

65. Swan SK, Lasseter CK, Ryan CF, Buechel LJ, Lambrecht LJ, Pinto MB et al. Renal effects of multiple-dose rofecoxib (R), a Cox-2 inhibitor, in elderly subjects. *J Am Soc Nephrol.* 1999;10:641A [Abstract].

66. Kargman SL, O'Neill GP, Vickers PJ, Evans JF, Mancini JA, Jothy S. Expression of prostaglandin G/H synthase-1 and -2 protein in human colon cancer. *Cancer Res.* 1995;55:2556–9.

67. McLemore TL, Hubbard WC, Litterst CL, Liu MC, Miller S, McMahon NA et al. Profiles of prostaglandin synthesis in normal lung and tumor tissue from lung cancer patients. *Cancer Res.* 1988;48:3140–7.

68. Rigas B, Goldman IS, Levine L. Altered eicosanoid levels in human colon cancer. *J Lab Clin Med.* 193;122:518–23.

69. Abulafi AM, Williams NS. Local recurrence of colorectal cancer: the problem, mechanisms, management and adjuvant therapy. *Br J Surg.* 1994;81:7–19.

70. Watson AJM, Dubois RN. Lipid metabolism and APC: implications for colorectal cancer prevention. *Lancet.* 1997;349:444–5.

71. Sano H, Kawahito Y, Wilder RL, Hashiramoto A, Mukai S, Asai K et al. Expression of cyclooxygenase-1 and -2 in human colorectal cancer. *Cancer Res.* 1995;55:3785–9.

72. Crofford LJ, Lipsky PE, Brooks P, Abramson SB, Simon LS, van de Putte LBA. Basic biology and clinical application of specific cyclooxygenase-2 inhibitors. *Arthritis Rheum.* 2000;43:4–13.

73. Aisen PS. Inflammation and Alzheimer Disease. *Mol Chem Neuropathol.* 1996;28:83–8.

74. Adams J, Collaco-Moraes Y, de Belleroche J. Cyclooxygenase-2 induction in cere-

bral cortex: an intracellular response to synaptic excitation. *J Neurochem.* 1996;66:6–13.

75. Aisen P, Davis KL. Inflammatory mechanisms in Alzheimer's Disease: implications for therapy. *Am J Psychiatry.* 1944;151:1105–13.

76. Abramowics M, Rizack AM, Goodstein D, Faucard A, Peter D, Hansten DP et al. Rofecoxib for osteoarthritis and pain. *The Medical Letter.* 1999;41:59–62.

77. Bombardier C, Laine L, Reicin A et al. Comparison of upper gastrointestinal toxicity of rofecoxib and naproxen in patients with rheumatoid arthritis. *N Engl J Med.* 2000;343:1520–8.

26 | The future of cyclooxygenase-2 inhibitors

ZUNAID KARIM AND PAUL EMERY

Rheumatology and Rehabilitation Research Unit, University of Leeds School of Medicine, 36 Clarendon Road, Leeds LS2 9NZ, UK.

The discovery of the two different forms of cyclooxygenase (COX) enzymes (COX-1 and COX-2) expanded on the original concepts of Sir John Vane[1] and led to the hypothesis that non-steroid anti-inflammatory drug (NSAID) toxicity was related to COX-1 inhibition. This resulted in the rapid development of targeted molecules specifically designed to inhibit COX-2, and the licensing of the first two selective COX-2 inhibitors belonging to the chemical class of coxibs within the NSAIDs. These two, celecoxib and rofecoxib, have now been used extensively in phase IV studies, which have allowed the testing of the primary hypothesis of the COX-2 story, namely that the selective drugs would retain the efficacy of NSAIDs without their COX-1 mediated side effects.

Prior to the advent of these two new inhibitors, some COX-1 sparing NSAIDs were already available, including etodolac (see R. A. Jones, Chapter 22), nimesulide (see A. Bennett, Chapter 24) and meloxicam. Of these, meloxicam received the most extensive clinical trials and its therapeutic efficacy and safety are well attested (see F. Degner et al., Chapter 23).

THE STORY THUS FAR

Gastrotoxicity has been the greatest source of NSAID-associated morbidity and mortality, and this was the major rationale for the development of COX-2 selective drugs. So, have coxibs lived up to their promise of equal efficacy with reduced toxicity?

In terms of analgesic efficacy, single doses of celecoxib[2,3] and rofecoxib[4,5] are superior to placebo and equally as effective as aspirin, ibuprofen or naproxen, respectively, for pain relief following dental extraction. Rofecoxib also has anti-pyretic activity in humans[6].

Celecoxib[7] and rofecoxib[8,9] are as effective as naproxen, ibuprofen or diclofenac, respectively, in the treatment of knee or hip osteoarthritis (OA). Both significantly improve[10,11] all physical and mental health domains (except general health) of the SF-36 Health Survey in patients with OA. Celecoxib is as effective as naproxen[12] and diclofenac[13] for symptomatic relief in rheumatoid arthritis (RA). Rofecoxib is not licensed for use in RA.

NSAID associated dyspepsia is important in that it leads to discontinuation of treatment in more than 10% of patients[14]. The current evidence suggests patients experience less dyspepsia with coxibs than with non-selective NSAIDs. The exact relationship between dyspepsia and gastrointestinal (GI) bleeding, however, is unclear. Most patients who present with ulcer complications give no antecedent history of dyspepsia[14,15], and paracetamol, which has not been established as a cause of peptic ulcers, causes as much dyspepsia as non-selective NSAIDs.

Concerning gastrotoxicity, celecoxib causes levels of gastric mucosal injury similar to placebo and less than naproxen in acute studies[16], and is similar to placebo and reduced compared with naproxen and diclofenac in 3–6 month studies[12,13]. Rofecoxib, at ten times the recommended maximum dose, causes levels of gastric mucosal injury similar to placebo and less than ibuprofen or aspirin[17]. Rofecoxib does not increase faecal blood loss[18] and has no effect on gastric mucosal prostaglandin (PG) E_2 synthesis[19] or on small intestine permeability[20].

The important question as to whether these findings translate to a reduction in clinical upper GI events has recently been addressed by long-term safety studies comparing celecoxib (the 'Celebrex' Long-term Arthritis Safety Study: CLASS) and rofecoxib (the 'Vioxx' Gastrointestinal Outcomes Research: VIGOR) with non-selective NSAIDs.

Two to four times the maximum therapeutic dose of celecoxib or rofecoxib was compared with the standard dose of conventional NSAIDs in each study. The studies were broadly similar in design, patient numbers and duration of treatment (see Table 1). They differed in that CLASS included patients with OA and RA, and allowed concomitant aspirin use, whilst in VIGOR only patients with RA were included and aspirin use was not allowed. CLASS and VIGOR had primary end-points of complicated upper GI events and clinical upper GI event rates, respectively.

CLASS

In the CLASS trial[21] the primary end-point of the annualized incidence of complicated upper GI events did not reach significance overall, but this was achieved when aspirin users were excluded (see Table 2). There were, however, significant reductions in all patients with celecoxib use for the secondary (clinically valid) end-points of complicated upper GI events plus symptomatic

Table 1 Design of the CLASS and VIGOR studies

	CLASS	VIGOR
Coxib	Celecoxib 400 mg b.i.d.	Rofecoxib 50 mg o.d.
Comparator NSAID	Ibuprofen 800 mg t.i.d.	Naproxen 500 mg b.i.d.
	Diclofenac 75 mg b.i.d.	
Patients enrolled	8059	8076
Patient diagnosis	OA (72%), RA (28%)	RA only
Mean age (years)	60	58
Corticosteroid use	30%	> 50%
Concomitant aspirin use	Yes (21%)	No (but 4% significant cardiovascular risk)
Duration of study:		
Median	9 months	9 months
Maximum	13 months	13 months
Study design	Randomized, controlled double-blind	Randomized, controlled double-blind
Analysis	Intention to treat	Intention to treat
Primary end-point	Upper GI ulcer complications	Clinical upper GI events
Secondary end-point	Upper GI ulcer complications plus symptomatic ulcers	Complicated upper GI event

Table 2 Results of CLASS and VIGOR trials. All results are presented as incidence rates in percentages for coxib versus comparator NSAID

	CLASS (all patients)	CLASS (excluding aspirin users)	VIGOR
Primary end-point	0.76% versus 1.45% (ns)	0.44% versus 1.27% ($P = 0.04$)	2.1% versus 4.5% ($P < 0.001$)
Secondary end-point	2.08% versus 3.54% ($P = 0.02$)	1.40% versus 2.91% ($P = 0.02$)	0.6% versus 1.4% ($P = 0.005$)
Withdrawal due to GI intolerance	8.7 % versus 10.7% ($P < 0.05$)	8.0% versus 10.1% ($P < 0.05$)	3.5% versus 4.9.% ($P < 0.05$)
Myocardial infarction	0.3% versus 0.3% (ns)	< 0.1% versus 0.1% (ns)	0.4% versus 0.1% ($P < 0.05$)
Myocardial infarction[*]	nr	nr	0.2% versus 0.1% (ns)
Cerebrovascular accidents	0.1% versus 0.3% (ns)	< 0.1% versus 0.2% (ns)	0.2% versus 0.2% (ns)
Deaths due to cardiovascular events	nd	nd	0.2% versus 0.2% (ns)
All deaths	nd	nd	0.5% versus 0.4% (ns)

nr = not relevant; ns = not significant; nd = not discussed; [*] = excluding patients with baseline cardiovascular risk (VIGOR).

ulcers, overall GI, hepatic enzyme, renal and cutaneous adverse effects. There were also significant reductions in overall withdrawals due to adverse effects, and withdrawals specifically due to hepatic enzyme, GI and cutaneous adverse effects.

Low dose aspirin use had a significant effect on the primary end-point. This may be attributed to the high event rate with aspirin use and the higher than expected concomitant use (21%) of aspirin. Aspirin use had a significant effect in the celecoxib group with a relative risk (RR) of 4.5 ($P = 0.01$), however the effect was not significant in the NSAID group with a RR of 1.7 ($P = 0.29$). Corticosteroid use was not associated with any significant increase in upper GI complications in either treatment group. There was no significant difference in cardiovascular events such as cerebrovascular accidents and myocardial infarction in this trial.

VIGOR

The completed trial[22] achieved its primary and secondary end-points with significant reductions of 54% in clinical upper GI events and 57% in complicated upper GI events with rofecoxib compared with naproxen (see Table 2). Rofecoxib also reduced the risk of GI bleeding by 62% ($P < 0.001$) and had less discontinuation of treatment due to GI adverse events ($P < 0.05$) compared with naproxen. A significant reduction in GI events was seen in all patient categories with rofecoxib including concomitant corticosteroid use and *Helicobacter pylori* presence. This benefit extended to the lowest risk factor group (under 65 years, no previous history of clinical GI event, *H. pylori* negative and no corticosteroids).

While overall there was no significant difference in cardiovascular mortality or cerebrovascular accidents, there was a significant difference seen between rofecoxib (0.4%) and naproxen (0.1%) in the myocardial infarction incidence rates. Once patients with cardiovascular disease that met Food and Drug Administration, USA, criteria for aspirin prophylaxis were excluded (4% of all patients) the difference (0.2 versus 0.1%) was no longer significant.

These two studies highlight the beneficial and toxic effects of low dose aspirin. The impact of aspirin on the primary end-point in CLASS is consistent with its COX-1 effect. There is no *a priori* reason why celecoxib should prevent this toxicity, although endoscopic studies with celecoxib and concomitant aspirin have suggested there may be a small risk reduction compared with conventional NSAIDs and concomitant aspirin use. The VIGOR trial excluded aspirin use and therefore precludes comparison, although the impact of aspirin is likely to be the same across the class of coxibs.

It is notable that the myocardial infarction rate in most studies is around 0.4%, and celecoxib (0.3%) and rofecoxib (0.4%) in these studies have similar rates. An interesting finding was the reduction in the naproxen group

(0.1%). Naproxen is a non-selective and long-acting NSAID and it is possible that for the first time the beneficial COX-1 'aspirin like' effect of non-selective NSAIDs on myocardial infarction has been demonstrated. This would be consistent with the fact that a large proportion of the reported myocardial infarctions (38%) seen with rofecoxib were in a small group of patients (4%) who should have been receiving aspirin for secondary cardiovascular prophylaxis. Furthermore, the overall incidence of thromboembolic events and cardiovascular mortality in a review of nine OA clinical trials of rofecoxib, involving more than 5000 patients, revealed rates similar to placebo and comparator NSAIDs[23], albeit at a lower dose of rofecoxib.

Common adverse effects of NSAIDs in the kidney are reductions in glomerular filtration rate (GFR), renal blood flow, and sodium and potassium excretion. Prostaglandins in the kidney are important in maintaining GFR and renal blood flow, especially in salt-depleted states. Since GFR is reduced with age, the elderly are more susceptible to these renal adverse effects. COX-1 seems to produce vasodilating prostaglandins that maintain GFR and renal medullary blood flow. COX-2 is constitutively expressed in the kidney in the macula densa and afferent arteries, and is more evident in the kidneys of older adults[24,25].

Recent studies in healthy elderly subjects have suggested a sparing of GFR with celecoxib and rofecoxib over conventional NSAIDs; however, a transient reduction in sodium excretion and reduced prostaglandin synthesis was seen for both coxibs and conventional NSAIDs[26,27]. These results differ from studies in salt-depleted elderly subjects (where prostaglandin mediated regulation is more important), which do not demonstrate any advantage with celecoxib or rofecoxib over conventional NSAIDs[28,29].

These results would suggest that GFR is predominantly COX-1 mediated in healthy states, but that COX-2 becomes increasingly important in salt-depleted states. This indicates that coxibs may have an advantage over conventional NSAIDs in healthy states. In patients with salt-depleted states, such as congestive cardiac failure or diuretic use, there may be no renal benefit from using coxibs.

So what will this mean for future prescribing?

THE FUTURE

It is likely that most new prescriptions for NSAIDs will be for selective COX-2 inhibitors. It will be hard to justify giving a drug with greater toxicity when a less toxic one with equal efficacy is available. In the light of the CLASS and VIGOR studies, further work will need to be carried out to quantify reliably any cardiovascular risk, and the effect on it of concomitant aspirin. Any risk will then need to be assessed against the documented GI benefit. In the meantime cardiovascular risk should be assessed separately and treated with concomitant low-dose aspirin, if indicated. Some non-selective NSAIDs may be mildly cardioprotective and their role in patients with mild cardiovascular risk will require clarification (see Table 3).

It is likely that the aetiology of dyspepsia is multifactorial, although patients on selective COX-2 inhibitors experience less of this side effect. The commonest reason for changing to a selective inhibitor will be the higher incidence of dyspepsia on a non-selective drug rather than the history of a recent bleed. The newer, even more selective, COX-2 inhibitors may well reduce dyspepsia rates closer to that of placebo. The role that all NSAIDs may have in masking dyspepsia and allowing 'silent' peptic ulcer formation is unclear. In the meantime physicians may well continue patients with dyspepsia on a selective COX-2 inhibitor, treating the dyspepsia symptomatically, because of the reassuring data on peptic ulcer disease. However, it is advisable that patients at high risk of ulcer complications are treated with a proton pump inhibitor, which should provide both symptomatic relief and ulcer protection.

It is hoped that the widespread use of selective COX-2 inhibitors will reduce to a background or placebo level the incidence of GI bleeds with NSAID use. This will hopefully allow a clearer understanding of the aetiology of peptic ulcer disease, in particular whether *H. pylori* and non-selective NSAIDs account for the majority of current bleeds.

Extrapolating the data from VIGOR, the numbers needed to be treated with rofecoxib as opposed to naproxen to prevent one clinical upper GI bleed per year would be 41. The cost efficacy of these drugs will require further investigation.

Rheumatoid arthritis

NSAIDs remain the cornerstone of symptomatic treatment in RA. Although clinical experience has shown that NSAIDs do not appear to influence radiographic progression, preliminary evidence from our group suggests they improve Health Assessment Questionnaire (HAQ) scores and reduce swollen and tender joint scores in RA. Imaging studies, using magnetic resonance imaging and ultrasonography, of early RA in our group have also demonstrated the ability of NSAIDs to reduce synovial volume.

Table 3 Possible NSAID indications in the future

- Selective COX-2 inhibitors
  - Analgesia (central, peripheral)
  - Corticosteroid, anti-TNF sparing
  - Prevention and treatment of GI/breast/skin malignancies
  - Prevention of Alzheimer's disease
  - Delaying premature labour
- Non-selective NSAIDs
  - Analgesia in patients with mild cardiovascular risk factors

Whether or not selective COX-2 inhibitors at high doses given in early disease could influence RA disease progression remains to be tested in a formal programme. In RA, upregulation of tumour necrosis factor (TNF) is associated with increased COX-2 production. One of the features of anti-TNF therapy is the quick response in terms of reducing synovitis[30]. This suggests that downregulation of COX-2 may be involved, implying a speculative anti-TNF sparing role for selective COX-2 inhibitors. Another potential benefit is that COX-2 is expressed in endothelial cells particularly in situations of shear stress and angiogenesis. If inhibitors have an effect on angiogenesis then clearly there would be a potential role in inhibiting growth of synovium.

Osteoarthritis

Osteoarthritis (OA) presents practical difficulties with current NSAID use in that it is prevalent in that group of patients most at risk of GI toxicity, namely the elderly. Patients often find NSAIDs the most effective pain relievers in OA[31], creating a major conflict between efficacy and toxicity. It is worth noting that pain is the major reason a joint replacement is undertaken and that COX-2 is involved in pain transmission both peripherally and centrally.

Again, there are potential advantages to using selective COX-2 inhibitors rather than current NSAIDs in OA subgroups with synovitis. The effects of COX-2 inhibition on PG-mediated bone turnover and chondrocyte biology are yet to be determined and further studies with selective COX-2 inhibitors will help delineate the role of the COX isoenzymes in bone biology.

Other rheumatological conditions

The potential role of selective COX-2 inhibitors in controlling synovitis may also be relevant in systemic lupus erythematosus (SLE). Again, high dose inhibition may result in better symptom relief and, importantly, a steroid sparing effect. COX-2 is upregulated in mesangial cells in lupus nephritis, and selective COX-2 inhibition in particular, without any COX-1 related loss of GFR, may well prove beneficial in this group.

Again the anti-synovitic role may be important in other inflammatory arthritides such as ankylosing spondylitis (AS) and psoriatic arthritis, where COX-2 upregulation in synovitis has also been demonstrated[32]. In AS, adequate analgesia, coupled with exercise, is the mainstay of treatment to minimize loss of spinal movement. NSAID use has been associated with flares of skin lesions in psoriasis, which is thought to be secondary to an increase in lipoxygenase pathway products as a result of COX inhibition[33]. Selective COX-2 inhibition may change the balance of PG/lipoxygenase products resulting in less aggravation of skin lesions.

Other clinical advantages

There is growing evidence that COX-2 has an important role in pain modulation, parturition, the development of Alzheimer's disease (AD) and certain malignancies.

Recent evidence suggests that NSAIDs are effective in ameliorating the progression of AD[34]. Although the roles for the two COX isoenzymes in neurophysiology are unclear, there are reports of increased COX-2 expression in AD. In contrast, other work suggests COX-2 is important in cerebral function and development. Current prospective randomized studies in AD are already underway.

Another area of potential benefit is in large bowel carcinoma. There is firm epidemiological evidence of reduction in prevalence of this carcinoma with aspirin use[35]. Studies have confirmed a high expression of COX-2 in bowel tumours and demonstrated that COX-2 selective drugs are more effective than conventional NSAIDs at inhibiting disease progression[36]. Celecoxib has recently been licensed, in combination with usual care, as prophylaxis to reduce the number of adenomatous colorectal polyps in familial adenomatous polyposis. Increased COX-2 expression has been documented in upper GI, lung, breast and skin cancers with a potential modulating role for COX-2 inhibition.

If the proposed benefit of selective COX-2 inhibitors is realized in AD and certain malignancies we may well see prophylactic use of these drugs in high-risk groups, like tamoxifen in breast cancer, especially if post-marketing surveillance reaffirms a low toxicity index.

COX-2 expression has a key role in the onset of premature labour. Indomethacin delays onset of preterm delivery[37] but its use is limited by side effects, usually within 48–72 h, namely oligohydramnios and premature closure of the ductus arteriosus. Nimesulide is similarly effective, but the development of oligohydramnios takes longer and is thought to be due to accumulation in the fetus leading to greater COX-1 inhibition. Selective COX-2 inhibitors may therefore be effective in preventing premature labour without the current adverse events. COX-2 is also involved in ovulation and implantation and in theory may act as a contraceptive. Selective COX-2 inhibitors and conventional NSAIDs should therefore be avoided if possible in those planning pregnancy.

A third COX enzyme has recently been proposed[38], which is perhaps of importance in the resolution of inflammation, inadvertent inhibition of which may prolong the inflammatory process.

Already a dual inhibitor of COX and lipoxygenase has been used that is effective in models of inflammation. As cost efficacy becomes a bigger issue in management decisions, combinations of non-selective NSAIDs with a standard gastroprotectant, or standard NSAIDs containing a nitric oxide releasing moiety, may well compete with selective COX-2 inhibitors for the same market. It is difficult to predict the outcome of this but pricing will no doubt be crucial.

In summary, the advent of selective COX-2 inhibitors has been the largest and most successful drug launch to date, and is a model for the development of targeted therapy in the modern era. Many of the theoretical benefits await further clarification. Only time will tell just how good (and safe) these drugs really are.

REFERENCES

1. Vane JR. Inhibition of prostaglandin synthesis as a mechanism of action for the aspirin-like drugs. *Nature*. 1971;231:232–3.
2. Hubbard RC, Mehlisch DR, Jasper DR, Nugent MJ, Yu S. SC-58635, a highly selective inhibitor of COX-2, is an effective analgesic in an acute post surgical pain model. *J Invest Med*. 1996;44:293A.
3. Mehlisch DR, Hubbard RC, Isakson P, Karim A, Weaver M, Mills S et al. Analgesic efficacy and plasma levels of a highly selective inhibitor of COX-2 (SC-58635) in patients with post-surgical dental pain. *Clin Pharmacol Ther*. 1997;61:195 [Abs PIII–2].
4. Ehrich E, Mehlisch D, Perkins S, Brown P, Wittreich J, Lipschutz K et al. Efficacy of MK-966, a highly selective inhibitor of COX-2, in the treatment of postoperative dental pain. *Arthritis Rheum*. 1996;39(suppl 9):S81 [Abs 329].
5. Mehlisch DR, Mills S, Sandler M, Yuan W, Dury W, Ehrich E et al. *Ex vivo* assay of COX-2 inhibition predicts analgesic efficacy in post-surgical dental pain with MK-966. *Clin Pharmacol Ther*. 1998;63:139 [Abs PI–8].
6. Schwartz J, Mukhopadhyay S, McBride K, Jones T, Adcock S, Sharp P et al. Antipyretic activity of a selective cyclooxygenase (COX)-2 inhibitor, MK-966. *Clin Pharmacol Ther*. 1998;63:167 [Abs PI–123].
7. Hubbard RC, Geiss GS, Woods EM, Yu JS, Zhao W. Efficacy, tolerability, and safety of celecoxib, a specific COX-2 inhibitor, in osteoarthritis. *Arthritis Rheum*. 1998;41(suppl):S196.
8. Saag K, Fisher C, McKay J, Ehrich E, Zhao P-L, Bolognese J et al. MK-0966, a specific COX-2 inhibitor, has clinical efficacy comparable to ibuprofen in the treatment of hip and knee osteoarthritis (OA) in a six-week controlled clinical trial. *Arthritis Rheum*. 1998;41(suppl):S196 [Abs 984].
9. Cannon G, Caldwell J, Holt P, McLean B, Zeng Q, Ehrich E et al. MK-0966, a specific COX-2 inhibitor, has clinical efficacy comparable to diclofenac in the treatment of hip and knee osteoarthritis (OA) in a 26-week controlled clinical trial. *Arthritis Rheum*. 1998;41(suppl):S196 [Abs 983].
10. Ehrich E, Bolognese J, Kong S, Watson DJ, Zeng Q, Seidenberg B. Improvements in SF-36 mental health domains with treatment of OA: a result of decreased pain and disability or independent mechanisms? *Arthritis Rheum*. 1998;41(suppl):S221 [Abs 1134].
11. Zhao SZ, Hatoum HT, Hubbard RC, Koepp RJ, Dedhiya SD, Geis SG et al. Effect of celecoxib, a novel COX-2 inhibitor, on health-related quality of life of patients with osteoarthritis of the knee. *Arthritis Rheum*. 1997;40(Suppl 9):S88 [Abs 348].
12. Geiss GS, Hubbard RC, Callison DA, Yu JS, Zhao W. Safety and efficacy of celecoxib, a specific COX-2 inhibitor. *Rheumatol Eur*. 1998;27(suppl 1):118.

13. Geiss GS, Stead H, Morant SV, Nandin R, Hubbard RC. Endoscopic and tolerability results from a study of celecoxib, a specific COX-2 inhibitor, in patients with rheumatoid arthritis. *Rheumatol Eur.* 1998;27(suppl 1):118.

14. Singh G, Ramey DR, Morfeld D, Shi H, Hatoum HT, Fries JF. Gastrointestinal tract complications of nonsteroidal anti-inflammatory drug treatment in rheumatoid arthritis. A prospective observational cohort study. *Arch Intern Med.* 1996;156:1530–6.

15. Armstrong CP, Blower AL. Non-steroidal anti-inflammatory drugs and life threatening complications of peptic ulceration. *Gut.* 1987;28:527–32.

16. Lanza FL, Rack MF, Callison DA, Hubbard RC, Yu SS, Talwalker S et al. A pilot endoscopic study of the gastroduodenal effects of SC-58635, a novel COX-2 selective inhibitor. *Gastroenterology.* 1997;112(suppl):A194.

17. Lanza F, Simon T, Quan H, Bolognese J, Rack MF, Hoover M et al. Selective inhibition of cyclooxygenase-2 (COX-2) with MK-0966 (250 mg qd) is associated with less gastrodoudenal damage than aspirin (ASA) 650 mg qid or ibuprofen (IBU) 800 mg tid. *Gastroenterology.* 1997;112:A194.

18. Hunt R, Bowen B, James C, Sridhar S, Simon T, Mortensen E et al. COX-2 specific inhibition with MK-0966 25 or 50 mg qid over 4 weeks does not increase fecal blood loss: a controlled study with placebo and ibuprofen 800 mg tid. *Am J Gastroenterol.* 1998;93:A247.

19. Cryer B, Gottesdiener MD, Gertz B, Hsieh P, Dallob A, Feldman M. Effects of a novel cyclooxygenase(COX)-2 inhibitor on gastric mucosal prostaglandin (PG) synthesis in healthy humans. *Am J Gastroenterol.* 1998;93:A104.

20. Bjarnason I, Sigthorrsen G, Crane R, Simon T, Hoover M, Bolognese J et al. COX-2 specific inhibition with MK-0966 25 or 50 mg qd does not increase intestinal permeability: a controlled study with placebo and indomethacin 50 mg tid. *Am J Gastroenterol.* 1998;93:A246.

21. Bombardier C, Laine L, Reicin A, Shapiro D, Burgos-Vargas R, Davis B et al. Comparison of upper gastrointestinal toxicity of rofecoxib and naproxen in patients with rheumatoid arthritis. *N Engl J Med.* 2000;343:1520–8.

22. Silverstein FE, Faich G, Goldstein JL, Simon LS, Pincus T, Whelton A et al. GI toxicity with celecoxib vs NSAIDs for arthritis. *J Am Med Ass.* 2000;284:1247–55.

23. Daniels B, Seidenberg B. Cardiovascular safety profile of rofecoxib in controlled trials. *Arthritis Rheum.* 1999;42(suppl):435.

24. Komhoff M, Grone HJ, Klein T, Seybert HW, Nusing R. Localisation of cyclooxygenase-1 and -2 in adult and fetal human kidney: implication for renal function. *Am J Physiol.* 1997;272:F460–8.

25. Nantel F, Meadows E, Denis D, Connolly B, Metters KM, Giaid A. Immunolocalization of cyclooxygenase-2 in the macula densa of human elderly. *FEBS Lett.* 1999;457:475–7.

26. Catella-Lawson F, McAdam B, Morrison BW, Kapoor S, Kujubu D, Antes L et al. Effects of specific inhibition of cyclo-oxygenase-2 on sodium balance, hemodynamics, and vasoactive eicosanoids. *J Pharmacol Exp Ther.* 1999;289:735–41.

27. Whelton A, Schulman G, Wallemark C, Drower EJ, Isakson PC, Verburg KM et al. Effects of celecoxib and naproxen on renal function in the elderly. *Arch Intern Med.* 2000;160:1465–70.

28. Rossat J, Maillard M, Nussberger J, Brunner HR, Burnier M. Renal effects of cyclooxygenase-2 inhibition in salt-depleted subjects. *Clin Pharmacol Ther.* 1999;66:76–84.

29. Swan SK, Rudy DW, Lasseter KC, Ryan CF, Buechel KL, Lambrecht LJ et al. Effect of cyclo-oxygenase-2 inhibition on renal function in elderly persons receiving a low-salt diet: a randomised controlled trial. *Ann Intern Med.* 2000;133:1–9.

30. Elliott MJ, Maini RN, Feldmann M, Kalden JR, Antoni C, Smolen JS et al. Randomised double blind comparison of chimeric monoclonal antibody to tumour necrosis factor alpha (cA2) versus placebo in rheumatoid arthritis. *Lancet* 1994;344:1105–10.

31. Emery P. COX-1, COX-2: so what? *Scand J Rheumatol.* 1999;28:6–9.

32. Amin AR, Attur M, Patel RN, Thakker GD, Marshall PJ, Rediske J et al. Superinduction of cyclooxygenase-2 activity in human osteoarthritis-affected cartilage, influence of nitric oxide. *J Clin Invest.* 1997;99:1231–7.

33. Griffiths CEM. Therapy for psoriatic arthritis: sometimes a conflict for psoriasis. *Br J Rheumatol.* 1997;36:409–10.

34. Stewart WF, Kawas C, Carrada M, Metter EJ. Risk of Alzheimer's disease and duration of NSAID use. *Neurology.* 1997;48:626–32.

35. Reddy BS, Rao CV, Seibert K. Evaluation of cyclooxygenase-2 inhibitors for potential chemopreventive properties in colon carcinogenesis. *Cancer Res.* 1996;56:4566–9.

36. Peleg II, Maibach HT, Brown SH, Wilcox CM. Aspirin and nonsteroidal anti-inflammatory drug use and the risk of subsequent colon cancer. *Arch Intern Med.* 1994;154:395–9.

37. Bennett P, Sawdy R, Slater D. The role of cyclooxygenase-2 in reproduction. In: Vane JR, Botting RM, editors. *Clinical Significance and Potential of Selective COX-2 Inhibitors.* London: William Harvey Press; 1998:171–83.

38. Willoughby DA, Moore AR, Colville-Nash PR. COX-1, COX-2, and COX-3 and the future treatment of chronic inflammatory disease. *Lancet* 2000;355:646–8.

Index